healthy ~
for the world's poorest communities

The Working Equid Veterinary Manual

Whittet Books

Whittet Books Ltd
1 St John's Lane
Stansted
Essex CM24 8JU
UK

mail@whittetbooks.com

www.whittetbooks.com

First published 2013

© The Brooke 2013

This publication is in copyright. Subject to statutory exception and to the provisions of relevant collective licensing agreements, no part of this publication may be reproduced, transmitted or stored in a retrieval system, in an form or by any means, without the prior permission of Whittet Books Ltd.

Whittet Books Ltd has no responsibility for the persistence or accuracy of URLs for external websites referred to in this publication, and does not guarantee that any content on such websites is, or will remain, accurate or appropriate.

A catalogue record for this publication is available from the British Library.

ISBN 978 1 873580 87 5

Designed by Lodge Graphics

This book is printed in Europe on paper manufactured to ISO 14001 and EMAS (Eco-Management & Audit Scheme) international standards, minimising negative impacts on the environment.

Contents

	Preface	vii
1	The consultation process and responsibilities of a veterinarian	1
2	Welfare, behaviour and handling of working equids	23
3	Pain – Indicators and management	51
4	Clinical techniques	71
5	Medicines	97
6	Dehydration and fluid therapy	121
7	Sedation and anaesthesia	133
8	Euthanasia	163
9	Ophthalmology	175
10	The teeth – Ageing and a practical approach to dentistry	223
11	The gastrointestinal system	253
12	The respiratory system	293
13	The urinary and reproductive systems	329
14	The musculoskeletal system	351
15	The integumentary system	421
16	The neurological system	457
17	Parasitology	469
18	Foal diseases	501
	Index	511

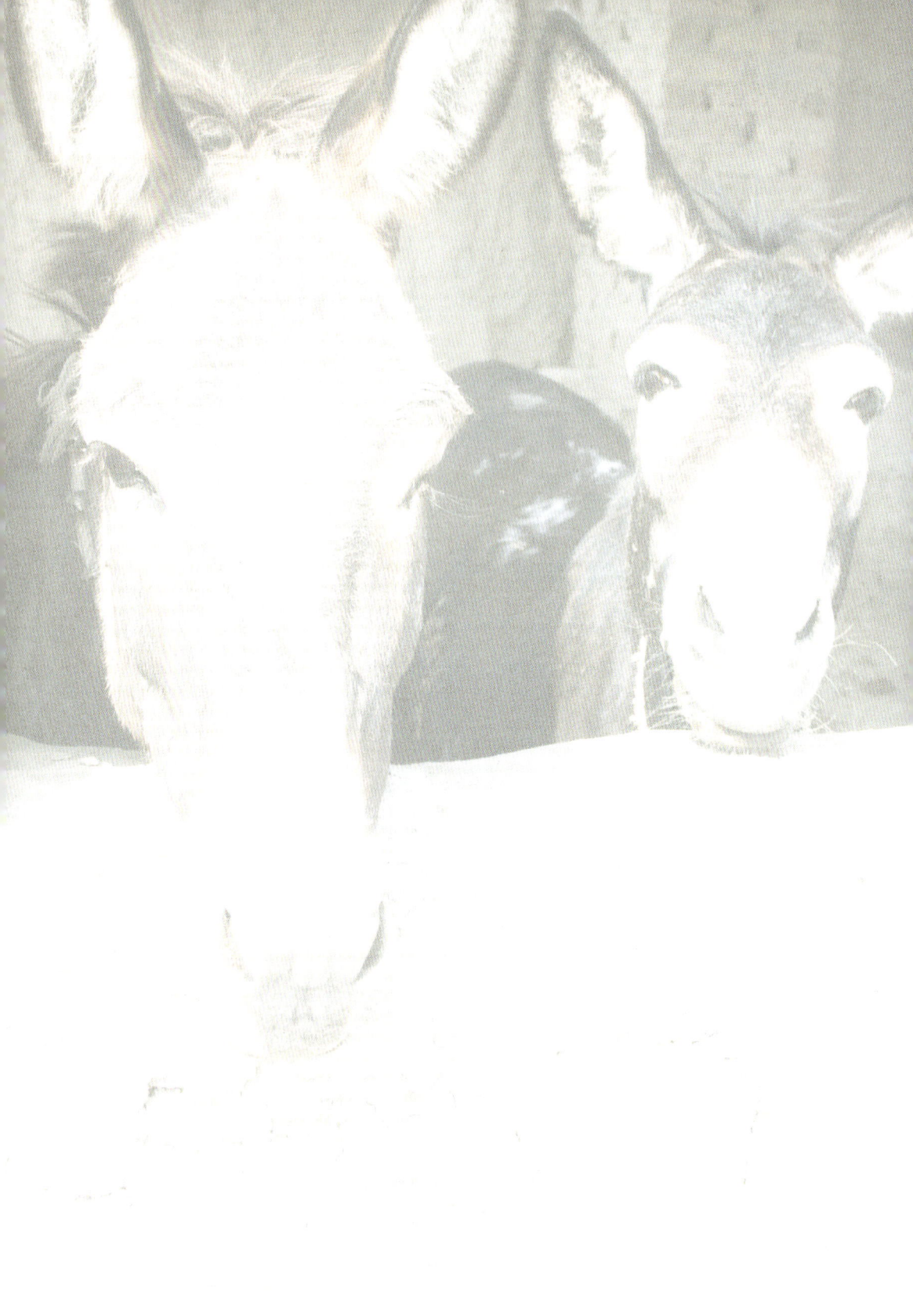

Preface

The work of the Brooke

The Brooke is an international animal welfare organisation dedicated to improving the lives of working horses, donkeys and mules in the poorest parts of the world. There are around 100 million working equids across the world and, during the course of their lives, it is estimated that more than half of these animals suffer from exhaustion, dehydration and malnutrition as a result of excessive workloads, difficult climates and owner poverty. This results in suffering for the animals and insecure livelihoods for the people relying on them. Limited equine health services in many less developed regions lead to prolonged distress and inappropriate treatment of diseased and debilitated working equids. Some of these problems can be avoided.

The Brooke provides veterinary training and treatment as well as community programmes around animal health and well-being, across Africa, Asia and Latin America. We work with communities so they understand how to care for their animals, ensuring they have regular rest, shade and water. Establishing the root cause of a health problem and preventing it from happening in the first place is the most effective way to ensure sustainable fitness and well-being. We train local veterinarians as well as service providers such as farriers, saddlers, harness and cart makers. By working with animal owners they become aware that healthier animals can be more productive.

Working animals can be happy and healthy if they have the care and respect they deserve. This year, we will reach more than a million working horses, donkeys and mules, benefiting around six million of the world's poorest people who rely on these animals to earn a basic living.

The Working Equid Veterinary Manual

This manual has been created from the Brooke online vet wiki (a web application, which allows people to add or modify content). Brooke vets across our programmes have developed the content by editing the text and also by submitting photographs and case studies. This was supported by technical checking and evidence-based referencing to ensure the accuracy and reliability of the information. This groundbreaking book represents a truly international collaboration. This has brought direct experience from the field and also ensured that the content was written with a focus on the hard-working horses, donkeys and mules in developing countries. The Brooke vet wiki continues to evolve online.

The manual will be distributed to Brooke and other veterinarians in developing countries to be used as a reference manual for the direct treatment of working equids. Within the Brooke there is a strong ethos of knowledge transfer and it is anticipated that this manual can also be used as a training aid. This manual will be a vital resource as the Brooke moves towards more sustainable solutions in the long term by training animal health practitioners and improving local systems to deliver quality healthcare to working horses, donkeys and mules.

The consultation process and responsibilities of a veterinarian 1

Introduction	1.1
The responsibilities of an animal health provider	1.2
Taking a good, complete history	1.3
The clinical examination process	1.4
Formulate a list of differential diagnoses	1.5
Further diagnostic tests	1.6
Owner communication and determining the prognosis for return to work	1.7
Zoonotic disease	1.8
Case study – Communication and prognosis	1.9
References	1.10

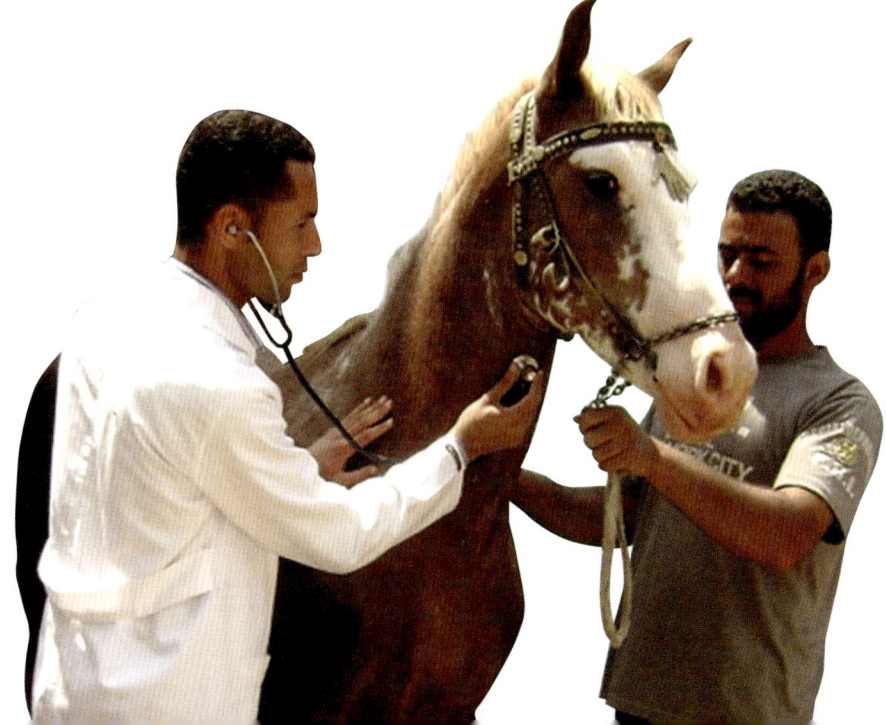

1.1 Introduction –
What is meant by an 'integrated' consultation process?

A thorough consultation process will provide the opportunity for **maximum impact** on that animal's life. Whilst obtaining the most likely diagnosis, diligent communication with the owner also increases the likelihood that the **long-term welfare** of that animal will improve through good management and prevention principles (Figure 1.1.1).

Consider the following three aspects of the animal's life:

Past	'What has happened in this animal's life up until now?'
Present	'How can I help this animal at this moment?'
Future	'How can I make a long term, sustainable difference to the welfare of this animal?'

Why is it important to conduct an integrated consultation?

The **animal** is the primary stakeholder, but ultimately the **owner** is the stakeholder who can make the biggest positive difference to that animal throughout its lifetime – good communication is essential.

The diagram below (Figure 1.1.1) shows the links between animal, owner and veterinarian. At the junction of various stakeholders, aspects for the consultation process can be seen; these link to the three phases of the animal's life – past, present and future.

> Ultimately all phases lead to the central goal of improving the welfare of the animal.

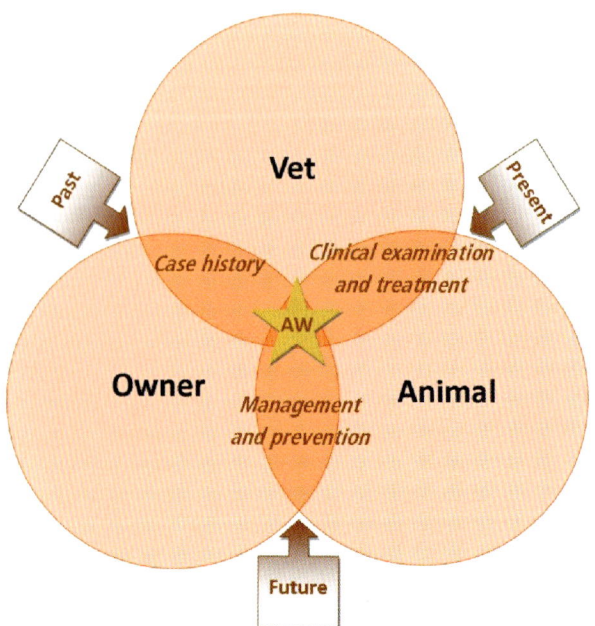

Figure 1.1.1 An Integrated Consultation Process is the complete interaction between animal, owner and veterinarian. (AW = Animal Welfare)

The responsibilities of an animal health provider 1.2

Working equine veterinarians are accountable to the animals, to owners/communities, to the profession, and to society.

This section outlines **five** main competencies expected of working equine veterinarians:

1. Animal welfare advocate	4. Clinical governance
2. Veterinary expert	5. Lifelong learner and trainer
3. Communication	

1. Animal welfare advocate

As a veterinarian, act as an animal welfare advocate at all times, ensuring the following:

- **Welfare-friendly consultation process** Practical application of the five freedoms relating to handling, restraint, distress and pain (Korte *et al.* 2007). For a full description of the five freedoms see Section 2.1.
- **Accurate diagnosis and treatment** following diagnostic procedure, with correct drug and treatment choice.

In all cases, ensure that the benefit outweighs the harm caused to the animal through appropriate technique or treatment choice (Figure 1.2.1).

2. Veterinary expert

- Integrate medical knowledge, professional attitudes and clinical skills under the principles of evidence-based veterinary medicine.
- Always make the best choice of treatment available for the condition in that individual animal.
- Ensure best practice at all times in the areas of technical veterinary skills, preventive medicine, therapeutic medicine, population medicine and clinical pathology (Figure 1.2.2).

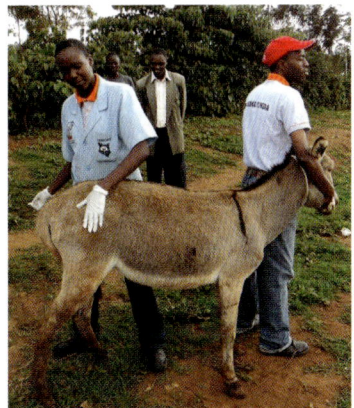

*Figure 1.2.1 In decisions with working equids ensure that **benefit** outweighs **harm**.*

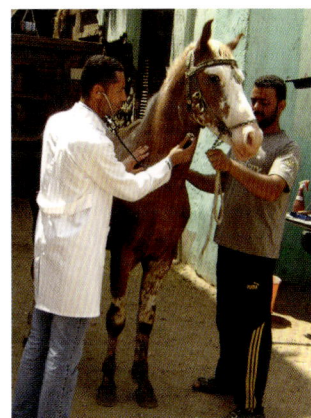

Figure 1.2.2 Veterinary skills, knowledge and attitude are all equally important.

1 THE CONSULTATION PROCESS AND RESPONSIBILITIES OF A VETERINARIAN

3. Communication

The owner and community should be the first point of contact (Figure 1.2.3).

> Avoid examining an animal before interacting with the owner/community if at all possible.

- **Good communication** with all parties involved in the care of the animal
  - explanation of treatment and follow-up/nursing
  - management and prevention advice to ensure long-term improvement in animal welfare.
- **Safety** Ensure people and animals do not get hurt.
- **Drugs**
  - good instructions to the owner on handling and responsible storage
  - proper labelling of prescribed medicines.

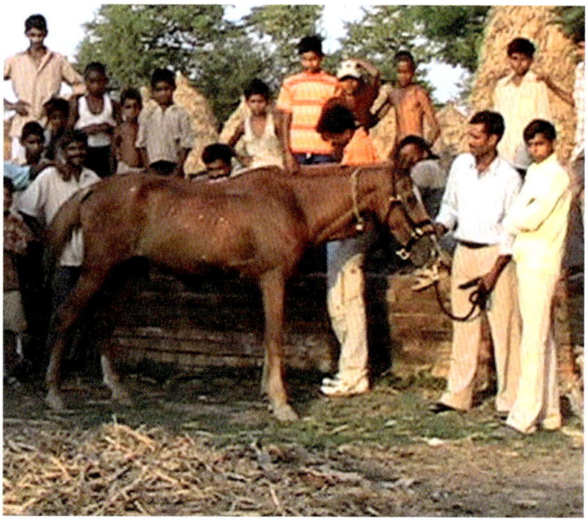

4. Clinical governance

- **Record keeping** This provides accountability, monitors the efficacy of treatment and directs drug procurement choices.
- **Registration** It is mandatory that all veterinarians are registered with the veterinary body of their country (and often state/territory/province). Although the requirements differ between countries, compliance with veterinary notifications is non-negotiable. The same applies for paraprofessionals; they must abide by the laws of their country.
- **Dispensing of drugs** All veterinary procedures should have minimum standards for drug prescription and dispensing. It is the responsibility of the veterinarian to set an example to other stakeholders regarding responsible use of medicines to ensure that resistance and poor compliance is not perpetuated (more information in Chapter 5 *Medicines*).
- **Biohazard waste and carcass disposal** Ensure equipment is always clean and/or sterilised and that needles, syringes and drugs are effectively stored and disposed of correctly (Figures 1.2.4 and 1.2.5). Carcass disposal should adhere to local laws and, if buried, waste matter must be deep enough so that other animals will not be able to gain access. Ensure post-mortem/euthanasia areas are always cleaned appropriately. Ideally there should be a clearly outlined protocol describing the disposal procedure in order to aim for the responsible and legal disposal of waste.

Figure 1.2.3 The owner and community are the first point of contact.

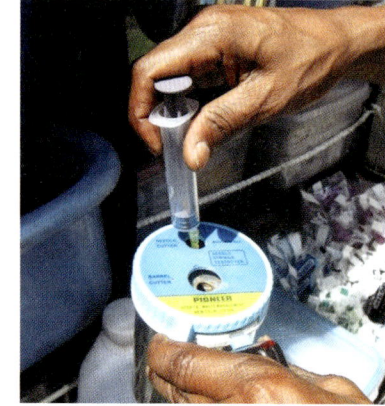

Figure 1.2.4 Correct disposal of used needles and syringes.

THE RESPONSIBILITIES OF AN ANIMAL HEALTH PROVIDER 1.2

> Ensure a clean working environment.

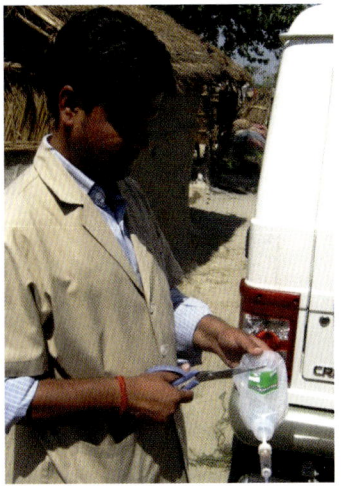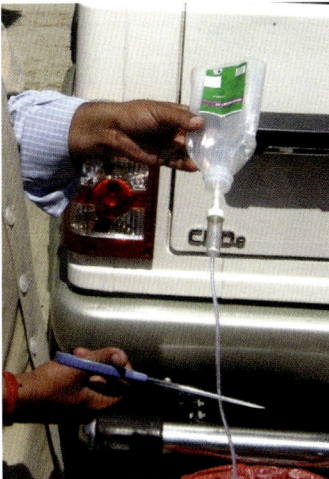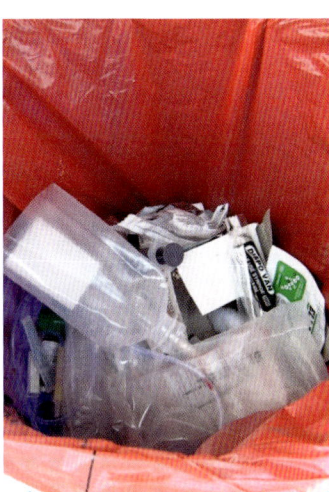

Figure 1.2.5 Correct disposal of a used fluid bag.

5. Lifelong learner and trainer

It is the responsibility of a veterinarian to keep up-to-date with recent advances in veterinary knowledge. This can be achieved in a number of ways, including being a learner and a trainer of others:

- private study/reading
- attending conferences or lectures
- professional discussions with colleagues
- distance learning (webinars, e-modules)
- practical training sessions as either a trainee or a trainer
- research
- studying for a qualification

1.3 Taking a good, complete history

> Taking a good history is a skill that requires practice and development.

Direct and indirect questions

History questions should be asked with care, so that the answer given will help with the diagnosis. Questions can be asked either directly or indirectly, depending on what information is sought and the clinician's relationship with the owner (Figure 1.3.1).

1 Indirect questions These are usually predominant at the start of a consultation, help to establish rapport with the owner and relax the animal prior to examination. Indirect questions help to reveal facts about the illness/treatment which the owner may not wish to disclose. The same question may need to be asked in a number of different ways to establish the whole story. However, be careful the owner does not become frustrated.

2 Direct questions (different from 'leading' questions) Often specific technical information is required to help obtain the correct diagnosis although the owner may not understand unless asked explicitly. The following scenario is a common example of an occasion when only a direct question can elicit the correct information:

> Vet: *'Is your horse passing faeces/droppings?'*
>
> Owner: *'Yes'*.

However, the owner does not necessarily know normal faecal amount and consistency so something may be missed if specific questions are not asked. It is the clinician's responsibility to elicit exactly the information required. For example:

> Vet: *'Does your horse show signs of diarrhoea?'* or *'What consistency and colour are the faeces?'*, and *'How are often are faeces passed?'*

> Questions such as these help to determine the exact behaviours and clinical signs the animal is showing. It takes a little longer but will ultimately help with diagnosis.

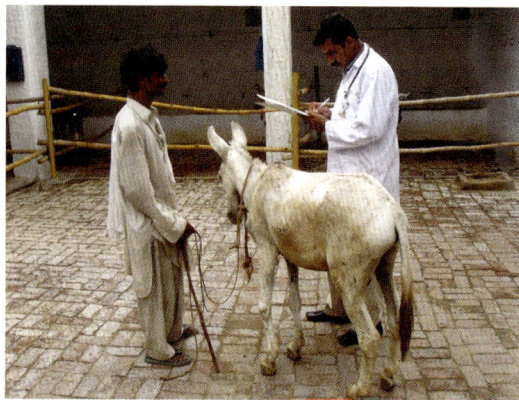

Figure 1.3.1 Taking the time to listen to the owner demonstrates care. Clinicians must ensure they record this information to maintain good clinical records.

TAKING A GOOD, COMPLETE HISTORY   1.3

> Taking the time to listen to owners demonstrates care. They are more likely to trust the clinician's skills and listen to advice if they feel they have been listened to.

Considerations when taking the history from an owner

- Avoid scientific words the owner may not understand.
- Avoid questions that will 'lead' the owner to answer in a particular way: *'Is there a nasal discharge?'*, if so *'What colour is it?'* is preferable to *'Have you seen a yellow nasal discharge?'*

> Misleading histories are common. Owners often have their own diagnosis in mind, or do not want to admit how long their animal has had a problem.

- If in doubt about what the owner has told you, ask the same question in a different way later on in the consultation. Getting an owner to describe the symptoms that have been noticed can be helpful. For example, if the owner has noticed a nasal discharge, having the owner describe the appearance and volume of this may be helpful and is not leading in any way.
- Try to learn and understand the local or traditional names of diseases, equipment, etc.

What questions should be asked?

Here are some examples of initial information that might be requested:

- **Signalment** – age, sex, work type, pregnancy status, breeding history
- **Length of time** the owner has had the animal and history of previous illness
- **Living arrangements** – bedding, shelter, other animals kept together
- **Feed** – appetite, quantity/quality of food, frequency, food type, difficulty eating (quidding), faeces (appearance and amount)
- **Water** – thirst, quantity/quality of water, frequency, difficulty swallowing, urine appearance and amount
- **Work pattern** – lameness, weakness, or loss of vigour and for how long. New or increased work activities for the animal
- **Breathing** – discharge from eyes/nose, coughing, wheezing, tiredness
- **Abnormal behaviours**

Once a good understanding of the animal's life and general signs has been gained then ask more specific questions about the presenting problem:

- Why did the owner present the animal?
- When did the problem start? Was there a specific incident that started it?
- Is the problem getting better, worse, or staying the same?
- Are any other animals affected?
- Has there been any treatment already given? If so, who administered it, what did they give and for how long/how many times? What was the response of the animal to this treatment?

1.4 The clinical examination process

> A good clinical examination, when coupled with a good history, helps formulate an idea of the most likely diagnosis. Developing communication skills is central to good veterinary practice.

'I can see the problem, it's obvious...'

Even so, it is **good practice** to do a full clinical examination, providing the opportunity to:

- pick up other problems
- bond with animal and owner
- assess improvement over time
- speak with the owner about husbandry issues while you are working
- demonstrate care.

Things are not always what they seem – a skin lesion may indicate underlying liver disease; weight loss may be a sign of dental disease.

Initial observation of the animal – No hands

Always observe the animal from a distance to start with (Figure 1.4.1). This can provide some interesting information that would be missed by starting the physical examination too soon and gives initial clues to inform the diagnostic work-up.

While taking a history, always **watch** the animal, taking into account the following:

- Temperament/demeanour
- Body condition
- Stance
- Head position
- Symmetry/limb conformation
- Swellings
- Shifting of weight
- Breathing abnormalities
- Signs of pain
- Hair loss or scabs

Observe from the front, rear and both sides, if possible, so as not to miss anything on initial examination (Colahan *et al.* 1999).

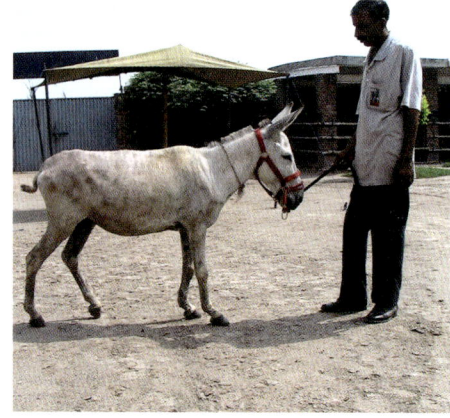

Figure 1.4.1 Observe the animal from a distance initially.

Offer water (Figure 1.4.2) – this is the most reliable way to diagnose and treat dehydration in adult working horses (Pritchard *et al.* 2008).

> Compare and contrast what the animal looks like with what the owner is describing. How well does the information from both sources fit together?

THE CLINICAL EXAMINATION PROCESS 1.4

> When carrying out the clinical examination it is always useful to complete the exam in a logical order so that nothing is missed out.

A logical order may be starting at the nose and finishing at the tail, or working through each body system one at a time. With practice a systematic approach can be developed.

The approach described below starts from the head:

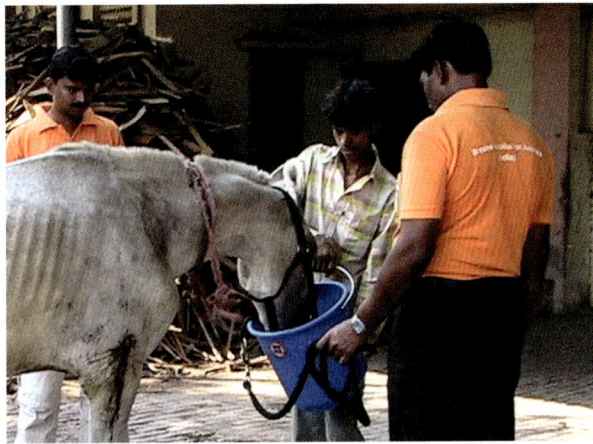

Figure 1.4.2 Offer water to assess hydration status as well as to provide one of the five freedoms (Pritchard 2005, Korte et al. 2007).

Head and neck

1 **Mucous membrane colour** indicates the level of tissue oxygenation and perfusion of the capillary bed. Severe disturbances will induce a colour change, even when a haemogram is normal. Look inside the mouth, nostrils, or eyelids (see Chapter 9 *Ophthalmology*). For the mouth, insert a thumb or finger into the corner of the lips and lift the top lip until the gums are visible. **Ignore the darker line immediately around the base of the teeth.** Abnormal colours are **pale/white, yellow, red,** or **purple**. Each of these changes can be significant, so it is important to assess in conjunction with other clinical signs (see Table 1.4.1).

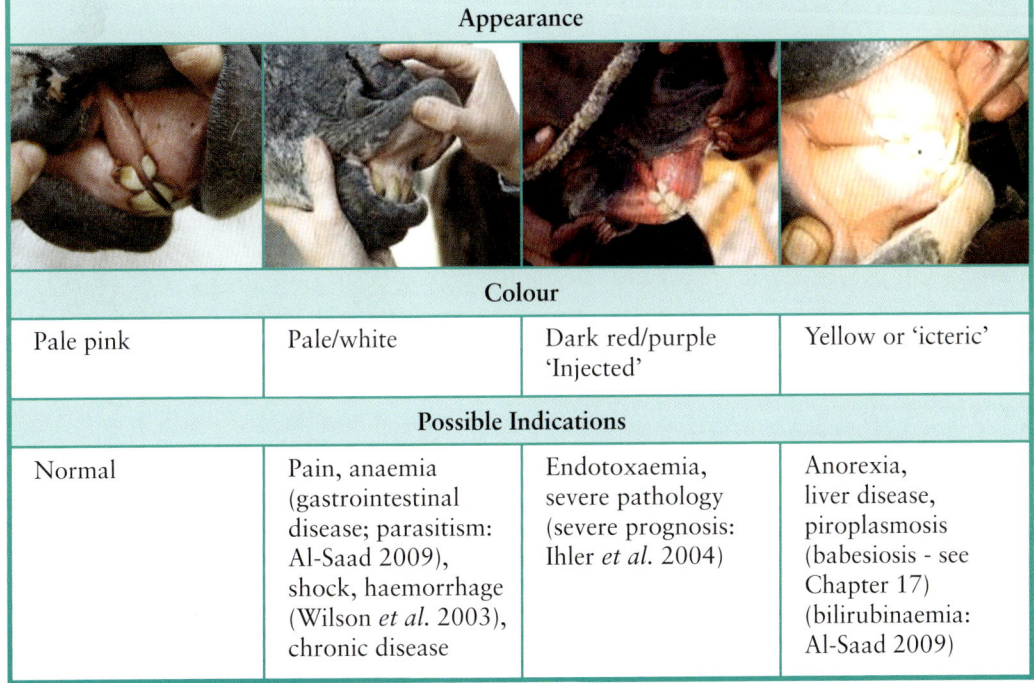

Appearance			
Colour			
Pale pink	Pale/white	Dark red/purple 'Injected'	Yellow or 'icteric'
Possible Indications			
Normal	Pain, anaemia (gastrointestinal disease; parasitism: Al-Saad 2009), shock, haemorrhage (Wilson *et al.* 2003), chronic disease	Endotoxaemia, severe pathology (severe prognosis: Ihler *et al.* 2004)	Anorexia, liver disease, piroplasmosis (babesiosis - see Chapter 17) (bilirubinaemia: Al-Saad 2009)

Table 1.4.1 The range of mucous membrane colours with their interpretation relating to disease status.

1 THE CONSULTATION PROCESS AND RESPONSIBILITIES OF A VETERINARIAN

2 Capillary Refill Time (CRT) CRT measures the degree of peripheral perfusion, thus indicating the strength of blood flow to the extremities. Press firmly on the gum until it goes pale under the finger, then release and count how many seconds pass before normal colour returns to the area. **Normal CRT is 1-2 seconds.** CRT is prolonged with decreased peripheral perfusion e.g. shock.

3 Pulse Feel the pulse from the mandibular artery – note strength, rate and regularity (Figure 1.4.3). Pulse can be taken before opening the mouth which may distress the animal.

4 Nostrils Discharge can indicate upper or lower respiratory tract infection or inflammation and is **always significant** even if very little. The colour can range from clear (usually indicating viral or allergic condition) to blood-tinged or yellow/green, which is more likely indicative of bacterial infection. **Smell** can indicate infection of the nasal passages, sinuses, guttural pouches, or the lower respiratory tract. Also feel for inequality of air flow or asymmetry between the two sides.

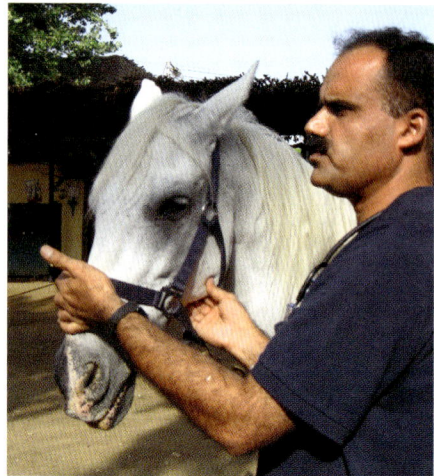

Figure 1.4.3 Palpation of the pulse from the mandibular artery.

5 Eyes Always take time to examine the eyes as they can provide useful information both on health status and on husbandry practices:
   a. discharge – colour, consistency, amount
   b. conjunctivae – colour, inflammation, foreign bodies
   c. third eyelid – apply digital pressure to the eyeball via the upper eyelid to view this. Look for protrusion, swellings, petechiae, or granulation tissue.
   d. cornea – opacities, ulcers, or evidence of a previous ulcer that has healed, often detected by a white plaque on the eye and opacities
   e. globe – signs of recurrent uveitis, colour changes, opacities, or cataracts (see Chapter 9 for more detail on the ocular examination procedure).

6 Ears Always stand in front of the animal to assess head symmetry. A tilt to one side could indicate a problem/pain in the ear on that side. Look for signs of external damage, scratching, wounds, or discharge.

7 Incisor teeth (See Table 1.4.2) Inspect briefly at this stage, since the incisors can give a preliminary indication of age and function of the alimentary system. An estimation of the age of the animal can also help shape the list of differential diagnoses. For example, younger animals are often prone to injury, ingestion of inappropriate substances (foreign objects, plastic bags), toxicities and acute contagious viral or bacterial infections, whereas older animals are more likely to have chronic conditions such as arthritis, systemic diseases involving organs (such as liver and kidney), or tumours. (See Chapter 10 *The teeth* for more information on the ageing process.)

> Remember the eruption times of the incisor teeth of donkeys has been reported as later than that of horses by up to one year (Muylle *et al.* 1999); the presence of hooks and Galvayne's groove for ageing are unreliable in donkeys.

THE CLINICAL EXAMINATION PROCESS 1.4

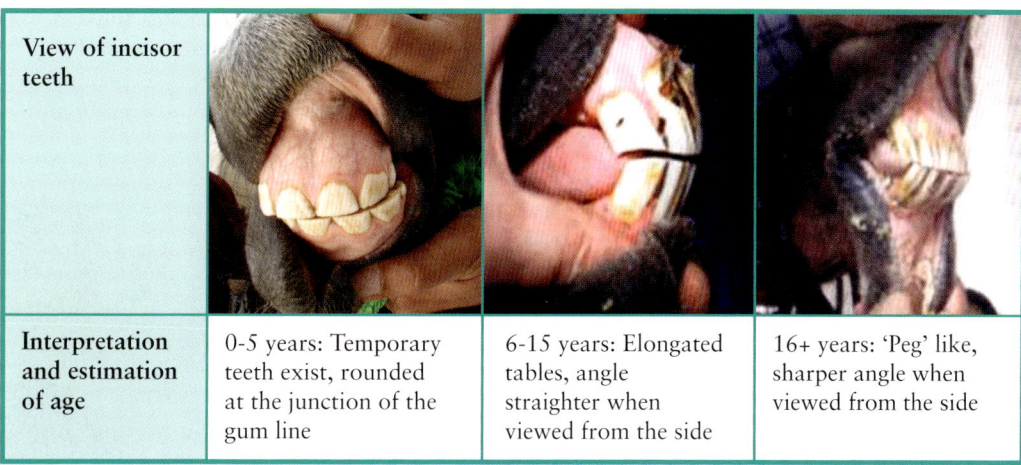

View of incisor teeth			
Interpretation and estimation of age	0-5 years: Temporary teeth exist, rounded at the junction of the gum line	6-15 years: Elongated tables, angle straighter when viewed from the side	16+ years: 'Peg' like, sharper angle when viewed from the side

Table 1.4.2 Estimating the approximate age of an equid by examining the incisor teeth.

8 Submandibular lymph nodes Palpate between the rami of the mandibles and in the region of Viborg's Triangle (borders are vertical ramus of the mandible rostral, tendinous insertion of sternomandibularis muscle dorsal and linguofacial vein ventral) to determine whether the lymph nodes are enlarged. Lymph nodes will be hot and painful if abscessed, or there may be fibrosis if the animal has had Strangles (*Streptococcus equi var. equi*) previously. This could be significant if there are systemic signs which could indicate Bastard Strangles (see Chapter 12).

Thorax

> Heart (pulse) and respiratory rates are most accurate if taken at rest when the animal is calm.

Pain is an important factor that can have an effect on these indicators.

1 Auscultation of the heart Primary heart disease is uncommon in equids compared to other species. Signs of cardiovascular disease include ventral oedema, prominent jugular pulse (when the head is raised) and altered respiratory rate and effort. Listen to the heart for at least 1 minute on **both** sides as this allows time for the heartbeat to settle if the animal is nervous. Note regularity of the heartbeat and any murmurs (Figure 1.4.4).

2 Auscultation of the lungs Auscultate both right and left lung fields in at least **four** places each side, taking in both dorsal and ventral areas of the lung field. Listen for both rate and effort; lung sounds should be clear and the animal should not show any signs of increased effort.

Note the large size of the lung fields as depicted by the triangle in Figure 1.4.5. The borders are as follows: a caudoventral line from the 17th intercostal space level with the tuber coxae, past

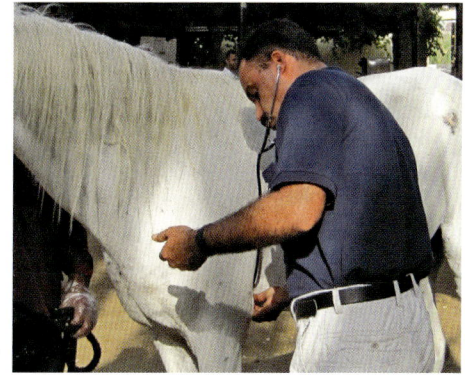

Figure 1.4.4 Auscultation of the heart with recording of heart rate in a horse.

1 THE CONSULTATION PROCESS AND RESPONSIBILITIES OF A VETERINARIAN

the 11th intercostal space level with the point of shoulder, to the point of the elbow; cranial border is the scapula/shoulder; dorsal border is the epaxial muscles/thoracic spinal transverse processes (Colahan *et al.* 1999).

Listen for crackles, wheezes, or evidence of fluid in the lungs (see Chapter 12 for details).

> **Remember to listen for abnormalities in the tracheal and laryngeal areas too in case of upper respiratory tract disease (Figure 1.2.2).**

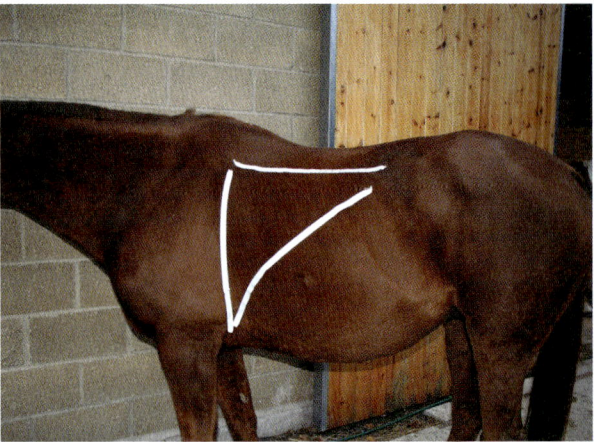

Figure 1.4.5 Area of lung fields depicted by outline of white tape.

Reported values for the heart and respiratory rates of working horses, donkeys and mules are shown in Table 1.4.3. Adult horses and mules show similar values for resting heart rate (29–41 beats per minute), whilst donkeys and foals may show higher values (up to 60 beats per minute for donkeys and over 100 beats per minute for foals); resting respiratory rate for adult horses and mules may range from 8 to 28 breaths per minute and up to 40 breaths per minute in donkeys.

> ### What is a 'heaves' line and how is it significant?
>
> A 'heaves' line is a sharp demarcation of the abdominal muscles along the lower border of the lung fields (Figure 1.4.6.), indicating that the animal has been taking deeper 'abdominal' breaths over a period of time. Presence of a heaves line is most likely due to a chronic respiratory condition where the lung capacity is decreased, thus the animal needs to take deeper breaths in order to get enough oxygen for circulation.

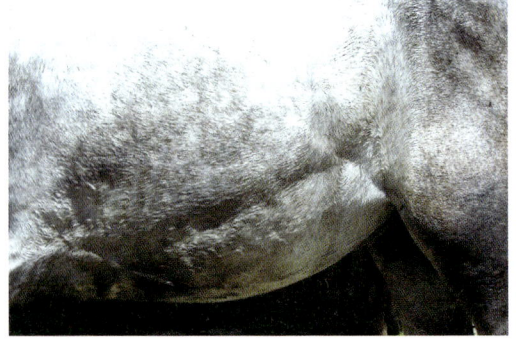

Figure 1.4.6 Heaves line seen in a horse.

Abdomen

> **Auscultate the abdomen in at least four areas on both the right and left sides.**

Auscultate from the caudal edge of the ribs, from the paralumbar fossa to the ventral abdomen (see Figures 1.4.7, 1.4.8 and 1.4.9). Even if the animal is not presenting with colic, it is important to listen in case of abnormalities, either increased or decreased sounds (White and Edwards 1999).

THE CLINICAL EXAMINATION PROCESS 1.4

Listen for sounds associated with the *ileocaecal* valve in the area of the right paralumbar fossa. This classically sounds like 'water down a drainpipe' and there should be about 1–3 per minute; absence of this noise is significant (Colahan *et al.* 1999). It is important to be able to know whether the gut sounds are normal, increased, or decreased. See Chapter 11 for gastrointestinal problems.

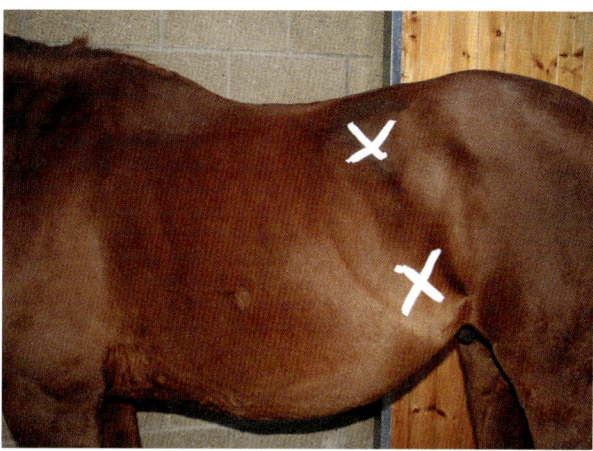

Figure 1.4.7 *The white crosses indicate focal areas for auscultation of the left paralumbar fossa (upper) and left ventral abdomen (lower). However, it is good practice to auscultate over a wide area of the abdomen.*

> **Confidence in lung or abdominal auscultation can only increase by listening to many different animals over time, thus building up a picture of the range of normality.**

Always consider the safety of the handler, the animal and any other persons present. Ensure safe positions for all and responsible, welfare-friendly handling at all times. If the animal is unhappy with any examination procedure allow more time to relax and try again.

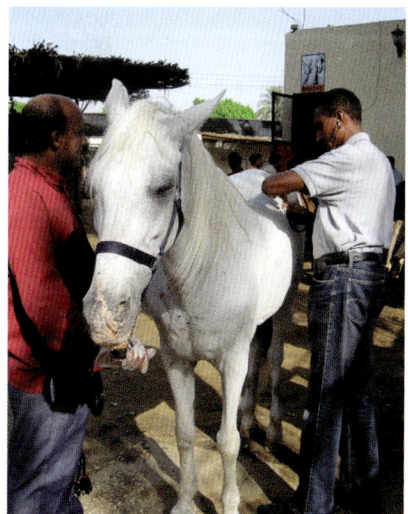

Figure 1.4.8 *Auscultation of the abdomen at the left paralumbar fossa.*

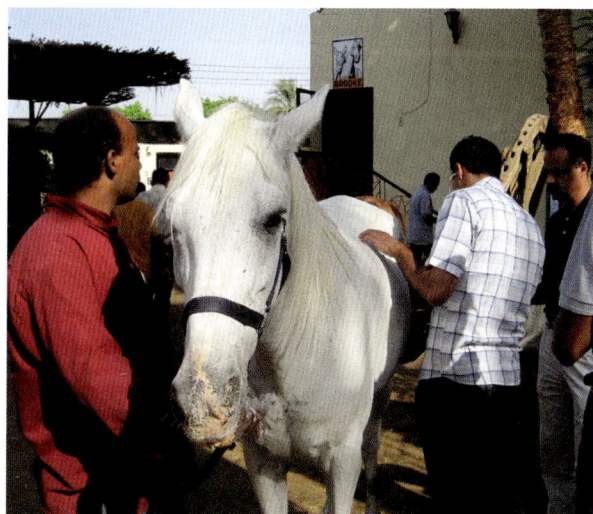

Figure 1.4.9 *Auscultation of the abdomen at the left lower flank region.*

Urogenital system

Examine briefly for evidence of swelling, discharge, or injury. Do not forget to look at the mammary glands in females, especially if nursing (see Chapter 13 for more details).

Musculoskeletal system

> A brief assessment of the musculoskeletal system is ideal in all cases, even if it is not the presenting problem, as so many welfare issues stem from an incorrect gait (Pritchard *et al.* 2005, Broster *et al.* 2009).

A specific lameness examination is covered in Chapter 14; however, it is important to note any swellings, lumps, or gait abnormalities (Figure 1.4.10).

In the hindlimbs the hock is a common site of chronic lameness. Assess hindlimb symmetry and whether there is atrophy of major muscles such as the gluteals. The forelimbs often show evidence of swelling below the carpus in working equids, particularly of the flexor tendons, and lower limb joint swelling (Broster *et al.* 2009).

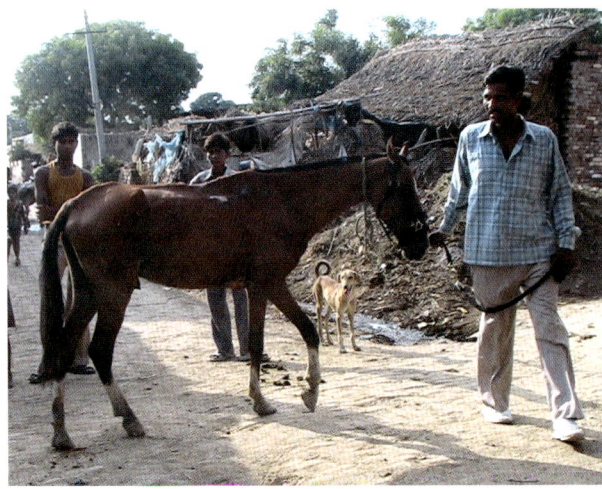

Figure 1.4.10 Examine the gait for lameness.

Assess the hoof walls for signs of cracking and wear which may indicate poor hoof quality or poor hoof management. Look over the soles of the feet to check for any foreign bodies, bruising, or smell which may indicate an infection such as thrush. Assess the condition of the frog and the quality and state of wear of the shoes, if present.

Rectal temperature

Body temperature is referenced as a range around the physiological normal value and has an acceptable deviation by 0.5–1.0 degree either side depending on age, weather, working conditions and other effects such as showering or drugs.

> Remember: one parameter alone (e.g. temperature) will not give the full story; put the whole picture together to make an accurate assessment.

Reported values for rectal body temperature of working horses, donkeys and mules are shown in Table 1.4.3. The temperature range does not vary more than 1.5 degrees from 37.5°C; however, foals, especially newborn, may have temperatures as high as 39°C.

How to take the rectal temperature:

1. Shake/flick the thermometer until the mercury falls down to the bulb (with a digital thermometer this is not necessary).
2. Lubricate the bulb (vaseline, jelly, or water).

THE CLINICAL EXAMINATION PROCESS 1.4

3. Slide bulb gently into and along the side of the rectum, avoiding insertion into faeces which results in an inaccurate reading.
4. Wait at least 60 seconds (or until the beeping sound with a digital thermometer).
5. Remove thermometer gently and keep it horizontal whilst reading the temperature.

N.B. Note the correct positioning of the examiner's body is close to the animal at the side of the hindquarters (Figure 1.4.11), reaching around to the rectum; neither the safety of the person nor the animal's welfare is compromised.

> Always consider the welfare of the animal, correct calm handling and good technique. Do not continue if there is a risk to human or animal safety.

Summary

With all the findings from the clinical examination, start creating a list of differential diagnoses, or identify further examination or diagnostic tests to aid diagnosis.

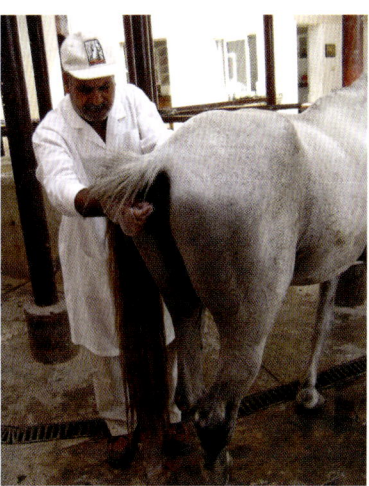

Figure 1.4.11 Safely taking the rectal temperature of a horse.

Reported values

	Heart (pulse) rate (beats per minute)	Respiratory rate (breaths per minute)	Rectal temperature (°C)	Reference
Horse (adult resting)	Range 20–80 (mean 38.2)	Range 12–60 (mean 31.5)	Range 33.5–39.6 (mean 36.6)	Upjohn 2013 (personal communication): 852 apparently healthy working horses from Lesotho
Donkey (adult resting)	38–48	14–26	36.0–38.3	Lemma and Moges 2009: 85 working donkeys from Ethiopia
	39–56	21–42	36.6–38.0	Canacoo et al. 1991: 27 apparently healthy donkeys from Ghana
Mule (adult resting)	29–37	8–16	37.1–38.1	Ali and Anjum 1998: 700 mules from 7 farms over 3 regions of Pakistan

Table 1.4.3 Reported values for heart, respiratory rates and rectal temperature of healthy working horses, donkeys and mules.

1.5 Formulate a list of differential diagnoses

Think about the following list of **potential causes** of illness, disease or injury. By comparing the history and clinical signs, a clinician can identify which are the **most likely possibilities** for the case presentation and define a list of differential diagnoses according to the primary cause(s):

- Developmental, degenerative (e.g. arthritis)
- Allergic
- Metabolic (e.g. hypocalcaemia)
- Neoplastic
- Inflammatory, infectious (bacterial, viral, fungal, protozoal)
- Toxic
- Parasitic
- Iatrogenic (e.g. aspiration pneumonia)
- Genetic

1.6 Further diagnostic tests

Diagnostic work-ups should not be undertaken lightly. Many diagnostic procedures compromise the animal's welfare in some way, with some even leading to risk of death. Always ensure a valid scientific justification and an ability, either in the clinic or a laboraory, to analyse the results.

> *Never* undertake a procedure unless it is the logical sequence of steps that should be followed to obtain a diagnosis.

Assess each case individually. If diagnostic services are not available it is better that no further work-up procedures are conducted. For example, there is no point doing a rectal examination if the clinician does not know the gastrointestinal tract anatomy well enough to detect abnormalities. There is little use in taking samples if a laboratory cannot analyse them. Always know where to seek advice or refer the animal if necessary.

No procedure should be done unless the benefit outweighs the harm.

Ensure that by further compromising the animal's welfare there will ultimately be an improvement, otherwise the diagnostic tests cannot be justified.

FURTHER DIAGNOSTIC TESTS **1.6**

Specific diagnostic procedures can be found in the relevant chapters:

- Chapter 4 *Clinical techniques*
    Taking blood samples
    Making a blood smear
- Chapter 9 *Ophthalmology*
    Nasolacrimal Flushing
    Vision Testing
    Fluorescein and Rose Bengal staining tests
    Ophthalmic nerve blocks
- Chapter 10 *The teeth – Ageing and a practical approach to dentistry*
    Nerve blocks – mental and infraorbital
- Chapter 11 *The gastrointestinal system*
    Insertion of a nasogastric tube
    Rectal examination
    Abdominocentesis
- Chapter 12 *The respiratory system*
    Nasal swabbing for viruses
    Use of a re-breathing bag
- Chapter 13 *The urinary and reproductive systems*
    Urinary catheterisation
    Urine examination
    Pregnancy diagnosis
- Chapter 14 *The musculoskeletal system*
    Lameness work-up
    Hoof testing
    Palpation
    Cleaning the hoof
    Nerve blocks
    Taking a synovial fluid sample
    Flushing an infected joint
- Chapter 15 *The integumentary system*
    Skin scrapings and smears
    Fluid aspiration
    Biopsies, tumour removal
- Chapter 17 *Parasitology*
    Faecal egg counts

1.7 Owner communication and determining the prognosis for return to work

Why is good communication so important to animal welfare improvements?

> Good owner communication is just as important as obtaining the most likely diagnosis.

Effective communication is essential to avoid owner confusion. By increasing owner understanding the animal will benefit. Even if a clinician does an excellent job, insufficient communication could give the impression that they do not know what they were doing, or even, do not care.

> Always include the owner in the consultation process, in as many stages as safely possible.

Listen carefully to owners when taking a history and include them in the treatment process, as this encourages their interest in the case and good compliance.

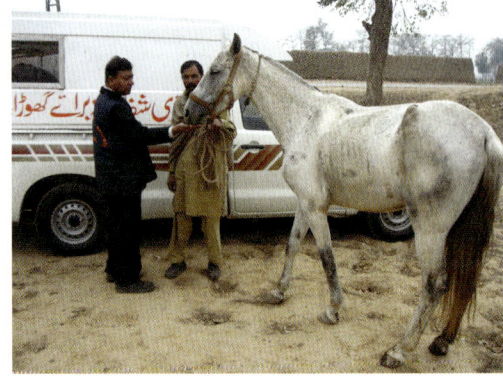

Figure 1.7.1 Good communication with the owner is an essential component of the consultation process.

- Teach them how to clean eyes and wounds, pick out feet, or change dressings. Demonstrate first, do not just describe because, unless they see it, they may not have the confidence to do it. Even better, once demonstrated, have the owner perform the task while observing before leaving them to continue at home, e.g. dressing a bandage on a wound.
- Let them help to medicate the animal the first time. An owner will often be more successful later since they have practised, especially with oral treatments.
- Speak with owners about all aspects of the animal's management and husbandry even if they are not directly related to the presenting problem.
- Encourage owners to see and feel the pathology, e.g. let them feel a swollen leg compared to the other one. This will help them to understand the problem.
- Encourage the owner to empathise with the animal and understand the pain or discomfort it is in.

> It is the responsibility of the clinician to advise on as many issues as possible, given the time limitations of a consultation. Speaking with owners is an art form and will only improve with practice (Figure 1.7.2).

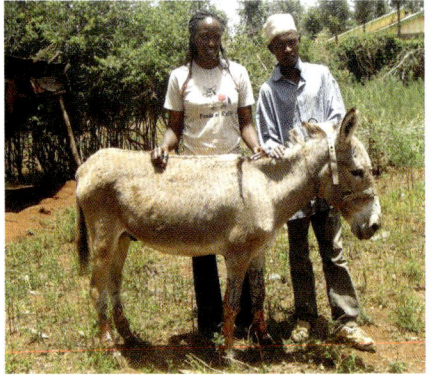

Figure 1.7.2 Good communication with the owner is key to a successful outcome.

Prognosis

Prognosis is a **prediction** of how the presenting condition/disease will progress and the likely degree of recovery if the animal is given appropriate treatment and managed well in terms of owner compliance. Remember, in chronic cases the aim may not be total recovery but return to work. The two things are very different and it is important to be realistic about how the animal will perform in the future.

The ability to determine prognosis accurately often comes from previous experience. However, this improves dramatically with the correct diagnosis. This is where the clinical examination, history taking and owner communication all come together, and gives the clinician a chance for the owner to build up trust and confidence.

There are some generalities, but each individual case is different. As a veterinarian, there is a responsibility to examine the animal thoroughly and explain the potential outcome to the owner.

> It is not always possible to obtain the exact diagnosis, but it *is* always possible to use a knowledge of biological principles and make an *informed decision* about that animal's potential to return to work.

1.8 Zoonotic disease

Presented below is a list of zoonotic infections that can spread from horses to humans. It is important when attending cases of suspected zoonotic disease that precautions are taken to protect your safety and also that the owners are informed of the risks. In many countries suspicion of certain zoonotic infections must be reported to the government authorities.

Anthrax See Section 11.5

Brucellosis See Sections 13.4 and 14.10

Cryptosporidium See Section 18.1

Dermatophilosis See Section 15.3

Glanders See Sections 12.7 and 15.3

Leptospirosis See Sections 9.6 and 13.4

Rabies See Section 16.1

Ringworm See Section 15.3

Salmonella See Section 11.6

Togaviral encephalitis See Section 16.1

Vesicular stomatitis See Section 11.4

West Nile Virus See Section 16.1

1.9 Case study – Communication and prognosis

Signalment A 9-year-old mare; has been in owner's possession 3 years. Used for transportation of people by cart.

History This animal presented with massive carpal swelling and chronic arthritis, whereby the owner requested the veterinarian to cut off the 'tumour'.

Clinical examination The carpus of the left forelimb was extremely enlarged, particularly on the dorso-medial aspect (Figure 1.8.1). The horse was 5/10 lame on the left forelimb at the walk. There was reduced range of motion on flexion of the carpus with a pain response from the horse (pulling the limb away from the examiner).

Diagnosis Carpal osteoarthritis with severe surrounding soft tissue swelling.

> *How should this case be managed?*
> Owners do not necessarily understand the underlying mechanisms as to why a condition presents *visually* the way it does. It should be explained in simple terms that the swelling on the carpus is not a tumour than can be surgically removed. If the owner does not understand this they may belive that the vet has not done a good job.

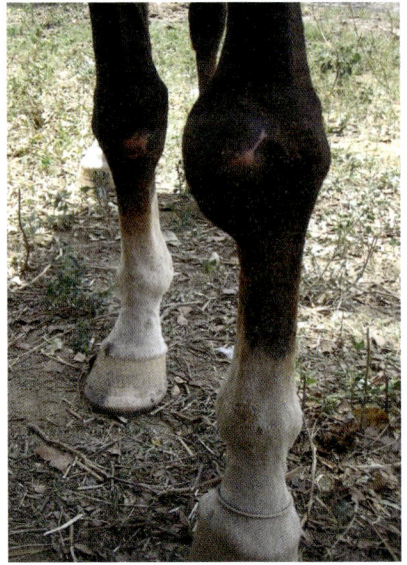

Figure 1.8.1 Carpal growth on the left foreleg.

Treatment Pain relief (non-steroidal anti-inflammatory drugs) short term IV, then long-term PO. Advice on resting the horse until improvement is seen in the condition. Follow-up phone calls and visits by the veterinarian to check on progress and alter advice and management as necessary.

Prognosis If chronic changes are already present then chances of improvement are reduced. In this case a prognosis of 'return to normal' is not likely. Instead, this animal's lifestyle and pain must be correctly managed in order for her to have some relief and potentially 'return to work'. However, if the underlying, long-term mechanisms for arthritis are not explained (chronic work on hard roads, possible previous injury, poor foot trimming, etc.) the owner will not understand why it cannot be fixed. Worst of all, if they brought their animal for a 'cure' which cannot be provided, the owner will not trust the expertise of the clinician, and consequently may not follow up any management advice which has been offered. The worst case scenario is that the owner will seek an even more damaging treatment such as firing (see Chapter 2).

Discussion See Section 1.1 of this chapter on the consultation process:

'How can I make a long term, sustainable difference to this animal?'

> The answer lies strongly with the concept of owner communication (Figure 1.8.2) – therefore ensure to invest in this every time!

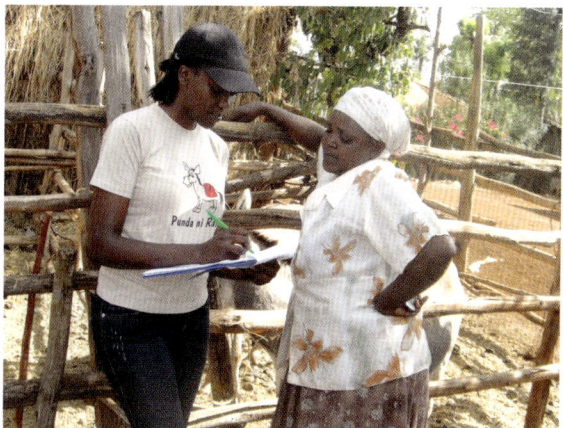

Figure 1.8.2 Spending time in creating good vet-owner relationships will reap rewards for the animal.

References 1.10

Ali, R., Anjum, A. (1998) Rectal temperature, pulse rate and breath rate in mules. *Pak. J. Biol. Sci.* 1 (4), 271–273.

Al-Saad, K.M. (2009). Acute Babesiosis in foals. *J. Anim. Vet. Adv.* 8 (12), 2585–2589.

Broster, C.E., Burn, C.C., Barr, A.R.S., Whay, H.R. (2009) The range and prevalence of pathological abnormalities associated with lameness in working horses from developing countries. *Equine Vet. J.* 41 (5), 474–481.

Canacoo, E.A., Eliis-Sackey, G.J., Quashie, B.S., (1991) Some physiological values of apparently healthy donkeys in Ghana, Proceedings of the international Colloquium, Edinburgh, Scotland, 3rd - 6th September, pp. 98–102.

Colahan, P.T., Mayhew, I.G., Merritt, A.M., Moore, J.N. (1999) Manual of Equine Medicine and Surgery. Mosby, Inc. Missouri, pp. 17–22.

Ihler, C.F., Venger, J.L., Skjerve, E. (2004) Evaluation of clinical and laboratory variables as prognostic indicators in hospitalised gastrointestinal colic horses. *Acta. vet. scand.* 45, 109–118.

Korte, S.M., Olivier, B., Koolhaas, J.M. (2007) A new animal welfare concept based on allostasis. *Physiol. Behav.* 92, 422–428.

Lemma, A., Moges, M. (2009) Clinical, hematological and serum biochemical reference values of working donkeys *(Equus asinus)* owned by transport operators in Addis Ababa, Ethiopia. *Livest. Res. Rural Dev.* 21 (8), 127.

Muylle, S., Simoens, P., Lauwers, H., Van Loon, G. (1999) Age determination in mini-shetland ponies and donkeys. *J. Vet. Med. A.* 46, 421–429.

Pritchard, J.C., Lindberg, A.C., Main, D.C.J., Whay, H.R. (2005) Assessment of the welfare of working horses, donkeys and mules, using health and behaviour parameters. *Prev. Vet. Med.* 69 (3–4), 265–283.

Pritchard, J.P., Burn, C.C., Barr, A.R.S., Whay, H.R. (2008) Validity of indicators of dehydration in working horses: A longitudinal study of changes in skin tent duration, mucous membrane dryness and drinking behaviour. *Equine Vet. J.* 40 (6), 558–564.

White, N.A., Edwards, B. (1999) Handbook of Equine Colic. Reed Elsevier plc. p.11.

Wilson, D. V., Rondenay, Y., Shance, P.U. (2003) The cardiopulmonary effects of severe blood loss in anaesthetised horses. *Vet. Anaesth. Analg.* 30 (2), 81–87.

Further Reading

Colahan, P.T., Mayhew, I.G., Merritt, A.M., Moore, J.N. (1999) Manual of Equine Medicine and Surgery. Mosby, Inc. Missouri. 17–22.

White, N.A., Edwards, B. (1999) Handbook of Equine Colic. Reed Elsevier plc. p. 11.

Welfare, behaviour and handling of working equids

2

Welfare	**2.1**
Behaviour	**2.2**
Handling and restraint	**2.3**
Harmful traditional practices	**2.4**
Case study – Firing	**2.5**
References	**2.6**

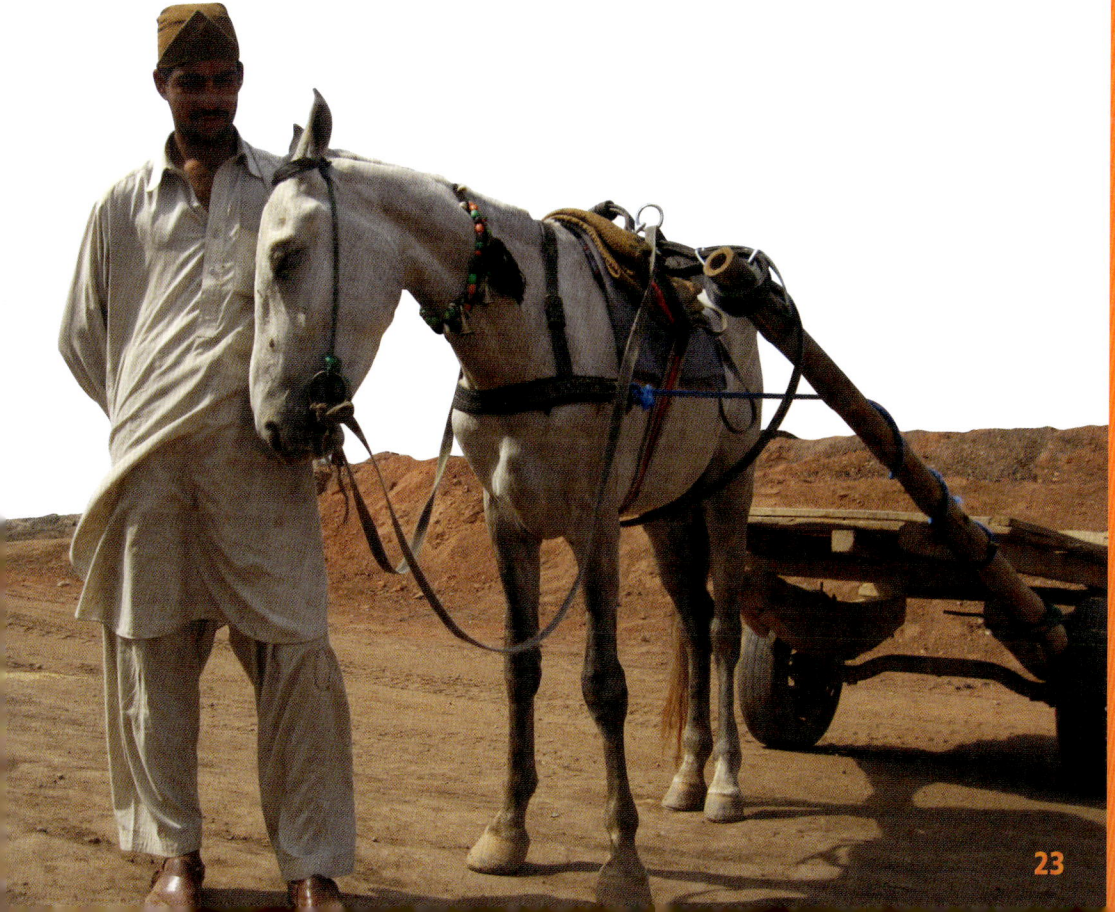

2.1 Welfare

Animal welfare and sentience

What is 'animal welfare'?

'Animal welfare' is not a purely scientific concept but one based on values of what is *better* or *worse* for an animal (Fraser et al. 1997). 'Animal welfare' is a term used to explain consideration towards an animal's life experiences, their needs and how they feel, both physically and mentally. Information that we gather on working horses, donkeys and mules when we observe them (Figure 2.1.1.) can be applied to different welfare frameworks (see glossary, page 33) to help reach a consensus about an animal's welfare state.

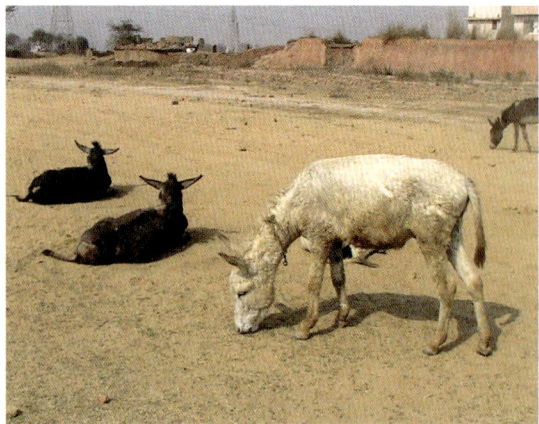

Figure 2.1.1 Observing working equids at the end of a working day.

What is 'sentience'?

'Sentience' is a term often used in discussions on animal welfare. Animals (vertebrates and cephalopod invertebrates) are sentient beings, meaning they have the capacity for sensing or feeling. This includes perceptions of their surroundings, awareness of what is happening to them, positive feelings such as joy and happiness, and negative feelings such as pain and loneliness.

'Animal welfare' is a complex concept designed to help observation and consideration of the animal's experience, its needs and feelings. This should determine the course of action: what can, should and must be done for the animal in any particular context.

> In the working equid context, rarely is a working horse, donkey, or mule experiencing perfect welfare. Make a judgment about the animal's welfare which takes into consideration human behaviour towards the animal, its environment, available resources and aspects of the animal itself (e.g. age).

The animal's welfare may be:

- **Good** The animal is physically fit; mentally the animal feels well and enjoys positive life experiences. The animal appears strong, healthy and happy because its basic needs are met and its feelings are considered in daily life. There is an absence of actions and conditions which result in unnecessary harm for the animal.

- **Between good and bad** Some aspects of the animal's welfare may be good and some need improvement. There may be opportunities to provide alternatives to the conditions the animal is currently experiencing.

- **Bad** The animal is not physically fit; mentally it feels bad and does not enjoy life experiences. The animal appears weak, unhealthy and sad because its basic needs are not being met, nor are the animal's feelings considered. There is an absence of actions and resources which result in good for the animal.

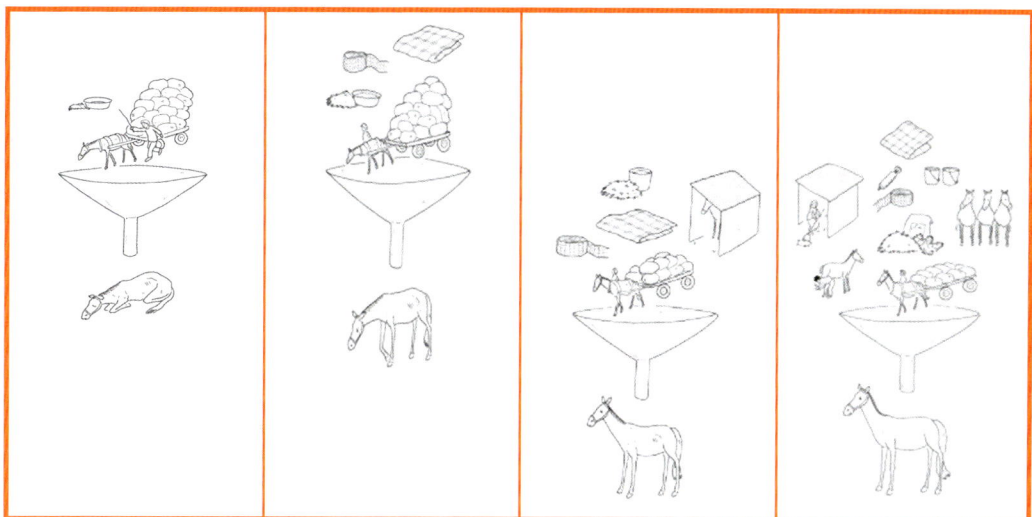

Figure 2.1.2 Visualising welfare inputs and outputs as a continuum. © Martha Hardy at GCI

Figure 2.1.2 shows the inputs at the top of the diagrams, such as food and shelter. From left to right the animal has more and more inputs available to them (going into the funnel). The outputs are the welfare state of the animal seen at the bottom of the diagrams.

> The focus on inputs should be the inclusion of good practices, as outlined by the Five Freedoms (Passantino 2011) and also the absence of bad practices (e.g. overloading, poor handling).

How do animal welfare concepts fit into daily veterinary work?

A veterinarian will develop routines; it is equally important that there is flexibility to meet the needs of individual animals.

> To capitalise on opportunities to create a better state of well-being and better life for the animal, it is necessary to spend time observing, thinking and practising 'listening to the animal'.

Consider the following four points at each interaction with a working equid:

Observe the animal and its surroundings.

Feel what the animal is feeling e.g. anxiety, confusion, struggle, contentment, pain, distress, comfort, or playfulness.

Reflect Think 'in this situation I would...'

Action Try something. If successful, great; if not, reflect and adjust the plan.

2 WELFARE, BEHAVIOUR AND HANDLING OF WORKING EQUIDS

Just as years were spent learning and practising veterinary knowledge and skills in university, learning how to understand the animal, its language, and how to provide for its needs takes continuous learning and practice. Creativity is required to overcome challenges faced in the field. Approaches that work for one animal may not work for another. With time, this process becomes automatic.

Contributing towards an animal's 'Five Freedoms'

> The 'Five Freedoms' looks at welfare outputs in terms of 'freedoms'. This is a compact of rights for animals under human control.
>
> Keep the Five Freedoms of Animal Welfare at the forefront of veterinary work.
>
> Aim to apply them practically as much as possible during the consultation process.

- Consider what can be arranged in advance of a field visit. For example, what should be brought, what can be arranged to benefit the animal? Some examples include: water, shelter, handling equipment and arranging for a community member to prepare the field/environment.
- During the consultation process consider the opportunities to meet the animals' welfare needs.

Observe the animal, its behaviour and environment (Figure 2.1.1).

Feel what the animal is feeling e.g. is it thirsty, hot, scared, in pain, exhausted, dull, depressed, alert, confused?

Reflect 'In this situation I would...'

Action Try something; make adjustments if needed.

- Reflect on the animal's future life. What advice is a priority? Check that the person receiving the advice understands and feels confident to comply with it.

Consider each of the Five Freedoms when 'listening to the animal'

- Freedom from hunger and thirst
- Freedom from discomfort
- Freedom from pain, injury and disease
- Freedom from fear and distress
- Freedom to express normal behaviour

1. Freedom from hunger and thirst

As a minimum, provide water (carry water in the vehicle or arrange beforehand with the community) and give the animal time to drink (Figure 2.1.3). Advise on nutrition.

Observe e.g. body condition, ability to eat/drink, quidding, sunken eyes, sharp teeth, mucous membranes.

Feel what the animal is feeling in its environment and working routine e.g. thirst, dehydration, exhaustion, respiratory distress, hunger, pain.

Reflect 'In this situation realistically I can...'

Action e.g. rasp the teeth, show owner what to feed and what not to feed (Figure 2.1.4).

> Offering water is important; we might not always know when the animal last had the chance to drink. If the animal drinks it can help to diagnose and treat dehydration simultaneously (Pritchard *et al.* 2008).

Equids need time to drink undisturbed; there may be an initial delay before drinking and time must be allowed for this.

2. Freedom from discomfort

Look for opportunities to make the animal more comfortable physically.

> At a minimum, pay special attention to the effect of environmental conditions and equipment on the animal.

Observe e.g. animal hobbled so it cannot move, wounds present under equipment, equipment itself (Figure 2.1.5), objects on the ground animal could injure itself on, natural shade options (Figure 2.1.6).

Feel what the animal is feeling in its environment and working routine e.g. hot, tired, in pain, unable to move, agitated by flies (Figure 2.1.7).

Reflect 'In this situation realistically I can...'

Action e.g. advise on equipment maintenance or fly control, remove stones/debris from hooves.

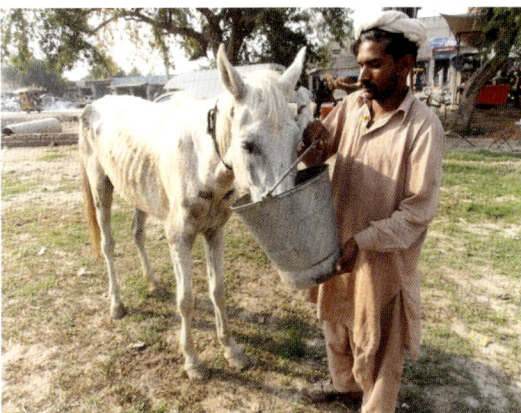

Figure 2.1.3 This animal has had the opportunity to drink.

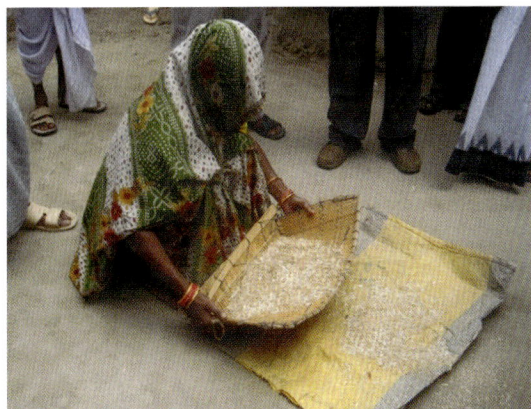

Figure 2.1.4 An owner was advised on how to clean and sort feed to remove sharp objects; she demonstrates what she has learned.

2 WELFARE, BEHAVIOUR AND HANDLING OF WORKING EQUIDS

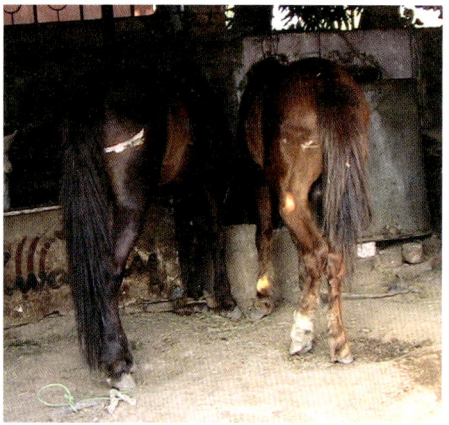 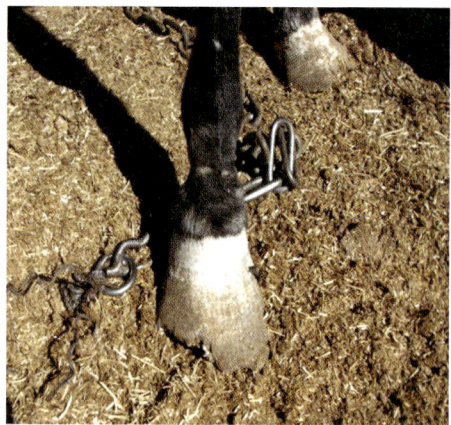

Figure 2.1.5 The wounds and scars caused by equipment (harness and chain hobble).

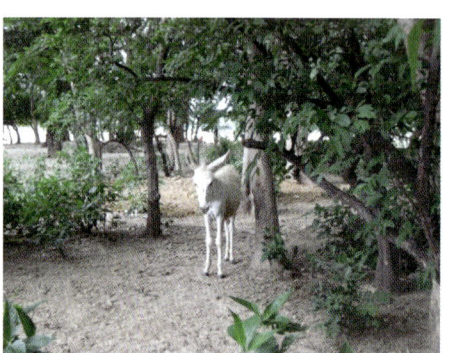 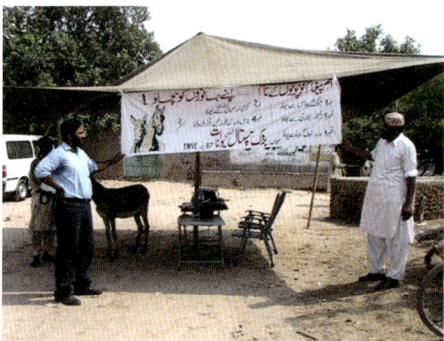

Figure 2.1.6 Use natural or man-made shade when preparing to work with animals.

Consider how owners could be advised on handling and equipment choices which are causing animals injury and distress (e.g. best material, correct fit, cleanliness and maintenance).

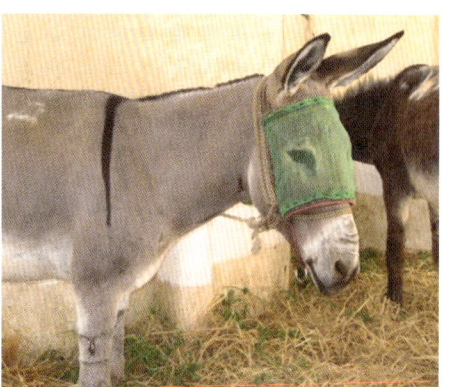 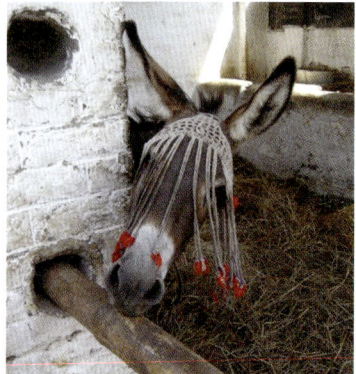

Figure 2.1.7 A fly fringe helps manage the animal's response to flies; this gives animals a further opportunity to rest.

3. Freedom from pain, injury and disease

This is partly achieved when a veterinarian attends to assist the animal. Further opportunities are always present.

When treating sick animals there is a high potential for disease to be spread by veterinarians, animal handlers and owners/users.

> Pay special attention to the treatment environment, minimising transmission of pathogens and disease by keeping hands and equipment clean and disinfected.

Observe e.g. animal's temperament, physical marks on its body, other animals present that are also ill. This will help to spot trends.

Feel what the animal is feeling in its environment and working routine e.g. alert, dull, scared, sick, uncomfortable, blind, lethargic.

Reflect 'In this situation realistically I can...'

Action e.g. advise on equipment maintenance or fly control, treat priority health issues.

Harmful objects should be removed (e.g. those an animal could injure itself on, attempt to eat) and a safe, clean space should be set up in order to treat animals quickly, securely and calmly. This is especially important when high numbers of animals are waiting for treatment. Ensure work is conducted in a hygienic manner.

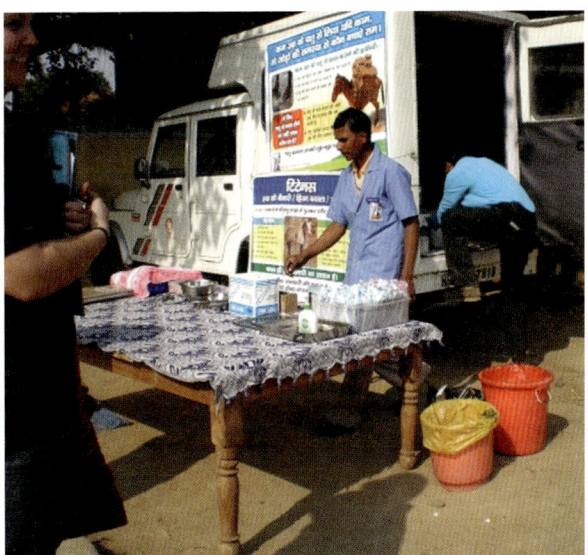
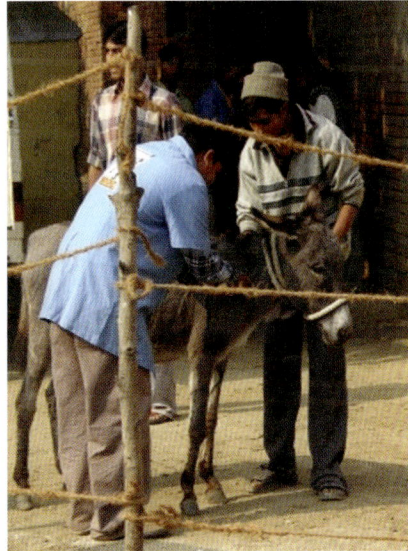

Figure 2.1.8 How an organised treatment and waiting area for animals and owners has been created.

2 WELFARE, BEHAVIOUR AND HANDLING OF WORKING EQUIDS

> **Encourage future prevention of welfare issues, particularly issues prioritised as affecting the animal the most.**

For example, the practice of *seton* where foreign material is stitched under the skin of an animal, or other unnecessary mutilations such as firing, needs owner education to bring about the end of such harmful practices.

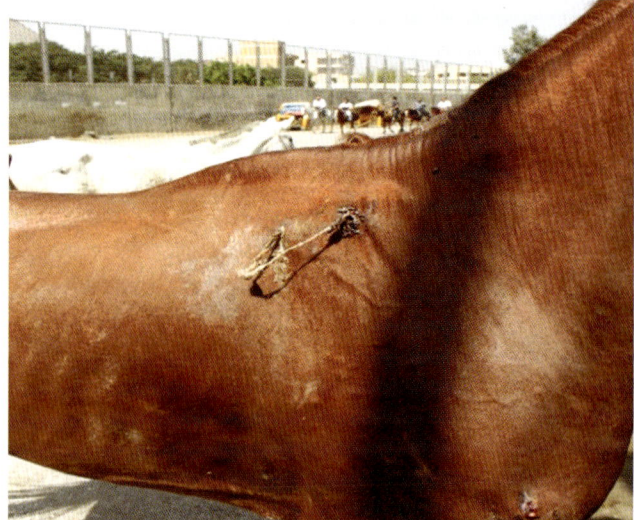

Figure 2.1.9 The harmful practice of seton.

4. Freedom from fear and distress

> **Look for opportunities to avoid causing unnecessary suffering and minimise stress during human-animal interactions.**

At a minimum, work with an experienced handler and give the animal an opportunity to calm down and accept the presence of strangers before proceeding with diagnostic tests or treatment (Figure 2.1.10).

Observe e.g. how does the animal react to its owner or other handlers; is the animal protective towards any part of its body?

Feel what the animal is feeling in its environment and working routine e.g. is it alert, happy, scared, unsure, accepting, or fighting the interaction?

Reflect 'In this situation realistically I can...'

Action e.g. work as quickly as possible, or take more time (according to the individual animal), spend a few minutes comforting the animal (using a calm voice, stroking the neck, etc.)

Be vigilant of other animals, children, vehicles and onlookers, all of which can contribute to a chaotic environment and may frighten the animal.

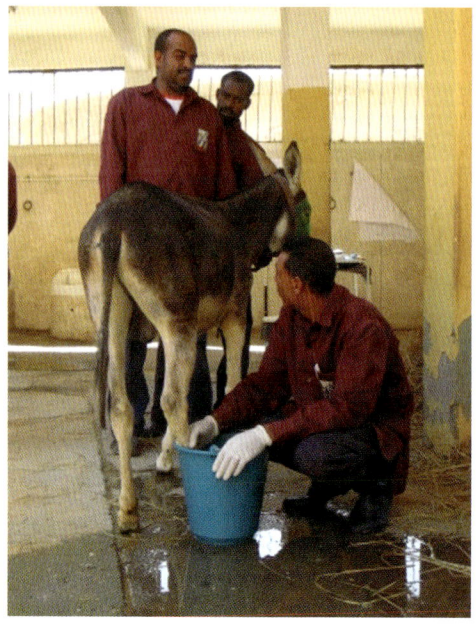

Figure 2.1.10 An animal accepting foot soaking, even with several people nearby.

Consider options for engaging with members of the community to demonstrate treatments and good welfare (Figure 2.1.11). Allow yourself enough space to work safely with the animals being treated.

Consider adjusting the approach to an individual animal (Figure 2.1.12). This might include: treating with a companion nearby, having only one person restrain rather than more, or moving the animal to a different area.

If the animal appears highly stressed, allow it time and space to calm down (Figure 2.1.13).

> **Only carry out actions which prove necessary and useful.**

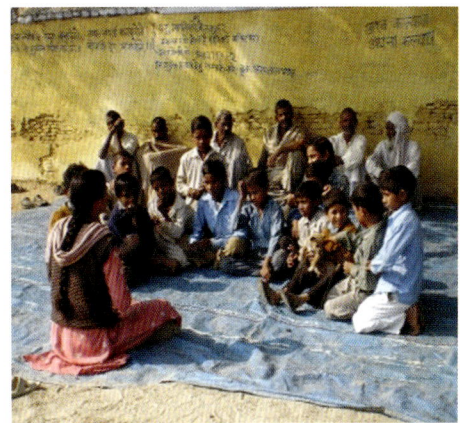

Figure 2.1.11 A team in India engage the children from a community in field activities, away from the animal.

For example, if conducting a diagnostic test (e.g. taking the rectal temperature) on a highly stressed animal, question whether the result will be accurate. It is good practice to evaluate how necessary the diagnostic result is and how to obtain it in the best way.

5. Freedom to express normal behaviour

Working equids can be restricted from exploring their environment and behaving as they would choose to because they are working and/or have restricted movement during rest.

> **During a veterinary consultation, the animal can still enjoy opportunities to carry out normal behaviours during handling and treatment.**

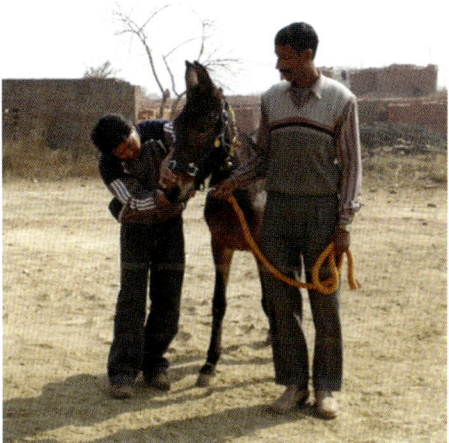

Figure 2.1.12 Examining the animal from the side.

Remember, observing the animal from a distance prior to the clinical examination contributes to the diagnosis and approach to treatment (see Chapter 1).

As a minimum, using a correctly fitting halter and lead rope will allow control of the animal. This means the handler can feel confident to allow the animal to move its head, shift its weight, roll, vocalise, sniff and explore when it is an appropriate time to do so. Also the handler is easily able to position the animal when veterinary treatment is required.

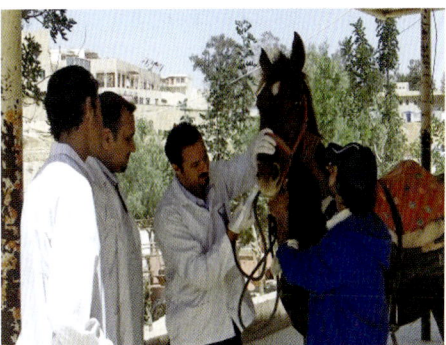

Figure 2.1.13 If an unpleasant treatment is to be administered allow time for the animal to become accustomed to the situation.

2 WELFARE, BEHAVIOUR AND HANDLING OF WORKING EQUIDS

> **Do not punish the animal by using force. Immediately cease investigation if the animal expresses aggressive behaviour.**

The animal may be frightened, distressed, in pain or be unclear as to what a person is asking it to do. Can something be adjusted: human behaviour, equipment, environment, method of physical or chemical restraint?

Observe e.g. easy or difficult to handle, sweaty, positive or negative interactions with other animals such as grooming or fighting.

Feel what the animal is feeling in its environment and working routine e.g. itchy, nervous, hot, annoyed by other animals, or wanting to play.

Reflect 'In this situation realistically I can...'

Action e.g. allow the animal to roll (Figure 2.1.14), release restraint, bring a companion animal close-by (Figure 2.1.15).

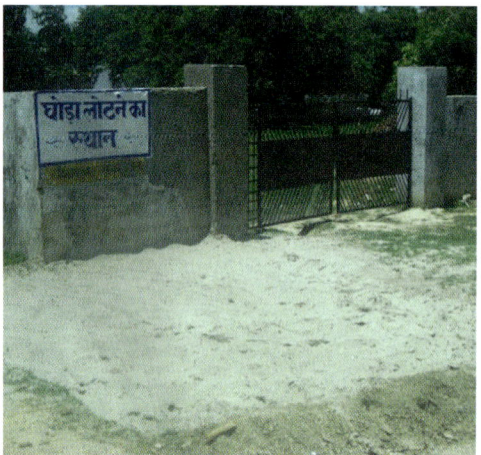

Figure 2.1.14 A community created this sand pit specifically to give their animals a safe place to roll before and after work, or after veterinary interventions.

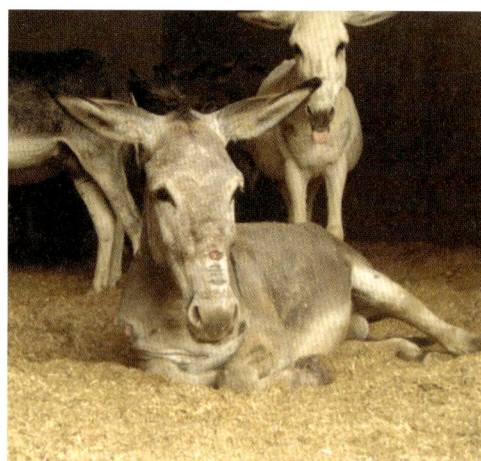

Figure 2.1.15 Patients may be more relaxed if they are near other animals.

WELFARE 2.1

Glossary

Animal welfare science, ethics and law

> - **Animal welfare science** investigates the effect on the animal (this informs ethics and law).
> - **Animal welfare ethics** investigates how humans should treat animals.
> - **Animal welfare law** states how humans must treat animals.

Recognised animal welfare frameworks which can be applied to working equids

- **Five freedoms** This framework looks at welfare outputs in terms of *'freedoms': the ideal situations for animals which we should work towards achieving.* Each freedom is then linked to the inputs (resources and management practices) which are needed to achieve that freedom.

- **Physical welfare, mental welfare and naturalness** This view of animal welfare emphasises three components, such as 'fit and feeling good'. It recognises that both physical and mental welfare are important. It also includes *'naturalness': the ability of an animal to do what it would choose to do in a natural or wild state.* For example, the opportunity for a working donkey still to be a donkey – grazing, braying, socialising in a herd with other donkeys – rather than just being a machine for people's benefit.

- **Fit and feeling good** *This definition says that an animal has good welfare if it is 'fit and happy' or 'fit and feeling good.'* Fitness means that the animal can sustain health and vigour throughout an effective working life. 'Feeling good' recognises that animals are sentient; in other words they have feelings that matter. We should aim to ensure that animals do not suffer and have the positive feelings gained from comfort, companionship and security.

- **Four principle ethics** This is an ethical framework developed and used extensively in human medicine, which may also help with thinking about animal welfare. It is a useful checklist to apply when making any ethical decision. The four principles are:

> 1. **Non-malfeasance** 'Do no harm', or at least 'minimise the harm'.
> 2. **Beneficence** 'Maximise the good' (once the harm has been minimised).
> 3. **Autonomy** The ability of people (or animals) to be self-governing, or at least to make choices about their lives and their medical treatment. For animals, take into account what the animal would choose in a certain situation.
> 4. **Justice** Treat all people (or animals) fairly and equally.

3 R's – Refinement, Reduction and Replacement These have developed from laboratory animal protection law. They can be very usefully applied after making any ethical decision, in order to minimise or mitigate any negative effects; for example when deciding whether to use animals in training courses.

2.2 Behaviour

What do we mean by 'behaviour'?

Behaviour is an animal's way of expressing its feelings and experiences, positive or negative. In order to work with animals, it is important to understand their feelings.

> **Interpreting equine body language will improve the assessment of the health of an animal as well as allowing safe management of actions and reactions.**

Opportunities to improve the welfare of animals enjoy interactions with them, will be missed if assessment of behaviour is skipped.

Getting to know the patients involves:

- understanding traits and general behaviours, e.g. natural history, evolution of equids, anatomy, categories of behaviour
- observing the animal; understanding what it might be feeling based on its behaviour
- questioning and interpreting what is seen, e.g. indicators of good or poor welfare.

Understanding traits of equids

Below are some key traits of equids. Appreciation of these can help explain some of the animal's actions or reactions.

1. Equids are a 'prey' species.

> **In a natural prey-predator relationship, prey animals are vulnerable to predators and therefore are focused on survival.**

Equids are very perceptive. They have evolved to be aware of and react to experiences or objects they find threatening; this includes humans!

- Their eyes are positioned on either side of their head (Figure 2.2.1.) enabling an 'almost full circle of horizontal vision' (Hanggi 2012), which provides a strong scanning capability, useful in defence. There are believed to be two 'blind spots' or areas where the animals cannot see: immediately in front of the animal (anterior to the forehead and below the nose), and immediately behind them (Hanggi 2012). Their long noses allow them to have their heads down for grazing whilst still maintaining surveillance of their surroundings.

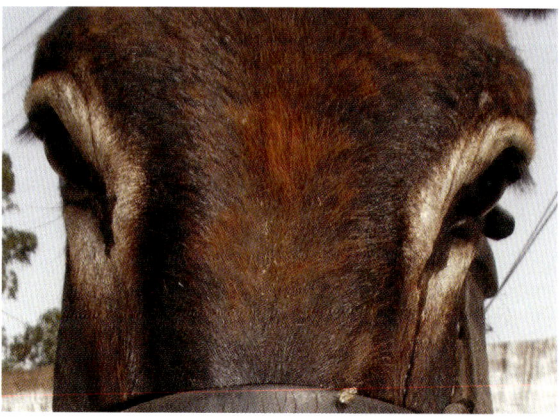

Figure 2.2.1 Equid eyes are situated on the sides of the head, enabling almost a full circle of vision.

BEHAVIOUR 2.2

> **Prey species do not like restraint or feeling 'trapped'.**

- Equids are cautious and use their speed and agility as a means of self-preservation. Restricting their movement can cause fear, distress or displays of unwanted behaviour, demonstrating that they are upset; restraint must be done with consideration.
- They are able to stand for long periods of time, enabling them to move swiftly to escape from predators. Equids usually only lie down for short periods of time; normally when other equids are standing or grazing nearby.

> **Extended periods of trotting and cantering are unnatural for equids and they should be trained and conditioned for work slowly.**

- They need to conserve their energy in order to have it available for survival situations – to escape from predators ('fight or flight'). So their natural instinct is to move slowly and regularly as they graze.
- In a working relationship, humans must use behaviour which shows that we mean no harm. By making the animal feel safe and allowing it enough freedom to carry out small movements, we can expect to see less unwanted behaviour, such as kicking and biting.

> **The goal should be for an animal to have a good experience every time it is with the veterinarian.**

2. Equids adopt a 'flight or fight' response to threatening stimuli.

> **An equid's main aim is survival, it will adapt its behaviour to suit the circumstance and remain safe; flight is an escape response.**

The stimulus for provoking a flight response may be visual, olfactory (smell), tactile (touch), auditory (sound), or a combination of any of these. Fight is an aggressive social interaction involving potentially harmful actions through physical contact. Fight responses occur when animals cannot escape; thus these responses are often secondary to flight attempts.

- Something which does not cause fear – the animal's reaction will be to ignore or explore the person, animal or object. It is in its nature to be curious.
- Something to fear – the animal's first reaction to the person, animal or object they fear will be to move away from it. This is the animal's 'flight response'.

> **If the animal does not feel it is able to escape the threat, it will send warning signals that it is prepared to fight. This is the animal's 'fight response'.**

- Flight responses (e.g. turning head away, moving away) are attempted before fight responses (e.g. kicking, biting, or rearing).

> **If the animal shows a fight response, this usually means that it tried a flight response first and this was either ignored or prevented – equid fight responses are triggered by our own behaviour towards them so we should take responsibility for these.**

2 WELFARE, BEHAVIOUR AND HANDLING OF WORKING EQUIDS

- In a working relationship equids will give behavioural warning signs when they are fearful or distressed and those handling or treating working animals should be aware of these and alter approaches as necessary.

In Figure 2.2.2 the donkey was startled by the movements of the examiner. In this case the examiner should stop, the donkey should be allowed to calm and another attempt should be made using a soothing voice and slow movements, with gentle but firm touch. Do not tickle.

3. Equids are herd species or social herbivores.

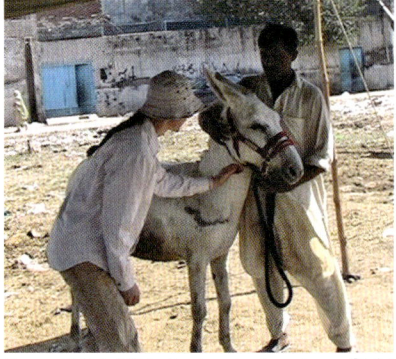

Figure 2.2.2 This donkey is showing a flight response when touched by the examiner.

> **Equids benefit from, and have an innate preference for, the companionship of other animals of the same species for added safety and mutual comfort.**

Tactile communication between equids (along with olfactory, auditory and visual communication) is important. They can feel insecure or stressed as a result of being isolated.

> **In a working relationship, a greater success in handling and treating equids is attained with a calm and patient manner. Adjust the environment to suit the individual animal.**

- There is an expression that 'horses are mirrors'. This means that the animal's behaviour reflects what it sees, both from humans and other animals around. Calm behaviour from humans will lead to calmer animals; rushed or agitated behaviour from handlers will lead to agitated or fearful responses from horses, donkeys and mules. Bringing another calm, controlled animal into the treatment environment may help comfort the animal receiving treatment.
- To show an equid that no harm is intended, try not to act like a predator – looking directly at its face, grabbing it quickly and holding on – because the instincts of the horse, donkey or mule will tell it that it is about to be hurt or killed. Instead, when approaching for the first time, lower the eyes, move close to the animal and/or touch it, and then immediately move away a few steps, turning sideways to the animal. Repeat this two or three times before examining or treating the animal.

> **A predator always faces the animal straight on, looks at it intently, and never just touches its prey and walks away, so this technique helps the horse, donkey or mule to understand that the veterinarian is not a predator.**

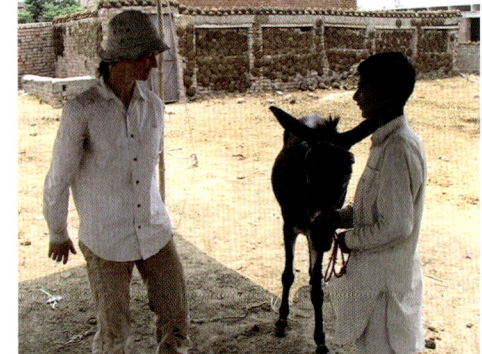

Figure 2.2.3 A non-threatening approach. As the examiner retreats a few steps the donkey shows non-fearful interest.

4. Equids learn and make associations all the time. They may not respond well to unfamiliar or confusing commands.

   ▮ In a working relationship, we should not assume that the animal knows what we want it to do, e.g. stand still for an injection or wound cleaning. We should also not assume that the animal knows when an experience will end, e.g. during a leg lift used as a means of further restraint.

> **If the equid acts in an unexpected way, it is actually reacting to whatever we are doing, or to something else in the environment.**

   ▮ To prevent or minimise an unwanted behaviour we need to look for the action that led to the reaction in the horse, mule or donkey.
   ▮ Equids do not have the higher cognitive ability to be stubborn, deliberately naughty, jealous, vicious, annoy people, or indulge in other human behaviour. If we give their behaviour these labels, it can lead us to treat them in a way that does not take their real motivations into account and therefore help us to reduce the unwanted behaviour.

> **If we always think of equine behaviour in terms of the natural need for survival – to protect themselves from harm and to find food, water and other horses/donkeys/mules – then we will understand their true motivations and be able to reduce any unwanted behavioural consequences of these survival instincts.**

   ▮ Useful questions to consider when dealing with unwanted equine behaviour (almost all unwanted behaviours have one of these four root causes):
     - Is the animal frightened?
     - Is the animal in pain?
     - Is the animal reliving a negative experience from the past?
     - Is the animal not understanding (or confused by) what it is being asked to do?

Understanding their language

Equids communicate to humans in the same way that they communicate to other equids.

   1. Look and listen to the overall picture: **what combination** of vocalisations, breathing, posture, facial expressions, and muscle tension can be seen?

> **Observe the animal from a distance in the same manner as conducting a clinical examination.**

   ▮ Does the animal appear bright, alert, responsive or dull, depressed, excited, stressed, in pain?
   ▮ Is the animal behaving normally? Or is the animal exhibiting unwanted or concerning behaviour?

   2. Further information

   ▮ Further reading can be found in the References list at the end of this chapter.
   ▮ For information on the behavioural signs of pain refer to Chapter 3 *Pain – Indicators and management in working equids* and the review article by Ashley *et al.* (2005).

2.3 Handling and restraint

> Handling of equids for any reason should be carried out in a calm and gentle manner with consideration for the animal's experience in the process.

The principle objective of restraint is to limit an animal's movement for its own safety, while it is receiving some form of attention (Fraser 2010), this may be an examination or treatment. No handling procedure should be based on infliction of pain on the animal and the principle of **'do no harm'** should be practised. Even for very experienced veterinarians and assistants, handling and restraint of working equids can at times be difficult. While many patients will accept handling and treatment, some others may display unwanted defensive behaviours such as moving away, biting, rearing or kicking.

Ideally those coming in contact with working equids should:

- understand equine behaviour and appropriate communication methods. For example, be aware of natural behaviours and senses, and develop the ability to appear non-threatening from the animal's point of view.
- understand how to keep safe during any interaction. For example, be aware of danger zones and warning signs shown by the animal (Table 2.3.1).
- apply understanding of animal behaviour, needs and feelings when creating a treatment environment and preparing to work with each individual animal
- always use the minimum level of restraint needed to carry out a procedure safely
- have a willingness to adjust technique to the individual animal's needs and behaviours.

> **The aim should be appropriate treatment without force.**

Table 2.3.1 identifies the six main body parts of equids (zones) which can cause injury to humans or other animals, and the ways in which injury could be caused (dangers). Veterinarians, assistants and handlers should remember these at all times when working around equids, and communicate between each other if warning signs are displayed.

Zone	Dangers
Head	Butting with the animal's nose or top of its head
Teeth	Biting
Front legs	Striking in front, standing on human feet, pawing, stamping, and kicking towards the belly
Body	Crushing the handler against something solid (e.g. fence, wall)
Hind legs	Kicking behind, kicking towards the belly, kicking to the side
Tail	Whipping in the face or eyes (particularly with horses, less so with donkeys)

Table 2.3.1 The six main danger zones of equids and the potential source of injury.

HANDLING AND RESTRAINT 2.3

Approaching and examining a working equid

When considering the approach and examination of a working equid reflect on the following aspects of good practice in Table 2.3.2 (below).

> Think about how the animal will perceive human actions and reactions, and be aware of the environment, other people, animals and distractions.

Good practice	Why
Remember to observe the animal, assess its feelings and anticipate how to work with the animal.	Behavioural assessment is valuable in determining the best approach to the consultation process.
Approach the animal from the side (same approach for left or right side). If the animal is blind in one eye, approach from the opposite side.	Equids' eyes are on either side of their heads (See Section 2.2). They are unable to see directly behind or in front ('blind spots').
Do not make direct eye contact, look at the neck and breast instead, and allow the animal to investigate (i.e. sniff).	Equids are prey species and feel threatened by predators. Predators approach with direct eye contact so this should be avoided.
Be aware of other stimuli (e.g. vehicles, children). Approach with your arms down or to your side, making a little noise (e.g. talking softly).	Horses, donkeys and mules have keen senses and startle easily. To minimise unfavourable reactions avoid approaching too fast, with sudden movements or loud noises (e.g. waving or outstretched arms, shouting, using mobile phones).
Observe the animal's response to an approach. Continue to do this throughout the interaction, moving with calm purpose around the body.	If the animal appears excited, nervous, frightened or aggressive, further time should be spent putting it at ease and making it feel calm and accepting the interaction.
Identify an area where the animal is comfortable having someone standing close (e.g. shoulder). Rather than retreating too quickly if the animal reacts negatively, return to this position to calm the animal before continuing.	It is often better to stay with the animal. Retreating too quickly will demonstrate fear. The animal will learn that it can control human movements in this way, making future attempts at handling and treatment less successful.
Use hands and voice to reassure the animal while working. Always try to maintain contact with the animal.	The use of hands and voice lets the animal know the position of the clinician and reduces the potential to startle. This is particularly useful if the animal is blind in one or both eyes.

2 WELFARE, BEHAVIOUR AND HANDLING OF WORKING EQUIDS

Good practice	Why
Use the minimum amount of contact necessary to assess/treat the animal, particularly in areas which are sensitive (e.g. girth/belly, limbs, equipment contact points, wounds, scars).	Animals may be more sensitive and reactive around areas where there tends to be little contact normally or where there is evidence of physical trauma or pain. Equids tend to be more sensitive over areas of bone than muscle. Scars are evidence of a previous painful occurrence. Typically once the tissues have healed, the animal will no longer feel pain. However, negative experiences can make animals more difficult to handle. This can be overcome by showing the animal non-threatening behaviour.
When unwanted behaviours (e.g. moving away, biting, rearing or kicking) are observed, stop the examination or treatment. Together with the handler, assess the situation and make adjustments.	Equids have evolved systems of behaviour to help them successfully detect, avoid and react to threats. Potentially these are justified behavioural responses due to the animal experiencing pain, distress or fear. Manage these behaviours to achieve the best welfare outcome for the animal.
Where sedatives and analgesics are not available, painful procedures should not always be attempted. Consider the harm versus benefit.	The consequences from any immediate course of action should be investigated from the animal's point of view.

Table 2.3.2 List of good practice relating to approaching and examining a working equid.

Methods of restraint

Physical restraint

Restraint is a necessary part of a meaningful consultation process. The whole veterinary team should ensure they are prepared with the knowledge and tools to handle the animal in a calm and gentle manner. When using methods of physical restraint, look out for signs of pain and distress in working equids. It is important to know when to stop and re-evaluate the situation should the interaction be difficult.

1. Halter, headcollar or rope halter

Equids use their head and neck as a way of resisting handling; it is essential to secure the head as a first step in control (Fraser 2010). While other methods may be used by owners (e.g. neck rope, head lock only) this is rarely a sufficient or acceptable way to control the animal during a veterinary procedure.

HANDLING AND RESTRAINT 2.3

> With control of the animal's head, the handler is able to manoeuvre the whole body of the animal more easily, thus achieving greater safety for the animal and person.

- Ensure the headcollar is well-fitting (Figure 2.3.1).
- A device can be made easily out of a 4–5 metre long, 15 mm thick, piece of rope, when a halter or headcollar is not available.
- Many working equids, especially donkeys, may not be used to wearing a headcollar. They may require more time and patience to become accustomed to it. Allow the animal to see/sniff the rope first, or place it on over existing work equipment.
- Ask for assistance from the owner if necessary.

To make a rope halter

Tie two knots in the rope ensuring each knot has a loop which the remaining rope can fit through. Feed the remaining rope through the first knot (this creates the part over the ears), then through the second knot (this creates the part under the chin). The rope halter can now be placed over the animal's muzzle, then behind the ears (see Figure 2.3.3). Use a long enough piece of rope so that the free end can serve as a 2-metre lead rope. There are many descriptions and videos available, outside of this text, showing this process in detail.

2. Leg lift

This is a useful alternative form of restraint, which can be used in addition to a halter or headcollar to help keep an animal still for a short period of time while an examination or treatment is carried out. It limits the animal's opportunity to move but the animal is able to balance on its other legs.

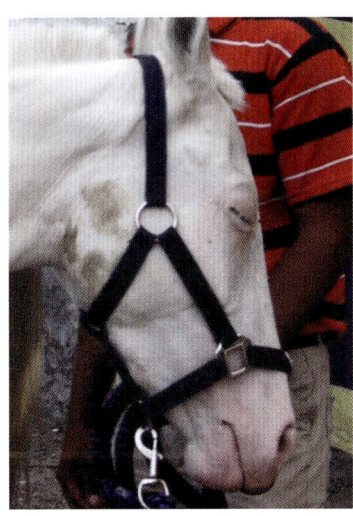

Figure 2.3.1 An example of a well-fitting headcollar.

Keep the leg up only for the duration needed to examine or treat the animal.

- To prevent the animal from moving around or kicking with a back leg, lift the front leg on the same side.
- Use a light grip and move with the animal, both will prevent the animal from snatching the leg away. Avoid letting the animal lean into the handler.
- If the animal is struggling to balance with one leg raised, place the leg back on the ground and give the animal time to regain its balance before lifting again.
- Raise the leg in line with the body. Avoid raising it too high or too far to the side as this prevents the animal from being able to balance.
- Working equids often have painful arthritis in their joints (Broster *et al.* 2009) – always bear this in mind with this form of restraint as it could be causing unnecessary pain; advise owners of this.
- This technique may not work with very nervous or difficult animals. In that case avoid repeat attempts of this form of restraint, particularly if the animal is rearing up. Decide when it is best to leave all four feet on the ground.

41

2 WELFARE, BEHAVIOUR AND HANDLING OF WORKING EQUIDS

Good lifting technique Lift the leg straight up to a comfortable height for the animal. The animal should stand without struggling once it has balanced (Figure 2.3.2).

> **Lifting the leg too high or out to the side (i.e. against normal movement) can result in an animal losing its balance and fighting against this method of restraint. Allow the animal to regain balance before proceeding.**

Figure 2.3.2 shows a right foreleg being lifted to aid examination of the contralateral forelimb. Ensure that a competent handler is present, with a halter or headcollar, and a good lifting technique is used. Notice the animal in the photograph appears attentive but relaxed.

3. Upper lip twitch

> **Avoid use with donkeys. Never twitch the ear, jaw or tongue.**

A twitch is a loop of rope threaded through a hole in a wooden pole (50 cm long). This is a more extreme form of restraint but may be used

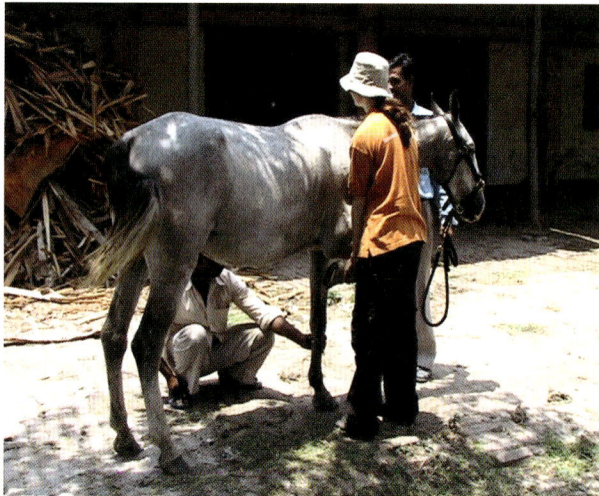

Figure 2.3.2 Leg lift restraint using the right forelimb.

in certain circumstances. Use in addition to a halter and lead rope with a competent handler. A twitch is used to divert attention and to control the animal's reaction to aid further necessary diagnostics or treatment.

Two main hypotheses have been proposed to explain the twitch's mode of action on a horse: a sedative effect through the release of endorphins (McCarthy *et al.* 1993) and a distraction (McGreevy 2004). **Either effect is controversial as discomfort and pain occur first.** In fact, McCarthy *et al.* (1993) showed that the beta-endorphin release which occurs when a twitch is applied to the upper lip of a horse also occurs when a horse undergoes prolonged air transport or has severe abdominal pain (colic).

> **This evidence demonstrates that the beta-endorphin release when a twitch is applied may be due to the stress/pain associated with the technique.**

Application of a twitch The decision to use a twitch should be taken carefully, not automatically. It may be appropriate when performing a short, non-painful procedure where the use of sedatives would be inappropriate as the effect would be too long-lasting. If a procedure will take some time, or a twitch is applied and the procedure takes longer than anticipated, stop. Take the twitch off and use chemical restraint where possible or re-assess the acceptability of performing the procedure.

Not every animal will accept the twitch. Only a few attempts should be made to place the twitch and force should not be used, particularly with highly stressed animals.

HANDLING AND RESTRAINT 2.3

- The handler should be experienced in this technique. Judge the time and pressure based on the animal's behaviour and remain vigilant towards the animal, the examiner, the handler, and the twitch itself during procedures.
- The handler should stand on the same side as the veterinarian (examiner), slightly to the side, so that if the animal kicks forwards with its forelegs nobody will be injured.
- The twitch should calmly be applied to the upper lip only. It should be done quickly but not excessively tightly. **Do not tighten the twitch any more than is necessary.** The initial response of the animal will vary but may include: rigidity, tension and a freeze in posture.
- Start the procedure once the animal shows signs of relaxing and calmness.
- Keep the duration of application as **short as possible** (5–15 minutes).
- Use caution when removing the twitch, keep control using the halter and lead rope.
- Release the twitch as soon as the procedure has finished.
- Gently rub the muzzle once the twitch is removed to aid circulation.

Check that the twitch is made from strong, natural rope with a smooth finish that will not damage the animal's skin, and has a long handle. Longer handles provide greater safety for the handler as well as the animal.

Twitch use in donkeys Less evidence is available for twitch use in donkeys, but what does exist suggests it is less effective (Vreeman *et al.* 2009).

- Donkeys have smaller, more rounded noses, so twitches slip off and are difficult to maintain in position.

The twitch is not advisable for use with donkeys.

- Equine professionals who have experience with donkeys state that twitches are less effective, particularly when the animals are stressed. Individuals may choose to use a 'head-restraining' approach with donkeys in addition to a halter and lead rope (Figure 2.3.3). With this approach the handler lightly cradles the donkey's head in their arms, approximately following the lines of the headcollar, and with one hand holding the nose or lower jaw. Be careful not to restrict breathing and do not use force. Handlers should use caution for their own health and safety with this approach. Halters are preferred.

4. Skin twitch – neck only

This is an additional form of restraint to a halter and lead rope. A fold of skin on the neck is held lightly (without force) to distract the animal (Figure 2.3.4, on page 44). This technique can be useful when giving an injection, but like all methods of restraint should be carefully thought through and not automatic. Release the pressure immediately after the procedure and stroke the area.

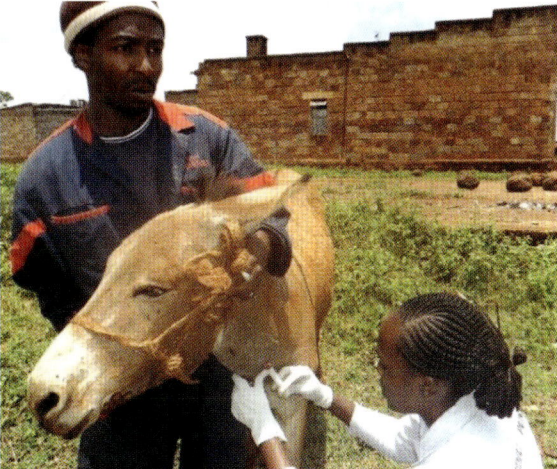

Figure 2.3.3 Use of a rope halter. Restraint of the head of a donkey for a brief treatment procedure (injection).

5. Limiting the animal's sight using a cupped-hand

This is an additional form of restraint to a halter and lead rope. The handler stands on the same side as the veterinarian. Using the hand in a cupped-shape, the handler blocks the animal's view of the veterinarian. This technique can often prove useful.

> Be flexible and creative when restraining an animal – what works for one animal may not for another.

Each individual animal is different. It may be helpful to utilise structures, spaces or other animals within the environment. These methods are anecdotal and based on field experience, what works for one animal may not work for another. Always remember '**do no harm**'. This means pay attention to the animal's experience (e.g. behavioural indicators of stress) and avoid the use of excess pressure.

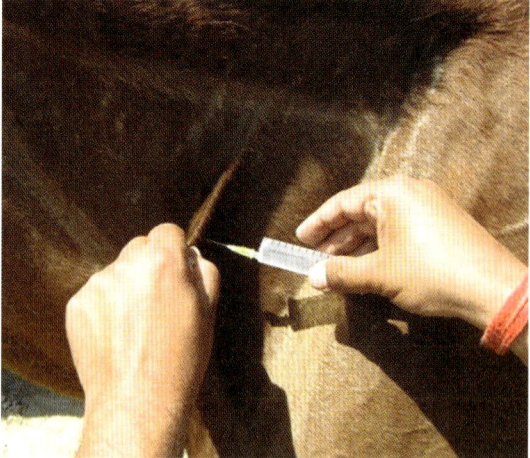

Figure 2.3.4 *Taking a fold of skin to distract from an injection.*

> **Having a companion nearby who is also well restrained with a halter and lead rope may calm or reassure the animal requiring treatment.**

Consider any of the following:

- Move the animal to stand near a corner, so it cannot back up. This limits an option for movement in one direction but the animal will still perceive that it can move forwards and won't feel trapped.
- Move the animal to a more open space, so the animal perceives it can move in more directions. This may be enough to make the animal feel safe so it remains still.
- Examine and treat the animal with its working equipment on. Working equids often suppress their natural behaviour when in their working equipment, so whilst it is normally best practice to remove everything to enable a proper examination, it might be better to try keeping working equipment on, or take it on and off in sections.

> **Ensure that pain, fear and stress are minimised at all times during the consultation.**

Be aware of how owners are using restraint and encourage them to try alternatives. For example, showing an owner how to use a halter and lead rope rather than ear twitching could be an immediate welfare improvement for the animal now and in the future.

Chemical restraint

Chemical restraint refers to the use of drugs for sedation, local/regional anaesthesia or general anaesthetic, all of which is discussed over various sections in Chapter 7.

> **Chemical restraint reduces fear, makes the procedure faster, easier, safer and, depending on the drug combinations used, may have an analgesic effect.**

Considerations with chemical restraint

1. Although very effective and commonly used in veterinary practice, no form of chemical sedation will improve animal welfare if the wrong drug/dosage is used, or if the risks have not been accurately assessed beforehand.

2. The importance of having a *plan* has already been mentioned: the earlier chemical restraint is given, the more beneficial it is to the animal. So planning will also help with making early decisions as to whether sedation will be necessary.

3. Drugs require time and a quiet, calm environment to work most effectively; they are not as effective in situations where an animal has become distressed. In such cases, allow the animal to calm down first before administering the chemical sedative.

4. The veterinarian is responsible for the animal until it fully recovers. If something happens during recovery it will be the veterinarian's responsibility, not that of the owner, the veterinary assistant or anyone else who happens to be there. Leave enough time to supervise recovery, and warn the owner beforehand that the animal will not be able to work until fully recovered from the sedative, which can be a number of hours; ensure 'informed consent'.

> **Drugs are always preferable over force but they must be used responsibly. Always ensure that the owner is aware of why the animal needs to be sedated, understands the risks involved, and knows how to manage the animal in the recovery phase.**

2.4 Harmful traditional practices – Firing and nostril slitting

Firing

Firing (thermocautery) is practised in many parts of the world, particularly in poorer, rural areas where access to health services (both animal and human) are scarce (Figure 2.4.1). In many countries local healers have a long family tradition of firing animals, and are supported and respected by their communities for the role they play in animal health service provision.

Firing patterns are a combination of points and lines. Points penetrate deeper into the tissues and lead to scarring, reduced blood supply and contraction especially over joints. Lines usually penetrate less deeply and cause cutaneous inflammation and scarring (Auer and Fackelman 1981).

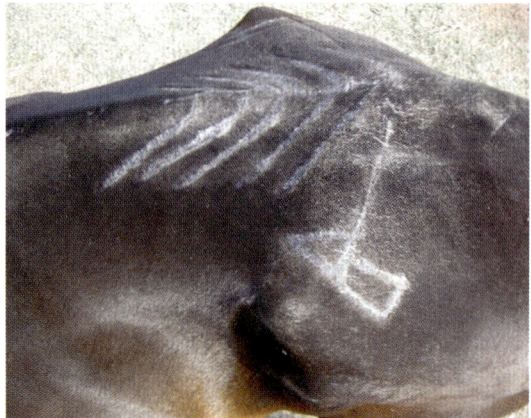

Figure 2.4.1 Firing of the pelvic and lumbar areas.

> **To prevent the use of these practices, veterinarians must work with local communities to look at the reasons why people fire and why they feel it helps their animals.**

- **Raising owner awareness** starts with looking at the root causes of why animals are ill or lame in the first place (nutrition, overloading, irregular hoof care) and helping owners to understand that, scientifically, firing cannot prevent or resolve conditions since it is merely the burning of the outer skin layers, and does not address the root cause (McCullagh and Silver 1981).

- **Training days for local practitioners** comprise discussions and practical sessions based on preventative practices such as correct drug administration routes, farriery, good harnessing and saddling techniques, wound management and hair clipping. These aim to provide alternatives to firing, and offer alternative sources of income for the local healers.

Nostril slitting

> Nostril slitting occurs in many countries due to the belief that it increases an animal's air intake, and therefore increases the capacity to work.

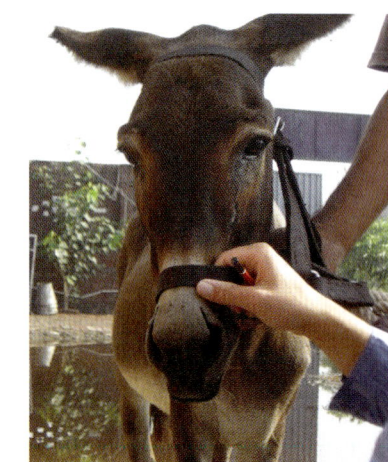

Figure 2.4.2 A donkey with slit nostrils.

Alternatively, signs of pain such as experienced during colic are often thought to indicate that an animal is having difficulty breathing; this is another reason why nostrils are slit (Figure 2.4.2.).

To prevent this practice, simply 'persuading' the owners not to do these things is difficult and not effective. Use knowledge of anatomy and physiology to find a way to describe the airways which makes sense to owners, and thus convince them from a scientific viewpoint why slitting the false nostril will have no impact on the speed or volume of air intake.

Case study – Firing

2.5

Signalment This 15-year-old mare has been in the owner's possession for 2 years, and is used to transport goods by cart.

History The mare has had recurrent bouts of lameness over the first year of ownership. The owner took her to a traditional healer who fired both her forelimbs (Figure 2.5.1). The lameness did not improve.

Clinical examination The mare has a body condition score 2 and appears dull and depressed. On gait assessment she is lame on both forelimbs with a shortened stiff stride. On flexion of the forelimbs there is reduced flexion of the metacarpophalangeal joints in both forelimbs and signs of pain on flexion as the mare pulls her limbs away. There is bony enlargement around these joints and distension of the synovial pockets of the metacarpophalangeal joints.

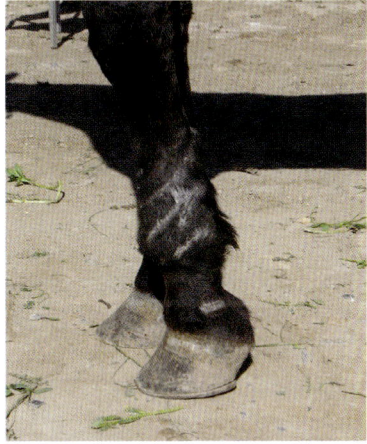

Figure 2.5.1 Firing of the distal metacarpus and metacarpophalangeal joints of both forelegs.

Treatment The mare is given an injection of flunixin meglumine and the owner given phenylbutazone to continue giving orally daily for the next 5 days before a follow-up visit. The owner is advised to rest the animal. The owner said this was not possible, so the advice was to reduce the work load or work speed of the animal to allow the inflammation within the joints to subside. The owner is advised that the bony growth around the joint is permanent and no treatment can reduce this. The thickening of the skin around the limb has been made worse by the scarring resulting from the firing. The owner is made aware that the practice of firing was detrimental to the animal and should not have been carried out.

Follow-up The joint swelling had reduced slightly but the rest of the pathological changes had not altered as these are permanent.

Discussion The owner was made aware that the firing process does not cure the problem, but causes more pain to the animal and should not be carried out. The owner was advised that, due to the permanent changes in the metacarpophalangeal joints, only reducing the work pattern combined with analgesia would keep her from suffering too much.

Ideally the mare would stop work, but due to financial reasons the owner is not able to do this. Long term analgesic drugs can lead to side effects on the body (see NSAIDs in Chapter 5) and should be managed carefully. Correct shoeing can go a long way to ameliorate the condition. Gentle therapies, such as massage of the limbs, can be carried out by owners. The mare should have regular check-ups by a veterinarian to assess any progression or deterioration of the condition and advise the owner as necessary.

> Cases of degenerative joint disease need to be treated individually, formulating a management plan that suits both animal and owner (Auer and Fackelman 1981).

2.6 References

Appleby, M.C., Hughes, B.O. (1997). Animal Welfare. Cabi Publishing. Cambridge, USA.

Auer, J.A., Fackelman, G.E. (1981) Treatment of degenerative joint disease of the horse: a review and commentary. *Vet. Surg.* 10 (2), 80–89.

Broster, C.E., Burn, C.C., Barr, A.R.S., Whay, H.R. (2009) The range and prevalence of pathological abnormalities associated with lameness in working horses from developing countries. *Equine Vet. J.* 41 (5), 474–481.

Fraser, D., Weary, D.M., Pajor, E.A., Milligan, B.N. (1997) A scientific conception of animal welfare that reflects ethical concerns. *Anim. Welfare*, 6 (3), 187–205.

Fraser, A.F. (2010) The Behaviour and Welfare of the Horse. 2nd Ed. CABI USA. pp. 182–195.

Hanggi, E.B., Ingersoll, J.F. (2012) Lateral vision in horses: A behavioural investigation. *Behav. Process.* 91 (1), 70–76.

McCarthy, R.N., Jeffcott, L.B., Clarke, I.J. (1993) Preliminary studies on the use of plasma beta-endorphin in horses as an indicator of stress and pain. *J. Eq. Vet. Sci.* 13 (4), 216–219.

McCullagh, K.G., Silver, I.A. (1981) The actual cautery – Myth and reality in the art of firing. *Equine Vet. J.* 13 (2), 81–84.

McGreevy, P. (2004) Equine Behaviour: A guide for veterinarians and equine scientists. Saunders, Elsevier Ltd. pp. 318–319.

McGreevy, P. (2007) Firm But Gentle: Learning to Handle with Care. *J. Vet. Med. Educ.* 34 (5), 539–41.

Passantino, A. (2011) Welfare issues of the donkey *(Equus asinus)*: a checklist based on the five freedoms. *J. Verbr. Lebensm.* 6, 215–221.

Pritchard, J.P., Burn, C.C., Barr, A.R.S., Whay, H.R. (2008) Validity of indicators of dehydration in working horses: A longitudinal study of changes in skin tent duration, mucous membrane dryness and drinking behaviour. *Equine Vet. J.* 40 (6), 558–564.

Van Dijk, L., Pritchard, J.C., Pradhan, S.K., Wells, K. (2010). Sharing the Load: a guide to improving the welfare of working animals through collective action. Practical Action Publishing, Rugby, UK.

Vreeman, H.Z., van der Kolk, J.H., van Brenda, E., de Graaf-Roelfsema, E. (2009) The effectiveness of the twitch in donkeys. PhD Faculty of Veterinary Medicine Universiteit Utrecht. *(This paper advised use of a twitch in donkeys but this is not a peer-reviewed paper and the sample size was only five animals.)*

Webster, A.J.F., Main, D.C.J., Whay, H.R. (2004). Welfare assessment: indices from clinical observation. *Anim. Welfare* 13, S93–98.

Webster, J. (2006) Animal sentience. *Appl. Anim. Behav. Sci.* 100 (1–2), 1–3, 1–152.

WSPA (2012) Sentience Mosaic – Why Sentience Matters. World Society for the Protection of Animals. (Online) Available at http://www.animalmosaic.org/sentience/ (accessed on 24 October 2012).

Further Reading

For information on the behavioural signs of pain refer to Chapter 3 *Pain – Indicators and management* and the review article by Ashley *et al.* (2005).

Appleby, M.C., Hughes, B.O. (1997) Animal Welfare. Cabi Publishing. Cambridge, USA.

Ashley, F. H., Waterman-Pearson, A.E., Whay, H.R. (2005) Behavioural assessment of pain in horses and donkeys: application to clinical practice and future studies. *Equine Vet. J.* 37 (6), 565–575.

Fraser, A.F. (2010) The Behaviour and Welfare of the Horse. 2nd Ed. CABI USA. pp. 182–195.

McGreevy, P. (2004) Equine Behaviour: A guide for veterinarians and equine scientists. Saunders, Elsevier Ltd. pp. 318–319.

Van Dijk, L., Pritchard, J.C., Pradhan, S.K., Wells, K. (2010). Sharing the Load: a guide to improving the welfare of working animals through collective action. Practical Action Publishing, Rugby, UK.

Pain – Indicators and management

3

Pain – Introduction	3.1
Indicators of pain	3.2
Management and treatment of pain	3.3
Case study – Chronic pain	3.4
References	3.5

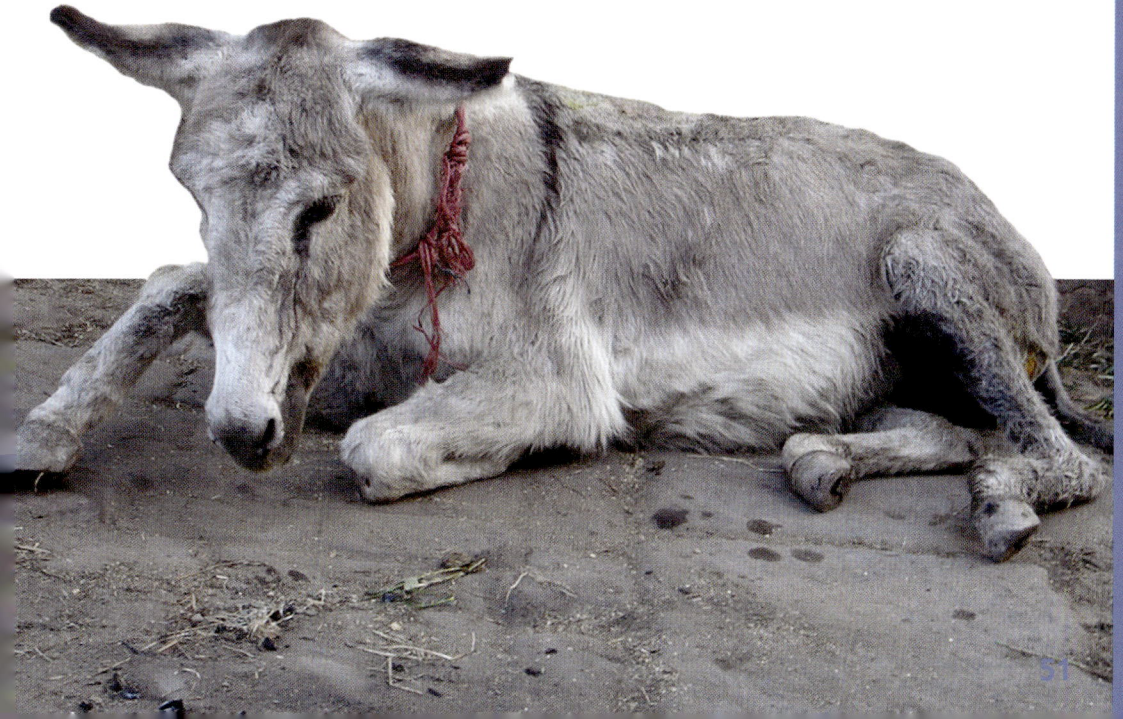

3.1 Pain – Introduction

Introduction and definition of pain

What is pain?

> **Pain is an unpleasant sensation and comes in many forms, all of which cause suffering to the animal.**

Molony and Kent (1997) defined pain as: '*An aversive, sensory experience which represents awareness (by the animal) of damage or threat to the integrity of its tissues*'.

In other words, pain can be thought of as a sensation resulting in the activation of protective mechanisms of an animal.

Why is it important for a veterinarian to recognise pain?

Pain is a sign of disease in an animal. Pain is exhausting and may lead to secondary complications such as weakness, unwillingness to eat (Dobromylskyj *et al.* 2000, Almeida *et al.* 2008), drink or sleep and increased susceptibility to disease and accidents.

> **It is the responsibility of a veterinarian to be able to recognise and alleviate any pain that the animal is experiencing.**

It is also necessary to be able to assess when pain has been relieved and treatment has been successful.

How can pain be diagnosed and managed?

Although the animal cannot tell a clinician about its pain experience, physiological and behavioural changes can be observed which help you to diagnose that pain is present.

> **Always consider whether pain may be present during a consultation.**

Refer to Section 1.1 for a detailed explanation of the 'integrated consultation process'.

- Recognise that an equid may be in pain.
- Where is the pain coming from?
- Consider how to alleviate the pain, if present.
- Explain pain to an owner who may not see pain as a problem.
- Minimise any pain caused during the consultation process.

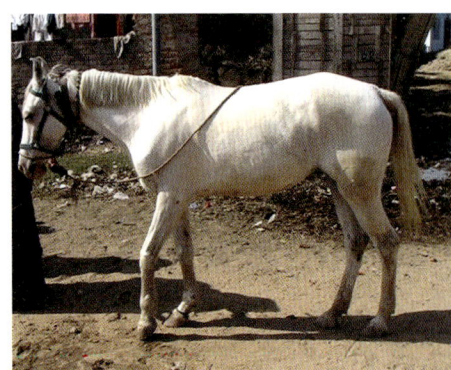

Figure 3.1.1 Assessment of pain is a part of every veterinary consultation.

PAIN – INTRODUCTION 3.1

Protective mechanisms when an animal is in pain occur for the following reasons:

> 1. To reduce or avoid the damage
> 2. To reduce the likelihood of pain recurrence
> 3. To promote recovery

Physiological mechanisms of pain production

There are two physiological mechanisms which enable an animal to feel pain: peripheral and central.

Peripheral mechanisms (tissue stimulation)

Skin, muscle, bone and other tissues have thousands of nerve endings. Stimulation of these nerves generates signals which travel to the spinal cord and brain within seconds.

> **If the signal is 'pain' an appropriate physiological and/or behavioural response occurs, such as withdrawal of the affected limb.**

Tissues can be stimulated in two ways

- **Non-noxious (non-painful) stimulation** (e.g. touch) is used by the animal to make it aware of its immediate surroundings. This rarely produces pain unless the nerve fibres are sensitised, for example by chemicals released during the inflammatory process ('hyperalgesia' – see below).

- **Noxious (painful) stimulation** (mechanical, thermal, electrical, chemical) is detected by pain receptors called nociceptors which convert painful stimuli into electrical impulses. These electrical signals (action potentials) are transmitted to the spinal cord by thinly myelinated (A delta) and unmyelinated (C) sensory nerve fibres. The A delta nerve fibres transmit electrical impulses much faster than the C fibres and are responsible for the rapid onset of sharp pain that triggers aversion and withdrawal from the stimulus. This is often an immediate reflex that is the result of a local neuronal path which doesn't go via the brain (unconscious). Alternatively, activation of C fibres results in a slower onset pain (second pain) that in humans is associated with a dull throbbing or burning sensation. It is worth noting that visceral pain (internal pain from internal organs) is transmitted exclusively by C fibres which travel with the nerves of the **autonomic nervous system**.

> **This may help explain the exaggerated physiological responses (tachycardia, hyperpnoea, hypertension, sweating) associated with visceral pain.**

- There are some very short neuronal paths, that do not go via the brain, which result in unconscious responses, such as a withdrawal reflex from noxious stimuli, and are immediate, e.g. if you touch a hot surface you withdraw your hand without thinking about it. Other neuronal pathways, especially from C fibres, go via the brain and produce more complex defensive responses, such as behavioural adaptations to pain, e.g. protecting a wound from further trauma.
- Chemical substances (prostaglandins, leukotrienes, bradykinin, nerve growth factors, histamine) produced by tissue damage and inflammation, activate and sensitise these nociceptors resulting in increased sensitisation to pain.

3 PAIN – INDICATORS AND MANAGEMENT

> An exaggerated and prolonged response to noxious stimuli is called hyperalgesia (Whay *et al.* 2005) and the sensation of pain by normal innocuous stimuli is called allodynia (Muir 2010a) (e.g. if a wound is touched even gently it hurts).

- Moreover, severe or prolonged pain can result in central sensitisation, which again is characterised by hyperalgesia, allondynia and hypersensitivity.
- Nociceptors respond to high intensity mechanical or thermal stimulation, for example pricking or stretching the skin, or extreme temperatures. Chemical mediators released during the inflammatory process will also sensitise nociceptors. This is important to remember when choosing appropriate analgesia (see Chapter 5 *Medicines*).

> This increased sensitisation to painful stimuli has been referred to as pain 'wind up' (Muir 2010b). It can be reduced if analgesics are given pre-emptively wherever possible, e.g. if a painful procedure is going to be performed, always give the analgesic before the procedure. This will inhibit this sensitisation of pain wind up and give more effective pain control.

Remember that pain responses will vary between individual animals. As with pain thresholds in humans, what one animal accepts as mildly painful may not be felt in the same way by another animal. This is important to remember when carrying out diagnostic examinations and procedures using sedatives and local anaesthetics.

> A dose rate that works for most cases may not be sufficient in some individuals due to increased pain or stress responses.

The physiological and behavioural effects of pain will vary according to whether the skin/tissue is normal, damaged, infected or inflamed. It is important to understand the effects or lack of effects on these peripheral mechanisms when two different types of pain modifying drugs are used: aspirin-like (NSAIDS) and morphine-like (opioids).

Central mechanisms: Unconscious processing by the brain and spinal cord

Pain mechanisms utilising central pathways result in a pain response from the spinal cord and brain. Nerve fibres from nociceptors reach the grey matter of the spinal cord, and contribute to local spinal reflex responses such as withdrawal from the stimulus. Alternatively the response may progress to the brain, leading to complex defensive responses.

Pain duration

Acute pain

> Acute pain occurs immediately with injury or trauma and disappears when the injury heals.

Pain can usually be attributed to either the 'somatic' (musculoskeletal system) or 'visceral' (smooth muscle) systems. Acute pain is detected as being one of the five signs of acute inflammation (see Chapter 5) and is usually easy to detect if external (somatic). It is often accompanied by heat, swelling, redness and loss of function in the affected area.

Chronic pain

> **Chronic pain occurs when an animal's physiological and behavioural responses are unsuccessful in alleviating the pain.**

Attempts to overcome such pain can often result in permanent structural or physiological changes. This is important to consider when attempting to provide an equid with medicinal relief from chronic pain, for example that seen with osteoarthritis.

Chronic pain is usually a lot harder to recognise or evaluate. However, the following signs should alert a clinician to the possibility that the animal has been in pain for some time:

- Changes (decreases) in responses to outside stimuli (depression) (see Figure 3.1.2)
- Changes in eating and drinking
- Changes in sleeping or recumbency times
- Changes in social behaviour
- Weight loss
- Other signs such as hard swellings of joints and tendons

Mechanisms for coping with pain

> **When animals are experiencing chronic pain, they may reduce the severity in a phenomenon known as a 'coping mechanism'.**

It is unclear how such mechanisms work and when they are used although it is thought to involve the central nervous system.

Such 'coping mechanisms' in chronic pain can be so effective that physiological and behavioural changes of the animal are only detected when these mechanisms are suppressed or temporarily overpowered. This is sometimes referred to as **'breakthrough pain'**.

Stress-induced analgesia has been demonstrated but its significance for pain relief in different species is unclear.

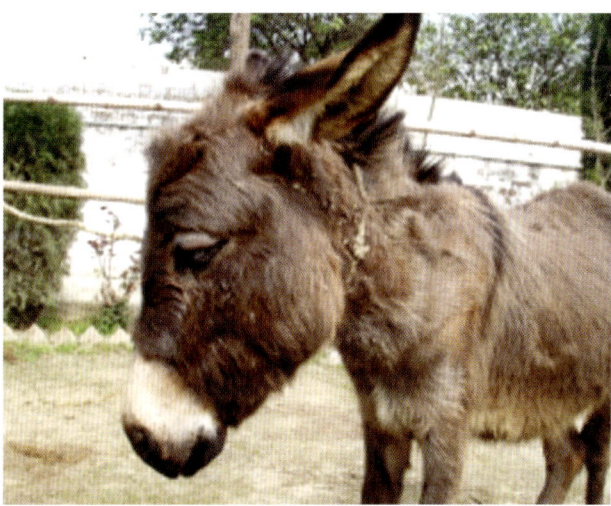

Figure 3.1.2 Chronic pain can be hard to evaluate.

3 PAIN – INDICATORS AND MANAGEMENT

Types of pain responses

An animal may adopt one or more of the following in an effort to cope with pain:

1. **Behavioural changes** in which the animal reduces or avoids the recurrence of the pain experience. This involves emotional experiences and learning, for which high-level central nervous functions are required. Examples include running away, or trying to remove or reduce the cause by licking, biting or attacking its source.

2. **Automatic reflex responses/reactions which protect the animal** This is common with thermal stimuli, for example the automatic withdrawal from a hot firing iron.

3. **Responses which minimise pain and assist healing** e.g. lying down, standing very still or by adopting some other characteristic posture. To enable this, the animal may move away or hide.

4. **Protective responses** These are designed to elicit help or to stop another animal (including human) inflicting more pain. For example, communication via vocalisation, posture or smell.

5. **Absence of well-established behavioural responses** due to the continuing pain being predominant. This may lead to failure of social interactions, unresponsiveness to commands and inattention.

3.2 Indicators of pain

Pain assessment

How to determine how much pain an animal is suffering

When we first observe any working equid the question of whether the animal is experiencing pain, and how much, should always be considered.

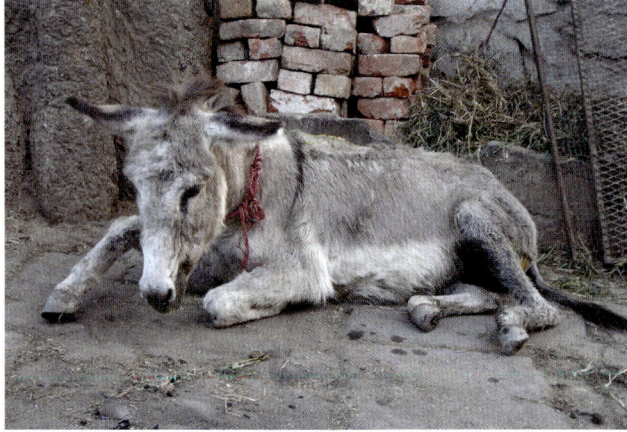

Figure 3.2.1 Is this animal in pain?

INDICATORS OF PAIN 3.2

Subjective assessment

This is an assessment of pain levels based on what the clinician thinks the animal is feeling, rather than any measurable indicators. Evaluation of pain will improve with:

- an acceptance that animals do feel and experience pain
- knowing the species, breed, work-type and individual animal well
- learning the characteristics of pain-associated behaviour
- treatment experience
- considering the possibility that pain is present in all consultations with working equids and taking the appropriate action to alleviate it

Objective assessment

This uses *specific measurements* to identify the animal's level of pain

1. Measures of **general body function** such as food and water intake

- Sudden decreases in eating/drinking in the period before the owner presented the animal can be significant
- Changes in eating/drinking patterns with the commencement of analgesia
- Changes in normal grazing behaviour

2. Measures of **behaviour** (Figure 3.2.2)

- Anxiety
- Restlessness
- Flehmen response (upwards curling of the upper lip)
- Depression
- Aggression

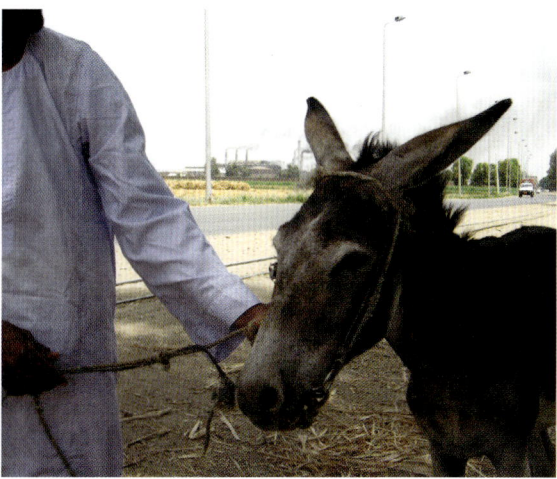

Aggression has been strongly associated with pain (Ashley *et al.* 2005), as a genuine response to pain on palpation, as a fear response in anticipation of a pain related stimulus, or through a learned association.

> **The instinctive response of an equid to an aversive stimulus is flight; however, if confined, the only possible defence for the animal is to attack the source of the pain.**

Figure 3.2.2 Observe the behaviour of each animal before examination.

Equids in severe, unrelenting pain can become difficult to handle with little consideration for other people and animals. This should always be considered in aggressive animals, and a careful clinical examination should be performed. If in doubt, administer analgesics.

3 PAIN – INDICATORS AND MANAGEMENT

3. Measures of **physiological responses**

These can be unreliable so do not base decisions on these alone; always consider in the context of a complete examination. In the field, it is extremely difficult and unnecessary to rely on invasive testing to determine pain levels.

▮ Heart rate	▮ Corticosteroid
▮ Respiratory rate	▮ Beta-endorphines
▮ Catecholamines	▮ Cortisol

Cortisol is often measured to assess pain responses in animals under experimental conditions; however, measurement of this hormone in a clinical context is impractical and it has shown to be an unreliable indicator of pain as many other factors can affect it (Molony and Kent 1997).

> **It is important to remember that increased cortisol levels as seen in pain and stress will have a detrimental effect on an animal's immune system.**

Cortisol not only inhibits healing and repair but also inhibits the animal developing an appropriate immune response to pathogens and makes it more susceptible to opportunistic infections.

Practical assessment

For practical assessment of pain under field conditions, assess individuals or groups of equids on the following points:

- Look at the **interaction** of animals and their individual demeanour.
- Assess any abnormal **activities** or **postures**, including the position of limbs (Figure 3.2.3), head, neck, ears and tail.
- Identify and assess any changes in **gait**.
- **Approach** the individual animal to observe the response to disturbance (evoked behaviour). Look for decreased flight distances and the speed of response to the threat.

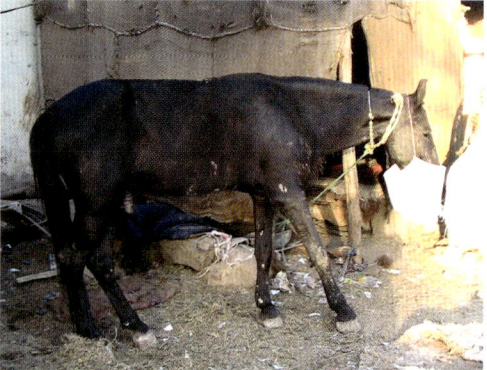

Figure 3.2.3 Observe the posture of all limbs from a distance.

> **Equids showing reduced responses may be in pain.**

- Look for signs of poor body, skin and coat condition, presence of external parasites, wounds, or other **signs of disease**.
- Look for **physiological signs** such as altered respiratory effort (including increased rate, depth, gasping, open-mouthed breathing, panting), sweating, trembling, increased muscle tone, dilated pupils, wide-open eyes, depression and aggression towards observer, particularly in response to touch.
- Note any **physiological, environmental or husbandry conditions** that could also account for any of the observed signs, e.g. pregnancy, heavy rain.

INDICATORS OF PAIN 3.2

▪ Seek the **owner/carer's assessment** of the animal and note his/her competence and co-operation.

Why is it important to recognise pain-associated behavioural changes?

> **The recognition of pain-associated behavioural changes is a vital tool for pain detection and management.**

Knowledge of normal versus abnormal equine behaviour is necessary. However, it can often be difficult to detect altered demeanour in working equids as they typically follow a restricted schedule that is different from the activities they would engage in if they had free choice.

> **An owner will know his animal better than anyone else so, if an owner says the animal is acting abnormally, they should, generally, be taken seriously.**

Clinical examination must prioritise pain assessment and help owners see and believe that pain is real. Good communication is the key. Below are descriptions of different pain signs, also refer to Ashley *et al.* (2005).

▪ **Generalised signs** These may include excitement, circling, pacing, depression, fear, reluctance to be handled, reduced social behaviour, reduced movement, reduced food or water intake, playing with food and water, 'snapping' jaws or grinding teeth, difficulty or reluctance in standing up or lying down, increased or decreased lying down times, rigid stance, tension evident in face or muzzle, staring or rolling eyes, flared nostrils, increased respiratory rate, muscle tremors or sweating.

> **Changes in normal behaviour often indicate pain, although this varies greatly between species and individuals.**

▪ **Head/dental pain** Signs include difficulty picking up, holding or swallowing food, retaining food in the cheek pouches, dropping uneaten food from mouth (quidding), standing over food or water but not eating or drinking, chewing on one side, head-shyness, reluctance to open mouth, reluctance to work or accept the bit, scratching or rubbing the face, head-pressing or head-shaking, depression, and inappetence (lack of appetite).

▪ **Abdominal pain (colic)** Signs include looking at flanks (Figure 3.2.4), pawing the ground, kicking the belly, rolling, collapsing, leaning against walls, stretching, grunting, grinding teeth, lying on back (especially foals), depression, inappetence, and anorexia. Abdominal pain can lead to quite violent behaviour.

▪ **Skin pain** Itching, rubbing and other signs of self-trauma, swelling and redness, exudate, secondary infection and alopecia or thickening of skin. There could be evidence of reluctance to move or other gait abnormalities due to tension of the skin over certain areas of the body, depression inappetence, guarding/protecting the area when attempts are made to touch/examine it.

▪ **Ear pain** Dropping or swelling of the pinna (Figure 3.2.4), discharge, wet hairs, shaking or rubbing of the head and evasion when the head area is handled, depression, inappetence, guarding/protecting the area when attempts are made to touch/examine it.

3 PAIN – INDICATORS AND MANAGEMENT

- **Eye pain** Wet eyelashes, excessive tear production, ocular discharge (Figure 3.2.4), blepharospasm (holding eye closed), drooping eyelid, head-shyness, fear of handling, photophobia (light avoidance), rubbing eye or side of the head, depression, inappetence, guarding/protecting the area when attempts are made to touch/examine it.

- **Limb pain** Signs include overt lameness (limping), shortened stride length (especially when turning), uneven weight distribution, pointing or resting a forelimb, pointing a hindlimb, shifting weight, lifting foot off ground (Figure 3.2.4.), dropping hip/stifle or elbow/shoulder when moving, reluctance to stand or move, reluctance to work, kicking when limb handled, limb withdrawal on palpation or with hoof testers, head nod or rigid head and neck, depression, and inappetence.

Pain assessment in donkeys

It is documented that donkeys demonstrate more subtle pain behaviours than horses; perhaps due to our current inability to interpret the more subtle behavioural changes they present with (Ashley *et al.* 2005). It is interesting that a similar problem has been noted in semi-feral and wild horses, where the ability to hide pain is a valuable survival technique for animals that are naturally predated.

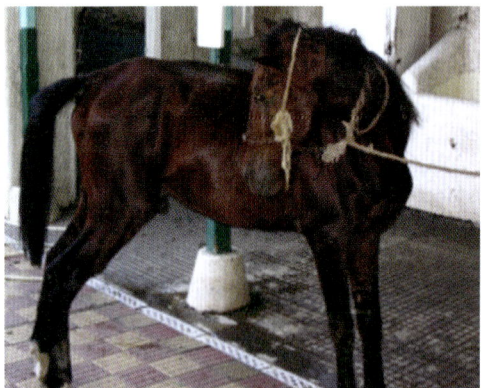
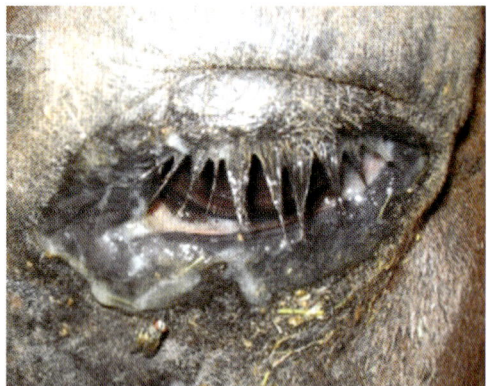
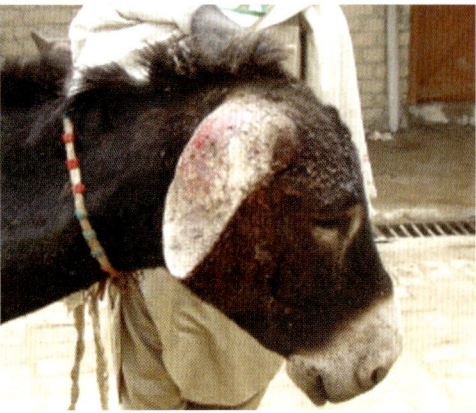
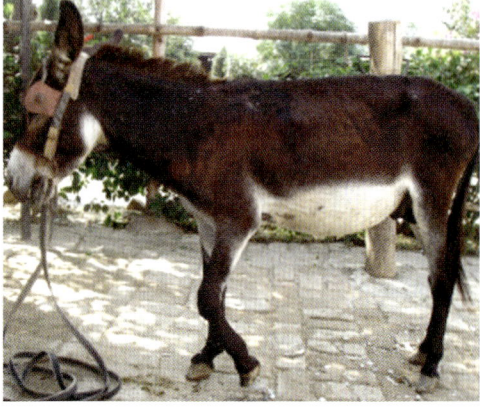

Figure 3.2.4 Examples of: abdominal pain (top left); eye pain (top right); ear pain (bottom left); limb pain (bottom right).

INDICATORS OF PAIN 3.2

> More subtle pain behaviours do not mean that donkeys do not feel pain.

Non-specific behavioural indicators of pain in donkeys

- In horses, restlessness, anxiety and agitation are characteristic of severe/acute pain. This cannot be relied upon in the donkey and more subtle behaviours may be shown.
- A rigid stance and reluctance to move (likely to be a protective behaviour) has been recognised in donkeys. However, this can be over diagnosed.
- Lower head carriage is difficult to interpret in donkeys.
- Fixed stare and flared nostrils described in horses as indicators of chronic pain have not been described in donkeys.
- Aggression towards handlers, harness and other animals is strongly reported for horses and this has been described in the donkey, but tends to be more subtle (Ashley *et al.* 2005).

Behavioural indicators for abdominal pain in donkeys

- Vocalisation is well described in horses, but not reported in donkeys.
- Rolling is well described in horses. It is reported in donkeys but not reliable; i.e. just because a donkey is not rolling does not mean abdominal pain can be ruled out.
- Kicking abdomen is well described in horses, but not reported in donkeys.
- Flank watching is well described in horses, but not reported in donkeys.
- Dullness and depression is well described (Ashley *et al.* 2005).
- Lying down is commonly reported in the field.
- Stretching out whilst standing is also reported in the field (see Chapter 11).

> Dullness and depression is commonly reported as the *only* observable behaviour change caused by abdominal pain in donkeys.

Behavioural indicators for limb and foot pain in donkeys

> Weight shifting between limbs is a reliable indicator in horses and donkeys.

- The donkey may guard the affected limb.
- Abnormal weight distribution: abnormal/altered posture to alleviate limb loading e.g. placing the front feet forward of the body in laminitis. This is reported as much more subtle in donkeys.
- Abnormal movement is reported in donkeys.
- Reluctance to move is slightly associated with limb pain in donkeys (Ashley *et al.* 2005).

These lists are not exhaustive and as more evidence emerges we should get a greater understanding of how to recognise and interpret pain in donkeys.

With every examination consider whether the donkey is in pain or whether the condition could be painful, even if no overt signs of pain are noted.

> If there is any possibility of pain, analgesics should be included in the treatment regime. Owners should be made aware of the signs of pain so that they recognise them and will be more inclined to manage pain appropriately in the short and long term.

3.3 Management and treatment of pain

Pain alleviation

What to do if an animal is in pain

> Veterinarians have a responsibility to alleviate pain and suffering.

Remember in some cases, euthanasia may be the only choice in order to achieve this (see Chapter 8). The best approach to pain is to remove the cause of the pain rather than mask it (e.g. with analgesics), where this is possible.

Owner communication, nursing and management

These aspects are of primary importance since, long term, it is the owner/carer who is responsible for ensuring the animal is comfortable, and remains that way, once the vet leaves the consultation.

- **Rest** Pain is exhausting and the nervous system of an animal in pain is hyper-sensitised to further pain (Whay *et al.* 2005). Rest allows healing to take place, minimises painful movement and helps to prevent further knocks and injuries that will increase the level of pain.

- **Warmth and comfortable lying conditions** Animals in pain need to be kept comfortable in order to allow them to lie for longer periods of time; minimising movement and maximising the healing process. The lying area should be clean and comfortable to cushion pressure points and prevent pressure sores, as well as protecting the animal from cold. The best way to tell if the lying area is suitable is to watch lying and rising behaviour; if the animal does not want to lie down or get up, or if it is not lying for long periods, the area is not warm or comfortable enough (unless the condition is so severe as to prevent this behaviour).

- **Assisted feeding/drinking** Animals in pain may need help with feeding and drinking, either by placing food and water within easy reach when they are lying down, or by hand-feeding small amounts at frequent intervals. This requires time and attention to detail by attendants in order to make sure enough food and water is consumed.

- **Physiotherapy and massage** Rest and extended lying periods may lead to joint stiffness, muscle cramp or congestion and oedematous swelling of the limbs. Gentle daily massage or physiotherapy can aid circulation and flexibility, enabling a faster return to normal movement when the pain

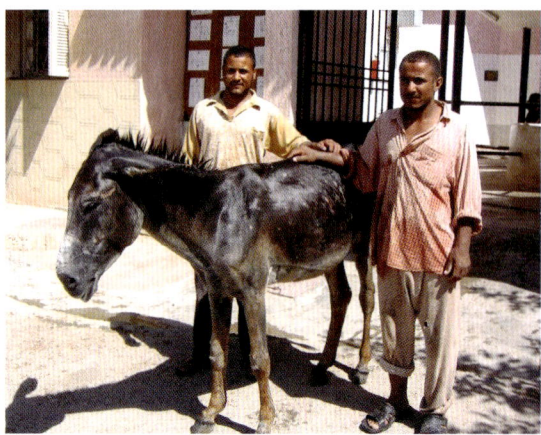

Figure 3.3.1 Good relationships and communication with owners are the key to successful nursing care and therefore a positive outcome for working equids.

MANAGEMENT AND TREATMENT OF PAIN 3.3

has subsided. Care should be taken to look for signs of pain that may be exacerbated by physiotherapy or massage; if this occurs, avoid the painful area and focus on other body regions.

> Good communication with owners and carers of working equids is essential if effective nursing and management of sick patients is to occur (Figure 3.3.1).

Analgesic drugs

In many circumstances, pain alleviation requires the use of **analgesic drugs**, especially in the acute stages. It is important to remember that drugs alone do not give maximal improvement in the animal's comfort.

> Effective pain relief also requires management of the animal's environment (as discussed above).

There are three main groups of medicines available to relieve pain and suffering:

1. Opioids
2. Anti-inflammatory drugs
3. Local anaesthetics

Refer to Chapter 5 for more information on specific drug actions.

> The administration of analgesics must be an informed decision. Know the drugs that are available and the pharmacological and physiological effects they induce. Knowledge of expected efficacy will greatly improve the ability to alleviate an animal's pain and suffering.

Remember that removing the source of the pain is the first priority. Analgesics will mask signs of pain and will make an animal feel temporarily better, but will not cure the cause of pain. In some instances it is not possible to remove the cause of pain, e.g. with chronic joint arthritis. However, the effects can still be minimised through good foot trimming and farriery, reduced work load and improved working conditions.

> Owner education and compliance is the key to success.

Remember that, even if there is no other option than the provision of long-term pain relief medication to make an animal comfortable, all analgesics have detrimental side effects that become more evident with increasing dose and duration of treatment. Additionally, by masking the pain, the animal will no longer protect the affected region meaning that further damage is more likely. Both of these facts should be considered when long-term pain relief treatment is advised and they should be fully explained to owners.

> Effective pain management is absolutely critical in improving working equid welfare.

3 PAIN – INDICATORS AND MANAGEMENT

Pain management should be at the fore of every veterinarian's mind. No painful veterinary procedure should be performed without careful consideration as to whether it can be avoided (harm-benefit analysis) and, if it is essential, how the pain can be ameliorated during the process.

Response to analgesia

> All animals requiring pain relief must be monitored carefully and their pain control plan re-evaluated regularly, either through re-examination or owner communication.

1. **Observe behavioural changes** once analgesics have been administered to confirm that the presence of pain has been alleviated. Assess pain levels, e.g. if an animal becomes much brighter following pain relief this is a good indication that the animal was in pain before this medication and that the medication has helped to alleviate the pain.

2. **The volume, route and potency** of the selected analgesia will determine how quickly a response to treatment can be expected, and can help assess original pain levels.

3. **Remember to be aware of the duration of action.** Most drugs which alleviate pain are only effective for a few hours. Ensure that the animal is reassessed before the analgesia wears off, and then decide on the next step.

4. **Be aware of the deleterious side effects** associated with analgesics. Side effects should be minimised by ensuring that the correct dose, preparation, dose frequency and route of administration is followed for each drug (see Chapter 5).

> Ensure a long-term treatment plan exists if you intend to use analgesia. Is it practical in the long term?

In the case of chronic pain in working equids, consideration of the use of long-term analgesia has to be monitored carefully (Figure 3.3.2). See Section 3.4 of this chapter for a case study on chronic pain management.

It is the ultimate responsibility of the veterinarian to relieve pain and suffering.

> In acknowledging that equids have the capacity to experience pain, a veterinarian is obligated to minimise its occurrence through prevention and treatment.

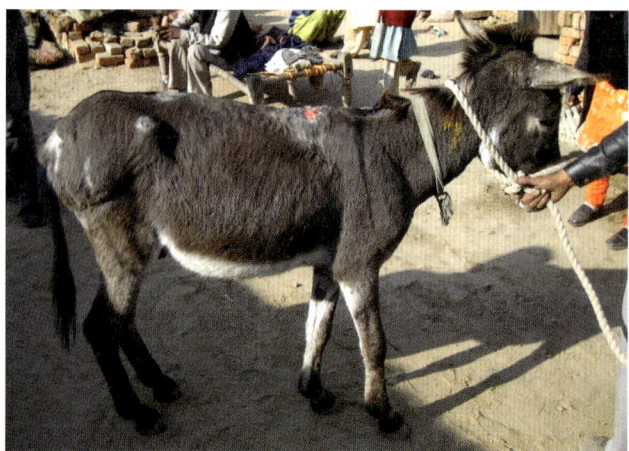

Figure 3.3.2 In all examinations consider chronic pain management.

If it is possible that an animal is in pain give the animal the benefit of the doubt. Administer appropriate treatment and advice to the owner to protect its welfare.

MANAGEMENT AND TREATMENT OF PAIN 3.3

Veterinarians can promote:

1. Refinements in animal care

   ▍ Discuss general use/care of the animal with owners/users.
   ▍ Advise on appropriate management practices:
   - Water provision
   - Best possible diet based on what is available
   - Regular removal of faeces and urine-soaked bedding
   - Dry and clean equipment
   - Comfortable environment (stable, bedding, quiet, light, good ventilation)
   - Fly control

2. **Provision of anaesthetics and analgesics** Bearing in mind what is locally available always do what is best from the animal's viewpoint, minimising the pain of diagnostic and treatment procedures.

3. **Refinements in local procedures intended to improve animal welfare** Is the owner performing procedures/mutilations that are painful and detrimental to the animal (see Figure 3.3.3)? What actions can be taken if it is known that painful practices are occurring? In what way does the community feel that they benefit from adopting these painful practices? These are all important issues to raise in veterinary or programming meetings. It is also beneficial to work with community development teams in order to address such matters. See Section 2.4 for ways to overcome harmful practices.

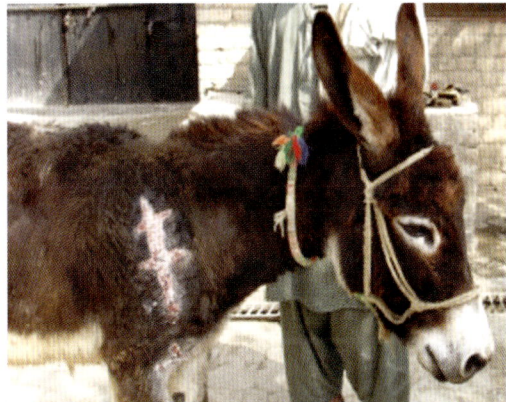

Figure 3.3.3 Firing, which causes pain and suffering, is a common practice in many parts of the world.

Pain management in donkeys

> Physiological differences exist between donkeys and horses which affect the pharmacokinetics of certain drugs.

Donkeys have a different metabolic capacity for specific drugs compared with horses (Scarth *et al.* 2012). For some drugs, e.g. phenylbutazone (PBZ), an increased frequency of dosing is required as PBZ is cleared from the body of donkeys 5–15 times faster than horses (Cheng *et al.* 1996a, Lizarrago *et al.* 2004). (See Chapter 5.)

> Always check species' specific dosing regimens.

Unfortunately, dosing regimens for many drugs for donkeys and mules are currently extrapolated from horse data, due to lack of research into all species.

3 PAIN – INDICATORS AND MANAGEMENT

Fewer adverse drug reactions are noted in donkeys compared to horses; however, there have been reports of injection site reactions to oil-based formulations, unbuffered solutions, and suspensions (Lizarrago *et al.* 2004).

Differences in drug metabolism and dosing in donkeys for the common non-steroidal anti-inflammatory drugs (NSAIDs) available in the field

Refer to Table 3.3.1 and Chapter 5 for differences between dose rates for some commonly used NSAIDs.

> It is very important for effective pain relief that dose rates and frequencies are appropriate for the species.

NSAID	Dosing frequency
Phenylbutazone (PBZ)	Data suggests dosing should be more frequent for donkeys than horses, as donkeys eliminate PBZ faster than horses (Cheng *et al.* 1996a). However, take care to avoid toxicity.
Flunixin meglumine	Dosing should be more frequent for donkeys than horses. (Cheng *et al.* 1996b).
Ketoprofen	Dosing should be more frequent for donkeys than horses, due to the increased clearance of the drug from donkeys' bodies and the fact that they have larger volume distribution than horses. However, the same dose of 2.2 mg/kg IV produced similar pharmacokinetics results in both species (Oukessou *et al.* 1996).
Carprofen	Donkeys require a reduced dosing rate than horses as they metabolise this drug more slowly than horses (Coakley *et al.* 1999).

Table 3.3.1 *Information on commonly used NSAIDs for which frequency of dosing differs between horses and donkeys.*

Case study – Chronic pain   3.4

Case of a burnt donkey

Location Mwea, Kenya

Attending veterinarian Dr Mary Gichure

History
The owner, Salim, reported that his two donkeys had been burned. In this area of Kenya, January is the harvesting season for rice. The by-products of rice (straw, hay and husks) do not fetch a good price at market hence farmers burn them to prepare the land for the next planting season. A burning heap looks greyish (like ash) from the outside yet inside the heap is red hot. Salim's two donkeys were left loose after a days' work and they strayed into a burning heap, sustaining serious burn wounds.

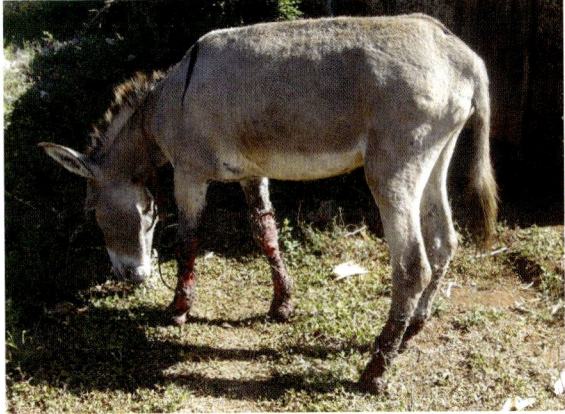

Figure 3.4.1 Salim's donkey with the burn wounds; the donkey is in a poor body condition.

Examination
One donkey was burnt on all the ventral body areas (abdomen and genital areas as well as limbs). The other donkey had burn wounds on the limbs only (Figure 3.4.1).

After examination, the veterinarian recommended euthanasia of both donkeys. The main reasons being:

- the degree of pain that the donkeys were suffering
- the poor hygiene and open wounds that would pre-dispose the donkeys to infections (considering the donkeys are not housed)
- complications that would arise due to this condition like tetanus, arthritis, and wound contracture
- shock due to the large area with open wounds that were bleeding.

Salim denied consent for euthanasia and requested the veterinarian to *'do anything to save these donkeys besides putting them down. They were given to me as a present and I am ready to take care of them in whatever way. In case they die, during treatment, then, I will be comfortable knowing that at least I did something to help them. As long as they are feeding, it means they still have the will to live'*.

Outcome
The first donkey with the more severe ventral abdominal wounds died the following day. A course of treatment was commenced for the second surviving donkey.

3 PAIN – INDICATORS AND MANAGEMENT

Treatment
- Daily washing with a solution of Povidone Iodine
- Application of Clotrimazole/Gentamycin/Betamethasone ointment to wounds
- Amoxicillin trihydrate 15 mg/kg injection for the first 3 days
- Flunixin meglumine injection for the first day and during follow-up visits

> Salim was taught home-based daily wound care. This involved daily examination of the wounds, cleaning the wounds with a solution of Povidone Iodine and topical application of ointment. He was also to note any changes and report the progress of the donkey to the veterinarian.

The donkey was rested and Salim was able to get another donkey to work with (as a donation from one of his group members), in order to sustain his income.

Follow-up
The wounds were slow to heal (Figure 3.4.2). One of the reasons for this was due to the location of the wounds over the joints. Every time the donkey flexed and extended his joints, the skin stretched which resulted in delayed healing.

Figure 3.4.3 shows a closer view of the limbs during a follow-up visit 3 months later. The wounds were still not fully healed. Notice the left hind hoof which shows re-growth since the initial hoof fell off after burning. Notice also the swollen joints – evidence of arthritis.

Figure 3.4.4 shows the donkey 5 months after initial treatment. Notice the rice husks stuck to the wounds on the limbs, evidence that the wounds have not completely healed, although there is good progress. The arthritis complication is evident.

Discussion
Salim's readiness to take care of his donkey went a long way in prevention of other complications and aided the healing of the wounds. Today, the donkey has recovered and has acquired a new walking style (like tip-toeing) due to the chronic arthritis as a complication of this case and is not used for work.

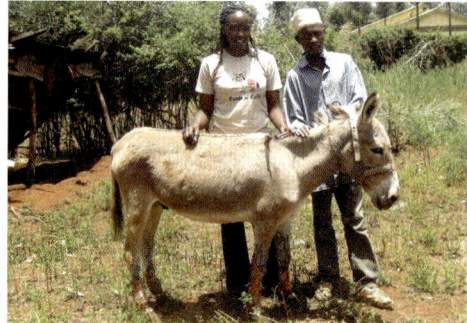

Figure 3.4.2 Salim with Dr Mary during a follow-up visit to review progress.

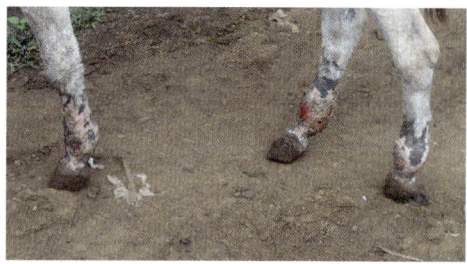

Figure 3.4.3 The wounds on the limbs showing delayed healing.

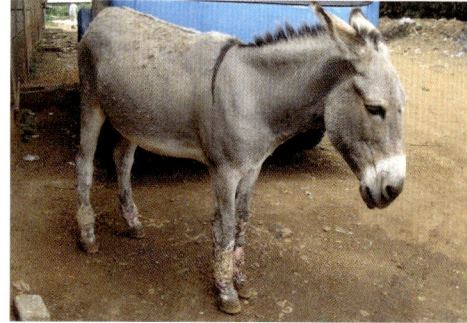

Figure 3.4.4 The donkey in June 2012 (5 months after the burning incident). Notice the improved body condition compared to the Figure 3.4.1.

CASE STUDY – CHRONIC PAIN 3.4

Challenges of dealing with this case

> - The owner did not necessarily understand the extent of pain experienced by his donkey, hence leaving the animal to suffer from chronic pain.
> - The value of the donkey after recovery is reduced, because of the remaining condition; it cannot be used for work. In this case, the owner did not seem to mind this; according to him, he saved his donkey.
> - The donkey nowadays is left to roam around the town since it is not housed; therefore it is exposed to the danger of road accidents which are very prevalent in this area.

The veterinarian advised the owner to provide a place to shelter his donkeys so that they do not stray into danger again. Housing is a major issue in this small urban centre since most donkey owners only go there to work. The accommodation in which they live does not have any provision for donkeys to shelter at night, and hence they are left to roam.

This case study focuses on a number of issues that many working equid veterinarians are faced with daily:

> - Poor management of working equids resulting in serious injuries (e.g. roaming)
> - Refusal of owners for euthanasia (ignorance, economic, cultural, religious, social, peer-pressure) (see Chapter 8 for more discussion on euthanasia)
> - Management of chronic pain (animals still working)
> - Management of non-healing wounds
> - Owner compliance (communication and relationship), see Chapter 1

3.5 References

Almeida, P.E., Weber, P.S.D., Burton, J.L., Zanella, A.J. (2008) Depressed DHEA and increased sickness response behaviours in lame dairy cows with inflammatory foot lesions. *Domest. Anim. Endocrin.* 34, 89–99.

Ashley, F. H., Waterman-Pearson, A.E, Whay., H.R. (2005) Behavioural assessment of pain in horses and donkeys: application to clinical practice and future studies. *Equine Vet. J.* 37 (6), 565–575.

Cheng, Z., McKellar, Q.A., Nolan, A., Lees, P. (1996a) Pharmacokinetics and pharmacodynamics of phenylbutazone and oxyphenbutazone in the donkey. 149–151. *J. Vet. Pharmacol. Therap.* 19, 149-151.

Cheng, Z., McKellar, Q.A., Nolan, A., Lees, P. (1996b) Preliminary pharmacokinetic and pharmacodynamic studies on flunixin meglumine in donkeys. *Vet. Res. Commun.* 20, 469–472.

Coakley, M., Peck, K.K., Taylor, T.S., Mathews, N.S., Mealey, K.L. (1999) Pharmacokinetics of flunixin meglumine in donkeys, mules, and horses. *Am. J. Vet. Res.* 60 (11), 1441–1444.

Dobromylskyj, P., Flecknell, P.A., Lascelles, B.D., Livingston, A., Taylor, P., Waterman-Pearson, A. (2000) Pain assessment. In: *Pain Management in Animals*. Eds: P.A. Flecknell and A. Waterman-Pearson, W.B. Saunders, London. pp. 53–80.

Lizarrago, I., Sumano, H., Brumbaugh, G.W. (2004) Pharmacological and pharmacokinetic differences between donkeys and horses. *Equine vet Educ.* 16 (2), 102–112.

Muir, W. (2010a) Pain mechanisms and management in horses. *Vet. Clin. N. Am. – Equine.* 26, 467–480.

Muir, W.W. (2010b) NMDA receptor anatagonists and pain: Ketamine. *Vet. Clin. N. Am. – Equine.* 26 (3), 565–578.

Molony, V., Kent, J.E. (1997) Assessment of acute pain in farm animals using behavioural and physiological measurements. *J. Anim. Sci.* 75 (1), 266–272.

Oukessou, M., Bouljihad, M. Van Gool, F., Alvinerie, M. (1996) Pharamacokinetics of ketoprofen in the donkey *(Equus Asinus)*. *J. Vet. Med. A.* 43, 423–426.

Scarth, J.P., Teale, P., Kuuranne, T. (2012) Drug metabolism in the horse: a review. *Drug Test. Analysis.* 3, 19–53.

Whay, H.R., Webster, A.J.F., Waterman-Pearson, A.E. (2005) Role of ketoprofen in the modulation of hyperalgesia associated with lameness in dairy cattle. *Vet. Rec.* 157, 729–733.

Further reading

For behavioural indicators of pain in equids refer to:

Ashley, F. H., Waterman-Pearson, A.E., Whay, H.R. (2005) Behavioural assessment of pain in horses and donkeys: application to clinical practice and future studies. *Equine Vet. J.* 37 (6), 565–575

For further definition of terms relating to pain refer to:

Muir, W. (2010a) Pain mechanisms and management in horses. *Vet. Clin. N. Am. – Equine.* 26, 467–480.

Clinical techniques 4

Drug administration techniques	**4.1**
Clinical pathology	**4.2**
Blood sampling	**4.3**
Blood smears and staining	**4.4**
Haematology and biochemistry	**4.5**
Sterile skin preparation	**4.6**
References	**4.7**

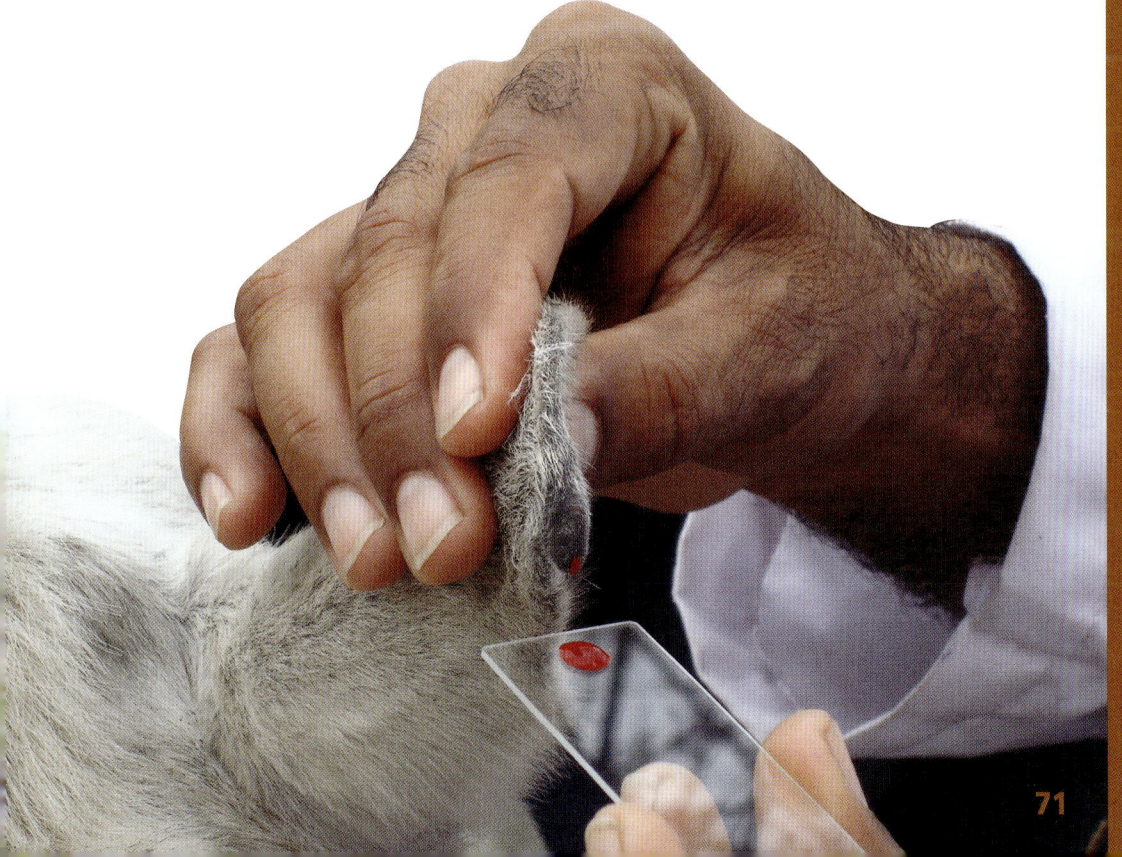

4.1 Drug administration techniques

Drug administration to equids is a routine daily task for veterinarians, but care must be taken to do it correctly every time. All drug administration routes have the potential for negative consequences.

> Remember: In the first instance, cause no harm!

Veterinarians can have a large positive impact on equine welfare by ensuring medicines are administered properly.

When using any drug, ask the following questions:

1. Is it the correct drug?
2. Is it the correct dose?
3. Is it the correct route?
4. Is it a welfare friendly administration technique?
5. What are the possible complications?

Oral administration

> Drugs given by mouth are designated as 'Per Os' (p/o or PO).

Many drugs are designed for use in tablet, bolus or powder form, given directly into the mouth or mixed in food. Other routes of oral administration include using a stomach tube or drench technique.

Always ensure that the handler is competent and that the person administering the drug has the equipment and drug ready to ensure that the procedure takes as short a time as possible for the animal. The head will need to be raised until the animal swallows to ensure that the drug is ingested. Figure 4.1.1 shows a calm, competent person administering a drug PO. The owner is present to reassure the donkey. It is an unpleasant experience, but it is possible to make it as quick for the animal as possible whilst still ensuring correct dosage.

Ensure there is no food in the mouth before starting the administration technique. Ensure the full dose is consumed; if any amount of drug is lost or dropped from the mouth, re-dosing will be necessary.

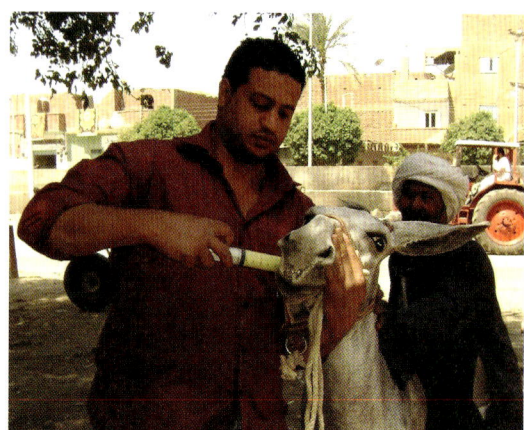

Figure 4.1.1 Administering oral medication to a donkey.

Administering tablets or powder

Two techniques are as follows:

1. **Form a paste** by mixing the powder with water. Draw this mixture up into a plastic syringe. Raise the head, open the mouth and deposit the drug on the back of the tongue or in the cheek pouch. If a smaller amount is to be administered it might be possible to deposit this under the tongue. Close the mouth and keep the head raised until the paste has been swallowed.
2. **Roll a bolus** by mixing tablets or powder with thick molasses, jaggery (unrefined cane sugar) or other locally available palatable substances. Offer the mixture to the animal to eat and supervise until finished.

Administering liquids

Drenching

Drenching is the technique of administration of liquid products directly into the back of the mouth and down the throat. This carries a risk of aspiration pneumonia; liquid paraffin is best avoided and powder suspensions are especially risky. If drenching is essential, allow the animal to swallow more easily by letting it close its mouth regularly and pouring the liquid **very slowly**.

> *Never* pour liquids directly into an animal's nose: this will result in severe inflammation of the nasal cavity and pharynx and most likely result in aspiration pneumonia.

The following drugs are available as preparations for drenching:

- Antacids (magnesium carbonate and sodium carbonate, and omeprazole)
- Laxatives (magnesium sulphate) **Take care!** These can cause aspiration pneumonia if they go down the trachea.
- Anthelmintics (fenbendazole, oxfendazole, ivermectin)

Nasogastric (stomach) tube insertion

If large volumes or potentially irritating fluids such as liquid paraffin are to be given orally, it is recommended to use a stomach tube (Figure 4.1.2). This is also used to aid in diagnosis of colic cases (see Section 11.5 *Colic*).

Equipment required

- **Stomach tube** designed for equids. Ensure the end of the tube is rounded and the tube is smooth, so as not to damage the delicate nasal mucosa. Soaking in hot water before use will make the tube more flexible.
- A large **funnel** which should fit the other end of the tube tightly.

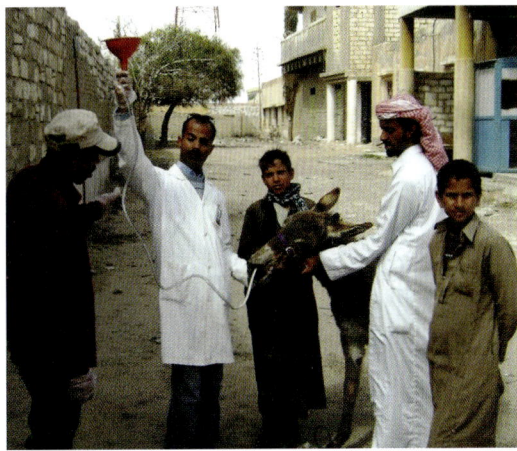

Figure 4.1.2 Administering fluids by a nasogastric tube.

4 CLINICAL TECHNIQUES

To pass a stomach tube

1. **Restraint is important** Use a head collar. If a twitch is necessary, ensure that the animal can breathe freely and the nostrils are not distorted (see Section 2.3). Over-restraint will cause the animal to become nervous which will make the procedure much more difficult.

> Sedation can interfere with the swallowing mechanism making intubation more difficult and it can also lead to a decreased cough reflex if the tube is in the trachea, so try to avoid this if possible.

2. **Mark the tube** Hold one end at the position of the stomach on the outside of the animal and trace along the outside of the oesophagus to the nostril, mark the tube at the nostril and throat. When introducing the tube the marks will show how far into the animal the tube has reached, when the animal should swallow the tube and when it should have reached the stomach.

3. **Lubricate** the end with liquid paraffin, water or obstetrical lubricant.

4. **Introduce the tube slowly** and gently into the ventral meatus (lower part of the nostril). It helps to keep the thumb of the hand introducing the tube pressed firmly down on to the tube to keep it directed ventrally in the nostril and prevent it moving dorsally in the nasal cavity where it will cause bleeding as it comes into contact with the ethmoid turbinates. Keep the animal's head flexed and advance the tube slowly. When the tip is at the pharynx, the animal may swallow, cough or move its head. Some resistance is encountered as the tube passes over the epiglottis; do not force it. Try to pass the tube on the first swallow, if this is not possible wait until the animal swallows again to pass the tube. Do not force it down.

5. **Continue advancing the tube into the oesophagus.**

> Visualise the tube going down the left-hand side of the neck in the region of the jugular groove (and/or feel it).

If the tube is in the correct position there will be negative pressure when sucking air back. If the tube is in the trachea it is possible to suck and blow freely down the tube and the tube cannot be visualised in the left jugular groove. Ensure that the tube can be seen on the left side of the neck – do not rely on the animal coughing if the tube is incorrectly placed in the trachea. Once in the stomach, gas that smells like ingesta will be emitted and a bubbling noise from the stomach may be heard.

The information in Table 4.1.1 may help to ensure that the tube is placed correctly into the stomach and not the lungs.

Check for gastric reflux

Once the tube is placed correctly in the stomach, pour a small volume of fluid (< 500 mls) into the tube via a raised funnel connected to the end. Once it has gone in under the influence of gravity lower the free end of the tube to the ground, which allows any excess gastric fluid to be siphoned off. This can be encouraged by rapidly withdrawing the tube by 10 cm, and then repositioning it. Repeat this process a number of times – repositioning the tube within the stomach to ensure that the stomach is not distended before liquid is added in a greater volume.

DRUG ADMINISTRATION TECHNIQUES 4.1

> **Failure to detect gastric reflux can lead to gastric rupture if a large volume of fluid is added to an already full stomach.**

Pour the liquid into the funnel and hold it as high as possible.

TIP If medicating with liquid paraffin this will run in more easily if mixed with warm water.

Removal of the tube

This is achieved by bending the end of the tube over and withdrawing it slowly and in one smooth movement. Kinking the tube helps prevent any residual fluid from entering the lungs as the tube passes the larynx. Try to prevent the animal from throwing its head up as the tube is removed, as this can cause bleeding from the nose.

How to manage possible complications of using a stomach tube

- **Nosebleed (epistaxis)** This is a common complication, especially if the animal moves its head a lot, the tube is too big or is not in the ventral meatus. It looks alarming but will stop in a short time. Keep the animal quiet until the bleeding stops.

- **Aspiration of fluid into the lungs** This is a much more serious complication compared to epistaxis. It can occur if the tube is placed in the lungs instead of the stomach, and can result in death within minutes. Alternatively, despite correct placement of the tube, careless or over-zealous fluid administration or tube removal may still result in some of the fluid entering the lungs, causing aspiration pneumonia. See Section 12.7 for treatment of this condition.

Sign	Tube in oesophagus (correct)	Tube in trachea (incorrect)
Resistance	Slight resistance to passage of the tube	No resistance to passage of tube in early stages
Left jugular groove	Tube visible and palpable as it passes down the oesophagus	Tube not palpable or visible in left jugular groove
Coughing	No coughing after the tube passes the pharynx	Repeated spasmodic coughing as tube is advanced
Breathing	No breath (air movement) felt when end of tube held near the handler's cheek	Regular breathing movements felt when end of tube held near the handler's cheek
Blow down the tube	Smell of stomach contents and gurgling sounds from the end of the tube when it reaches the stomach	No smell of stomach contents No gurgling sounds
Stress	Little or no distress seen in the animal as the tube is advanced	Animal is very uncomfortable and resists handling. (A very sick or painful equid may not react a lot to the procedure even if the tube is in the trachea, so rely on the other parameters.)

Table 4.1.1 Signs that can help determine if a nasogastric tube is in the oesophagus or trachea.

4 CLINICAL TECHNIQUES

Injections

All injections carry a risk of infection and can cause pain, fear and distress to some extent. They should never be given unnecessarily. Use paraprofessional training opportunities to demonstrate correct techniques to others. The following rules apply for all injections:

- **Always** use a sterile syringe and needle (Figure 4.1.3) to avoid creating an injection site abscess (see Section 15.3). Wipe the top of the medicine bottle with surgical spirit if it is dirty (Figure 4.1.4).
- **Always** use the narrowest gauge (G) that allows smooth injection of the drug, i.e. 20G or 21G for watery drugs and vaccines, 16G or 18G for oily drugs or suspensions.
- **Always** ensure the injection site is clean and free from mud or dirt.

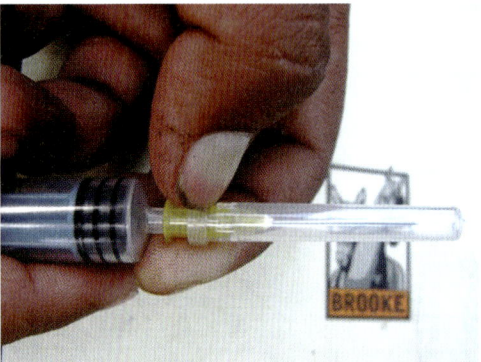

Figure 4.1.3 Selection of a correct sterile needle.

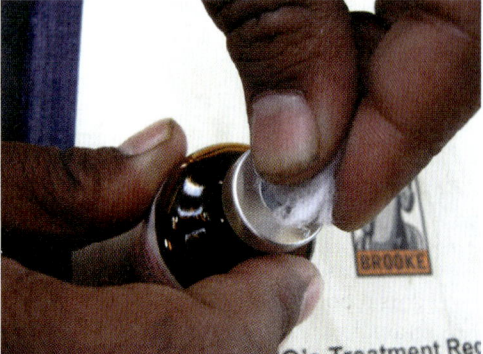

Figure 4.1.4 Wiping clean the top of a drug bottle.

Subcutaneous injection

Drugs given by subcutaneous injection are designated as s/c or SC.

Ensure that the drug is formulated to be given subcutaneously. Many drugs are poorly absorbed from subcutaneous tissue or can give a bad reaction, especially if large volumes are given.

Any skin site may be used, but preferred areas are the neck (see Figure 4.1.5) and pectoral regions where there is looser skin covering the body. Using a short needle (one inch), pinch the skin and introduce the needle almost parallel to the skin surface to avoid placement in underlying muscle, there should be little resistance to injection. The depot of drug under the skin leaves a small swelling, which disappears as the drug is absorbed.

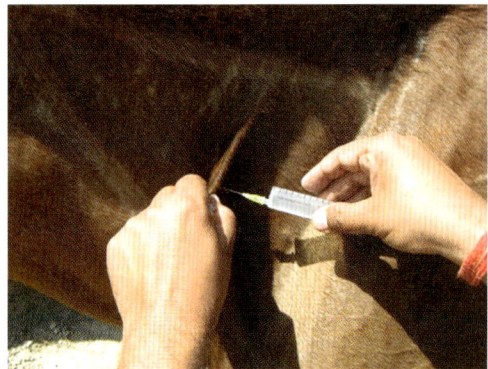

Figure 4.1.5 Subcutaneous injection in a horse.

DRUG ADMINISTRATION TECHNIQUES **4.1**

Intramuscular injection

> Drugs given by intramuscular injection are designated as i/m or IM.

Ensure that the drug is formulated for intramuscular use. Some drugs cause severe inflammation when injected intramuscularly. As a precaution never give more than 20 ml in any one site. Malignant oedema is a rare, often fatal, infection caused by *Clostridial* bacteria, typically caused by activation of dormant spores within the muscle; a possibility if IM injections are not given cleanly and carefully or if an irritant drug (e.g. flunixin meglumine) is used.

> Ensure a competent handler and consider the safety of the handler, the animal and the administrator of the drug at all times.

Ensure that all drugs are ready and drawn up and all equipment (needles and syringes) are sterile. Suitable needles for IM injections in equids are 18–21G depending on the viscosity of the solution (e.g. 18G for penicillin). The length of the needle for adult horses and mules and well-muscled adult donkeys should be 1.5 inches, for foals and thin donkeys one inch would suffice, to inject the drug deep into the muscle mass.

There are three preferred sites for intra-muscular injections:

1. **Neck** – in the triangle of muscle demarcated by the nuchal ligament, the dorsal border of the cervical spine and the cranial border of the scapula. Alternatively a hand can be placed on the neck with the base at the junction of the neck and the shoulder, half-way between the crest and the ventral side of the neck: the hand will be covering the area suitable for injection (Figures 4.1.6 and 4.1.8).

2. **Gluteal muscles** – in the centre of the muscular square bordered by the *tuber coxae, tuber ischii*, sacrum and base of tail. **Do not** inject caudal to the femur as this may damage the sciatic nerve (Figures 4.1.7 and 4.1.9). For gluteal injections ensure safety when administering the injection by maintaining body position as close to the animal as possible; use a spare hand on the animal's body to detect sudden movements.

3. **Pectoral muscle (horses only)** – in thickest part. Maximum volume is 5 ml per site and do not inject potentially irritating drugs in this area as it will affect movement.

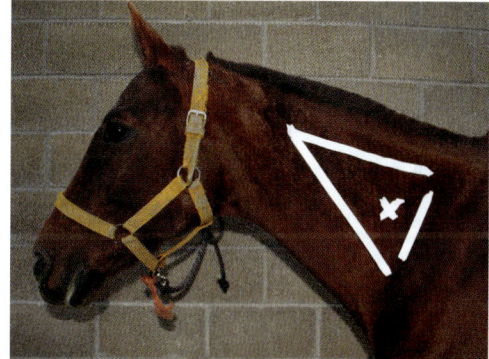

Figure 4.1.6 The white tape outlines the area safe for IM injection of the neck. The cross indicates the position a hand would occupy if placed with the base at the junction of the neck and shoulder, half-way between the crest and ventral neck and would be the ideal place for IM injection.

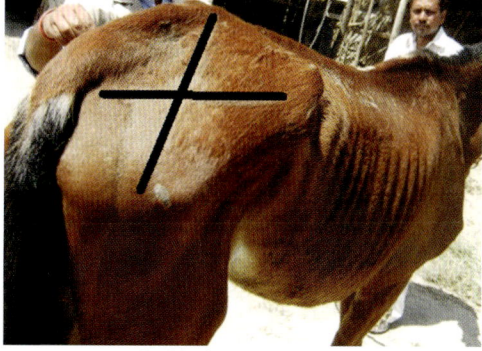

Figure 4.1.7 The black cross indicates safe placement of IM injection in the gluteals.

4 CLINICAL TECHNIQUES

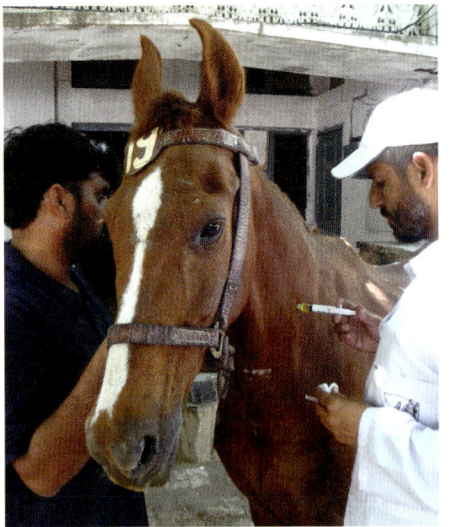

Figure 4.1.8 IM injection of the neck.

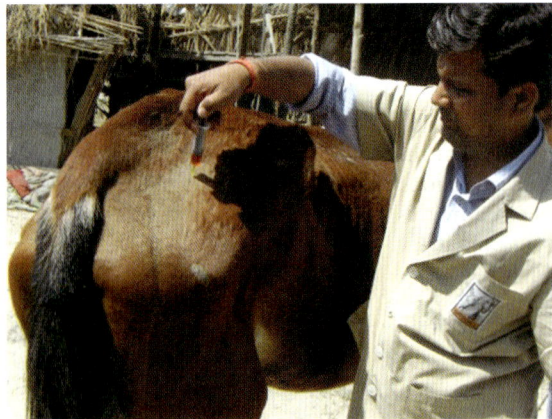

Figure 4.1.9 IM injection of the gluteal muscle.

For foals, donkeys, or when using potentially irritant drugs, keep the injection volume small (maximum 10 ml per site) in order to minimise adverse reactions. If necessary, divide the dose into two or three syringes and inject at different sites.

How to give intramuscular injections – two suggested techniques

1. For the neck, grasp a small fold of loose skin close to the injection site with a free hand. This distracts the animal and enables the clinician to move with it if it jumps away from the needle. With the other hand, introduce the needle smoothly into the adjacent muscle, at right angles to the skin. Inject drug into the deepest part of the muscle before withdrawing needle.

or

2. For the gluteals and pectorals, detach the needle from syringe, hold it between thumb and forefinger and mildly slap the muscle twice with the back of the hand. On the third slap turn the hand over and introduce needle quickly and firmly up to the hub. Attach syringe and inject. This action again distracts the animal's attention from the procedure.

Important consideration when injecting intramuscular procaine penicillin: Always pull back to check there is no blood in the syringe before injecting into the muscle.

> **Severe reactions, possibly death, can occur if white procaine penicillin formulated for IM injection ends up directly in the bloodstream.**

See Section 5.2 *Antibiotics* for the indications and recommendations on how to act when a penicillin reaction of this nature occurs.

DRUG ADMINISTRATION TECHNIQUES 4.1

Intravenous injection

> Drugs given by intravenous injection are designated as i/v or IV.

Ensure that the drug formulation is suitable for intravenous use. Many drugs (including almost all suspensions and some oily preparations) cause severe systemic reactions or death when injected by this route. Check that the drug is within the expiry date and contains no particles or contamination.

The correct site for IV injection is the **cranial third** of the jugular vein, where there is less risk of hitting the carotid artery. Inject slowly over 5–10 seconds.

> Do not inject drugs into the carotid artery!

Venous blood is dark red and flows in a steady drip or trickle. If the blood is bright red and flows in spurts, then the needle is in the carotid artery.

Always ensure that a competent handler is present and use safe positions when injecting. Ensure all drugs are drawn up ready in syringes and all equipment is sterile. Suitable needles for IV injection are 21–18G, the larger for more viscous or larger quantities that need administering more quickly; a 19G would suffice for most routine IV injections. A 1–1.5-inch length needle can be used depending on the size of the animal.

Two techniques for IV injection

1. **Detached needle** Raise the jugular vein by occluding it with a thumb at the base of the neck; it should be visible in all but the fattest animals. Insert the needle into the vein and check that venous blood is flowing freely. Once satisfied, attach the syringe and inject slowly. Always draw back regularly on the syringe to check that the needle is still in the vein. The advantages of this technique are that it is easy to see if the needle is in the jugular vein, and that nervous animals usually settle once the needle is in. When inserting the needle imagine following the line of the vein up the neck, i.e. once through the skin, angle the needle upwards and do not insert it at an acute angle. This avoids inserting the needle too deeply through the vein and into the carotid artery.

or

2. **Needle attached** Raise the vein and insert the needle whilst attached to the syringe. Draw back and check for dark (venous) blood entering syringe (Figure 4.1.10). If the blood is bright red and/or under pressure it means that the needle may be in the carotid artery. When satisfied, proceed as described above. It is more difficult to ensure that the needle is not in the carotid artery with this method.

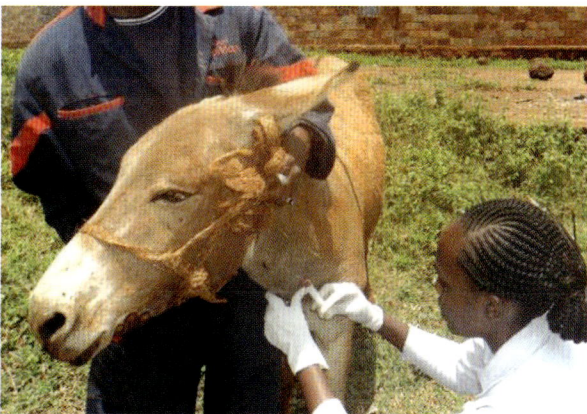

Figure 4.1.10 IV injection in a donkey.

4 CLINICAL TECHNIQUES

Possible complications of intravenous injection

1. **Intra-arterial injection** A serious complication occurs when the drug is injected into the carotid artery. The risk is highest if the needle is too long or is inserted accidentally low down in the neck. Typically, intra-arterial injection will cause the animal to collapse before the injection is finished. Seizures, twitching and coma may occur. Recovery depends on the type and volume of drug injected and the degree of cerebral inflammation caused. Some animals recover spontaneously in a few minutes. Others may die or have residual neurological damage.

2. **Peri-vascular injection** If the needle comes out of the vein and drugs are injected into the surrounding tissue, local irritation and inflammation may occur which can damage surrounding nerves. The severity depends on the type and volume of drug and the structures affected. Treat local swelling symptomatically and dilute the drug by infusing normal saline around the area and massage.

> If the animal is extremely fractious, and when using medication which is particularly irrititant when injected perivascularly, insert a catheter to administer the medication.

3. **Phlebitis/thrombophlebitis** Inflammation and partial or total occlusion of the jugular vein can occur as a complication of repeated IV injections or venous catheterisation, especially if the technique is not sterile. Thickening of the vein is visible and palpable, being hot, painful and swollen in acute cases. Raising the vein makes the site of occlusion more obvious. If the vein is totally occluded, there may be oedema of the head, which normally resolves over time as collateral circulation is established. Treat phlebitis with warm compresses, massage and NSAIDs. Prevent by using a sterile technique and avoiding multiple injections or long-term catheterisation of the same vein.

Placing an intravenous catheter

An IV catheter should be used:

- for IV fluid therapy or slow infusion of drugs (Figure 4.1.11)
- when repeated blood sampling or IV injections are needed such as during a general anaesthetic
- for safer administration of irritant drugs (minimises possibility of complications described above)
- for euthanasia if multiple drugs are to be used, large volumes need to be given, and to allow venous access throughout the procedure.

In most cases with working equids, IV catheters will not be left in the animal ('indwelling') for long periods of time as this increases the risk of infection. Any animal requiring daily IV injections should also be monitored by a veterinarian. Do not leave IV drugs for the owner to inject. If catheters are not available, the only other option is a long (2-inch) 14 or 16G needle. However, remember never to leave a needle in an animal, they always need to be taken out.

Catheter placement

1. Shave the skin over the cranial third of the jugular vein and prepare it aseptically. This eases catheter placement and minimises the risk of infection. See Section 4.6 of this chapter for explanation of how to carry out a sterile scrub of an area.

2. For wide-bore catheters or nervous animals, inject a subcutaneous bleb of local anaesthetic (LA) before catheter placement. See Section 7.2 for use of LAs.

3. Raise the vein. With the stylet (metal needle) in place, introduce the catheter at 45 degrees to the neck until blood is seen at the hub. Insert a further 2–3 mm, then flatten the catheter out almost against the neck, keep the stylet still while continuing to advance the plastic catheter up to its hub following the course of the vein underneath the skin. The catheter should advance without resistance. Remove the stylet and attach a bung or extension set to avoid introducing air into the jugular vein.

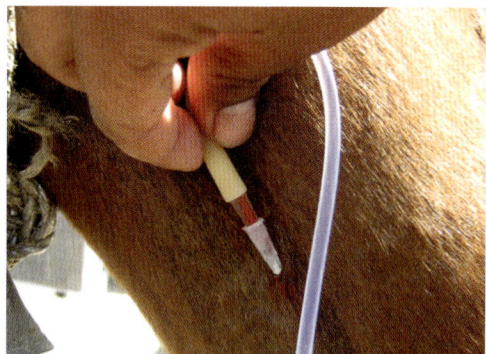

4. Secure the catheter with a piece of tape around the hub and the neck (Figure 4.1.11), or attach to the skin with two skin sutures. LA is placed subcutaneously in two blebs, one either side of the hub of the catheter, and then two simple skin sutures placed and tied onto the placement doles on either side of the catheter hub. A needle and forceps are not required to do this; simply thread two strands of suture material through two sterile needles and use the needle to place the thread through the skin. Ensure a sufficient length of thread to be able to tie the knots easily by hand.

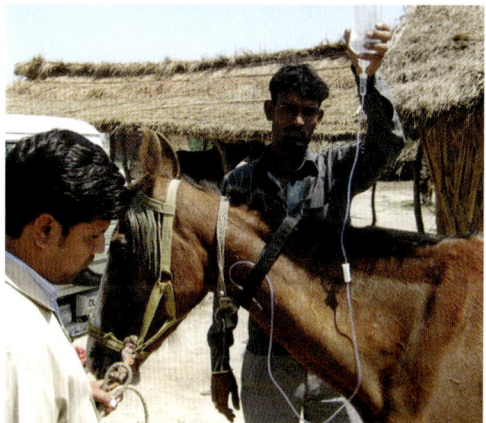

5. Ensure any giving set or extension set that is being attached to the catheter has been flushed with sterile saline so that air is not administered intravenously.

6. Each time the catheter is used, ensure it is still in the vein. To keep it patent, flush with normal saline before and after each injection. For long-term use, change the catheter every 48 hours, alternating between the two jugular veins to minimise the risk of thrombophlebitis.

> **Handle the catheter as aseptically as possible, even once it is in place, to reduce the risk of thrombophlebitis.**

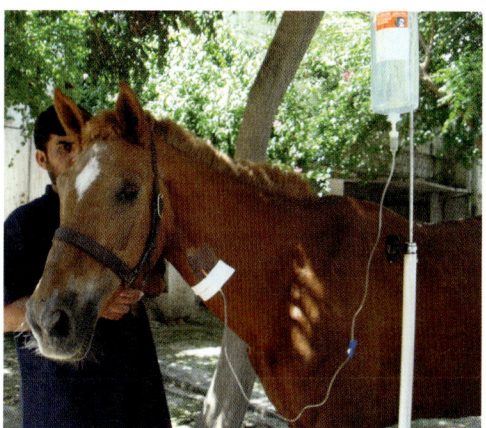

Figure 4.1.11 IV catheter in place and administration of fluids. Both down-the-vein (top and centre) and up-the-vein positioning of the catheter (bottom) are shown.

4 CLINICAL TECHNIQUES

Complications of intravenous catheterisation

1. **Thrombophlebitis** – as discussed on page 80.

2. **Air embolism** – If a catheter is placed pointing in a downward direction (down-the-vein), and is not covered by an injection cap, it will suck air into the jugular vein. This can be fatal – and therefore catheters should never be left open.

3. **Embolisation** of a piece of the catheter can occur if it is severed (when an animal struggles) or if it is cut when being removed. Never leave an owner to inject through or remove a catheter; this should only be done by a trained veterinarian.

> For further information on fluid therapy refer to Chapter 6.

Intra-articular injection

Introducing a needle into the joint of a working equid may occasionally be necessary in order to:

- take a sample of synovial fluid from a joint, if infection (septic arthritis) is suspected
- flush an infected joint
- inject antibiotics into an infected joint
- inject anti-inflammatory drugs into an inflamed joint.

> Aseptic preparation and knowledge of anatomy is paramount to avoid creating unnecessary harm.

Procedure

1. Sedation is recommended to minimise the likelihood of the animal flexing the joint and breaking the needle during injection. In nervous animals, it may be necessary to inject a subcutaneous bleb of local anaesthetic. Flushing the joint can be painful and may require general anaesthesia.

2. Shave the hair 3–5 cm above and below the joint, all the way around the limb – as it may be necessary to move the needle to a different site during the procedure.

3. Scrub the site from the centre outwards (as for a surgical operation – see Section 4.6 of this chapter) using sterile cotton wool or swabs and antiseptic: chlorhexadine gluconate (CG) or povidone iodine (PI). The antiseptic should be left on the skin for a minimum of 2 minutes for CG and 3 minutes for PI, to ensure all the bacteria are killed (Stinner *et al.* 2011).

4. Scrub hands in the same way and wear sterile surgical gloves if available. Always use a new, sterile syringe and needle.

> The correct sites for joint injection should be studied carefully.

Refer to equine anatomy and lameness textbooks for details; see also Chapter 14 *The musculoskeletal system*.

The decision to administer drugs intra-articularly should be made after considering the potential complications of entering a synovial structure. If bacteria or dirt inadvertently contaminate a synovial structure during an injection, this can lead to an incurable lameness potentially ending an equid's working life and requiring euthanasia on welfare grounds.

Direct intra-synovial administration produces higher drug levels in a joint than systemic administration which is useful for the treatment of certain conditions, e.g. joint infection or arthritis. However, anything injected intra-articularly should be chosen carefully to prevent further inflammation or irritation of the joint. Only drugs labelled for intra-articular use should be used.

Clinical pathology

What is 'clinical pathology'?

> Clinical pathology aims to diagnose disease using laboratory testing of blood and other bodily fluids, tissues, and microscopic evaluation of individual cells.

Within this chapter techniques for sampling, examining and testing (haematology and biochemistry) are described. For urinalysis see Chapter 13 *The urinary and reproductive systems*), for faecal analysis see Chapter 11 *The gastrointestinal system*, and Chapter 17 *Parasitology* gives further information on faecal egg counts, as well as referring to other clinical pathology texts where more information can be found.

What to consider when choosing a test?

Always remember the following when deciding on which test to undertake:

- Think carefully about the history of the case.
- Think about the presenting problem and the possible underlying causes.
- Ensure the test fits in with the clinical signs, not the other way round.
- What is the likelihood the animal is suffering from a particular disease?
- Negative results do not necessarily rule out a disease process and equally a positive result does not confirm it.
- Will doing the test compromise animal welfare?
- Will the treatment change depending on the results, i.e. is a diagnosis necessary?

What factors can affect the reliability of a test?

- Problems with the 'marker' of disease, e.g. antibody levels may vary at different stages of the disease
- Differences between individual animals
- Problems with sample collection or storage, e.g. not stored at the correct temperature
- Problems with the testing procedure, e.g. not carried out correctly

4 CLINICAL TECHNIQUES

What to consider when submitting a sample to a laboratory?
- Telephone the laboratory and ask for advice about what to submit.
- Follow their instructions, i.e. keep the sample cool, freeze, or air-dry as instructed.
- Package the sample safely.
- Label with details of the animal and date collected.
- Provide a history to the laboratory including any previous treatment.

> **Interpret all results in light of the clinical picture.**

Glossary

Below are some terms encountered when interpreting clinical tests:

Sensitivity The proportion of animals with disease which test positive

Specificity The proportion of animals without disease which test negative

Predictive value of a positive test How likely it is that an animal which tests positive actually has the disease

Predictive value of a negative test How likely it is that an animal which tests negative really is free from disease

True positive The animal has the disease and the test is positive.

False positive The animal does not have the disease but the test is positive.

True negative The animal does not have the disease and the test is negative.

False negative The animal has the disease but the test is negative.

Blood sampling

4.3

Taking blood samples

The number and nature of blood tests that are required will determine the volume and type of samples to be collected.

A blood sample is usually taken to assess the function of internal organs ('biochemistry'), and/or to look at the blood cells ('haematology'). See Section 4.5 for more details.

What blood tubes to use?

- **Plain tubes** Allow whole blood to clot. The serum layer is separated in the laboratory and tested for enzymes and proteins to assess organ function (biochemistry) or for specific antibodies against particular viruses and bacteria (serology).

- **EDTA tubes** Contain anticoagulant which stops blood from clotting. These samples are used to make blood smears, perform counts of different types of white blood cells (such as neutrophils or eosinophils) and red blood cells which give information on certain processes such as infection, inflammation, or anaemia.

- **Other tubes** Other sample tubes such as lithium heparin, sodium citrate, DNA sampling tubes and those for blood culture are used for specific tests (contact the local laboratory to discover which tests are available for equids and what sample tubes are required).

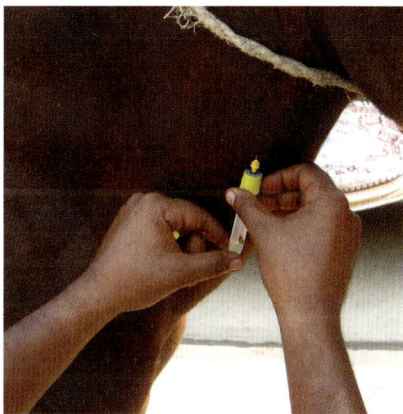

> Never compromise the welfare of an animal by taking a sample, blood or otherwise, without knowing *why*, *what* sample is required (volume and tube type) and *whether* the laboratory has the capacity to do the tests required. If the required information will not be gained, do not take a sample.

Two techniques for taking blood from major veins

1. Attach a one-inch, 19–20G needle to a syringe. Raise the vein and insert the needle. Keeping the vein raised, draw back steadily on the syringe until the required amount of blood is in the syringe (see Figure 4.3.1). Release the pressure on the vein before withdrawing the needle to avoid causing a haematoma.

or

2. Insert a double-ended vacutainer needle into the raised vein, then attach a vacutainer tube. Blood will flow into tube when the needle is correctly placed. Release the vein before withdrawing.

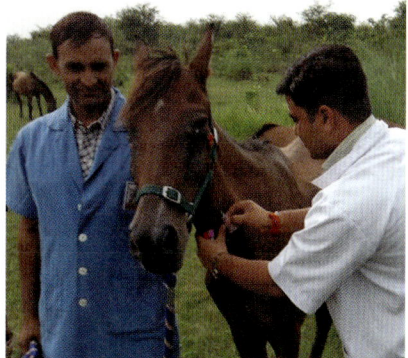

Figure 4.3.1 Collecting blood samples from the jugular vein.

4.4 Blood smears and staining

How to make a blood smear?

Learning the technique of good blood smear preparation is very useful. These are used to detect blood parasites (see Chapter 17) and perform differential white blood cell counts without having to send samples to the laboratory (refer to histology texts for further information on interpretation of smears).

Technique for making a blood smear

1. Acquire a blood sample. This is possible from a number of places including the ear tip. For the ear tip sample, clip a small area at the tip of one ear. Prick the skin with a 21G needle, squeeze a drop of blood directly onto a microscope slide and smear immediately before the blood clots; see Figure 4.4.1.

2. Use two glass microscope slides. Put a drop of fresh or EDTA tube blood at one end of one of the slides.

3. Holding the second slide (the 'spreader') at an angle of about 45 degrees, back it up against the drop of blood on the first slide until it runs (by capillary action along the short edge).

4. With an even motion, push the spreader along the whole length of the first slide so that the blood smears evenly; do not push the blood itself by having it ahead of the spreader. A good smear will have a thin, tapered, 'feathered' edge where the blood is less thick and looks thin and feathery.

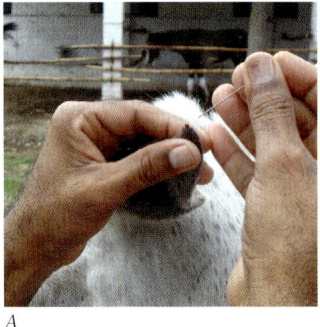

A

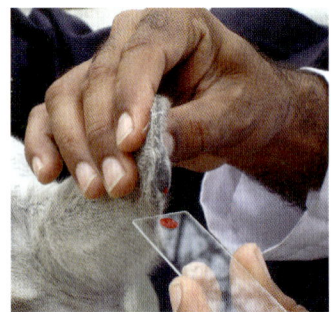

B

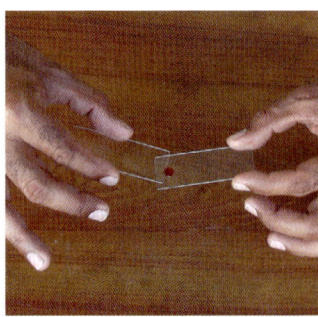

C

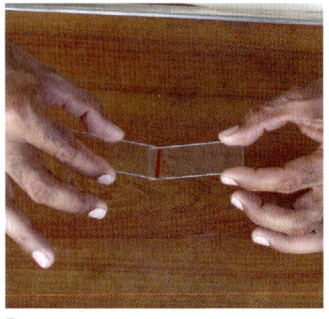

D

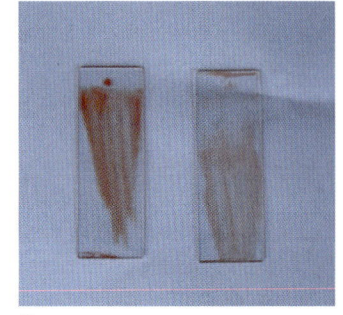

E

Figure 4.4.1. A) Prick the tip of an ear after clipping. B) Squeeze a drop of blood onto a glass slide. C) Blood smear preparation: Place the second slide at a 45 degree angle to the first. D) Touch the slide edge to the drop of blood to allow blood to spread along the leading edge, then push second slide along the first to create a smear. Ensure a good tapered, thin, 'feathered' edge. E) Air dry blood smears before staining and examination under a microscope.

BLOOD SMEARS AND STAINING 4.4

A good blood smear should:

- extend from one-half to three-quarters of the length of the slide
- have a thin, tapered, 'feathered' edge at the end of the smear
- be free of holes, lines or other defects.

If taking a blood sample from the jugular vein, ensure the following:

- Use a fresh sample mixed with EDTA.
- Mix the sample well before taking a drop for the slide.
- Air dry quickly before staining.
- Examine straight away.
- When sending it away to a laboratory do not stain but follow the above steps and put it into a slide container.

Staining techniques

The most common and easiest to perform are the Diff-quick and Gram staining techniques described below (RVC 2012).

Diff-quick staining technique

To perform this staining technique use the following three solutions:

1. Fixative (Fast green in methanol) – This is a **pale green** colour.
2. Stain solution 1 (Eosin G in phosphate buffer) – This is a **red** colour.
3. Stain solution 2 (Thiazine dye in phosphate buffer) – This is a **blue** colour.

Protocol

- Allow the smear to air dry.
- Dip the slide 5 times, for 1 second each time, into the fixative. Allow excess fixative to drain after each dipping.
- Dip the slide 5 times, for 1 second each time, into Stain solution 1. Allow excess stain to drain after each dipping.
- Dip the slide 5 times, for 1 second each time, into Stain solution 2. Allow excess stain to drain after each dipping.
- Rinse the slide in distilled water (or Weise's buffer, pH 7.2).
- Blot or allow to air dry.

Examine first at low power to identify structures and then at higher power under oil immersion. If a sample has been taken using a piece of sticky tape (see Section 15.2. *Diagnosis of skin abnormalities*) then allow this to dry and dip according to the protocol above. After rinsing, stick the tape to a slide (sticky side down) and continue with the protocol.

Observation. Note the following:

- Microflora and fauna present
- Morphology and organisation of squames (shed skin cells)
- Inflammatory cells
- Hairs, fibres, etc.
- Yeasts, bacteria and squames staining **blue**
- Inflammatory cells staining as follows: cell nucei – **blue**, cytoplasm – **red**.

4 CLINICAL TECHNIQUES

Gram staining technique

To perform this staining technique, use the following four solutions:

1. Crystal violet, 0.5% aqueous solution
2. Gram's iodine (Lugol's iodine)
3. Gram decolouriser (acetone/alcohol)
4. Safranin, 0.5% aqueous solution

Protocol

- Fix a thin smear by passing the slide through a flame for 3 seconds (e.g. a Bunsen burner).
- Stain with crystal violet for 30 seconds.
- Wash momentarily with water.
- Mordant with Gram's iodine for 30 seconds.
- Wash momentarily with water.
- De-colourise with acetone/alcohol. Allow de-colouriser to flow over the slide held at a 30-degree angle until the colour just ceases to flow from the smear for a few seconds.
- Wash immediately with water for 5 seconds.
- Counterstain with safranin for 15 seconds.
- Wash with water. Blot dry.

Examine under oil immersion at x 1000.

Observe

- Gram-positive bacteria will stain blue.
- Gram-negative bacteria will stain red.

4.5 Haematology and biochemistry

Always consider the following:

- Decide on the appropriate haematological diagnostic test and interpret the results in light of the clinical picture.
- Distinguish different cell types on a blood smear and morphological changes (see Section 4.4 of this chapter for the technique of making a blood smear).

Always interpret results in the light of the clinical picture.

HAEMATOLOGY AND BIOCHEMISTRY 4.5

Haematological analysis

Haematological evaluation consists of three components:

1. Automated analysis (by a laboratory)
2. Manual methods
3. Microscopic evaluation

Below are procedures described for manual techniques.

Manual Packed Cell Volume (PCV)

- PCV is a measure of the number of erythrocytes per cubic ml of blood.
- Manual PCV or micro-haematocrit is one of the most accurate, reliable and reproducible techniques for evaluation of the erythron (red blood cell).
- Important features are standardisation of spinning time and recognition of time necessary for maximum packing.
- **Technique:** Fill a capillary tube ¾ full and seal one end with clay or heat. Centrifuge for 6 minutes and read the PCV by placing the spun capillary tube against a haematocrit reader (Merck 2011).

Manual cell count

Manual counts for Red Blood Cell (RBC) and/or White Blood Cell (WBC) may be done using a haemocytometer. This is very time consuming and best left to the laboratories.

Errors inherent in manual cell counts include:

- random settling of cells within the counting chamber
- estimation of cell count from a very small volume of sample
- variation associated with filling of separate chambers for counts and inaccuracies of pipetting.

Differential cell count

Conduct a differential cell count just behind the feathered edge of a blood smear:

- WBC estimate
- Platelet estimate
- Morphology of leukcotyes (WBC), erythrocytes (RBC) and platelets

Observing a blood smear

View microscopically on x40 dry or x50 oil.

- View macroscopically to see if the smear is of a good quality.
- View microscopically behind the feathered edge to check individual cells are visible, not overlapping, smudged, etc.

4 CLINICAL TECHNIQUES

Estimate WBC

- Average number of leukocytes in dry high (x40) field is calculated by counting the total number of WBC in 10 fields ÷ 10 x 2000 = estimated total WBC.
- Go up to x100 oil immersion.
- Assess the morphology.
- Complete a **differential count**.

> **Differential WBC count technique:** Observe 100 WBC and express specific WBC types as a percentage of the total count (Fuentes-Arderiu and Dot-Bach 2009).

Estimate the platelet numbers

Estimation from the average number of platelets per high power field (x 1,000 oil immersion):

< 3–6 platelets on average – supports thrombocytopaenia.

10–25 platelets on average – suggests platelet count within normal limits.

> 25 – implies increased platelets (unusual).

Horses are prone to platelet clumping. They are also prone to rouleaux formation (stacking up of RBC like coins) which may be seen on this or the lower power.

White blood cells (leukocytes)

Refer to clinical pathology texts for images of normal and abnormal leukocytes. Below are listed a normal WBC differential and changes seen with certain abnormal states and diseases.

Normal differential WBC = neutrophils (45–55%), monocytes (0–3%), lymphocytes (35–50%), eosinophils (0–5%). NOTE: Basophils are very unusual. Ideally, actual numbers of each cell type per 10^9/L would be given rather than percentages. (This reference range is from the Department of Veterinary Pathology, University of Liverpool, UK. Values from other laboratories can vary – Knottenbelt 2006).

Toxic leukocyte changes

- There is an increased cytopolasmic basophilia and increased granularity of neutrophils; left shift, i.e. increased number of band cells.
- Equine band cells have slightly less chromatin clumping and are more U-shaped (less indentation).

Classic stress leukogram

- There is slight to moderate leukocytosis (WBC usually < or = 25 x 10^9/l) with neutrophilia and eosinopaenia (not the same thing as left shift), this is due to increased band cells.
- A stress leukogram where WBC count is < 25 x 10^9/l is likely to be due to inflammation or other reasons, not just due to stress.

Trypanosomiasis

- Trypanosomes can be seen free in the blood not intracellularly (see Section 17.8).
- Trypanosomes can be hard to find as the animal can have intermittent parasitaemia.
- Serial smears can be taken every 4 days for more accurate detection rates.

Piroplasmosis

- These are intracellular parasites (see Section 17.7).
- *Babesia equi* often clump together with four merozoites forming a cross shape (referred to as a Maltese Cross).
- Very low sensitivity as there will be lots of animals which are positive that this test does not pick up.

Thrombocytopaenia

Decreased platelet count may be the result of:

- platelet destruction
- platelet consumption
- sequestration
- blood loss
- decreased production.

Check smear for signs of clumping; this will result in an artificially low count. Less than $50 \times 10^9/l$ may result in bleeding.

A number of tests are available for testing platelet function, although these are unlikely to be used in practice.

- PTT (partial thromboplastin time) – a test for plasma clotting difficulties
- APTT (activated partial thromboplastin time) – assessment of haemostasis (Casella *et al.* 2009)

Saline autoagglutination: Dilute blood 1:4 in saline. If clumps remain this indicates true agglutination.

> **Donkeys!** A difference between prothrombin time and APTT has been found between donkeys and horses in a study by Mendoza *et al.* (2011), so always be cautious in diagnosing and unnecessarily treating coagulopathy in donkeys.

Biochemistry

The liver

A list of available tests is shown over; different laboratories my offer all or some of these.

> **Only SDH and GLDH are completely liver specific.**

4 CLINICAL TECHNIQUES

Hypoalbuminaemia is associated with liver problems especially if chronic in duration; no other signs may be seen and this may be the only change in the blood.

Tests

(Those in **bold** are most commonly seen elevated with **liver problems**.)

- **Alkaline Phosphatase (ALP)**
- **Aspartate Aminotransferase (AST)**
- **Gamma-Glutamyl Transferase (GGT)**
- Total Protein (TP)
- Albumin (Alb)
- Total Bilirubin (Tbili)
- **Direct** and Indirect **Bilirubin (DBili, IBili)**
- Bile Acids
- Glutamate Dehydrogenase (GLDH)
- Idiotal Dehydrogenase (IDH - formerly Sorbitol Dehydrogenase - SDH)
- Arginase (Arg)
- LDH, Isoenzyme 5

Increased **bilirubin** (especially indirect) is liver specific. Keep sample out of the sunshine and it will remain stable for 48 hours.

> **Serum bile acids may be raised with anorexia.**

The kidneys

The following tests assess kidney function:

- Creatinine
- Urea
- Total protein
- Albumin
- Urine protein
- Serum electrolytes
- Urinalysis

Elevations in urea and creatinine reflect decreased glomerular filtration rate. This may be associated with pre-renal, renal or post-renal conditions. Evaluation of urine specific gravity and urinalysis with ancillary tests to rule out concurrent disease that may affect the kidney provides the basis for determination of whether or not renal disease is present (see Chapter 13).

It is estimated that 65–70% of the nephrons must be dysfunctional before elevations of creatinine and urea and decreased urine specific gravity are detected in association with renal disease.

Urea may be decreased in liver disease.

Muscle

The following tests assess muscle damage:

- Asparate Aminotransferase (AST) – increases more slowly but stays high for longer
- Creatine Kinase (CK) – very high straight away
- Urine myoglobinuria

Serum proteins

- **Elevated Total Protein (TP)** with elevated albumin (and globulins) = likely dehydration
- Elevated TP with increased globulin and normal or decreased albumin = possible dehydration or possible inflammation
- Decreased TP with decreased albumin and globulins = protein losing disease (enteropathy or nephropathy)

Sterile skin preparation 4.6

Aseptic scrub procedure

Ensure that the animal is calm and handled by a competent person. If necessary the animal can be sedated for clipping the hair, depending on the condition of the patient and the forthcoming procedure.

Clipping hair

Depending on the procedure it may be appropriate to clip the hair from the area as this is a major potential contaminator. For surgeries and catheter placement it is advisable to clip the area; although some evidence from Hague *et al.* (1997) stated that after appropriate preparation there was no difference in bacterial numbers isolated in clipped and non-clipped sites prior to arthrocentesis.

> Know the anatomical boundaries and the essential area to clip.

Have all equipment to hand:

- Sterile gloves
- Sterile swabs/cotton wool
- Scrub solution: Povidone iodine (PI) or 4% chlorhexidine gluconate (CG)
- 70% surgical alcohol (e.g. isopropanol) or sterile saline

4 CLINICAL TECHNIQUES

The scrub solution is made up in a bowl in advance of the scrub procedure. Gloves are worn. A swab is soaked in scrub solution and squeezed to remove the excess, then starting from the central point of the procedure (e.g. point of proposed entry of catheter, or surgical site) the area is wiped in a circular motion working outwards. Once the outside edge is reached the swab is discarded and not returned to the central point. The next swab is taken and the procedure repeated, until the swab leaving the periphery is visually clean. A solution of 70% surgical alcohol is sprayed/poured over the area after a PI scrub, or sterile saline can be used after a CG scrub.

> **No difference in bacterial numbers has been seen between these two methods of PI and CG scrub preparation (Wilson *et al.* 2011).**

Scrub time

Studies looking at the effect of bacterial load and scrub time saw no difference between 10 minutes, 5 minutes, 3 x 30 seconds, and a one-step protocol of a surgical preparation of iodophor (solution was in skin contact for 2 minutes) (Zubrod *et al.* 2004).

For PI, the recommended contact time is 3 minutes.

However, always check for discolouration of the swabs. If at the end of 3 minutes the swabs are still showing signs of dirt, then continue scrubbing until they come away clean.

> **For CG the recommendation is a minimum of 2 minutes' skin contact time.**

Again, check on the state of the swabs to ensure all dirt is removed (Stinner *et al.* 2011).

References 4.7

Casella, S., Giannetto, C., Fazio, F., Giudice, E., Piccione, G. (2009) Assessment of Prothrombin time, activated prothrombin time, and fibrinogen concentration on equine plasma samples following different storage conditions. *J. Vet. Diagn. Invest.* 21, 674–678.

Fuentes-Arderiu, X., Dot-Bach, D. (2009) Measurement uncertainty in manual differential leukocyte counting. *Clin. Chem. Lab. Med.* 47 (1), 112–115.

Hague, B.A., Honnas, C.M., Simpson, R.B., Peloso, J.G. (1997) Evaluation of skin bacterial flora before and after aseptic preparation of clipped and non-clipped arthrocentesis sites in horses. *Vet. Surgery.* 26, 121–125.

Knottenbelt (2006) Equine Formulary. Saunders. Elsevier Ltd. pp. 4, 7.

Mendoza, F.J., Perez-Ecija, R.A., Montreal, L., Estepa, J.C. (2011) Coagulation profiles of healthy Andalusian donkeys are different than those of healthy horses. *J. Vet. Intern. Med.* 25, 967–970.

Merck (2011) Blood sample preparation and evaluation. (Online) Available at http://www.merckvetmanual.com/mvm/index.jsp?cfile=htm/bc/150216.htm (accessed 7 December 2012).

RVC (2012) Diagnosis in dermatology. (Online) Available at http://www.rvc.ac.uk/review/Dermatology/Tests/Diffquik.htm (accessed 12 November 2012).

Stinner, D.J., Krueger, C.A., Masini, B.D., Wenke, J.C. (2011) Time-dependent effect of chlorhexidine surgical prep. *J. Hospital infections.* 79 (4), 313–316.

Wilson, D.G., Hartmen, F., Carter, V.R., Klohnen, A., MacWilliams, P.S. (2011) Comparison of three preoperative skin preparation techniques in ponies. *Equine vet. Educ.* 23 (9), 462–465.

Zubrod, C.J., Farnsworth, K.D., Oaks, J.L. (2004) Evaluation of arthrocentesis site bacterial flora and after 4 methods of preparation in horses with and without evidence of skin contamination. *Vet. Surgery.* 33, 525–530.

Further reading

Consult texts on clinical pathology and veterinary laboratory medicine for more information on this subject.

Coumbe, K.M. (2012) Equine Veterinary Nursing. 2nd Edn. Wiley Blackwell. p. 417.

The Royal Veterinary College website has information on staining. (Online) Available at http://www.rvc.ac.uk/review/Dermatology/Tests/Diffquik.htm (accessed 12 November 2012).

Medicines

5

Introduction and nomograms	**5.1**
Responsible medicine use	**5.2**
Antibiotics	**5.3**
Non-steroidal anti-inflammatory drugs (NSAIDs)	**5.4**
Steroidal anti-inflammatory drugs (corticosteroids)	**5.5**
References	**5.6**

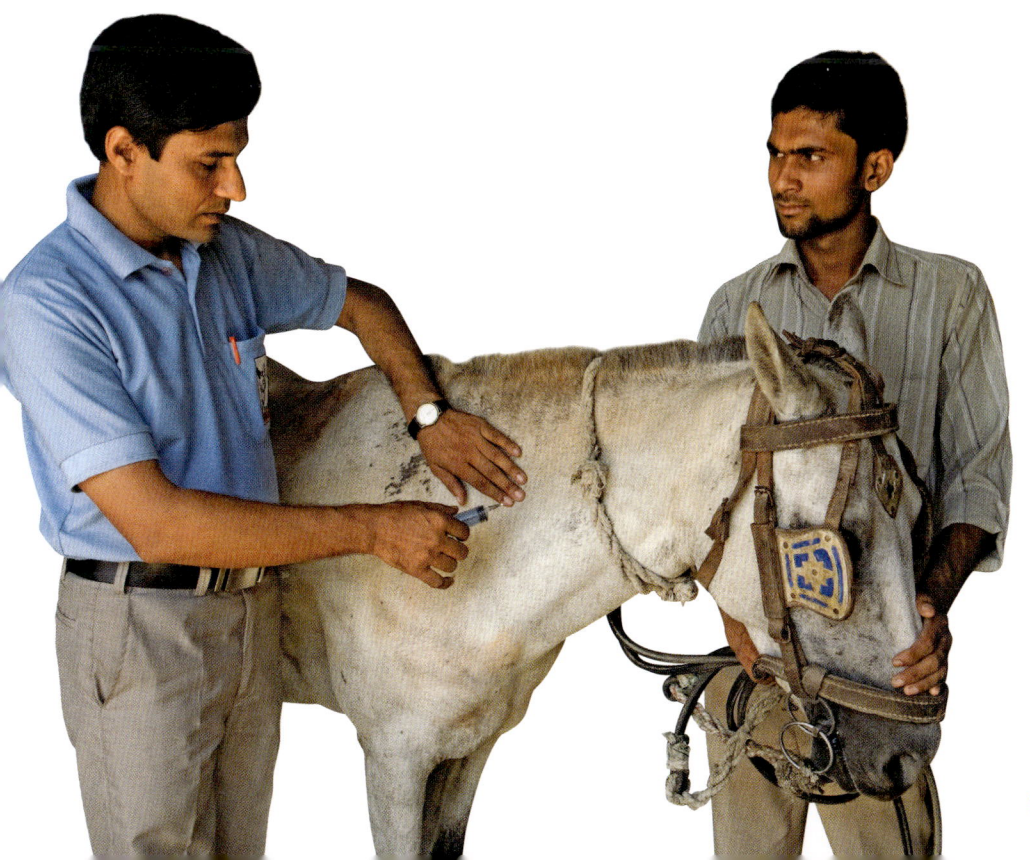

5.1 Introduction and nomograms

For the use of medicines for specific body systems or conditions, see the relevant chapters. For example, anthelmintics are discussed in Chapter 17 *Parasitology* and ocular therapeutics in Chapter 9 *Ophthalmology*.

Calculation of body weight (nomograms)

In any situation where drug doses need to be calculated, it is essential to be able to calculate the bodyweight of working equids accurately. If there is access to a weigh scale or bridge this is always preferable. Unfortunately this is not usually available.

There are a number of published calculations for estimating the weight of equids (Carroll and Huntington 1988 and Svendson 2008). However, remember that working equids often have low body weight in relation to their height or length compared with the sample populations that the calculations were made from, so take care in interpreting these calculations.

The equation used by Caroll and Huntington (1988) correlated well with the body condition score charts that they used: weight (kg) = $\dfrac{girth^2 \times length\ (cm)}{11900}$

5.2 Responsible medicine use

A veterinary qualification allows the legal right to dispense medication to animals. Although the levels of training required to dispense may vary between countries, veterinary undergraduate courses guarantee the teaching of pharmacological principles to an advanced level.

> As a veterinarian, set the standard of excellence for responsible medicine use in the working environment.

The dispensing of medication carries great responsibility. This is often forgotten or overlooked due to the frequency with which medicines are prescribed. The following paragraphs briefly describe some important considerations on this aspect.

Know the basic pharmacological principles of the medication

When administering a drug to an animal, there is an obvious responsibility that it should:

a) reach the affected area, and
b) be effective for the purpose required – a concept known as pharmacokinetics.

Although this concept sounds simple it encompasses five main principles which should be applied when choosing a drug regime:

1. **Absorption** How quickly will the drug leave the site of administration and get into the bloodstream? Is this appropriate for what is trying to be achieved? For example, to stop a per-acute anaphylactic reaction where the animal could die within minutes, an *instantaneous* effect is required, thus choose intravenous (IV) administration over oral (PO) or intramuscular (IM). On the other hand, if a drug needs to be absorbed more slowly and/or maintain effective concentrations in the body over a period of hours or days, intramuscular or oral drugs are best.

2. **Distribution** How rapidly will the drug reach the site of action and how long will it stay there? Drugs reach highly perfused organs (such as the kidneys and lungs) relatively quickly regardless of administration route, whereas they take longer to reach the skin, skeletal muscle and some other organs. Be aware how long effective drug concentrations will persist in the blood (the 'half-life'), as this may dictate how often the drug must be administered over a 24-hour period – once (SID), twice (BID), three (TID) or four times (QID).

3. **Metabolism** Be aware of how drug metabolism or 'breakdown' occurs for different substances, as this can alter the effectiveness. The majority of medicines are metabolised in the liver but some are metabolised in the kidneys, lungs or gastrointestinal system. Older animals or those with liver pathology may metabolise compounds more slowly than a young, healthy animal. This may have an effect on how fast the drug will work; for example, some drugs are administered in the form of a 'pro-drug' which first must be activated by liver metabolism. Consider whether long-term usage may have a negative effect on the liver or kidneys.

4. **Excretion** What goes in must come out. Medical compounds will be eliminated from the body either in the original form or as metabolites and it is important to know the routes. Most drugs are excreted through the kidneys although some are eliminated through the gastrointestinal system. Gaseous anaesthetics exit through respiration. Some drugs are excreted in milk; a very important consideration if a mare is lactating as metabolites could have side effects on the foal. The route of excretion also dictates the drug efficacy. Animals which are dehydrated or suffering from anuria may develop a toxic build-up of metabolites if they cannot excrete the drug through the urine.

5. **Drug Interactions** Interactions may be desirable with positive effects for the animal or undesirable with negative effects. An example of a positive interaction would be using smaller doses of two drugs which have a more profound effect when used in combination, e.g. combining an alpha-2 agonist (detomidine) and an opioid (butorphanol) to give a greater depth of sedation than a single larger dose of the alpha-2 alone would produce.

   In the case of undesirable effects there are two possibilities. The first is that some drugs interact, resulting in inactivation of them both, e.g. combining flunixin meglumine and gentamicin in the same syringe causes precipitation and inactivation. Secondly, certain drugs interact with a negative effect, e.g. if intravenous potentiated sulphonamides (sulphadiazine with trimethoprim, or sulphadoxine with trimethoprim) are administered to horses that have been sedated with the alpha-2 agonist drug detomidine, there is a risk of death from heart arrhythmia (Stack and Schott 2011).

The above has been included as something to think about. It is beyond the scope of this manual to cover the pharmacodynamics of all drugs used in equine practice so reference should be made to pharmacological texts when necessary. Moreover, the data sheet which accompanies most drugs should have pharmacokinetic information.

5 MEDICINES

The table below shows the common drug administration routes and some pharmacodynamic considerations for the use of each route.

Drug administration routes

See Section 4.1 for a full description of each route of administration.

Table 5.2.1 shows the pharmacodynamic considerations for various drug administration routes, outlining the main routes of administration of drugs for equids along with the absorption rates for each route, advantages of the route and any precautions that should be noted and stated to the owner.

Route	Absorption	Advantages	Precautions
Oral (PO) – direct, drench gun, stomach tube	+/- Variable, as must first pass through the gastrointestinal tract. Not possible for all drugs	Owner convenience (compliance), cheap, safe	Liquid may enter lungs Diarrhoea if gut flora upset Lack of absorption due to diet/other complications No guarantee animal will eat medication Depends on owner compliance of timing and correct administration
Intramuscular injection (IM)	+++	Good if drug unsuitable for IV use but a relatively fast onset of action is required	Requires a trained administrator Extreme pain and necrosis if drug is not meant for IM injection route Not > 20 ml/site Animal may show resistant behaviour if used for long term Injection sites may fibrose after time Accidental IV injection can be dangerous
Subcutaneous injection (SC)	++	Good for less soluble suspensions	Large volumes will not disperse Pain/irritation may result Poor absorption if animal is dehydrated

Route	Absorption	Advantages	Precautions
Intravenous injection (IV)	+++++ Immediate	Good for emergency situations or large volumes (absorption bypassed)	Risk of injection into carotid artery when attempting jugular vein injection, always check before injecting More skills required than other routes Systemic reaction/death if drug not suitable for IV Little time to act if adverse reaction or overdose Requires slow injection over 5–10 seconds Not suitable for owner administration
Topical	++	Easy compliance Good where systemic use may have side effects, e.g. steroids	Animal may lick/bite medication off Some preparations harmful to humans and require the use of gloves in application Absorption into skin of equids with hair cover may be variable

Table 5.2.1 *The rate of absorption, advantages and precautions of different routes of drug administration.*

Owner compliance

As a veterinarian, ensure that any dispensed drugs are adequately packaged and clearly labelled with the owner's name, drug name and instructions for use. Even in illiterate communities there are ways to devise instructions using pictures and symbols. Many community-based health programmes have successfully adopted this method (Hanson 1995, Daghio *et al.* 2010). If drugs are not dispensed in the correct packaging there is a risk they will be misused or accidentally consumed by children, with potentially devastating effects. Always ensure the owner thoroughly understands the prescription, how often it is to be given and any side effects to look out for.

5 MEDICINES

It is very important to give precise and clear instructions when dispensing drugs to owners.

> **State:**
> - The prescribing veterinarian's name and contact details
> - The owner's name and contact details
> - The identification of the intended animal
> - The dose rate – so the owner understands how much of the drug to give
> - The dosing interval – so the owner understands how often to give the drug
> - 'For animal treatment only'
> - 'Not for use in food production animals' (if required)
> - 'For external use only' with topical products
> - Any necessary warnings and special storage instructions
> - The date of supply and expiry date if applicable
>
> - Ensure the owner knows how to administer the drug – the best way to ensure this is to get the owner to administer the first treatment under direct observation.

Ensure that the owner understands if a drug is not to be used in animals intended for human consumption. Although the owner may not be intending to slaughter their equid for consumption, the drug may inadvertently be given to other livestock and owners must be made aware of potential consequences. If there are risks to humans from inadvertent consumption of the drug, these must also be explained to the owner.

> **Owner compliance is perhaps one of the biggest limiting factors in successful recovery of sick animals.**

There is a reliance on owners to carry out instructions once a consultation is finished. It is important to have owners report on the progress of treatment. If there is not a good relationship with the owner the outcome will most definitely be poor compliance, resulting in poor animal welfare.

Be aware of the wider consequences of medication.

Knowledge of pharmacology brings with it a broader understanding of the potential negative effects of drug usage, not just on the individual animal but on the surrounding human and animal populations, and the environment. Take note of the following guidance to limit the negative effect.

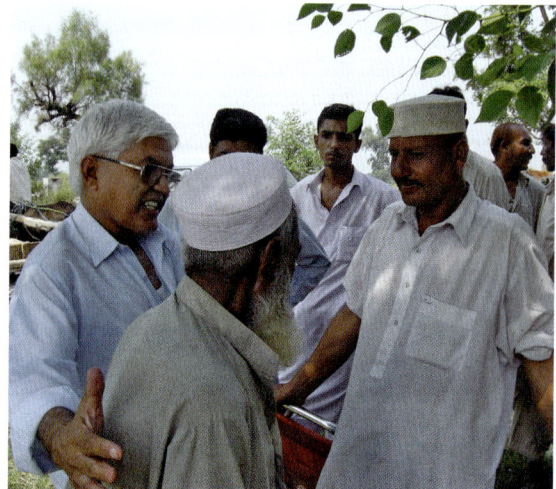

Figure 5.2.1 Developing good communication and rapport with owners is fundamental to a successful outcome.

- **Always prescribe the full course.** There are many examples of drug resistance, particularly in antibiotics and antiparasitics, and it is the responsibility of a veterinarian to avoid contributing to this as much as possible. Even if paraprofessionals, owners or markets

RESPONSIBLE MEDICINE USE 5.2

contribute to drug resistance in the locality, veterinarians should be setting the best standard, to avoid such practices. Use any available opportunity to guide government, paraprofessionals, pharmacists, other veterinarians and owners towards appropriate drug use.

▌ **Always administer the correct dose.** Overdosing can result in damaging side effects and toxicity, whereas under-dosing will encourage resistance and compromise animal welfare if it does not have the required effect. Body weight can be estimated using a simple tape measure. There are a number of nomograms published for calculating the body weight of horses and donkeys (Carroll and Huntingdon 1988, Svendson 2008).

▌ **Never administer a drug unnecessarily.** Veterinarians worldwide are unfortunately exposed to pressure from owners to administer medicines to animals against their better scientific judgement. Experience, confidence and having a good vet/owner relationship will soften the effect of such pressure. Remember, neither the animal's welfare, or in some cases the environment, will benefit from unnecessary treatments. Often drug resistance is the unfortunate result of over-prescription.

▌ **Think about the food chain.** Although not quite as pertinent in equine medicine as with production animal medicine, always be conscious of where the drugs prescribed may end up. Owners could use dispensed drugs for other livestock, and then consume the meat or milk without adequate withdrawal periods. A good example is the antibiotic metronidazole; banned in food-producing animals for its carcinogenic properties but often prescribed in equids. Other drugs, such as diclofenac, have resulted in devastation in local wild animal populations due to veterinary use in domestic animals (Oaks *et al.* 2004).

▌ **Take care when administering drugs that have not been licensed for equids** – there may be unpredictable results due to variations in absorption, metabolism and excretion compared to that in the species which the drug is licensed for. Also some drugs are toxic to equids.

The above examples only touch on the moral and ethical debates that may be encountered in daily practice. Capacity building of local paraprofessionals poses an opportunity for working equid veterinarians to emphasise the importance of responsible drug use in the community; leading by example is the first step.

> Always store drugs properly, maintaining the cold chain of those drugs for which this is required (see Figure 5.2.2).

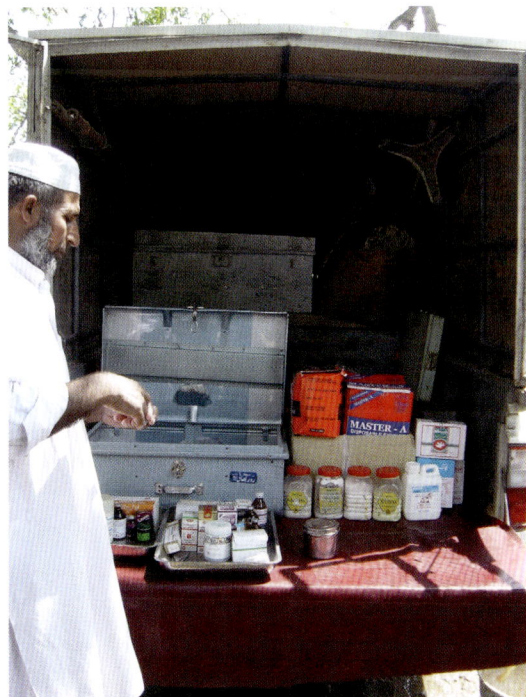

Figure 5.2.2 Ensure proper storage of drugs in mobile services.

103

5.3 Antibiotics

Rational use of antibiotics

> Antibiotics are used to treat infections caused by bacteria.

Antibiotics have no effect on other pathogens (including viruses). However, secondary bacterial infection is a common consequence of tissue damage from other causes.

There has been an increased awareness in recent years of the need for rational use and effective choice of antibiotics, given the escalation of bacterial resistance (Hollis and Wilkins 2009) and concerns over drug residues in consumable animal products and the environment.

Before dispensing any antibiotic therapy, consider the following:

Does bacterial infection actually exist, and is antibiotic treatment warranted?

Knowledge of pharmacological principles (see Section 5.2 of this chapter – *Responsible medicine use*) will help when making this decision; however, the use of antibiotics in **superficial wounds or as single doses** is unjustifiable. Superficial infections are usually due to commensal organisms which will be flushed away by adequate washing with water and careful attention to wound cleaning. 'One-off' dosages of antibiotics will usually not satisfy the pharmacological conditions necessary to overcome a bacterial infection, and will only encourage resistance. Look for alternatives in these situations.

> An increase in body temperature alone does not amount to a diagnosis of bacterial infection! Body temperature can be affected by environmental heat, working conditions, stress, pain, non-infectious inflammatory conditions and viral infections.

Where is the infection and how long has it been present?

Consider where the infection is in the body and whether antibiotics may penetrate the area. For example, antibiotics will not penetrate a walled-off superficial abscess so their use in this case is unnecessary.

Which bacteria are likely to be involved and which antibiotics are they likely to be sensitive to?

It may be possible to make an informed guess about which bacteria are the most likely cause of an infection, even without advanced diagnostics. Normal skin flora such as *Staphylococcus aureus* will be present in most traumatic skin wounds, whilst respiratory infections commonly involve *Streptococcus* species. Septic infections and toxaemias will most likely involve gram negative bacteria. Be aware of which antibiotics treat which types of bacteria and choose accordingly (see 'indications' under each antibiotic type in the following pages and other reference texts).

What dosage, frequency and administration route will ensure appropriate antibiotic concentrations at the site of infection?

As discussed earlier in this section, the formulation of a drug influences how quickly it enters the bloodstream and acts at the point of infection. Some antibiotics are formulated as 'long-acting' preparations, meaning they release slowly from the injection site and last for 48–72 hours. The duration of action may be affected by infection, inflammation or other pathology which may compromise the drug's metabolism, so shorter acting antibiotics are preferred whenever possible.

When deciding the frequency of administration required, consider the 'half-life' of the antibiotic in question, as this determines the inter-dosing interval (once per day – SID, twice per day – BID, three times per day – TID or four times per day – QID).

> If medication is not dosed according to the recommended frequency it will not combat the infection due to bacterial multiplication between dosages.

What adverse effects could arise from using antibiotics?

Decide whether the benefits of antibiotic therapy outweigh the risks. Equids are prone to drug reactions (e.g. procaine penicillin), and the use of IV potentiated sulphonamides have been known to cause fatal cardiac arrhythmias if used with the sedative detomidine (Stack and Schott 2011; see Section 7.1).

Additionally, equids are sensitive to changes in their gastrointestinal flora, to the extent that the use of antibiotics may cause diarrhoea and colic due to proliferation of potentially fatal pathogenic bacterial species such as *Salmonella* and *Clostridia*.

> Always weigh up the potential harm versus benefit of administering antibiotics in each situation to avoid unnecessary administration.

Consider the specific needs of the equid being treated.

Different animals have different pharmacokinetics which may influence which antibiotics are appropriate. For example, not all antibiotics used in adult horses are safe to use in neonatal foals – e.g. tetracyclines can result in flexor tendon laxity in foals. Similarly, horses with liver disease/liver failure can have greatly altered hepatic metabolism which can affect the pharmacokinetics of drugs. Antibiotics may have different pharmacokinetics in donkeys compared to horses (Lizarraga *et al.* 2004, Grosenbaugh *et al.* 2011).

Clinical use of commonly available antibiotics

Due to variations in availability of antibiotics in different countries the following list is certainly not exhaustive. Useful references are the review article by Haggett and Wilson (2008) on the use of antimicrobials in horses, and the paper by Grosenbaugh *et al.* (2011) on therapeutics in donkeys. Antibiotic formulations and their dose rates, which are suitable for equids, vary widely, so refer to recent texts and reliable formularies as well as the manufacturer's data sheets for specific dose rates for the preparation.

Procaine penicillin (Beta-Lactam)

Penicillins are part of the Beta-Lactam antibiotic group which act on enzymes in the bacterial cell wall. They are generally broad-spectrum, safe, effective drugs of low cost. Procaine penicillin is the white formulation for intramuscular use only. Refer to a formulary for IV and oral penicillin preparations for equids which may be available locally.

Indications
- *Streptococcal* spp. infections (first choice for equine respiratory infections), e.g. *Streptococcus equi* spp. equi infections (Hollis and Wilkins 2009)
- Anaerobes such as *Clostridial* spp., the obvious examples being tetanus (Section 16.1) or malignant oedema (Section 14.9)
- **Adverse penicillin reactions** are quite common in many species (including humans) especially after multiple doses. In equids they react to the procaine binder of the drug, and the chance of this occurring is greatly exacerbated if the penicillin is *injected into the bloodstream* by mistake (see Section 4.1. *Drug administration techniques*). Also the availability of procaine in the body is increased if the drug is overheated.

What does an adverse penicillin reaction look like, and how can this be managed?

> **An adverse penicillin reaction will usually occur as soon as, or shortly after, penicillin administration.**

In many cases the animal may have had a number of previous doses of penicillin without incident and the reaction will occur due to the cumulative effects of the drug over time. The animal will appear hypersensitive, with a range of signs including excessive muscle twitching/shaking, high head carriage, snorting, rigid stance, wide eyes and other manic behaviours. In severe reactions, collapse, seizures and death may occur – often within minutes.

Be warned that these reactions can be extremely violent, and ensure human safety if attempting any treatment. Although there is no antidote, adrenaline and intravenous corticosteroids can be given if it is possible to get access to a vein. Often the best thing to do is leave the animal in a quiet, dark place to recover, where it has minimal opportunities to further injure itself.

> **The potential severity of a penicillin reaction emphasises the importance of good IM injection technique.**

Owners must be made aware that a penicillin reaction has occurred. Emphasise that the animal should never be given penicillin or penicillin derivatives in the future. Note the reaction in veterinary records so that other veterinarians are aware of it.

Cephalosporins (Beta-Lactam)

Cephalosporins were developed in the 1950s due to concern over penicillin resistance in *Staphylococcus* spp. They have the same mechanism of action as penicillins. They are grouped into 'generations'. The more recent generations (3rd and 4th) should be used cautiously to avoid development of antibiotic resistance. They would not be considered a first-line antibiotic choice except in extremely ill animals. There are many different formulations available; if using them be aware of the dose rate and frequency.

Indications
- Gram +ve *Staphylococcus* species
- Some Gram -ve species such as *Pasteurella* (lung infections)
- *Pseudomonas* spp. (often associated with green-coloured pus) are **resistant**
- Not as effective against anaerobes as penicillin

Aminoglycosides (Gentamicin)

Aminoglycosides act by penetrating bacterial cells and disrupting protein synthesis, ultimately resulting in bacterial death. Besides being an injectable drug (usually IV), gentamicin is also suitable for intra-articular injection and is found in many topical eye preparations.

Aminoglycosides are important for the treatment of gram negative infections. If using gentamicin be aware that it is not as broad spectrum as some other antibiotics and must be used responsibly – never start a course unless sure the animal will be re-visited for subsequent injections *for at least 3 days*. It is administered only *once daily* (SID).

Streptomycin, another aminoglycoside, is commonly mixed with penicillin as 'Pen-Strep'; this combination product is formulated for ruminants. However, the streptomycin concentration in this mixture is not effective in equids, therefore its use is not recommended in this species.

Indications
- Gram -ve bacteria, including *Pseudomonas*
- Endotoxaemia from species such as *E. coli* species
- *Staphylococcus* spp. infections
- *Salmonella* and *Brucella* spp. are **resistant**
- **Do not use in suspected anaerobic infections** – aminoglycosides require oxygen for action.

> All aminoglycosides are nephrotoxic; carefully consider their use in dehydrated animals or those with suspected kidney or urinary problems, and weigh up the potential harm to the animal versus the benefit of using aminoglycosides in these cases.

Potentiated sulphonamides (Trimethoprim-Sulphur)

These drugs act on folic acid metabolism, disrupting nucleic acid synthesis in the bacteria. Sulphonamides are beneficial for a number of conditions as they penetrate the blood-brain-barrier and achieve high concentrations in liver, kidney and lung tissues. The action of potentiated sulphonamides is reduced in the presence of pus.

Although easily absorbed from the equine digestive tract, sulphonamides can be associated with causing **diarrhoea** (see Section 11.5). Therefore, be sure to advise the owner when dispensing oral tablets. If using IV, ensure slow injection as hypotension and collapse can occur – never use IV with detomidine as fatal cardiac arrhythmia can occur (Stack and Schott 2011).

Indications
- Gram +ve *staphylococcus* and *streptococcus* infections
- Some anaerobic infections including *C. perfringens*, *Fusobacterium* and *Bacteroides*
- Some Gram -ve strains of *E. coli* and *Pasteurella* (lung and gastrointestinal tract infection)
- **Do not** use in serious *Clostridial* infections such as malignant oedema
- First choice for infections of the skin, central nervous system and mammary/testicular tissues (mastitis, encephalitis) due to its ability to cross barriers and penetrate other tissues

Tetracyclines (Oxytetracycline)

Tetracyclines are bacteriostatic (they stop bacterial replication rather than kill the bacteria) and act via interference with bacterial protein synthesis. They are effective in most tissues. Injectable forms are recommended in equine medicine, as the absorption of oral products can be unreliable

5 MEDICINES

and has been associated with **diarrhoea**. Rapid IV injection can result in hypotension and collapse so inject slowly.

Long-acting cattle formulations are not licensed in equids and are **contra-indicated** as they can cause severe local irritant reactions and muscle necrosis in this species.

Indications
- Broad spectrum: effective against many Gram +ve, Gram -ve and anaerobic bacteria
- Good for tissue penetration due to high lipid solubility
- Some ability to get into mammary tissue
- Less effective against *Staphylococcus*, *E. coli* or *Pseudomonas*
- Reports of success in treating flexural limb deformities in foals (Haggett and Wilson 2008)
- Never use the long-acting cattle formulation (20%) in equids and advise paraprofessionals of the same (only use 10% or 5% in equids).

Macrolides (Erythromycin/Tylosin)

> **Macrolides are associated with potentially fatal colitis in adult equids so their use is not recommended.**

Indications
- *Rhodococcus equi* ('rattles') treatment of foals in specialist paediatric treatment centres (see Section 18.1)

Metronidazole

> **Metronidazole is a unique drug which has *specific action* against anaerobic bacteria and protozoal infections.**

It has little effect on Gram +ve and Gram -ve aerobic bacteria. It has good absorption from the digestive tract so is most often seen as an oral preparation.

Metronidazole is effective at penetrating those hard to reach places, such as anaerobic infections in bone, abscesses and the CNS. Alternatively, penicillin or cephalosporin-resistant infections can be treated with metronidazole, such as penicillin-resistant *Clostridium* spp. and malignant oedema cases.

Indications
- Penicillin-resistant anaerobic bacteria *Clostridium* spp., *Fusobacterium*, *B. Fragilis*
- Do not use in tetanus cases as penicillin is the prefered antibiotic for the treatment of *C. tetani* (see Section 16.1)
- Protozoal *Giardia and Trichomonas* spp.
- Polymicrobial infections with suspected beta-lactam resistant anaerobes such as peritonitis and pleuro-pneumonia
- Use is **prohibited in food-producing animals** due to carcinogenic (cancer-causing) properties, so ensure, when dispensing this drug, that the owner understands it is *solely* for use in equids.

ANTIBIOTICS 5.3

Summary of commonly used antibiotics in working equine practice

Below are tables showing reported dose rates for **horses** (Table 5.3.1), **donkeys** (Table 5.3.2) and **mules** (Table 5.3.3).

(SID = every 24 hours, BID = every 12 hours, TID = every 8 hours, IV = intravenous, IM = intramuscular, PO = per os (orally), SC = subcutaneous)

Horses

Trade name	Dose	Route	Frequency
Procaine penicillin	22,000 IU/kg	IM only	BID for 5 days
Cephalosporins	2.2–4.4 mg/kg	IM	SID
	2.2 mg/kg	IV/SC/IM	BID
	5–10 mg/kg – foal septicaemia	IV/SC/IM	TID/BID
Gentamicin	6.6 mg/kg	IV	SID
Trimethoprim-sulpha	15–24 mg/kg	IV slowly	TID/BID
	24–30 mg/kg	PO	BID
Oxytetracycline	5–10 mg/kg	IV	BID
Erythromycin *(Foals only!)*	20–25 mg/kg	PO	every 6–8 hours
Metronidazole	15 mg/kg – Clostridial enteritis	PO	TID
	20 mg/kg – anaerobic infections	PO/per rectum	TID
	20 mg/kg	IV	TID

Table 5.3.1 Dose rates for use of antibiotics in horses (Haggett and Wilson 2008).

Donkeys

Trade name	Dose	Route	Frequency
Procaine penicillin	20,000 IU/kg	IM only	BID/SID for 5 days
Cephalosporins (cefquinome – 4th generation)	1 mg/kg	IV	BID
Gentamicin	2.2 mg/kg	IV	TID
Trimethoprim-sulpha	2.5–12.5 mg/kg	IV	TID/BID (or SID)
Oxytetracycline	10 mg/kg	IV	SID (or every 48 hours)

Table 5.3.2 Dose rates for use of antibiotics in donkeys (Miller et al. 1994, Welfare et al. 1996, Widmer et al. 2009, Grosenbaugh et al. 2011).

5 MEDICINES

Mules

Trade name	Dose	Route	Frequency
Procaine penicillin	20,000 IU/kg	IM	–
Kanamycin	7.45–8.73 mg/kg	IV	BID
Oxytetracycline	15 mg/kg	IV	–

Table 5.3.3 Dose rates for use of antibiotics in mules (Muhammed et al. 2003, Reichmann et al. 2008).

5.4 Non-steroidal anti-inflammatory drugs (NSAIDs)

Clinical features of NSAIDs

> NSAIDs work to relieve pain, inflammation and fever which result from tissue injury, inflammation and/or infection.

Why do we want to control inflammation?

Inflammation is the body's natural response to injury. However, if this inflammatory response is excessive or prolonged, it can result in pain, loss of function, depression and anorexia. See Section 15.1 for a further explanation of the inflammatory process.

> Management of inflammation is therefore an important means of helping the body heal as well as relieving pain.

Inflammation in working equids is often a result of chronic stress and injury to the body (Figure 5.4.1). It is for this reason that a **holistic approach** is necessary for the long-term relief of pain – anti-inflammatory drugs alone are not sufficient. Refer to Chapter 3 for an in-depth look at pain management principles which should be adopted along with the use of any pain relieving drugs.

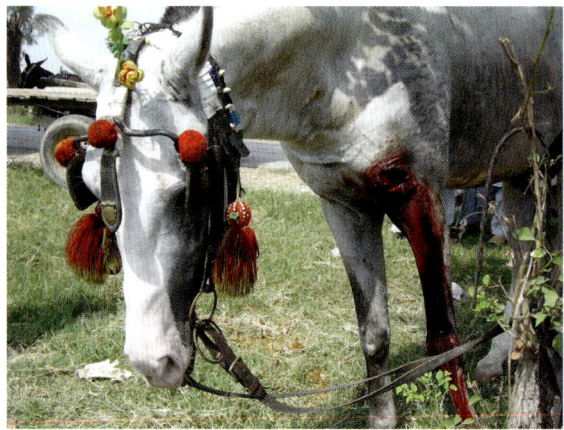

Figure 5.4.1 An example of a clinical condition where NSAIDs would form an important part of the treatment approach.

NON-STEROIDAL ANTI-INFLAMMATORY DRUGS (NSAIDS) 5.4

How do NSAIDs control pain and inflammation?

The inflammatory process is well described in pharmacology and physiology texts. The explanation below is a simplified overview. In order to understand how NSAIDs work, it is necessary first to remember the five clinical signs of acute inflammation:

1. **Heat** Increased blood flow
2. **Redness** Blood accumulation
3. **Swelling** Accumulation of exudate
4. **Pain** Sensitisation of nerve endings
5. **Loss of function** Pain, vascular disturbances

Blood supply is a key component of the inflammatory process.

> **When injury occurs, the body responds by *increasing blood supply* to the area, as blood carries substances which help fight infection and heal tissues.**

Chemical mediators responsible for the inflammatory process belong to the *eicosanoid* family, of which **Prostaglandin** (**PG**) is a member. Prostaglandins have many roles in the body (see adverse effects of NSAIDs below); however, during the inflammatory process, they work to cause vasodilation and nerve sensitisation. This makes it an important player in the five signs of acute inflammation.

Prostaglandin = vasodilation and nerve sensitisation

NSAIDs therefore work to decrease the production of prostaglandin and other inflammatory mediators, thus decreasing the signs of inflammation and pain. Prostaglandins are produced as a result of the COX-1 pathway.

> **NSAIDs work to block the synthesis of cyclo-oxygenase, thus resulting in decreased prostaglandin production.**

Are there any side effects of the use of NSAIDs in equids?

As mentioned previously, prostaglandins have many roles in the body so the side effects seen clinically often relate to decreased production or inhibition of natural prostaglandins.

- **Gastrointestinal** Prostaglandins protect the intestinal mucosa; therefore diarrhoea and gastrointestinal ulceration are two of the most common side effects seen in equids if NSAIDs are used in high dosages or for long periods of time. Be cautious when prescribing NSAIDs to an animal showing signs of gastrointestinal disease such as diarrhoea or melena (digested blood in faeces). This ulcerogenic effect is even greater in foals so ensure the correct dose is given for as short a time as possible in young foals. Treating foals less than 1 week old concurrently with omeprazole whilst on the NSAIDs will reduce the risk of forming ulcers.

- **Renal** Dehydrated animals have been shown to develop acute renal failure with therapeutic doses of NSAIDs. Always try to correct dehydration before administering NSAIDs; for example, before giving flunixin meglumine in a colic case.

5 MEDICINES

- **Plasma protein binding** NSAIDs bind to proteins in order to move around the body; however, so do drugs such as gentamicin and sulphonamides. If treating a case with one of these antibiotics together with NSAIDs, be aware that the gentamicin may not be as effective, or may require a slightly longer course.

- **Masking effects of anti-inflammatory drug use** Pain can work as a protective mechanism to stop the animal further injuring itself. The best example is in lameness where an equid may take weight off the injured limb. Another example is the masking of cardiovascular effects seen with flunixin meglumine administration in colic cases. Removal of the pain response with drugs may cause further damage if the animal subsequently works to full capacity or the owner works it harder thinking it is cured.

> NSAIDs must never be used in isolation – aim for full owner compliance in management of painful conditions.

Common NSAIDs used in working equids

Phenylbutazone (PBZ)

PBZ is available as IV or PO formulations, with the oral powder/tablet form often used at a low dose for chronic inflammatory conditions of working equids, particularly lameness. Despite being effective and relatively cheap, PBZ has a very narrow safety margin so ensure never to exceed the recommended dose rates below:

Horse Days 1–2: 4.4 mg/kg BID then as for chronic inflammation. For chronic inflammatory cases: 2.2 mg/kg BID, then SID after the first 5 days – this is a very effective dose rate for safe use over longer periods; however, remain aware of side effects with long-term use.

Donkey Donkeys metabolise PBZ 5–15 times faster than horses (Cheng *et al.* 1996a, Lizarrago *et al.* 2004), so a dose rate of 4.4 mg IV followed by twice-daily dosing of oral PBZ at 4.4 mg/kg is acceptable. Aim to achieve the lowest dose rate possible; 2.2 mg/kg orally BID may be adequate.

Flunixin meglumine

This NSAID is commonly used for visceral pain with its action thought to be comparable to many opioid analgesics without the negative side effects. Flunixin meglumine is anti-endotoxic at lower dose rates (refer to pharmacological texts for more information). Flunixin meglumine is normally given IV for instantaneous action in extreme cases, at the following dose rates:

Horses 1.1 mg/kg SID–BID (anti-inflammatory) or 0.25 mg/kg every 6–12 hours (anti-endotoxic)

Donkeys Again, donkeys metabolise flunixin meglumine at a faster rate than horses and will require a higher dosing frequency, but the same dose rate (Cheng *et al.* 1996b, Coakley *et al.* 1999)

Mules The same dose rate and frequency as for horses (Coakley *et al.* 1999)

Dipyrone

This is used primarily for its anti-spasmodic and analgesic properties in treating colic in equids. It has a fast onset of action and short clinical effect. Its anti-pyretic, anti-thrombotic and anti-inflammatory properties are poor.

NON-STEROIDAL ANTI-INFLAMMATORY DRUGS (NSAIDS) 5.4

Check the formulation before use, as dipyrone is often combined with other agents (e.g. dipyrone and hyoscine N-butylbromide); always check the dose and route of administration before use. Do not exceed the recommended dose.

Do not give IM, as this will result in localised tissue reactions. Do not use with phenothiazine ataractics (e.g. chlorpromazine) as this may cause hypothermia. Dipyrone may cause blood dyscrasia, hepatitis, nephropathy, colic and diarrhoea. There is an ulcerogenic action on the GI tract as a result of prostaglandin inhibition. Potential renotoxicity and hepatotoxicity is weak. Do not use if there is known hypersensitivity. See Table 5.4.1 for reported dose rates (Lees and Higgins 1985).

Acetylsalicylic acid (aspirin)

Although a good anti-inflammatory, the dose rates required for this effect in horses (10–100 mg/kg) are too large to be of any real practical use.

Aspirin is used at 10 mg/kg and is also a useful antithrombotic.

Diclofenamic acid (diclofenac)

Historically used as an anti-inflammatory in production animal medicine, this drug is now widely banned due to its adverse environmental effects in the food chain (Oaks *et al.* 2004).

The use of diclofenac is increasing in Africa, but should be discouraged.

Others

Meclofenamic acid, Ketoprofen, Carprofen may be available in some countries. Check manufacturer's recommendations for use of these drugs.

> The use of ibuprofen cannot be recommended as there is insufficient data for its use in equids.

Donkeys and Carprophen Donkeys require a reduced dosing rate to horses as they metabolise this NSAID more slowly than horses (Coakley *et al.* 1999).

Donkeys and Ketoprofen A higher dosing frequency is required; however, the same dose of 2.2 mg/kg as horses (Oukessou *et al.* 1996).

5 MEDICINES

NSAID	Presentation	Route	Dose	Frequency
PBZ	Injectable, or tablets	IV, PO	IV: 4.4 mg/kg q24h PO: Day 1: 4.4 mg/kg q12h Days 2–5: 2.2 mg/kg q12h, Thereafter: 2.2 mg/kg q24h	Donkeys require more frequent dosing than horses; however, more studies are needed for recommended dosing to prevent toxicity Present advice is to give the horse dose and monitor carefully for the need to re-administer sooner
Flunixin meglumine	Injectable, or granules	IV, IM, PO	**Anti-inflammatory** 1.1 mg/kg. (Toutain et al. 1994)	SID–BID
			Anti-endotoxic 0.25–0.55 mg/kg.	QID–TID
			Foal 0.5 mg/kg BID/SID – avoid if gastric ulceration is suspected (Holcombe 2003)	BID/SID Use lowest dose possible
			Donkey 1.1 mg/kg (Cheng et al. 1996b)	**Donkey** Dose frequency may be increased from that of horses due to faster body clearance (Coakley et al. 1999)
			Mule Same dose as horses (Coakley et al. 1999)	**Mule** The same dose frequency as horses (Coakley et al. 1999)
Dipyrone	Injectable, or tablets	IV, PO	22 mg/kg	Depends on formulation – check before use
Acetylsalicylic acid	Tablets	PO	100 mg/kg (Lees and Higgins 1985, Cambridge et al. 1991) **Antithrombotic** 10 mg/kg	SID
Ketoprofen	Injectable	IV	2.2 mg/kg of 10% solution	q24h for up to 5 days for musculoskeletal pain Single dose for abdominal pain

(IV = intravascular, IM = intramuscular, PO = orally, q = every, SID = once per day, BID = twice per day, TID = three times per day, QID = four times per day)

Table 5.4.1 *Reported dose rates, routes of administration and frequency of NSAIDs commonly used in working equids.*

Steroidal anti-inflammatory drugs (corticosteroids) 5.5

Corticosteroids can be used to treat a wide range of pathology in equine medicine:

- **Topically** Eye and skin inflammation
- **Intra-articular** Chronic joint pain/inflammation
- **Systemically** Either orally or injected, for chronic inflammatory disease such as recurrent airway obstruction (RAO), allergic dermatitis and many immune-mediated diseases

There are many corticosteroid formulations available for veterinary use, all with varying durations of action and concentration. Examples include prednisolone (short acting) and dexamethasone (long acting > 48h), see Table 5.5.1. Other corticosteroids used in equids are methylprednisolone for treating shock (Muir 1987) and intra-articular inflammation, although there is research showing its deleterious effects on the joint (McIlwraith 2010), and triamcinolone acetonide, commonly used for intra-articular inflammation, has been shown to be chondroprotective (Soma *et al.* 2011, McIlwraith 2010). See Section 14.7 for further information on treatment of joint disease.

The safe, effective use of corticosteroids in equids requires a good understanding of their mode of action and potential side effects. Equids are very sensitive to suppressive effects on the endocrine system from long-term systemic use, so it is advisable to use short-acting, less potent topical or local applications wherever possible.

Conditions where it is advisable not to use steroids

1. Laminitis
2. Corneal ulceration
3. Wound treatment

In working equids, corticosteroids should be considered in any immune mediated or hypersensitivity reaction (anaphylaxis, sweet itch, recurrent uveitis) or chronic respiratory illness (recurrent airway obstruction – RAO). Assess the local availability of different types of corticosteroid preparations and their recommendations. Always use them judiciously, remembering the adverse effects, especially from systemic use.

Serious potential side effects of corticosteroid use

- **Laminitis** Cause is unclear
- **Iatrogenic Cushing's syndrome** Due to adrenal insufficiency occurring with long-term use
- **Immunosuppression** Lowers the body's ability to fight off infections and may lead to secondary bacterial infection
- **Slows wound healing** Due to reduced collagen synthesis
- **Withdrawal response** It is advised that a decreasing dose is administered when

withdrawing treatment. When being treated with corticosteroid the body's endogenous corticosteroid production is lowered. Although in reality this is rare, always aim to taper treatment before stopping.

- **Gastric ulceration** A very rare complication

- During pregnancy Potential to induce **parturition or abortion in third trimester**, although single doses have been administered safely. **Potentially teratogenic in first trimester.** However, corticosteroid may be administered to mares at risk of pre-term delivery to aid maturation of the foal (Ousey *et al*. 2011). It is important when treating pregnant mares to consider the health of the mare versus that of the foetus.

- Joint injection can lead to **damage of cartilage and changes in synovial fluid, post injection flare (non-septic inflammation), septic arthritis, arthropathy (joint enlargement and increased rate of damage)** especially with high doses and high frequency of administration (see Sections 4.1 and 14.7).

STEROIDAL ANTI-INFLAMMATORY DRUGS (CORTICOSTEROIDS) 5.5

Drug	Duration of action (hrs)	Presentation	Route	Dose rate (mg/kg)	Frequency
Prednisolone	12–24	Tablet, or injectable	PO, IV	1 mg/kg	SID/BID Taper dose according to effect Use minimal effective dose to reduce side effects
Dexamethasone	> 48	Check formulation before injection to confirm dosing interval and route compatibility	IV, IM	0.1–0.5 mg/kg (lower end of range for anti-inflammatory, higher end of range for shock and hypersensitivity)	Dose frequency depends on preparation – so check this (Cornelisse and Robinson 2011, Ousey et al. 2011)
Methylprednisolone	12–24	Injectable	IV	Shock: 15–30 mg/kg	Administered as soon as possible after the onset of shock (Muir 1987)
Triamcinolone acetonide	Intra-articular (IA), IM: days to weeks IV: 36 hours	Injectable	IA, IM, IV	IA: 6–18 mg per joint; maximum 40 mg total dose per horse (McIlwraith 2010) IM, IV: 0.04–0.2 mg/kg	IA: Detected in synovial fluid for up to 10 days. Larger joints may require larger doses. IM: clinically effective for weeks (Soma et al. 2011)

(PO = orally, IV = intravenous, IM = intramuscular, IA = intra-articular, SID = once per day, BID = twice per day)

Table 5.5.1

5.6 References

Cambridge, H., Lees, P., Hooke, R.E., Russell, C.S. (1991) Antithrombotic actions of aspirin in the horse. *Equine Vet. J.* 23 (2), 123–127.

Carroll, C.L., Huntington, P.J. (1998) Body Condition scoring and weight estimation in horses. *Equine Vet. J.* 20 (1), 41–45.

Cheng, Z., McKellar, Q.A., Nolan, A., Lees, P. (1996a) Pharmacokinetics and pharmacodynamics of phenylbutazone and oxyphenbutazone in the donkey. *J. vet. Pharmacol. Therap.* 19, 149–151.

Cheng, Z., McKellar, Q.A., Nolan, A., Lees, P. (1996b) Preliminary pharmacokinetic and pharmacodynamic studies on flunixin meglumine in donkeys. *Vet. Res. Comms.* 20, 469–472.

Coakley, M., Peck, K.K., Taylor, T.S., Mathews, N.S., Mealey, K.L. (1999) Pharmacokinetics of flunixin in meglumine donkeys, mules, and horses. *Am. J. Vet. Res.* 60 (11), 1441–1444.

Cornelisse, C.J., Robinson, N.E. (2011) Glucocorticoid therapy and equine laminitis: fact or fiction? *Equine vet. Educ.* 16 (2), 90–93.

Daghio, M.M., Fattori, G., Ciardullo, A.V. (2010) Use of pictorial advice to promote compliance to diet and drugs among illiterate and migrant patients. Journal of Diabetology, 3, 3.

Grosenbaugh, D.A., Reinemeyer, C.R., Figueiredo, M.D. (2011) Pharmacology and therapeutics in donkeys. *Equine vet. Educ.* 23 (10), 523–530.

Hanson, E.C. (1995) Evaluating cognitive services for non-literate and visually impaired patients in community pharmacy rotation sites. *Am. J. Pharm. Ed.* 59, 48–55.

Holcombe, S.J. (2003) Current therapy in equine medicine. Elsevier.

Hollins, A.R., Wilkins, P.A. (2009) Current controversies in current antimicrobial therapies. *Equine vet Educ.* 21 (4) 216–224.

Lees.P, Higgins.A. (1985) Clinical pharmacology and therapeutic uses of non-steroidal anti-inflammatory drugs in the horse. *Equine Vet. J.* 17 (2), 83–96.

Lizarrago, I., Sumano, H., Brumbaugh, G.W. (2004) Pharmacological and pharmacokinetic differences between donkeys and horses. *Equine vet. Educ.* 16 (2), 102–112.

McIlwraith, C. (2010) The use of intra-articular corticosteroid in the horse: what is known on a scientific basis? *Equine Vet. J.* 42 (6), 563–571.

Miller, S.M., Mathews, N.S., Mealey, K.L., Taylor, T.S., Brumbaugh, G.W. (1994) Pharmacokinetics in Mammoth asses. *J. vet. Pharmacol. Therap.* 17, 403–406.

Muhammed, F., Hussain, F., Nawaz, M., Javed, I. (2003) Disposition kinetics in mules. *Vet. Arhiv.* 73 (4), 221–226.

Muir, W.W. (1987) Equine shock: the need for prospective studies. *Equine Vet. J.* 19 (1), 1–7.

Oaks, J.L., Gilbert, M., Virani, M.Z., Watson, R.T., Meteyer, C.U., Rideout, B.A., Shivaprasad, H.L., Ahmed, S., Chaudhry, M.J.I., Arshad, M., Mahmood, S., Ali, A., Khan, A.A. (2004) Diclofenac residues as the cause of vulture population decline in Pakistan. *Nature.* 427, 630–633.

Oukessou, M., Bouljihad, M., Van Gool, F., and Alvinerie, M. (1996) Pharamacokinetics of ketoprofen in the donkey (Equus Asinus). *J. Vet. Med. A.* 43, 423–426.

Ousey, J, Kolling, M., Kindhal, H., Allen, W. (2011) Maternal dexamethasone treatment in late gestation induces precocious fetal and delivery in healthy thoroughbred mares. *Equine Vet. J.* 43 (4), 424–429.

Reichmann, P., Lisboa, J.A.N., Araujo, R.G. (2008) Tetanus in equids: a review of 76 cases. *J. Equine vet. Sci.* 28 (9), 518–523.

Soma, L.R., Uboh, C.E., You, Y., Guan, F., Boston, R.C. (2011) Pharmacokinetics of intra-articular, intravenous and intramuscular administration of triamcinolone acetonide and its effects on endogenous plasma hydrocortisone and cortisone concentrations in horses. *Am. J. Vet. Res.* 72, 1234–1242.

Stack, A., Schott II, H.C. (2011) Suspect novel adverse drug reactions to trimpethoprim-sulphonamide combinations in horses: A case series. *Equine Vet. J.* 43 (1), 117–120.

Svendsen, E.D. (2008) The Professional Handbook of the Donkey, 4th Ed. Whittet Books, London, UK.

Toutain, P.L., Autefage, A., Legrand, C., Alvinerie, M. (1994) Plasma concentrations and therapeutic efficacy of phenylbutazone and flunixin meglumine in the horse: pharmokinetic/pharmacodynamic modelling. *J. vet. Pharmacol. Therap.* 17, 459–469.

Welfare, R.E., Mealey, K.L., Matthews, N.S., Taylor, T.S. (1996) Pharmacokinetics of gentamicin in donkeys. *J. vet. Pharmacol. Therap.* 19, 167–169.

Widmer, A., Kummer, M., Wehrli Eser, M., Furst, A. (2009) Comparison of the clinical efficacy of cefquinome with the combination of penicillin G and gentamicin in equine patients. *Equine vet. Educ.* 21 (8), 430–435.

Further Reading

Bertone J.J., Horspool, L.J.I. (2004) Equine Clinical Pharmacology, 1st Ed. Elsevier, Oxford, UK.

Grosenbaugh, D.A., Reinemeyer, C.R., and Figueiredo, M.D. (2011) Pharmacology and therapeutics in donkeys. *Equine vet. Educ.* 23 (10), 523–530.

Haggett, E.F., Wilson, W.D. (2008) Overview of the use of antimicrobials for the treatment of bacterial infections in horses. *Equine vet. Educ.* 20 (8), 433–448.

Knottenbelt, D.C. (2006) Equine Formulary. Saunders, Elsevier Ltd. p. 184.

Dehydration and fluid therapy

6

Anuresis, heat stress and dehydration	6.1
Fluid therapy	6.2
References	6.3

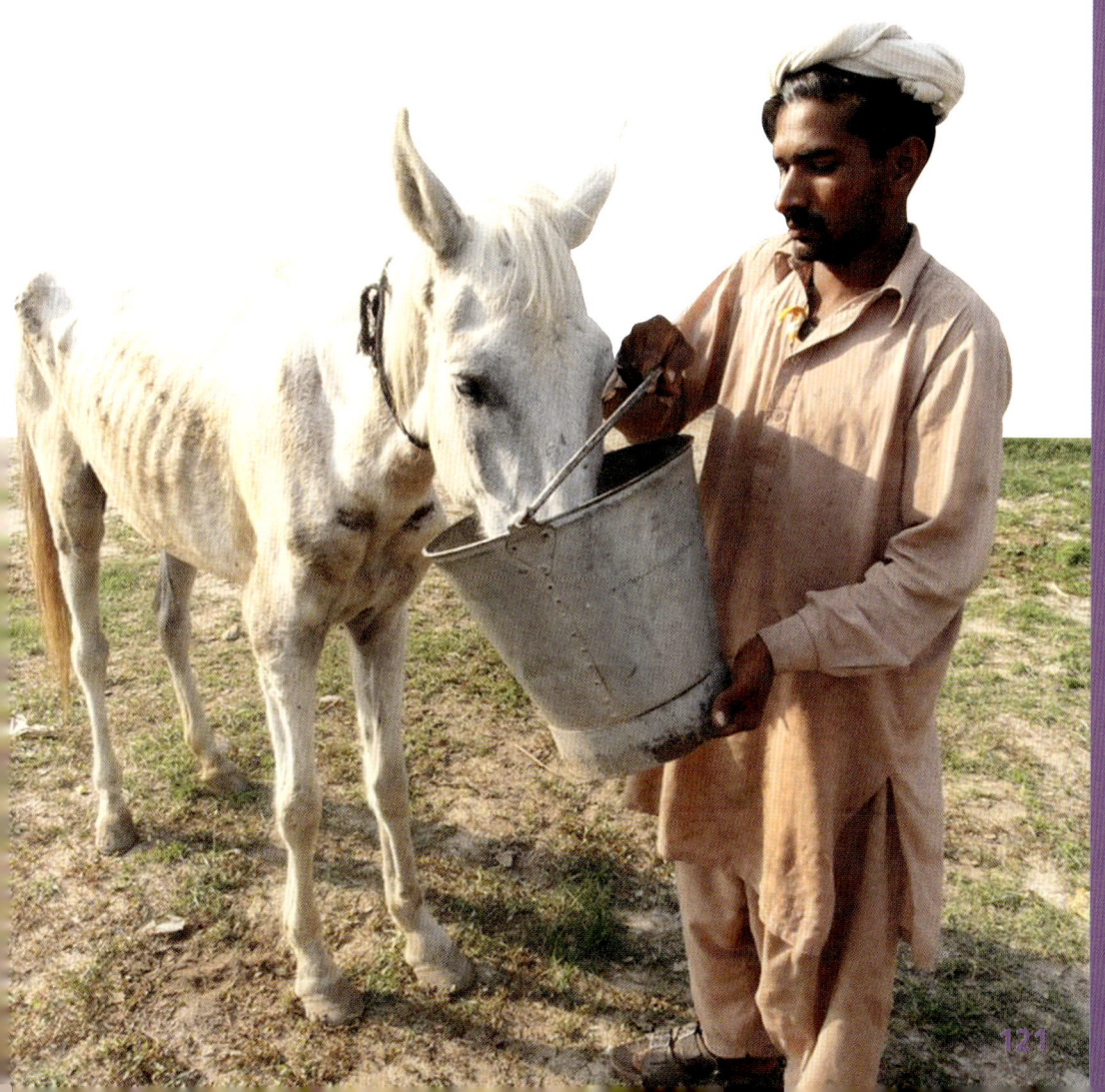

6.1 Anuresis, heat stress and dehydration

Anuria or 'lack of urine production'

> **Anuria** = absence of urination
>
> **Oliguria** = reduction in urination

Both of these describe symptoms and are not a diagnosis.

The pathophysiological mechanisms causing anuria/oliguria can be put into three different categories:

1. **PRE-RENAL** In response to hypoperfusion (decreased renal blood flow) of the kidney

   This can result from the following:

   a. Dehydration – which can be caused by an imbalance of fluid inputs versus outputs:
      i. A lack of water input: drinking water
      ii. Increased fluids outputs/loss: diarrhoea, sweating, respiration

   b. Cardiogenic shock, or sepsis (endotoxaemic shock) which affects blood distribution around the vascular system

2. **RENAL** In response to direct kidney damage (intrinsic renal failure), e.g. via damage caused by nephrotoxic drugs (NSAIDs/aminogylcosides)

3. **POST-RENAL** Caused by an obstruction to urinary output (e.g. urinary bladder rupture in foals, obstructing urinary calculi)

Anuria or 'failure to urinate' is a commonly encountered presentaion. Although it is important to consider obstruction any time an animal does not pass urine, often this is not the case; a primary blockage is rare in equids.

> In the majority of cases a good history will be able to identify the causes of anuria and allow the correct treatment.

This is really important because the wrong treatment may result in serious and permanent damage.

If an animal presents with anuria, the first thing to ascertain is whether it is pre-renal, renal or post-renal.

Pre-renal is the easiest to diagnose and is the most common cause of anuria. Post-renal is the next most common cause. Renal is the last and most unlikely cause.

- **Pre-renal causes** This can be very easy to assess – through offering water. Refer to the dehydration section below and 7.2 (Pritchard et al. 2008). Additionally a thorough clinical examination and history will help decide the underlying cause. Colic and other systemic factors are a common cause of anuria/dehydration as the animal is reluctant to drink. Observe the circulatory system for signs of shock, common in endotoxaemia, which may be the underlying cause.

ANURESIS, HEAT STRESS AND DEHYDRATION 6.1

- **Renal causes** Although not discussed at length in this manual, renal causes for anuria include acute renal failure or infection. Refer to diseases of the urinary tract in Section 13.2, and other equine texts.

- **Post-renal causes** Ascertain whether the animal has an obstruction or infection. This is relatively uncommon and will be diagnosed by history (straining to urinate or straining when urinating, passing small volumes of urine, blood in urine) and urinary catheterisation (unable to pass a urinary catheter past the blocked urethra). It is important to get a good understanding of the amount of water given/drunk, diet (increased mineral content of local water) and other possible causes, e.g. foaling. Refer to diseases of the urinary tract in Section 13.2 for more information.

Diuretics – Inappropriate use is a common contribution to poor welfare in many countries.

> The use Frusemide (Lasix) and other diuretics is strictly contra-indicated as a treatment for anuria.

This is very serious; owners may think that giving a Lasix injection will 'solve' the problem, and that making an animal urinate has fixed the problem. However, by understanding how the kidney works it is clear that *lack of urination is the **clinical sign**, not the problem itself*. A diuretic produces urine (thus fixing the 'sign') but **does not solve the underlying cause**.

> **N.B.** Administration of a diuretic is potentially lethal if there is an obstruction of any sort. If the animal is suffering from dehydration it can cause the animal to go into acute renal failure.

How diuretics work

Generally, all diuretics work to increase excretion of sodium and water leading to an increased urine output. There are many types with differing mechanisms of action; however, the most common in equine practice are the loop diuretics, e.g. frusemide. These have been comprehensively studied in equids due to widespread use in racehorses, and are the most likely diuretic available to veterinarians.

Diuretics have a dose-dependent increase in urine output, therefore the bigger the dose, the greater the urination.

Frusemide works by affecting the ion transport systems of the kidney's Loop of Henle, resulting in increased expulsion of sodium, potassium and chloride ions which causes the signs of urination.

> Although not indicated for anuria, diuretics can be very useful to decrease oedema associated with pulmonary or cardiac disorders, or consequences of trauma.

The historical practice of administering loop diuretics to bring about urination is no longer recommended; these drugs will worsen dehydration status.

Long-term diuretic use will have other effects. See clinical pharmacology texts for more information on the indications and correct usage of diuretic drugs in equine medicine. In general,

6 DEHYDRATION AND FLUID THERAPY

work to encourage owners and paraprofessionals to understand what causes urinary flow, i.e. the balance between the input (drinking) and outputs (urination, sweating, faecal loss, etc.), and help to decrease the inappropriate usage of diuretics to 'treat' anuria.

Heat stress in equids

Heat stress occurs when the body absorbs or produces more heat that it can lose. It will ultimately result in hyperthermia when the body temperature actually increases and this is a medical emergency that warrants immediate veterinary treatment. Simple cooling interventions can avoid hyperthermia altogether, and ensure that the welfare of working equids is not compromised. Although it is important to have reliable veterinary services available to treat sick equids with hyperthermia, it is even more important to educate owners how to stop their animals suffering from this entirely preventable condition.

> **Every equid treated should be offered water. Hot animals should be cooled while waiting to be examined. Aim to conduct examinations in the shade and provide shade to avoid further discomfort while animals are waiting.**

Heat stress is a common condition in working equids, especially in the hot, humid months. It is serious and may be fatal, but should be recognised as an abnormal physiological state, not a 'disease'. Treatment should be as simple as possible, focusing on measures which an owner can take at any time to prevent or reduce the severity of the condition.

> **The aim of management of heat stress is to show owners that it is both preventable and treatable without veterinary intervention. Education is critical to ensure that, in the future, owners are aware about how heat stress can be avoided. Also explain how to recognise the early stages of heat stress so treatment can be simple and intervention can be implemented before the animal develops more severe clinical signs.**

Clinical signs (may be unrelated to the presenting problem)
- Increased respiratory rate and effort
- Flaring nostrils
- Tripping when moving
- Lowered head, increased head movement
- Dullness, lack of response to environment (e.g. other animals nearby)
- Increased pulse and congested mucous membranes
- Raised rectal temperature

N.B. The behavioural signs indicating heat stress in this list are a valid diagnostic alternative to taking the rectal temperature. Therefore, although a clinician may need to take a temperature as part of a clinical examination, an owner does not need to do this to identify heat stress. Furthermore, the treatment for heat stress should not be delayed just to get the rectal temperature and an animal should not be overly stressed trying to obtain this reading as it is not essential for diagnosis.

In both horses and donkeys heat stress behaviour (as described above) is associated with an increased rectal temperature (Pritchard *et al.* 2006).

ANURESIS, HEAT STRESS AND DEHYDRATION 6.1

> If owners can recognise behavioural heat stress symptoms (Figure 6.1.1), they can use them to make judgements regarding rest and cooling.

Owner recognition of heat stress has a number of advantages:

- It will reduce the time it takes to improve the animal's condition – reducing the animal's suffering and avoiding progression. (If untreated, heat stress can progress to endotoxaemia, disseminated intravascular coagulation, renal failure, central nervous system disturbance, organ dysfunction and death.)
- It will prevent further heat load and fatigue while travelling to and waiting for veterinary attention.
- It will reduce the cost in both time and money for the owner and reduce dependency on external sources to improve animal welfare and management.

> All veterinary and animal health field staff, including community development workers, drivers and farriers, should be able to recognise the signs of heat stress and instruct owners on the necessary intervention if this is seen at any time.

Treatment of heat stress

Encourage owners and paraprofessionals to be able to recognise these signs and give the following first aid measures to the animal immediately:

- Pour two or three buckets of cool water over the animal's back, neck and belly. Rub the water into the hair so the skin is thoroughly wetted.
- Offer a bucket of water to drink. Leave it with the animal for 10 minutes, as it may be initially too overheated to drink. Allow the animal to drink in a quiet area if possible, as stress can deter drinking.
- Stand the animal in the shade.

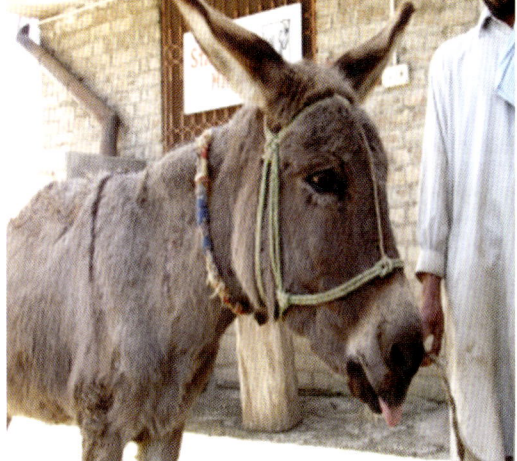

Figure 6.1.1 Clinical presentation of heat stress in a donkey.

Giving intravenous fluids/injections is not recommended for the majority of heat stress cases. They are not only unnecessary – as most animals can rehydrate themselves naturally through drinking – but involve needless veterinary intervention. Most importantly, aggressive veterinary treatment for heat stress may lead the owner to think that it can only be treated by a veterinarian, thus making them more likely to bring heat-stressed animals long distances to mobile or field veterinary clinics, instead of resting, watering and cooling the animal themselves.

> Prevention through extension and capacity building of paraprofessionals is better than cure.

6 DEHYDRATION AND FLUID THERAPY

If fluid therapy is required, for example the animal is unable or unwilling to drink, refer to the fluid therapy in Section 6.2 of this chapter. For more information refer to the paper by Pritchard *et al.* (2006) on behavioural measures of heat stress for dehydration in working equids.

Caution – Do not inject adrenaline. Adrenaline injected into a heat-stressed animal risks killing it by increasing the heart rate and metabolic oxygen demand in an already compromised circulation.

- Historically, intradermal (not IV) adrenaline has been used for the treatment of suspected cases of anhidrosis (the inability to sweat in response to normal stimuli). True anhidrosis (non-sweating) is an extremely rare condition and almost all animals that are not seen sweating are simply **too dehydrated** to produce sweat and do not have pathophysiology of the sweat gland requiring adrenaline as treatment. It is therefore recommended **never to inject adrenaline** in such cases.

6.2 Fluid therapy

Dehydration

Approach to an animal which is not drinking or urinating

Dehydration is a serious welfare concern in working equids and is known to be a contributing factor to exhaustion, heat stroke, reduced work capacity and work-related skin injuries.

Recognising dehydration

- The volume of water consumed and the number/duration of drinking bouts have been shown to be the most reliable guide to the hydration status in mature working horses (Pritchard *et al.* 2008).

  - **In the first instance give water.** Never assume a working equid is not dehydrated. Many owners say their animal is not drinking – but this is often because of stress or lack of time taken, an unsuitable or new environment, unfamiliar water container/trough, dirty water or bullying from other animals. All of these can be factors that prevent an animal from drinking.

    > Offering water is a recognised diagnostic test.

  - **Whether or not an animal drinks when offered water is a reliable test of dehydration in the majority of cases,** provided that there are no internal factors compromising their ability to drink, or external factors preventing them from drinking (e.g. fear of the environment, owner behaviour or water availability/quality).

FLUID THERAPY 6.2

Clinical signs of dehydration can be difficult to interpret as they can be affected by many other factors and do not become apparent in horses until they are at least 3–5% dehydrated.

Signs to look out for include:

- reduced or absent urination
- cool extremities – cool nose, ears (may not be see in heat stress)
- increased capillary refill time: CRT > 2 seconds
- heart rate increases as dehydration becomes more severe.

Caution

- Historically, skin tent time and mucous membrane dryness have been used as indicators of dehydration. However, these have been shown to be unreliable in working equids and therefore should not be used.
- Similarly, because of the confounding effects of sub-clinical disease, excessive sweat losses and poor nutrition on standard laboratory variables, the packed cell volume (PCV) and total protein (TP) are also unreliable measures of dehydration in working equids. (Pritchard *et al.* 2008).

> 'Offering palatable water to drink *ad libitum* (freely) provides both a simple diagnosis and a remedy for dehydration that can be implemented by any person in the field.' (Pritchard *et al.* 2008).

Refer to the full article by Pritchard *et al.* (2008) and ensure that daily clinical practices and future training reflect the conclusions of this work.

Treating dehydration

> **Offer fresh clean water and give the animal time and space to drink in a quiet environment, as stress can deter from drinking.**

- As part of a clinical examination, offer a bucket of clean water to drink (Figure 6.2.1). Allow the animal to drink in a quiet area if possible and leave water with the animal for 10 minutes to allow sufficient time for adequate water intake.
- Once the animal has drunk, monitor for urination. The best indication of adequate fluid therapy is an improved clinical status and, most notably, urine output. This is particularly important if the owner is concerned about anuria. It provides a good example to demonstrate to paraprofessionals/owners that an injection is not required to get the animal to urinate.

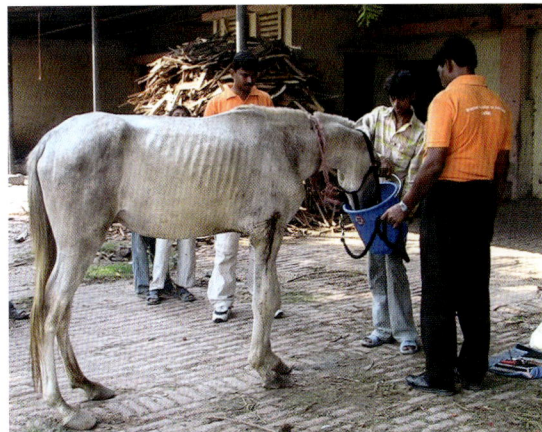

Figure 6.2.1 Offer fresh clean drinking water at each interaction with a working equid.

- **Clinical examination after urination has occurred** As previously stated, the evidence of urination has not necessarily solved the underlying cause of dehydration so it is important to ensure that the animal is showing no other signs of disease. However, if the anuria was caused by dehydration, the animal will be much improved following hydration and no further treatment is required. Then advise the owner about management to correct and maintain fluid input to prevent fluid deficits and dehydration in the future.

If the animal is unable or unwilling to drink, e.g. stressed by environment, very busy area, or recumbent, think about the following:

- Ensure there is no physical reason why the animal will not drink (e.g. choke, oral foreign body).
- If it is a behavioural response, and the animal has been left quietly and is still not drinking, then consider fluid therapy.

Fluid therapy

Estimate the volume of fluid that the animal requires to treat the fluid deficit.

Table 6.2.1 shows an estimation of the percentage dehydration of an equid related to clinical signs; these can be used to assess fluid balance.

(CRT = capillary refill time, PCV = packed cell volume)

Clinical signs	Percentage dehydration
- Strong desire to drink	0–4% – Subclinical
- Strong desire to drink - Cool nose, ears and extremities (useful to feel around fetlock regions) - Poor distensibility of the jugular vein - CRT 1–2 seconds	4–6% – Mild
- Strong desire to drink (may be subdued if very weak) - Thready, weak pulse - CRT 3–4 seconds	7–9% – Moderate
- Strong desire to drink (may be subdued if very weak) - Weak or no detectable pulse - CRT > 4 seconds - PCV may be increased (but if anaemic this will not be evident)	9–12% – Severe (over 15%; animal dies)

Table 6.2.1 Clinical signs related to percentage dehydration in equids.

FLUID THERAPY 6.2

The following calculation can be used to give the volume in litres of fluid needed to correct the hydration status of equids.

> Fluid deficit (litres) = % dehydration x bodyweight (kg)

Therefore, if a 300 kg horse is 8% dehydrated it will require 24 litres (L) of fluid to correct, i.e. 300 kg x 0.08 (8%) dehydration (Collatos 1999).

There is no point in giving a moderately dehydrated horse, donkey or mule 1–2 L of fluid. This is inadequate for rehydration and the animal will remain dehydrated after such treatment.

> Giving inadequate small volumes to dehydrated equids will not only compromise their welfare, by leaving them in a state of dehydration, but it is a waste of resources.

Route of administration

Enteral fluid therapy

> Oral fluid therapy is the most physiological and least invasive way to restore hydration.

The gastrointestinal mucosa acts as a natural selective barrier for absorption.

- **Plain water for drinking should always be offered first.** If this fails, fluids can be administered via a nasogastric tube. (Forced oral administration of large volumes is not recommended due to the risk of aspiration.)
- The stomach capacity of a 500-kg horse is approximately 18 L – remember working equids may be significantly lighter/smaller than this.
- Horses can tolerate oral fluids at a rate of 40 ml/kg bwt/hour. **Caution:** This is fine for continuous delivery, but take extreme care with bolus delivery of such an amount.
  - e.g. a 300-kg horse can receive a maximum of 12 L (40 ml x 300 kg) of fluids via nasogastric tube per hour if given continuously or in small boluses. Do not give such a large volume in one go. It can be split up into smaller doses at set intervals, e.g. 4 L every 20 minutes.

> Always ensure that there is no gastric reflux before enteral therapy is given.

- If gastric reflux is not checked for, the stomach can become distended and may rupture. Do not perform nasogastric intubation if in lateral recumbency as there is a risk of inhalation. If an animal can support itself in sternal recumbency then it is acceptable for fluid administration by stomach tube.

Fluid composition

- Equids with normal kidney function and adequate diet can tolerate even large volumes of oral fluids that are not of ideal composition. The diet provides a source of electrolytes and the kidney prevents severe imbalances developing.
  - Water is hypotonic. However, there is a risk of hyponatraemia (low sodium) and possible hypokalaemia (low potassium) if large volumes are given enterally.

6 DEHYDRATION AND FLUID THERAPY

- It is safe to use as a one-off in the dehydrated animal. However, it is better to make up isotonic fluid.
- ISOTONIC FLUID

> An isotonic solution is a better alternative to water and can be easily made in the field situation.

- Make up an isotonic solution by adding **4.5 g NaCl (table salt) and 4.5 g KCl (lite salt) per litre of water.** This provides sodium, which is important for water absorption in the gut, and potassium which can be low if a horse is anorexic or has an inadequate diet.
- Pre-weighed packs of salt can be prepared in advance (e.g. enough for 6 L of water) so that in a field situation these can be added directly to water without the need for weighing, etc.
- If repeated doses of enteral fluids are needed to restore hydration, the fluid should be as close to isotonic as possible.

Intravenous fluid therapy

- This should always be the last resort for fluid therapy – and only used if the other methods described above have failed or are not appropriate (e.g. very severe dehydration, hypovolaemia). See Figure 6.2.2.
- A jugular catheter and giving set should be placed aseptically (see Section 4.6).
- The volume of fluid required to correct the dehydration should be calculated – see above.

> **It is important to estimate the volume required, and to monitor the animal's response carefully, whilst delivering the first 75% of the total amount.**

- Once the volume has been calculated – start by giving 75% of this total volume, e.g. if 12 L is calculated as the volume needed to restore hydration, administer 8–9 L initially.
- **Sterile isotonic fluid should be administered, e.g. lactated ringers solution, 0.9% NaCl.**
- Monitor carefully the clinical effect this has on the animal and check for urination.
- Once hydration has been restored (e.g. animal urinates) stop the fluids.
- If after this initial therapy, the animal has improved but is still showing signs of dehydration, then deliver the last 25% slowly, monitoring carefully.

Glucose saline is not the most effective method of providing for an animal's energy requirements.

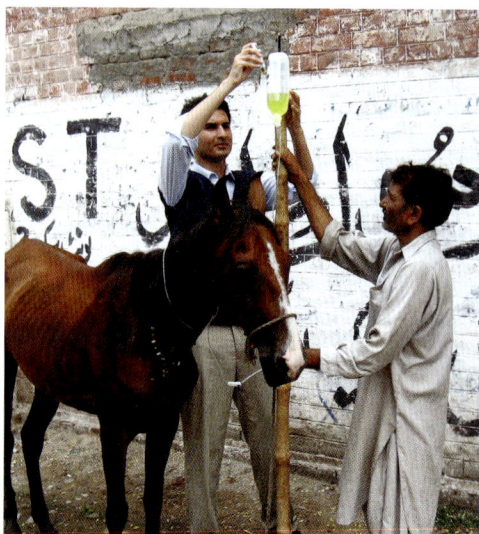

Figure 6.2.2 Intravenous fluids being administered to a working equid. Ensure the calculated volume required is given.

Historically, glucose saline has been administered in small volumes to heat-stressed or dehydrated animals in the belief that it provides energy. However, it should be remembered that giving 500 ml of 5% dextrose solution only contains 25 g (1 tablespoon) of dextrose which is not sufficient to replenish an animal's energy requirements.

> It is far more effective to supply energy by offering molasses/jaggery/green fodder or other energy sources after or while the animal is offered water. This will provide more energy for a more sustained period of time.

Monitoring fluid therapy

- **Monitor for urination** Many animals will pass dilute urine within 2 hours of fluids, although some may be slower. If an animal urinates this is a good indication that hydration has been restored and fluids should be stopped.

  - If an owner or paraprofessional is concerned about anuria it can be very useful to show them that an animal will urinate after just giving it water alone to drink and that it does not require aggressive veterinary intervention or drug therapy to resolve this problem. This is crucial to the education about this subject and will hopefully avoid incorrect diagnosis and unnecessary treatment in the future.

- **Monitor the animal's attitude and clinical parameters**

  - The animal should become brighter, more alert and responsive.
  - The extremities will feel warmer, and pulse quality will improve.

- **Monitor for signs of over-hydration**

  - Increased respiratory rate and effort. (**Note:** In adult horses this will only occur with very aggressive over-hydration.)
  - Abnormal, increased lung sounds on auscultation are suggestive of pulmonary oedema.
  - Provided an animal has normal kidney function, frequent and large volumes of dilute urine will accompany over-hydration.

Donkeys

Physiological differences exist between donkeys and horses. Donkeys are able to maintain their plasma volume even when 20% of their normal body water is lost compared with horses that are much less resistant to dehydration (Mathews *et al.* 1994).

6.3 References

Collatos, C (1999) Fluid therapy: when and where? Proceedings of the annual convention of the AAEP (45) 271–2.

Pritchard, J.C., Barr, A.R.S., Whay, H.R. (2006) Validity of a behavioural measure of heat stress and a skin tent test for dehydration in working horses and donkeys. *Equine Vet. J.* 38 (5), 433–438.

Pritchard, J.C., Burn, C.C., Barr, A.R.S., Whay, H.R. (2008) Validity of indicators of dehydration in working horses: A longitudinal study of changes in skin tent duration, mucous membrane dryness and drinking behaviour. *Equine Vet. J.* 40 (6), 558–564.

Mathews, N.S., Taylor, T.S., Hartsfield, S.M., Hayton, W.L., Jones, D.H. (1994) Pharmacokinetics of ketamine in mules and mammouth asses premedicated with xylazine. *Equine Vet. J.* 26 (3), 241–243.

Further reading

Lopes, M. (2002) Physiological aspects, indications and contraindications of enteral fluid therapy plan. *Equine vet. Educ.* 14 (5), 257–262.

Lopes, M. (2003) Administration of enteral fluid therapy: methods, composition of fluids and complications. *Equine vet. Educ.* 15 (2), 107–112.

Seahorn, J., Seahorn, T. (2003) Fluid therapy in horses with gastrointestinal disease. *Vet. Clin. N. Am. – Equine.* 19, 665–679.

Schott, H. (2006) Fluid therapy: A primer for students, Technicians, and veterinarians in equine practice. *Vet. Clin. N. Am. – Equine.* 22 (1), 1–14.

Sedation and anaesthesia

7

Sedatives and anaesthesia	**7.1**
Local anaesthetics	**7.2**
General anaesthesia in the field	**7.3**
References	**7.4**

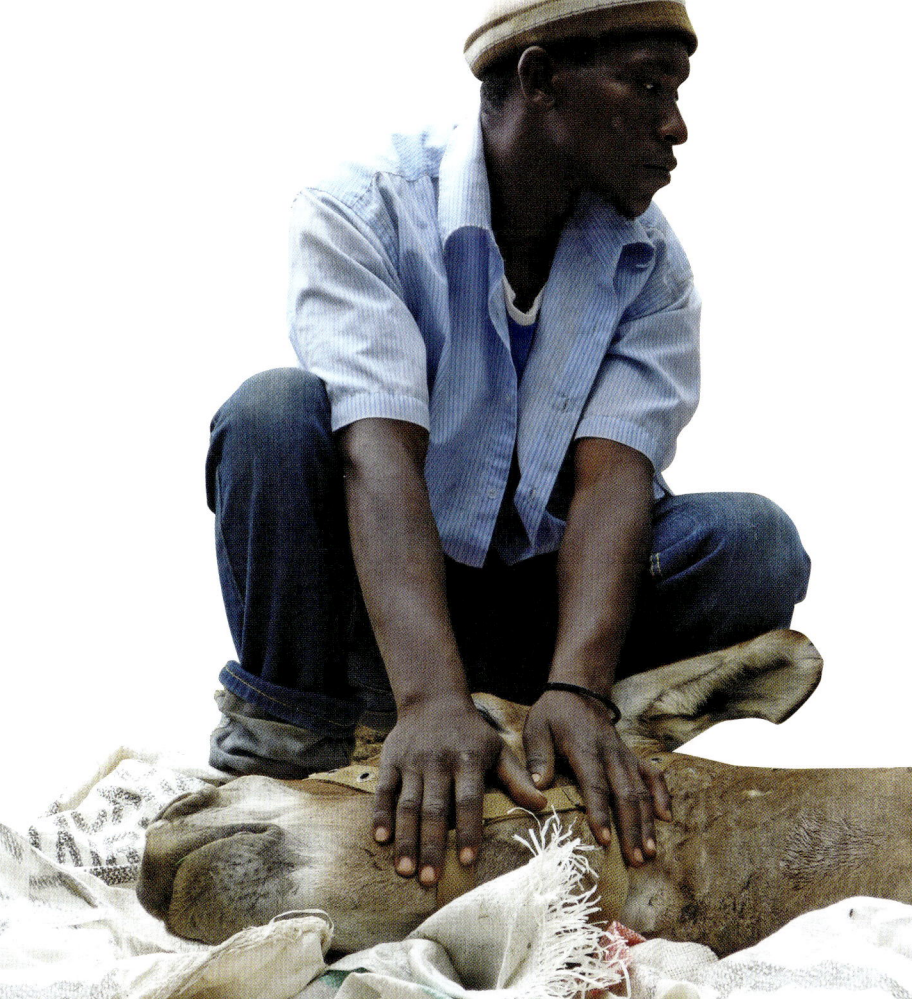

7.1 Sedatives and anaesthesia

There are now many safe, effective sedative drugs available and licensed which allow for less use of physical restraint. Assess the local markets to determine what is available.

Sedatives and tranquillisers alter mood, helping to calm the animal and make it less sensitive to external stimuli such as noise. The use of sedative or tranquillising drugs can also help animals to cope with fear or anxiety. This results in greater safety when carrying out examinations and treatment. These drugs are **never** a substitute for sympathetic handling (Section 2.3), correct usage of analgesia (Section 5.4) and local/general anaesthesia (Sections 7.2 and 7.3) where appropriate.

Considerations when using chemical restraint

Sedation of equids allows longer, more complex or painful treatment to be carried out and is often combined with local anaesthetic techniques or opioids for an enhanced effect. If performing any procedure where handling an animal is proving difficult due to its levels of pain and fear, sedation is required.

> **Consider sedation prior to attempting treatment, as this will decrease the dosage required and improve the animal's response to sedation.**

Considerations which will influence the choice and efficacy of sedation

- Available personnel and their ability to help
- Animal's temperament
- Type of procedure (length of time, pain level involved)
- Concurrent conditions/illness of the animal
- Behavioural factors – equids are flight animals and may panic when they feel the onset of ataxia or muscle weakness

> **Always respect a sedated animal as they can quickly be aroused and respond adversely – a safe, quiet environment is essential.**

Drugs commonly used for sedating equids

Phenothiazines

Commonly used agents (see Table 7.1.1)
- Acepromazine (ACP) 10%
- Chlorpromazine (There is very little information on its use in equids; use ACP as first choice.)

Onset and duration of action
- Effects of sedation are slow, seen after 30–40 minutes, regardless of administration route. Increasing the dose will only increase the duration of the effect, not the level of sedation itself.

Effect
- When used alone, ACP will act as a tranquiliser to calm the animal. It has **no analgesic or pain relief properties** so it is often used in conjunction with an opioid or NSAID.

SEDATIVES AND ANAESTHESIA 7.1

Key considerations

- **Profound hypotensive properties** Do **not** use in animals suffering from colic or haemorrhage.
- **Retractor penis muscle relaxation** Useful if examination of the penis is required. Prolonged exposure can result in trauma or paralysis, therefore use with caution in breeding stallions particularly if they are sick or debilitated; actual reported cases in the field are very low (< 1 in 10,000 cases), but do exist (Driessen et al. 2011).
- **Convulsions** ACP lowers the threshold for seizure activity and, although epilepsy is rarely diagnosed in equids, this is still a consideration.
- **Return to work** The cardiovascular effects last for up to 4–6 hours, long after any sedative effect has worn off. Warn owners not to work the animal for at least 4 hours after administration.

Route	Horse – dose	Donkey – dose	Mule – dose
IV	0.01–0.05 mg/kg (0.1–0.5 ml/100kg)	0.04–0.1 mg/kg	0.04 mg/kg IV (May require double dose compared with horses)
IM	0.03–0.1 mg/kg (0.3–1 ml/100kg)	0.03–0.1 mg/kg	*
PO	0.1–0.25 mg/kg	0.1–0.2 mg/kg	*

(Mathews et al. 1997, Carmona et al. 2007. *Information not available in the literature.)

Table 7.1.1 Reported dose rates and routes of administration for acepromazine in horses, donkeys and mules.

Alpha2-adrenoreceptor agonists (alpha2-agonists)

Commonly used agents (see Table 7.1.2)
- Xylazine
- Detomidine
- Romifidine

Onset and duration of action
- Maximal effect is usually within 5–10 minutes; however, **adrenaline overrides the effect** so the rate of onset may be slower or not occur at all if the animal is in a noisy environment, is very nervous, or has just stopped work.

Effect
- Level of sedation is dose-dependent (Lizarrago and Beths 2012). Predictable sedation occurs with the use of these drugs alone, although more often they are used with an opioid drug for an enhanced effect (see neuroleptanalgesia later).

Key considerations
- **Analgesia** **These drugs provide reasonable analgesia** for half to two-thirds of the time the animal is sedated, especially visceral analgesia, e.g. colic.
- **Decreased GIT Motility** Advise owners not to feed animals for a few hours after sedation with alpha2-adrenoreceptor agonists as there is a risk of choke.

7 SEDATION AND ANAESTHESIA

- **Pregnancy** Use with caution during pregnancy due to the effect of increased intra-uterine pressure (Schatzmann et al. 1994). Only administer if necessary, especially in the last trimester (check the data sheet).
- **IV sulphonamide antibiotics** Never use at the same time as these drugs as it can cause fatal cardiac arrhythmias (see Section 5.3).
- **Ataxia** Romifidine is preferred in many cases as it gives less ataxia and has the longest duration of action of the three; however, it cannot be given IM and is not available in all countries.
- **Bradycardia** is a common result of using these drugs. However, this is reversible with atipamezole at a dose of 0.1–0.2 mg/kg (Muir 1998) by slow IV/IM. Atipamezole may also be used if the sedation is prolonged or problematic; remember this will also reverse the analgesia effects.

Donkeys and mules

There are reports that **donkeys** are more resistant to alpha2-agonists and need higher doses for profound sedation; however, a study by Lizarrago and Beths (2012) concluded that various doses of xylazine (0.5–1.1 mg/kg) produced the same hypoalgesic effect in both horses and donkeys suggesting similar dose rates.

Studies of **mules** report that doses of 50% more drug are required compared with horses and donkeys (Mathews et al. 1997).

Drug	Horse – dose	Donkey – dose	Mule – dose
Xylazine	0.6–1 mg/ml	0.5–1.0 mg/kg IV 2.2–3 mg/kg IM (single dose)	1.1–1.6 mg/kg IV Mules require a 50% higher dose than horses or donkeys, and may even require up to double the dose compared with horses.
Detomidine	0.01–0.02 mg/kg – lower doses may be effective especially in young, old, debilitated or at-risk animals IM – dose 1.5/2 times greater than IV dose.	0.02–0.04 mg/kg IV or IM	0.03 mg/kg IV As for donkey, or 50% higher dose
Romifidine	0.04–0.12 mg/kg – onset of action 1–2 minutes Light sedation: 0.04 mg/kg Deep sedation: 0.08 mg/kg Deeper/prolonged sedation: 0.12 mg/kg	0.04 mg/kg IV	0.04–0.12 mg/kg IV or 0.12 mg/kg IM Note: Signs of sedation similar to other equids, but intensity less with same dose. IM route may be most efficient.

(Mathews et al. 1997, Alves et al. 1999, Portier et al. 2009, Carmona et al. 2007).

Table 7.1.2 *Reported dose rates and routes of administration of alpha2-adrenoreceptor agonists for horses, donkeys and mules.*

SEDATIVES AND ANAESTHESIA 7.1

Benzodiazepines

Commonly used medications (See Table 7.1.3)
- Diazepam

Note: Diazepam is not licensed for use in equids. The main use in adults is for induction of general anaesthesia in combination with ketamine. In foals diazepam is used for sedation and anti-seizure medication.

Onset and duration of action
- Rapid onset after IV administration due to high lipid solubility. Effects are short-lasting in adults (10–15 minutes). In foals the sedative effect is longer.

Effect
- Very mild sedation/sleepiness and muscle relaxation/ataxia in adult horses; more profound sedation in foals. Also used as an anti-convulsant.

Key considerations

> - **Foals** – Sole agent for sedation and restraint of young foals; however, will provide no pain relief when used alone.

- **Induction of general anaesthesia** Used in combination with ketamine as a general anaesthetic induction protocol in adult animals.
- **Reactions** Diazepam reacts with plastics, so never leave drawn up in a syringe – always use straight away.
- **Pain relief** None

Drug	Horse – dose	Foal – dose	Donkey – dose	Mule – dose
Diazepam	0.04–0.15 mg/kg	0.01–0.4 mg/kg slow IV	0.033–0.4 mg/kg slow IV	0.033 mg/kg IV

(Taylor 1985, Robertson 1997b, Mathews *et al.* 2005, Michou and Leece 2012a)

Table 7.1.3 Reported dose rates and routes of administration of diazepam in horses, foals, donkeys and mules.

Opioid analgesics

Opioid analgesics give **short-term pain control**. All drugs in this group are derived from the opium poppy, and have a similar effect by acting on μ (mu), k (kappa) and d (delta) receptors distributed widely within the CNS and periphery.

Commonly used medications (see Table 7.1.4)
- Butorphanol
- Buprenorphine
- Morphine
- Pethidine

Onset and duration of effect
- When used alone, the analgesic effects have been reported to last 30–90 minutes (Love *et al.* 2009). However, when used in combination with other sedative drugs the effects last

7 SEDATION AND ANAESTHESIA

longer and the negative side-effects are lessened (see neuroleptanalgesia below), for example buprenorphine and alpha2-agonist can provide analgesia for up to 12 hours (Michou and Leece 2012).

- As a result of the short duration of action they are not normally suitable for long term analgesia.

Uses

- Sedation and pain relief in combination with other drugs and short-term provision of analgesia

Drug	Horse – dose	Foal – dose	Donkey – dose	Mule – dose
Butorphanol	0.02–0.05 mg/kg IV (for sedation in conjunction with an alpha2-agonist – gives limited analgesia) 0.05–0.1 mg/kg IV (for improved analgesia)	0.02–0.05 mg/kg IV (0.1–0.2 mg/kg IM)	0.025–0.5 mg/kg IV (in combination with alpha2-agonist)	0.033–0.044 mg/kg IV (in combination with alpha2-agonist)
Buprenorphine	0.005–0.01 mg/kg IV/IM (IV in conjunction with an alpha2-agonist)	-	-	-
Morphine	0.1–0.2 mg/kg IV/IM (4–6 hours of good analgesia)	0.1 mg/kg IV	-	-
Pethidine *(IM only)*	1–3 mg/kg IM	-	2 mg/kg IM	-

(Mathews *et al.* 1992, Robertson 1997b, Mathews *et al.* 2005, Robert *et al.* 2008, Svendson 2008, Davis *et al.* 2012, Michou and Leece 2012) - where literature on opioids in some species is lacking.)

Table 7.1.4 Reported dose rates and routes of administration for opioids in horses, foals, donkeys and mules.

Key consideration

> - Side effects – The negative effect of the wide distribution of opioid receptors throughout the body is a wide range of potential side effects including excitement, manic behaviour and reduced gastrointestinal motility.

- Excitable behaviour is a widely reported side effect of some opioids, but is very rare with appropriate dose rates. The benefits of use in pain control far outweigh the small potential for side effects.

SEDATIVES AND ANAESTHESIA 7.1

- **Use in combination** with sedatives (see neuroleptanalgesia below). Intra-muscular administration further reduces the chance of excitation.
- **Opioids are controlled drugs**. They may have legal restrictions (e.g. a register to be kept of each purchase and use) and they should always be stored in a secure place.
- **Sourcing of opioids** Every effort should be made to keep at least one type of opioid in stock at the clinic at all times. Human pharmacists/hospitals may be valuable sources of opioids in areas where they are not available through veterinary suppliers. Check the local laws and regulations regarding the use of opioids locally.

Neuroleptanalgesia

Neuroleptanalgesia is the name given to a combination of sedative (usually an alpha2-adrenoreceptor agonist) and analgesic (opioid) which work together to give profound sedation and effective pain control.

> If there is any doubt about whether an examination, procedure or surgery may cause pain or fear to an animal, neuroleptanalgesia (opioid + alpha2-agonist) should be used to minimise distress and maximise safety of people and the anmal.

Commonly used medications (see Table 7.1.5)
- Butorphanol + alpha2-adrenoceptor agonist

Onset and duration of effect
- The onset is 5–10 minutes if given IV (may take longer if it is administered IM). Most combinations last between 20 and 60 minutes; however, as with all sedative effects, individual animals may vary in their response.

Key considerations
- **Combination with local or regional anaesthetic** This gives increased duration and effect of neuroleptanalgesia. For example, use with local anaesthetic for wound repair, or palmar digital nerve block for a foot abscess (see Section 7.2 of this chapter and Section 14.2 for details of the technique). This provides the best analgesia for the animal and the safest working environment for clinicians and handlers.
- **Other locally available drugs** This is not a complete list. Explore locally available options and consult the manufacturer or textbooks for appropriate dose rates where available.

When is the best time to use neuroleptanalgesia drug combination?

> Neuroleptanalgesia should be used for all painful procedures to minimise distress and maximise safety for all.

Examples include:
- cleaning, debriding and suturing wounds (see Section 15.1)
- examination of eye problems
- painful farriery or dental procedures
- minor (standing) surgery
- premedication before general anaesthesia (other options available see Section 7.3 of this chapter)

7 SEDATION AND ANAESTHESIA

- any procedure carrying a risk of being kicked. The addition of an opioid to sedation with an alpha2-adrenoreceptor agonist greatly reduces this risk.

Drug dose (mg/kg)	Horse	Donkey	Mule
Butorphanol	0.02–0.05 mg/kg IV	0.025–0.05 mg/kg IV	0.033–0.044 mg/kg IV
Combined with *one* of the following			
Xylazine	0.5–1.0 mg/kg IV	1.0 mg/kg IV	1.1–1.6 mg/kg IV
Detomidine	0.01–0.02 mg/kg IV	0.01–0.02 mg/kg IV	0.03 mg/kg IV
Romifidine	0.04–0.12mg/kg IV	0.08–0.12 mg/kg IV	0.04–0.12 mg/kg IV (higher dose gives more effective sedation)
ACP	0.02–0.05 mg/kg IM/IV	0.04 mg/kg IV	0.04 mg/kg IV

(Mathews *et al*. 1992, Mathews *et al*. 1997, Alves *et al*. 1999, Mathews *et al*. 2005, Michou and Leece 2012)

Table 7.1.5 *Neuroleptanalgesia dose rates for horses, donkeys and mules.*

Intramuscular administration of sedation

As discussed, sedation is very useful when examining a stressed or scared animal, or one in pain, as it improves the animal's mental state and improves the safety of the staff and owners who are dealing with the case. However, finding a vein in a stressed, frightened, possibly dangerous animal can be difficult.

A neuroleptanalgesia drug combination is a very useful IM alternative to IV sedation. The individual drug dose rates should be strictly adhered to (refer to drug data sheets):

- Butorphanol + Detomidine + ACP
- Mix together in the same syringe and inject into the muscle.

> Despite this neuroleptanalgesia drug combination being easy to administer, it is not to be used routinely as a substitute for finding a vein.

Being IM, it takes a lot longer to have effect, and the animal requires a very quiet environment for the medication to be effective. The addition of the ACP makes the hypotensive effects even more pronounced, so try to avoid this neuroleptanalgesia drug combination in animals with shock, haemorrhage, dehydration or any other condition in which a low blood volume or pressure is suspected.

Local anaesthetics

7.2

> Local anaesthetics (LA) remove all sensation in the area of administration (pain, touch, pressure and tension) whilst the animal remains conscious.

LA work by blocking conduction along sensory neurones by reducing sodium ion (Na+) influx via Na+ channels (Harkins *et al.* 1999) thus preventing action potentials and subsequently sensitisation or pain.

Commonly used medications (see Table 7.2.1)
- Lignocaine hydrochloride
- Bupivacaine hydrochloride
- Mepivacaine hydrochloride
- Proxymetacaine/oxybuprocaine (see Chapter 9 *Ophthalmology*)

Onset and duration of effect
- Most local anaesthetics take around 5–10 minutes to work (bupivacaine hydrochloride and mepivacaine hydrochloride take the longest at > 10 minutes).

> Always check the area to be desensitised with a needle/blunt-ended scissors to ensure the tissues are desensitised before commencing any procedure.

The duration can be from 30 minutes to 8 hours depending on the drug and procedure. Adrenaline prolongs the effect due to vasoconstrictive properties, thus preventing the LA dispersing from the area. Bupivacaine hydrochloride is four times as potent as mepivacaine (Harkins *et al.* 1999). Mepivacaine hydrochloride is less toxic than bupivacaine hydrochloride and produces less local tissue oedema, hence it is very popular for diagnostic analgesia of the limbs (Baller and Hendrickson 2002).

Uses
- Management of any painful procedure: eye examination (see Chapter 9), wound debridement/suturing (see Chapter 15)
- Peripheral nerve blocks
- Diagnostic tool, for example nerve blocks for lameness examination (see Chapter 14)
- Epidural anaesthesia
- Adjunct to sedation, neuroleptanalgesia and general anaesthesia for optimal pain control and to reduce the amount of sedation needed

Side effects and toxicity
LA solutions are mildly irritant to tissues, especially with compounds containing adrenaline. LA can cause sloughing of wound edges and delay healing. Excessive volumes may be absorbed systemically and lead to toxicity which is manifested by muscle tremors, seizures, and then coma. In some situations it may lead to respiratory arrest and coma.

7 SEDATION AND ANAESTHESIA

LA agent	Duration of action (minutes)	Dose (mg/kg)
Lignocaine hydrochloride	30–120	10–40 mg per site (for diagnostic limb analgesia: Harkins et al. 1998); highest safe dose rate is 4 mg/kg (Baller and Hendrickson 2002)
Bupivacaine hydrochloride	30–90 (reported up to 8 hours)	1–2 mg/kg (Baller and Hendrickson 2002), or 0.5–2 mg per site
Mepivacaine hydrochloride	60–120	30 mg per site (Midwell et al. 2004)

Table 7.2.1 *The duration of action and dose rates of local anaesthetics.*

Local or regional anaesthetic techniques for use in equids

See individual chapters for the LA techniques for specific areas: for the eye see Chapter 9, for face and teeth see Chapter 10 and for limbs see Chapter 14.

Topical – solutions without adrenaline

- Apply to mucous membranes for urinary catheterisation, examination and cleaning of wounds on gums and vulva.
- Proxymetacaine eye drops give corneal anaesthesia for 15–20 minutes. Use for eye examination, corneal ulcer debridement, washing or removal of foreign bodies (see Chapter 9).

Local infiltration

Local infiltration is a useful technique in equids.

> **However, it must be used carefully due to the potential for systemic toxicity if used over large areas or with large volumes of LA.**

The tissue irritation and delayed healing effects must also be taken into account.

- Inject subcutaneously close to a wound edge for skin suturing. Inject into one area and then perform further infiltrations through the previously anaesthetised area in a step-wise manner. This means the animal will only feel the first injection and is less likely to become fractious. Caution: Large volumes cause swelling and may impair healing.
- Inject 0.5–1 ml subcutaneously before placement of an IV cannula.
- Inject subcutaneously, into the body of the testicles and into the spermatic cord for castration.

LOCAL ANAESTHETICS 7.2

Possible complications

- Always draw back on the syringe to ensure that the LA is not injected inadvertently into a blood vessel. It can cause a decrease in cardiac electrical activity and contractility which may lead to cardiac arrest (Baller and Hendrickson 2002).

Nerve blocks (perineural anaesthesia)

> **Prepare all sites for nerve blocks in a sterile way to avoid the risk of possible infection post-injection (Section 4.6).**

Uses

- **Painful procedures** Extremely useful for analgesia of painful procedures, e.g. paring out foot abscesses or suturing muzzle or lower limb wounds. Wherever possible, use as an adjunct to sedation, neuroleptanalgesia or general anaesthesia to maximise pain control and reduce the amount of other drugs needed.
- **Lameness diagnosis** Useful for lameness diagnosis when performing nerve blocks from distal to proximal in a logical manner to pinpoint the site of pain (see Section 14.2 for details of palmar/plantar digital nerve block and abaxial sesamoid nerve block techniques).
- **Eye** For thorough examination of the eye and eyelids LA of the auriculopalpebral nerve block can be carried out (see Chapter 9 *Ophthalmology* for techniques). This nerve block blocks the motor function of the upper eyelid. This stops blinking. However, the surface of the eye is not desensitised, therefore ensure that topical ophthalmic LA is applied if required (sensory block). The sensory innervation to the medial (nasal) two-thirds of the upper eyelid can be eliminated by a supraorbital (frontal) nerve block. For examinations, suturing injuries of the eye and enucleations, administer the lacrimal, zygomatic and infratrochlear block leading to complete desensitisation of the eye and eyelids. (Full descriptions in Chapter 9.)
- **Distal face, jaw and lips** For examination and treatment of injuries of the distal face, jaw and lips, e.g. a suspected fractured mandible or mouth trauma, apply the mental nerve block (see Section 10.8 for full details of the technique). Further desensitisation of the upper lip and nose is provided by the infraorbital nerve block.

Caudal epidural anaesthesia

Caudal epidural anaesthesia provides analgesia of the perineum, rectum, vulva and vagina and can be useful in cases of dystocia as it helps with uterine relaxation. This technique allows surgical intervention in the standing animal without the risks and costs of general anaesthesia (Salmon *et al.* 1995).

> **Clipping and sterile preparation is mandatory for equine epidurals, unlike those performed on cattle.**

The aim is to produce regional anaesthesia **without** losing motor function to the hindlegs.

1. Sedate the animal, and clip and aseptically prepare the area cranial to the tail.
2. Ensure operator safety at all times – even with sedation, the animal can still react to the needle insertion so do not stand directly behind it.

3. With the animal standing square, locate the first inter-coccygeal space (Co1–Co2). This is the first obvious midline depression caudal to the sacrum, about 2½ inches (6–7 mm) cranial to the origin of the first tail hairs. Pumping/moving the tail up and down can assist in locating the depression. Place a bleb of local anaesthetic under the skin in this area (Figure 7.2.1).
4. Use a 2-inch, 19G needle. Before injecting into the space, place a few drops of sterile saline into the hub, for use as an indicator that the needle is in the right place (see next step).
5. Angling the needle perpendicular to the skin, direct it into the midline depression facing cranially. As the needle enters the right space, the saline in the hub will be sucked in quickly – the 'hanging drop' technique. Correct placement is also ensured by lack of resistance when injecting 5 ml of air. Always draw back before injecting to ensure a vein has not been inadvertently penetrated.
6. Inject – a combination of local anaesthetic and an alpha2-agonist is the most frequently used permutation of drugs for epidurals as this combination extends the period of action of epidural anaesthesia/analgesia: e.g. lidocaine 0.2 mg/kg and xylazine 0.17 mg/kg.

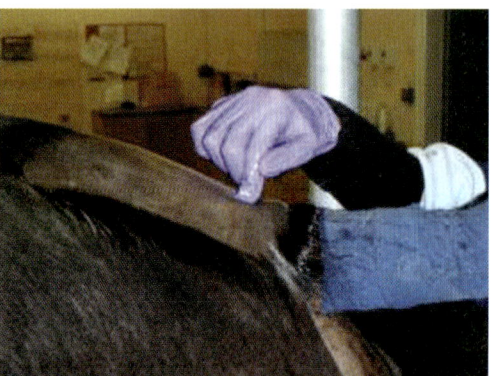 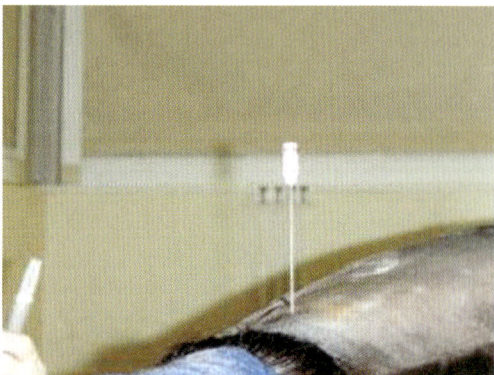

Figure 7.2.1 Site for caudal epidural anaesthesia (left) and placement of a needle (right). (Images provided by Avice O'Connor, University of Cambridge, UK.)

General anaesthesia in the field 7.3

Choice of anaesthetic agents

The choice is between:

(1) inhalants/volatile gases, such as halothane and isoflurane

(2) intravenous agents, such as thiopentone and ketamine.

> Field general anaesthesia (GA) is limited to procedures that can be done under short timescales.

It is also limited in the types of agents that can be used due to a lack of equipment for inhalant anaesthesia, which is expensive and impractical for the field (Robertson 1997a). Here only intravenous anaesthesia is described.

Intravenous agents can be given as:

- a single bolus for short duration procedures such as wound repair, tissue removal or castration. For example, a single dose of ketamine can give 10–27 minutes of GA time (Fisher 1984).
- repeated boluses administered when a longer GA time is required; the induction and anaesthetic agents are re-administered at intervals to maintain GA. However, it is difficult to maintain a steady plasma concentration of agents in the required therapeutic range, with peaks and troughs occurring (Robertson 1997a).
- a constant rate infusion. This is the ideal as the plasma drug rate will be constant within the therapeutic range. However, it does require extra equipment to administer the drugs: from higher technical computer-driven pumps to simple standard fluid-giving sets attached to a jugular catheter (Beths 2007).

Total Intravenous Anaesthesia

There have been advances in Total Intravenous Anaesthesia (TIVA) techniques in recent years based on the combination of two or three different drug types, usually involving a muscle relaxant, a sedative and an anaesthetic agent, without the need for inhalant anaesthetic facilities.

> Recent advances in the use of sedative combinations and local anaesthesia techniques also facilitate standing surgical procedures.

However, TIVA may still be necessary in some instances for short surgical interventions, painful diagnostic procedures and minor procedures in animals where pain or fear cannot be controlled by standing techniques.

> Field anaesthesia always carries some degree of risk, including fatality, which varies with the health of the animal and the skill and technique of the veterinarian.

The type of GA most applicable to working equine veterinarians is TIVA where equipment required is minimal and inexpensive.

Advantages of TIVA
- Applicable for the field situation
- Physiologically superior to gaseous anaesthetic agents: reports state that TIVA is less noxious than inhalant anaesthetic gasses and results in less cardiorespiratory depression (Robertson 1997a, Stanway 2001)
- Combinations of lower doses of several drugs reduce side effects of each individual drug (Muir and Scicluna 1998)

Disadvantages of TIVA
- Oxygen not always available
- Not suitable for lengthy procedures (greater than 90 minutes) as prolonged recoveries are then seen (Stanway 2001)
- Cannot remove any drug once administered (inhalant levels can more easily be adjusted)
- Anaesthetic depth harder to monitor, especially with ketamine as the usual signs of GA are not shown: the eye remains active with palpebral movements (nystagmus) and swallowing may also occur (Robertson 1997a)

> **Ideally, airways should be maintained with an endotracheal tube, and oxygen should be available from an oxygen cylinder (size E) and a demand valve (Brouwer 1985).**

Welfare cost versus benefit of GA

Animal welfare is paramount when considering GA.

Preparation for GA

Preparation must include a method of humane euthanasia close at hand in case the surgery fails or the animal injures itself severely during anaesthesia or recovery. Veterinarians must decide in advance the 'cut-off points' for failure of the procedure/irreparable injury and agree to destroy the animal humanely immediately if this occurs. This requires advance consent from owners for surgery and euthanasia if it becomes necessary. The field anaesthetic techniques described below are only suitable for short procedures. Some anaesthetic combinations can be maintained by 'top-up' doses or drip infusions.

> **In all cases the risk of side-effects increases with the duration of anaesthesia.**

The risk of fatality increases markedly after 1.5–2 hours.

Preparation is vital before any general anaesthetic procedure because situations can change rapidly and become dangerous to both the animal's welfare and that of the staff. All necessary equipment must be ready at hand, including spare equipment and a back-up plan in place if the first procedure fails or takes longer than anticipated. At least two experienced veterinarians should be present, of whom one must be responsible for anaesthesia at all times (not involved in surgery), and at least one trained assistant.

GENERAL ANAESTHESIA IN THE FIELD 7.3

Recumbent anaesthetised horses are anatomically, physiologically and pharmacologically susceptible to cardiorespiratory depression during anaesthesia leading to arterial hypoxaemia (low blood oxygen), hypercapnia (high blood CO_2), and hypotension (low blood pressure), which ultimately can produce skeletal muscle ischaemia and postanaesthetic myopathy.

> The risks should be fully explained to the owner, and GA should only be undertaken if there is sufficient time, resources and personnel to provide care for the procedure itself and for the post-op and recovery period.

Close consideration should be given to pre-, during and post-GA care to ensure that the animal's welfare is respected.

List of equipment for GA

- Anaesthetic consent form, signed after informed consent from the owner
- Head collar (with padding) and long lead ropes
- IV catheters
- Sedation and induction drugs and top-ups
- Ophthalmic lubricating ointment
- Towels

Pre-operative examination

The risk of a **healthy** equid dying under GA is approximately 1 in 100 (Stanway 2001).

This figure will rise dramatically if the animal is dehydrated, anaemic, in shock, has other cardiovascular compromise or any other sickness, due to the effects of anaesthetic drugs on the cardiovascular system. The importance of client communication and informed consent cannot be overstressed – always fill in a consent form for both anaesthesia and euthanasia.

Take a history and perform a thorough clinical examination, paying close attention to the heart (Figure 7.3.1) and respiratory rates, mucous membrane colour, capillary refill time (CRT) and lung auscultation – any signs of respiratory or cardiovascular distress should be taken seriously. Take the temperature.

> It is absolutely essential that an accurate weight is obtained prior to GA so that drug doses can be calculated accurately.

Information on estimating bodyweight can be found in the *References* (Section 7.4. of this chapter) and in Chapters 5 and 11.

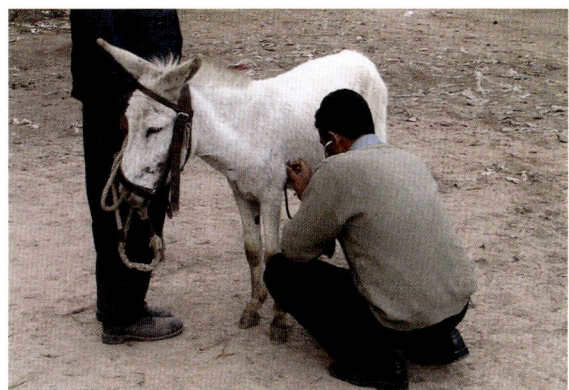

Figure 7.3.1 Perform a thorough pre-general anaesthetic clinical examination.

7 SEDATION AND ANAESTHESIA

Unsuitable conditions for GA
- Pyrexia
- Severe respiratory disease
- Diarrhoea
- Anaemia
- Cachexic or animals with BCS < 1.5 (on a scale of 1 = very thin, to 5 = very fat; see Section 11.1)
- Pregnancy (can be undertaken if essential, but should be avoided)

The environment for GA

> Sedation and general anaesthesia requires a quiet environment to be effective.

The ideal casting area is flat, dry and clean, free of other animals and unnecessary observers. The animal will need good grip to get up, so a grassy area is ideal (Figure 7.3.2).

Venous catheterisation

Always required – enables drugs to be administered IV rapidly and easily in the case of an emergency and it eliminates the risk of injecting into the carotid artery or extravascularly if the animal is lying down.

Phases of GA

There are four phases of GA:
1. Pre-anaesthetic
2. Induction
3. Maintenance
4. Recovery

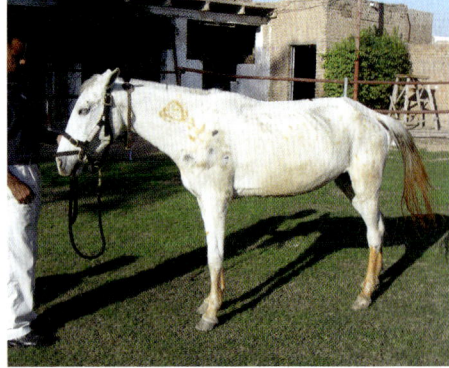

Figure 7.3.2 A good location for performing a general anaesthetic.

Pre-anaesthetic

> The aim of this phase is to produce an animal that is calm, sedated, free from pain and relaxed.

A pre-anaesthetic, or pre-medication, agent is a drug given **before** starting the GA to sedate the animal. Besides inducing muscle relaxation essential for a smooth induction, it reduces the total amount of each drug required. Certain combinations can also provide peri-operative analgesia.

Premedication drugs include acepromazine (ACP), alpha2-adrenoceptor agonists, opioids and NSAIDs, all of which have been discussed in Section 7.1. of this chapter and Chapter 5.

Do not be deterred by the combination of several drugs: this is safer and better for the animal than using only one anaesthetic agent.

Induction of GA

> The aim of induction is to get the animal from a standing to a recumbent position as smoothly, quietly and safely as possible for all involved.

It is essential that the animal is restrained quietly for induction and is not disturbed by noise or sudden movement as this can lead to a violent induction. The animal should be kept steady and not allowed to move around. It is not advisable to push an animal backwards as it will tend to push against the restraint and fall forward. With firm controlled restraint, the animal should buckle at the knees, thereafter sink back into sternal recumbency and then into lateral recumbency in a slow and controlled manner. Trained personal can aid the animal into lateral recumbency by keeping the head low and one hand on the front of the shoulder to guide the animal to the ground. Large equids may require two handlers, one either side of the head facing the shoulders with one hand on a lead rope either side and the other hand on the point of the shoulder; smaller equids can be controlled by a single person.

> Easy, safe induction is only possible with a calm animal that is well sedated – do not inject ketamine unless the animal is deeply sedated – top up with the same alpha2-adrenoreceptor agonist if necessary.

Maintenance of GA

The aims of this phase are to maintain a state of unconsciousness, analgesia and muscle relaxation, whilst minimising the physiological effects of the surgery. There are three planes of anaesthesia described by Geudel (1937): light, medium and deep.

Planes of GA

> 1. **Light** Decreased reflexes with no involuntary muscle movements. Palpebral, corneal reflexes and lacrimation are still maintained; swallowing reflex depends on GA agent used (absent with inhalants, present with TIVA).
> 2. **Medium** Ideal for most surgical interventions: absence of pain and palpebral reflexes, pupils dilated and corneal reflexes present. Local anaesthetic techniques required for ocular surgery (see Chapter 9).
> 3. **Deep** Signs of early overdose are seen. Respiration is depressed, bradycardia is present, all reflexes are absent.

Beyond this, cardiovascular and respiratory function cease and death will ensue.

Recovery from GA

> This is often the most crucial and yet forgotten stage of the GA.

The risks for the animal are increased. The aim is for a quiet, controlled transition from recumbency to standing. See later for more details.

7 SEDATION AND ANAESTHESIA

Injectable agents

Ketamine

Ketamine is a dissociative anaesthetic agent that produces a trance-like loss of consciousness whilst maintaining skeletal muscle tone and cranial nerve reflexes. The result is an animal with intact muscle tone, swallowing and ocular reflexes (blinking, nystagmus), which can be unnerving for the surgeon, and make anaesthetic monitoring difficult.

> **To reduce the excitement reactions which occur with ketamine induction it is vital the animal is well sedated with an alpha2-adrenoreceptor agonist.**

Many veterinarians combine ketamine with diazepam in the same syringe for induction to improve muscle relaxation. See Table 7.3.1 for protocols.

After injection of ketamine, lateral recumbency is usually achieved in 40–100 seconds; recumbency time is reported from 10 to 27 minutes, with 5–15 minutes surgery time (Muir 2010, Fisher 1984).

Thiopentone

This barbiturate anaesthetic is typically presented in 5-g vials, and is mixed with 100 ml sterile water for 5% solutions. It is a lot faster acting than Ketamine, often giving less than 10–15 minutes of surgical anaesthesia.

The disadvantages of thiopentone use is that, like all barbiturates, it has a cumulative effect and is generally not suitable for multiple top-up injections as this tends to cause prolonged, difficult recoveries with a higher risk of injury.

> **It is not suitable for use as a sole anaesthetic agent and premedication is vital.**

Rapid IV injections cause hypotension and respiratory depression. It is also an extreme irritant perivascularly, so do not use without an IV catheter. See Table 7.3.2 for protocols.

Recumbency is achieved 25–30 seconds after injection. Correct dosage is essential as under-dosage can lead to excitement on induction.

Drugs and doses for GA

Tables 7.3.1 and 7.3.2. show reported doses for pre-anaesthesia sedation and induction of GA. Always ensure that additional analgesia is given in the form of NSAIDs or opioids, as the analgesic effects of sedatives and induction agents are short-lived.

7.3 GENERAL ANAESTHESIA IN THE FIELD

Species (references)	Horse (Fisher 1984, Taylor 1995, Moens et al. 2003, Beths 2007, Muir 2010)	Donkey (Mathews et al. 1994, Mathews et al. 2005)	Mules (Mathews et al. 1992, Mathews et al. 2005)
Surgical/ recumbency time	5–15 minutes of surgical GA	15–30 minutes of surgical GA	5–20 minutes of recumbency time
Protocol	**Sedate with (optional):** ACP 0.04 mg/kg IM/IV (care with sick, dehydrated animals and entire males). **Wait 30–40 minutes if possible and then sedate with:** Alpha2-agonist, e.g. xylazine 1–1.1 mg/kg IV or romifidine 0.08 mg/kg IV (+/- butorphanol 0.02 mg/kg IV). **Wait 2–5 minutes (or to sedation effect) and then induce with:** Ketamine 2.2 mg/kg (+/- diazepam 0.04–0.1 mg/kg IV).	**Sedate with:** ACP 0.04 mg/kg IV. **Wait 30-40 minutes if possible and then sedate with:** Xylazine 1–1.1 mg/kg IV (+/- butorphanol 0.025–0.05 mg/kg IV). **Wait 5 minutes then induce with:** Ketamine 2.2 mg/kg IV (+/- diazepam 0.02–0.1 mg/kg IV).	**Sedate with:** Xylazine 1.6 mg/kg IV (Mules require 50% increased dose of xylazine and detomidine compared with horses and donkeys.) +/- butorphanol 0.044 mg/kg IV. **Wait 3-5 minutes then induce with:** Ketamine 2.2 mg/kg IV (Ketamine is cleared more quickly from the body of donkeys, followed by mules, then horses.) +/- diazepam 0.033 mg/kg IV.
Options	Depending on drug availability and patient, variations include: ■ Step 1 – Leave out ACP. ■ Step 2 – Leave out butorphanol and substitute romifidine **or** xylazine with detomidine 0.015–0.02 mg/kg. ■ Step 3 – Leave out diazepam and just use ketamine at 2.2 mg/kg.	Depending on drug availability, variations include: ■ Step 1 – Leave out ACP. ■ Step 2 – Instead of xylazine, sedate with detomidine 0.01–0.02 mg/kg, or romifidine 0.12 mg/kg IV; leave out butorphanol. ■ Step 3 – Leave out diazepam and just use ketamine at 2.2 mg/kg.	Options: ■ Step 1 – Detomidine 0.03 mg/kg IV +/- butorphanol 0.033–0.044 mg/kg IV ■ Step 2 – Leave out diazepam. ■ Mules following the protocol of xylazine/butorphanol/ketamine had smoother inductions, longer GA time, better analgesia, and better recoveries than those on xylazine/ketamine only.

Table 7.3.1 Reported protocols for ketamine induction in horses, donkeys and mules.

7 SEDATION AND ANAESTHESIA

Species (references)	Horse (Muir and Scicluna 1998, Stanway 2001)	Donkey (Mathews et al. 2005, Emami et al. 2006, Al-Heani 2010)	Mule (Grint et al. 2011)
Surgical time	-	17–24 minutes	-
Protocol	ACP 0.04 mg/kg IM/IV (Caution! – see above) **Wait 30–40 minutes then sedate with:** Detomidine 0.015–0.02 mg/kg IV, **or** romifidine 0.01 mg/kg IV, **or** xylazine 0.1 mg/kg IV. **Wait 2–5 minutes (or to sedation effect) and then induce with:** Thiopentone 4–10 mg/kg IV (+/- diazepam 0.04–0.1 mg/kg IV).	Romifidine 0.12 mg/kg IV

Wait 5 minutes then induce with: Thiopentone 4–10 mg/kg. | ACP 0.03 mg/kg IV

Wait 30–90 minutes then induce with: Thiopentone 10 mg/kg IV. |
| Options | Options:
■ Step 1 – Leave out ACP.
■ Step 2 – Select a more readily available or familiar sedative.
■ Step 3 – Leave out the diazepam. | Depending on drug availability, variations include:
■ Step 1 – Instead of romifidine, sedate with xylazine 1 mg/kg or detomidine 0.02 mg/kg.
■ Pre-step 1 – Administer atropine and ACP, then use xylazine sedation followed by thiopentone 7 mg/kg, maintained for up to 100 minutes with thiopentone 8 mg/kg in 500 ml normal saline. | – |

Table 7.3.2 *Reported protocols for anaesthetic induction with thiopentone in horses, donkeys and mules.*

Propofol

An alternative induction agent for GA is propofol. This has been used in foals (2–3 mg/kg IV) 5 minutes after xylazine sedation (0.5 mg/kg IV). However, it is very costly and this is generally prohibitive for adult equids due to the volumes needed. Respiratory depression has been reported in numerous cases (Robertson 1997a). For protocols using propofol refer to anaesthetic texts and the articles such as Robertson (1997b).

Guaifenesin

> **Guaifenesin is a centrally-acting muscle relaxant, causing no lack of consciousness or analgesia when used alone.**

It should be used **only** in conjunction with anaesthetic agents for TIVA in horses (Robertson 1997a, Beths 2007); providing GA for up to 90 minutes (Stanway 2001). It is used in combination with alpha2-agonists and ketamine ('triple-drip' combinations): guaifenesin/ketamine/xylazine, guaifenesin/ketamine/detomidine (Robertson 1997a, Stanway 2001) and guaifenesin/ketamine/romifidine (Beths 2007). Infusion rates can be altered depending on the depth of GA obtained; remember there is a 60-second delay in response to the combination (Stanway 2001); these techniques require catheterisation for a constant infusion of the mixture of drugs.

Guaifenesin availability is limited in some countries. Refer to the referenced papers for reported dose rates and protocols for infusion techniques.

Chloral hydrate

This has been used historically as an injectable agent for GA, alone and in combination with thiopentone (Crispin 1981); however, doses are close to the lethal limit and it is best used in combination. Reported doses of 100–120 mg/kg IV followed by thiopentone (10 mg/kg IV) have been used to produce GA for 5–40 minutes. Chloral hydrate is very cheap and may be considered if the safer alternatives (ketamine or thiopentone) are not available and a GA is absolutely necessary. (See Chapter 8 for use of chloral hydrate in euthanasia.)

Other important considerations for the induction of GA

1. Padding around metal rings of the head collar to protect the bony prominences and nerves of the head will prevent traumatic complications such as facial nerve paralysis.
2. Cover eyes with a towel to protect the upside eye from sunlight and the downside eye from the ground in lateral recumbency. Protect the eyes from desiccation during anaesthesia by applying lubricating ophthalmic drops/ointment.
3. Place cotton wool in the ears to minimise environmental stimulation and increase anaesthesia time.
4. Remember that local anaesthesia of the surgical site also helps decrease the painful stimulus and maintenance of smooth GA.
5. Atropine sulphate has been used in older protocols (and other species) to reduce airway and intestinal secretions during anaesthesia.

> **Atropine can cause gut stasis and impaction in equids so it is not recommended.**

6. Dorsal recumbency is physiologically a very stressful position for an equid, as breathing and circulation will be compromised. Lateral recumbency is better, although this, too, will eventually compromise the down-side lung and reduce oxygen availability.

> 7. All equids undergoing anaesthesia or a surgical procedure should receive appropriate analgesia – ideally given before induction (i.e. before the procedure is performed).

Pre-emptive analgesia (pre-induction) has been shown to be more effective than analgesics given after the painful stimulus has occurred as the cumulative pain cycle is inhibited, minimising the wind-up of pain receptors and mediators. The use of **butorphanol** and an **alpha2-agonist will not** provide adequate analgesia; the addition of an **NSAID** will provide longer and more effective analgesia.

Positioning an equid during GA

- Ensure the ground underneath the animal is well padded and soft (Figure 7.3.3).
- Extend the head and neck to maintain an open airway (Brouwer 1985).
- When in lateral recumbency ensure that the dependent forelimb (lower/downmost) is pulled rostrally (forwards) to take the pressure off the muscles of the shoulder and minimise the risk of compromise and post-anaesthetic myopathy. It may also be possible to support the uppermost foreleg with a bag of straw or similar. Hindlegs can be similarly supported.

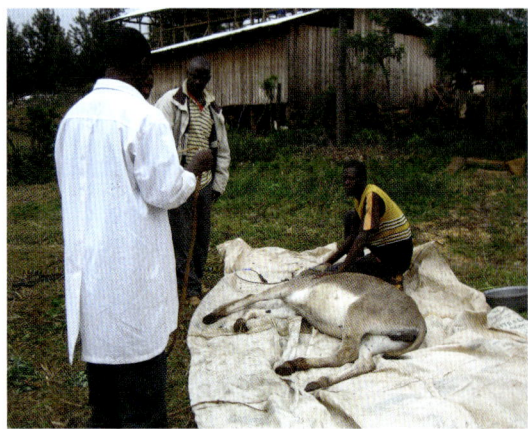

Figure 7.3.3 A sheet can be laid down to aid cleanliness of the operating site, and provide comfort for the animal.

Monitoring under TIVA

GA monitoring is difficult in field circumstances, especially if ketamine is being used because some ocular and motor reflexes are maintained which do not truly reflect the plane of anaesthesia (see earlier). It is important for the person monitoring the GA to record parameters and warn the surgeon of fluctuations in the plane of anaesthesia (see Table 7.3.3).

What if the animal has an adverse reaction or becomes unstable during TIVA?

This is the biggest problem with GA in the field. It is not possible to turn the anaesthetic down, turn the oxygen up, as with gaseous anaesthesia, or uninject medication that has already been administered. If there is a problem during anaesthesia warn the surgeon and monitor the animal. Prepare to administer reversal agents, if available. As the anaesthetic is metabolised the equid should become more stable.

> This emphasises the importance of choosing GA candidates wisely and only undertaking GA if it is entirely necessary.

GENERAL ANAESTHESIA IN THE FIELD 7.3

Parameter	GA too light	Surgical plane of GA (correct)	GA too deep
Respiratory pattern (Thiopentone may cause the animal to hold its breath for the first 2–3 minutes of anaesthesia – 'induction dyspnoea'.)	Change in respiratory *pattern* – a sudden, deeper breath may indicate the animal is lightening up. Equids do not increase their respiratory rate (RR) when lightening as do other species due to large respiratory reserves.	Strong and steady	Increasing periods of time between breaths
Pulse Palpate *every 5 minutes*. Mandibular (see Section 1.4), facial, metacarpal, metatarsal or digital pulses	The heart rate is *not* a good indicator of a lightening plane of anaesthesia due to the large cardiac reserve. However, use it to monitor overall cardiovascular system (CVS) function.	Strong and steady Mucous membranes pink with normal CRT (2 seconds)	Weak, irregular or slowing
Peripheral reflexes Corneal reflex and anal tone (Ketamine induction does not abolish cranial nerve reflexes – palpebral, gag and sometime skin twitch reflexes will remain making the monitoring of depth more difficult.)	Nystagmus Eye position is generally more unreliable in equids compared to other species.		A fixed, central, dry eye means the animal is too deep and may die.

Table 7.3.3 Anaesthetic monitoring parameters related to depth of GA.

7 SEDATION AND ANAESTHESIA

If a pre-operative check is not carried out there is an increased risk of anaesthetising an animal which is not fit enough to cope with a general anaesthetic. Remember the majority of working equids have at least one, if not more, factors which make them higher risk candidates for GA, as discussed earlier. The choice for GA should always be taken seriously.

Maintenance and 'top-ups' of TIVA

Once anaesthesia has been induced GA can be maintained if necessary by further intravenous 'top-up' techniques. These are easy to perform, but unlike continuous gaseous anaesthesia, will result in an undulating plane of anaesthesia.

Ketamine is the drug of choice to top-up with, even if thiopentone has been used as an induction agent. Thiopentone is less suitable for repeat administration due to the previously mentioned cumulative effects (the total dose given should not exceed 5 mg/kg). Draw up two or three top-up doses of ketamine (or thiopentone) before commencing the general anaesthetic. Ensure the drawn-up drugs are labelled and kept in a safe location. A second competent veterinarian, in addition to the surgeon, should be present to administer 'top-up' anaesthetic medication and to monitor the patient. Total GA time maintained via top-ups should not be longer than 90 minutes due to prolonged recovery times (Stanway 2001).

Top-up protocols

1. Ketamine

Donkeys and mules Boluses of ¼–½ the original dose can be administered (Mathews *et al.* 2005).

Horses Top-ups depend on the choice of alpha2-agonist used as pre-GA sedation (Stanway 2001), give boluses of either:

- xylazine 0.5 mg/kg + ketamine 1.1 mg/kg IV
- romifidine 0.025 mg/kg + ketamine 1.1 mg/kg IV
- detomidine 0.01 mg/kg + ketamine 1 mg/kg IV.

2. Thiopentone

Horses Repeated boluses of 1 mg/kg thiopentone can be given up to 5 times to maintain GA for a longer period (Stanway 2001).

Thiopentone works much faster than ketamine (which has a 60-second delay). If the animal is so light it starts moving, it is very useful to have a thiopentone 'top-up' drawn up. This agent will deepen the level of anaesthesia almost instantly.

> Use thiopentone after a ketamine induction and ketamine after a thiopentone induction, or even administer a bolus of thiopentone to deepen a 'triple drip' GA – whichever is available and desired at the time.

Recovery after TIVA

> Generally, recovery is smooth after TIVA, with less ataxia and fewer attempts to stand compared to gaseous anaesthesia.

A long line can be attached to the head collar to control the direction of the head upon standing, and caudal and downward pressure on the tail can also help with balance depending on the temperament of the animal.

Possible complications

- **Poor recovery** Animals may thrash or fall on recovery, causing injury which may be severe enough to require euthanasia. The risk is greater with thiopentone or if the animal is in pain as it recovers. When choosing a site for general anaesthesia, think ahead to the recovery and ensure a safe environment.

> Depending on the length of the GA the pre-anaesthetic dose of analgesia may need re-administering before the animal wakes up to avoid an excessive pain response.

- **Myopathy or neuropathy** GA time (> 1 hour) or abnormal positioning during general anaesthesia increases the risk of damage to muscles and nerves. Place large pads (e.g. bags of straw) between the front and back legs and under the head to reduce the risk. Make sure any animal being anaesthetised is normo-volaemic throughout the procedure to avoid low blood pressure which can predispose to myopathy. If myopathy occurs treat symptomatically with analgesics, anti-inflammatory drugs, IV fluids, massage, support and good nursing. The prognosis for recovery is often poor for these cases so prevention is paramount.

During recovery the animal should be discouraged from standing too early while it is still ataxic. Therefore, noise should be kept to a minimum and it can be useful to cover the animal's head with a blanket to prevent it from being visually stimulated.

Post-operative colic may very occasionally occur, due to reduced gut motility caused by anaesthetic drugs. Treat symptomatically and the prognosis is usually good.

Standing surgery

Continuous Rate Infusion (CRI) sedation with xylazine – a possible alternative to GA in some cases

> Standing sedation for a prolonged period of time, coupled with good analgesia and possibly local anaesthesia, can make standing surgery possible.

This CRI protocol involves xylazine (or romifidine) slowly administered by IV drip, resulting in prolonged standing sedation with a smoother level of sedation than that achieved by administering repeated boluses. Altering the drip rate gives a controlled sedative effect which may be feasible in the field for longer procedures in which a single injection of sedative may not be sufficient.

Maintain a constant plasma concentration of sedative drug which gives good sedation at the required level (the patient neither becoming ataxic nor moving unnecessarily). Nerve blocks are useful to reduce pain response during treatment which may lighten the level of sedation in the animal. Systemic NSAIDs and opioid analgesics are given to provide analgesia and reduce fluctuations in the sedation effect as a result of pain responses. Plan the procedure so that sedation can be increased during periods of more painful stimulation.

7 SEDATION AND ANAESTHESIA

A disadvantage is that CRI cannot be performed without a catheter and giving set, and the fluid bag cannot be reused. **Dispose** of unused fluid/drug mixture.

> CRIs should be approached the same way as a GA. Clinically assess the animal prior to anaesthesia and monitor carefully throughout and after the procedure.

If available, stocks and a head stand will support the animal and avoid the animal dropping its head excessively (due to the sedative) and stop the drug 'pooling' at the catheter site. If stocks are unavailable improvise to ensure that the animal is supported by using aspects of the environment and other objects, and by having experienced handlers. Always ensure the safety of the animal and handlers during this procedure. Doing this in the field will require the same supervision rate as a GA so be prepared to stay for an extended period of time whilst the animal recovers sufficiently.

Protocol for xylazine CRI sedation (Michou and Leece 2012)

1. Place IV catheter and administer **analgesia**.
2. Administer a loading dose of **xylazine 0.5 mg/kg IV**.
3. Connect fluid bag up to catheter and start infusion straight away xylazine 0.65 mg/kg IV (add **500 mg xylazine to a 500 ml bag 0.9% NaCl**).
4. Administer at 325 ml/hour; titre to the desired effect.

> Close supervision of the drip rate and sedation depth is mandatory – if the gauge on the giving set slips the animal will be over-sedated.

Reports advise to *start off slowly*, and then gradually increase the dose rate to 2 drops/second (assuming 20 drop/ml giving set) in the first 10 minutes. Once the desired level of sedation has been reached the drip rate can be halved for the remainder of the procedure. The animal should be able to walk within 10–15 minutes of stopping the drip.

There have been various other protocols for CRI with xylazine (Ringer *et al*. 2012a) and other drugs including romifidine (Ringer et al. 2012b), detomidine, butorphanol and ketamine. However, xylazine CRIs tend to be favoured amongst equid practitioners for its rapid onset.

Consult the literature to develop appropriate CRI protocols.

References

Al-Heani, W.A.Y. (2010) A comparative study of thiopental and thiopental-propofol admixture with xylazine premedicated donkeys. *Al-Anbar J. Vet. Sci.* 3, 2.

Alves, G.E.S., Faleiros, R.R., Gheller, V.A., Vieira, M.M. (1999) Sedative effect of romifidine in unmated mules (Equus asinus caballus) *Cien. Rural.* 29 (1), 51–55.

Baller, L.S., Hendrickson, D.A. (2002) Management of equine orthopedic pain. *Vet Clin Equine.* 18.

Beths, T. (2007) Total intravenous techniques for anaesthesia. *In Practice.* 29, 410–413.

Brouwer, G.J. (1985) Practical guidelines for the conduct of field anesthesia in the horse. *Equine vet J.* 17 (2), 151–154.

Carmona, J.U., Giraldo, C.E., Aristizibal, W., Garcia, A., Vallejo, L.G. (2007) Evaluation of the effects of the sedation with azaperone/acepromazine and immobilisation with guaiphenesin/thiopentone in mules. *Vet. Res. Commun.* 31, 125–132.

Crispin, S.M. (1981) Methods of equine general anaesthesia in clinical practice. *Equine Vet. J.* 13 (1), 19–26.

Davis, J.L., Messenger, K.M., LaFevers, D.H., Barlow, B.M., Posner, L.P. (2012) Pharmacokinetics of intravenous and intramuscular buprenorphine in the horse. *J. Vet. Pharm. Therap.* 35, 52–58.

Driessen, B., Zarucco, L., Kalir, B., Bertolotti, L. (2011) Contemporary use of acepromazine in the anaesthetic management of male horses and ponies: a retrospective study and opinion poll. *Equine Vet. J.* 43 (1), 88–89.

Emami, M.R., Seifi, H., Tavakali, Z. (2006) Effects of totally intravenous thiopental anaesthesia on cardiopulmonary and thermoregulatory system in donkeys. *J. Appl. Anim. Res.* 29, 13–16.

Fisher, R.J. (1984) A field trial of ketamine anaesthesia in the horse. *Equine vet J.* 16 (3), 176–179.

Grint, N.J., Lorena, S.E., Johnson, C.B., Luna, S.P., Whay, H.R., Murrell, J.C. (2011) Metabolic acidosis in healthy mules under general anaesthesia with halothane. *Vet. Anaesth. Analag.* 38 (5) 484–489.

Geudel, A.E. (1937) Inhalation anaesthesia: a fundamental guide. Macmillan Co. New York.

Harkins, J.D., Mundy, G.D., Woods, W.E., Lehner, A., Karpiesiuk, W., Rees, W.A, Dirikolu, L., Bass, S., Carter, W.G., Boyles, J., Tobin, T. (1998) Lidocaine in the horse: its pharmacological effects and their relationship to analytical findings. *J. vet. Pharmacol. Therap.* 21, 462–476.

Harkins, J.D., Lehner, A., Karpiesiuk, W., Woods, W.E., Dirikolu, L., Boyles, J., Carter, W.G., and Tobin, T. (1999) Bupivacaine in the horse: relationship of local anaesthetic responses and urinary concentrations of 3-hydroxybupivacaine. *J. vet. Pharmacol. Therap.* 22, 181–195.

Lizarrago, I., Beths, T. (2012) A comparative study of xylazine-induced mechanical hypoalgesia in donkeys and horses. *Vet. Anaesth. Analg.* 39, 533–538.

Love, E.J., Taylor, P.M., Clark, C., Whay, H.R., Murrel, J. (2009) Analgesic effect of butorphanol in ponies following castration. *Equine Vet. J.* 41 (6) 552–556.

Matthews, N.S., Taylor, T.S., Skrobarcek, C.L., Williams, J.D. (1992) A comparison of injectable anaesthetic regimens in mules. *Equine vet J.* 24 (S11) 34–36.

Matthews, N.S., Taylor, T.S., Hartsfield, S.M., Hayton, W.L., Jones, D.H. (1994) Pharmacokinetics of ketamine in mules and mammoth asses premedicated with xylazine. *Equine Vet. J.* 26 (3), 241–243.

Matthews, N.S., Taylor, T.S., Hartsfield, S.M. (1997) Anaesthesia of donkeys and mules. *Equine vet Educ.* 9 (4), 198–202.

Matthews, N.S., Taylor, T.S., Hartsfield, S.M. (2005) Anaesthesia of donkeys and mules. *Equine vet Educ.* 7, 102–107.

Michou, J., Leece, E. (2012) Sedation and analgesia in the standing horse 1. Drugs used for sedation and systemic analgesia. *In Practice.* 34, 524–531.

Midwell, L.A., Brown, K.E., Cordier, A., Mullineaux, D.R., Clayton, H.M. (2004) Mepivicaine local anaesthetic duration in equine palmar digital nerve blocks. *Equine vet J.* 36 (8), 723–726.

Moens, Y., Lanz, F., Doherr, M.G., Schatzmann, U. (2003) A comparison of the antinociceptive effects of xylazine, detomidine and romifidine on experimental pain in horses. *Vet. Anaesth. Analg.* 30, 183–190.

Muir, W.W., Scicluna, C. (1998) Anaesthesia and anaesthetic techniques in horses. *Equine Vet Educ.* 10 (1), 33–41.

Muir, W.W. (1998) Anaesthesia and pain management in horses. *Equine vet Educ.* 10 (6), 335–340.

Muir, W.W. (2010) NMDA receptor antagonists and pain: ketamine. *Vet. Clin. Equine.* 26, 565–578.

Portier, K.G., Jaillardon, L., Leece, E.A., Walsh, C.M. (2009) Castration of horses under total intravenous anaesthesia: analgesic effects of lidocaine. *Vet. Anaesth. Analg.* 36, 173–179.

Ringer, S.K., Portier, K.G., Fourel, I., Bettschart-Wolfensberger, R. (2012a) Development of a xylazine constant rate infusion with or without butorphanol for standing sedation of horses. *Vet. Anaesth. Analag.* 39, 1–11.

Ringer, S.K., Portier, K.G., Fourel, I., Bettschart-Wolfensberger, R. (2012b) Development of a romifidine constant rate infusion with or without butorphanol for standing sedation of horses. *Vet. Anaesth. Analag.* 39, 12–20.

Robert, C., Jacquet, S., Bertin, A., Denoix, J.M., Desbois, C. (2008) Romifidine-morphine combination for sedation of foals: clinical assessment of two protocols for administration. *J. Vet. Int. Med.* 19 (3), 485.

Robertson, S.A. (1997a) Total intravenous anaesthesia (TIVA) in the horse. *Equine Vet Educ.* 9 (1), 17–20.

Robertson, S.A. (1997b) Sedation and general anaesthesia of the foal. *Equine vet Educ.* 9 (1), 37–44.

Salmon, J., Blais, D. (1995) Caudal epidural anaesthesia in equine practice – anatomical and technical aspects. *Recl. Med. Vet.* 171 (10–11), 767–774.

Schatzmann, U. Josseck, H. Stauffer, J.L., Goosens, L. (1994) Effects of alph2-agonists on intrauterine pressure and sedation in horses: comparison between detomidine, romifidine and xylazine. *J. Vet. Med. A.* 41, 523–529.

Stanway, G. (2001) Anaesthesia for minor surgical procedures in the horse. *In Practice.* 23 (1), 22.

Svendson, E.D. (2008) The Professional Handbook of the Donkey. 4th Ed. Whittet Books Ltd. UK. pp. 222–238, 385–399.

Taylor, P.M. (1985) Chemical restraint of the standing horse. *Equine Vet. J.* 17 (4), 269–273.

Further reading

Staffieri, F., Driessen, B. (2007) Field Anesthesia in the Equine. *Clin.Tech.Equine.Prac.* 6 (2), 111–119.

Euthanasia

8

Introduction	8.1
Methods of euthanasia	8.2
Case study – Euthanasia	8.3
References	8.4

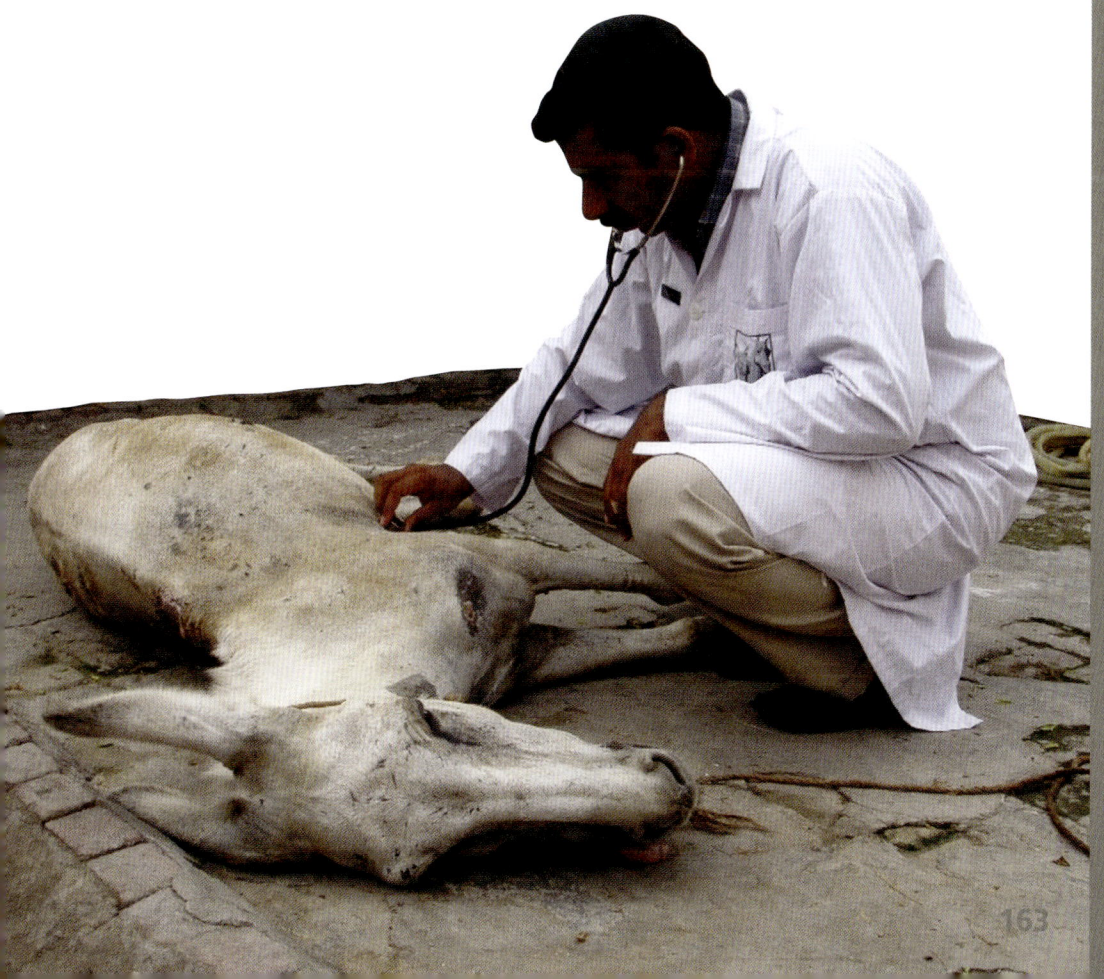

8.1 Introduction

What is euthanasia?

When suffering cannot be alleviated by any other means euthanasia is the only humane solution. Working equids may otherwise suffer a prolonged and painful death by abandonment, neglect or disease; an acute, painful death such as being eaten by wild animals (e.g. hyenas), or hit by a road vehicle. Euthanasia is therefore the humane method of ending an animal's life in the most pain-free and least stressful way possible.

> **Euthanasia is the humane method of alleviating animal suffering in cases of chronic or incurable disease, pain or injury.**

When making clinical decisions regarding euthanasia, consider the following:

- Owner involvement, discussion and consent
- Methods of humane destruction
- Disposal of animal carcasses
- Support for owners
- Staff support

In many cases the owner may refuse euthanasia for various reasons:

- Cultural
- Religious
- Economic
- Lack of recognition of the pain and suffering of the animal
- Peer pressure from family or neighbours
- Desperation at losing a work animal, a significant financial asset
- Belief that the animal will get better

It is the veterinarian's job to spend time with the owner explaining the animal's current welfare status and prognosis, and to educate the owner in understanding the reasons for proposing euthanasia.

The chosen method of euthanasia will depend on availability, country, the skill or preference of the veterinarian and options for carcass disposal.

Methods of euthanasia   8.2

Any method chosen must fulfil the following criteria (Jones 1992, Knottenbelt 1995):

1. Effect a quick reliable death without pain
2. Cause rapid loss of consciousness, with minimum stress
3. Be safe for human operators and the public
4. Be non-reversible
5. Be economic
6. Be easy to handle, store and administer

Physical methods

Free bullet

A properly placed gunshot can cause immediate insensibility and humane death. In some circumstances, a gunshot may be the only practical method of euthanasia.

> **Shooting should only be performed by highly skilled personnel trained in the use of firearms and only in jurisdictions that allow for legal firearm use.**

Personnel, public, and nearby animal safety should be considered. The procedure should be performed outdoors and away from public access.

When euthanasing an animal by a gunshot to the head, the firearm should be aimed so that the projectile enters the brain, causing instant loss of consciousness. The appropriate firearm should be selected for the situation, with the goal being penetration and destruction of brain tissue *without* emergence from the contra lateral side of the head. A .22-calibre long rifle, a 9 mm or .38-calibre handgun will be sufficient for most equids. The use of hollow-point or soft nose bullets will increase brain destruction and reduce the chance of ricochet.

Note the following advice:

- If the animal cannot be handled in a safe manner it should be sedated in advance of shooting.
- Have two spare bullets immediately available in case the first one does not kill the animal.
- Load one bullet at a time, do not preload all bullets into the gun in advance of shooting the animal because, if an animal is not killed with the first shot and in panic a second shot is fired inappropriately, this can be a major hazard to personnel.
- The person shooting the animal needs to be aware of his/her safety as he/she will need to be standing directly in front of the animal to ensure an accurate shot. The animal may fall forward when shot, so be ready to move quickly out of the way.
- The person firing the gun should also be in charge of holding the animal (e.g. via the lead-rope); there should be no other personnel or animals in the firing line.
- Imagine a line between the medial canthus of each eye and the base of each ear, forming a cross (Figure 8.2.1). The correct place to shoot a horse is around 2–3 cm above the point where the lines cross; 1–2 cm for a donkey.

8 EUTHANASIA

- The firearm should be aimed directly down the neck, perpendicular to the front of the skull, and held just away from the point of impact (Figure 8.2.2). It is important that the gun is not held in contact with the animal's head as this will not allow for the escape of muzzle gases.

Penetrating captive bolt

A penetrating captive bolt fires a retractable bolt several inches into the skull of an animal. Although it is reported that, when used properly, a penetrating captive bolt gun produces immediate brain tissue destruction and death in the animal, in practice this is not consistent. In other species it is normally recommended that pithing (destroying the brainstem mechanically using a rod inserted through the hole made by the captive bolt) should follow the use of a penetrative captive bolt.

> **It should be the standard requirement with this method of euthanasia in equids that pithing is always carried out following use of a penetrating captive bolt.**

Non-penetrative captive bolts (which have a mushroom-shaped end and do not make a hole in the skull) are *not* suitable for euthanasia of equids.

Before using the penetrative captive bolt for euthanasia, staff must be trained both in using and maintaining it, and in the technique of pithing. Furthermore, all those present during this procedure should understand the procedure and that the animal may show violent reactions while being pithed (although this is purely due to brainstem destruction and no pain is experienced by the animal).

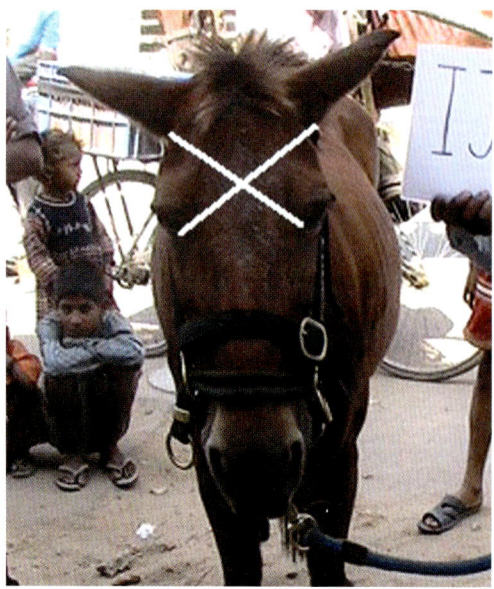

Figure 8.2.1 Imagine two lines drawn from the base of the ears to the medial canthi of the eyes. Aim to shoot a horse 2–3 cm above the place where the lines cross (white cross in photograph), and a donkey 1–2 cm above the cross.

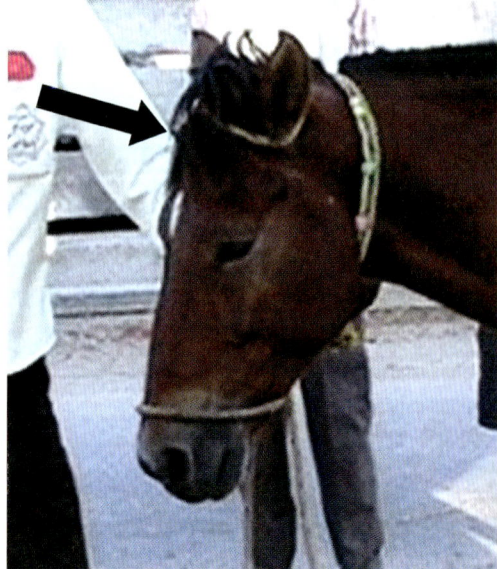

Figure 8.2.2 Black arrow showing the direction of aim of a firearm or captive bolt.

Captive bolts are powered by gunpowder, thus the selection of the cartridge strength should be appropriate for the size of the animal (adult versus foal); this varies among manufacturers. The penetrating captive bolt gun should be placed firmly against the skull at the same location previously described for gunshot. If the captive bolt is not in firm contact an incomplete stun may occur. Equids must be adequately restrained and, ideally, sedated to ensure proper placement of the captive bolt.

Pithing should be carried out immediately after firing the captive bolt. Animals will show spasms immediately following use of the captive bolt; however this must not delay the operator in pithing as quickly as possible. Ideally a specially designed pithing rod should be used. If this is not available a straightened metal coat hanger, a knitting needle, or other similar stiff rod of sufficiently small diameter to pass into the brain cavity through the captive bolt entry hole may be used. The pithing tool is introduced into the brain cavity and down into the spinal canal. Thrusting movements are used to ensure rapid and complete destruction of the brainstem. The animal may thrash violently while this is carried out: this is a result of the stimulation/destruction of nervous tissue rather than a sign of pain.

Severance of the aorta

This technique is not advocated as it can be highly dangerous for the operator as death may be violent. It involves cutting the aorta per-rectum and should only be attempted as a last choice if the animal is already anaesthetised (Knottenbelt 2006).

Pharmacological (chemical) euthanasia

In general this will consist of 2 steps:

> 1. Sedation or general anaesthesia of the animal
> 2. Administering an agent to kill the animal

Several different agents can be administered to kill the animal, and the depth of anaesthesia necessary for each agent varies.

> **It is essential that, before administering any agent that brings about death by cardiac arrest (e.g. saturated potassium salt solutions), the animal should be fully anaesthetised.**

Cardiac arrest is extremely painful and sedation alone is not sufficient.

When using pharmacological agents for euthanasia, it is important to consider the impact on **carcass disposal** as agents may present a risk to the environment and may also make the carcass toxic to any animal that might feed on it.

In all cases, it is important to ensure that all drugs are drawn up and ready before starting the euthanasia procedure. Pre-placement of a jugular catheter (preferably 14G) is also necessary due to the large volumes of drugs that need to be injected.

8 EUTHANASIA

Barbiturates

- Pentobarbitone sodium
- Thiopentone (see below in conjunction with KCl)

When properly administered by the intravenous route, barbiturate overdose depresses the central nervous system, causing deep anaesthesia progressing to respiratory and cardiac arrest. However, barbiturates can cause sudden or violent falls if administered too slowly or in insufficient quantities (see Table 8.2.1 for reported doses). Thus, the use of sedatives is advised (e.g. xylazine or detomidine) prior to the barbiturate overdose to minimise violent thrashing and provide more controlled progression to recumbency. Barbiturate overdose is less disturbing to observers (more aesthetically acceptable). It is relatively inexpensive.

> Ensure a catheter is placed as large volumes are needed.

In many countries, barbiturates may not be available or may be subject to specific legislation. Furthermore, carcass disposal after using them can be especially difficult as the drug persists in the carcass and may cause sedation or even death of animals that consume the body.

Drug	Dose	Reference
alpha2-agonist (e.g. xylazine)	See Table 7.1.2	See Table 7.1.2
pentobarbitone sodium	Range from 20–30 mg/kg to 40 mg/kg	Jones 1992, Knottenbelt 2006

Table 8.2.1 Reported dose rate of pentobarbitone sodium for euthanasia.

Potassium chloride

> Use of potassium chloride for euthanasia is unacceptable unless the animal is fully anaesthetised (Jones 1992).

The use of a supersaturated solution of potassium chloride injected intravenously (or, as a last course of action, intracardiac) **in an animal under general anaesthesia** is an acceptable method to produce cardiac arrest and death. For reported doses see table 8.2.2.

The high concentration of potassium ions is cardiotoxic, and rapid intravenous (or intracardiac) administration of 1–2 mmol/kg of body weight will cause cardiac arrest. This is the preferred injectable technique in situations where there is any risk that carcasses of euthanased animals may be consumed.

Potassium chloride is not a controlled substance. It is easily acquired, transported and prepared for use in the field. However, it is of the utmost importance that personnel performing this technique are trained and knowledgeable in anaesthetic techniques, and are competent in assessing the anaesthetic depth appropriate for administration of potassium chloride intravenously.

> **Administration of potassium chloride intravenously requires animals to be in a surgical plane of anaesthesia characterised by loss of consciousness, loss of reflex muscle response, and loss of response to noxious stimuli.**

Saturated potassium chloride solutions are effective in causing cardiac arrest following rapid intracardiac or intravenous injection. The residual tissue concentrations of general anaesthetics after anaesthetic induction have not been documented. No toxicoses have been reported in wildlife scavengers that might access and consume carcasses euthanased with potassium chloride in combination with a general anaesthetic. However, proper carcass disposal should always be attempted to prevent possible toxicosis by consumption of a carcass contaminated with general anaesthetics.

Drug	Dose	Reference
Thiopentone	5–11 g/kg	Abass *et al.* 1994, Muir and Scicluna 1998
Potassium chloride	1–2 mmol/kg	AVMA 2007

Table 8.2.2 Reported euthanasia protocol using thiopentone and potassium chloride.

Cinchocaine and quinalbarbitine

Available as a single preparation for use with or without prior sedation. Do not use with xylazine as violent reactions can occur which then negatively affect the procedure (Knottenbelt 1995). It is not available in all countries; however, when used correctly, injected over a period of 12–15 seconds, collapse occurs within 40 seconds and death within 2–3 minutes (Knottenbelt 1995).

Other injectable agents

- **Magnesium sulphate** Saturated solution administered after sedation (xylazine) and anaesthesia (thiopentone) has been induced – although condemned for use in equids by the AVMA (2007).

- **Chloral hydrate** Do not use as sole agent – large volumes are needed, at least three times the anaesthetic dose (Jones 1992).

- **Muscle relaxants** e.g. suxamethonium (succinylcholine at 0.1 mg/kg) – **Never** use in isolation, but it can be combined with or given shortly after barbiturates (thiopentone 10 mg/kg), or ketamine, to produce death (Jones 1992, Jones and Knottenbelt 2001, Knottenbelt 2006).

In some countries, none of the above agents is available and other agents will need to be sourced. In these cases, the considerations discussed above still apply. The methods should be discussed within the veterinary team with advice sought externally if required. Always consider the effectiveness of the agent, training of staff, the welfare and experience of the animal, and carcass disposal.

Confirmation of death

> Confirmation of death is essential.

Immediately following delivery of the euthanasia method a standing animal should collapse. It may experience a period of muscle contraction (usually no longer than 20 seconds). This may be followed by a period of relaxation and some poorly coordinated kicking or paddling movements. The pupils of the eyes will be fully dilated. The animal must be checked within 5 minutes to confirm death (Figure 8.2.3).

> Death may be confirmed by the absence of breathing, absence of a heartbeat (pulse), and absence of a corneal reflex (blinking).

To check the corneal reflex, touch the animal's cornea (surface of the eye). There should be no response if the animal is dead. The presence of any eye movement or blinking at this time is evidence of sustained or recovering brain activity; repeat the same or an alternative euthanasia procedure.

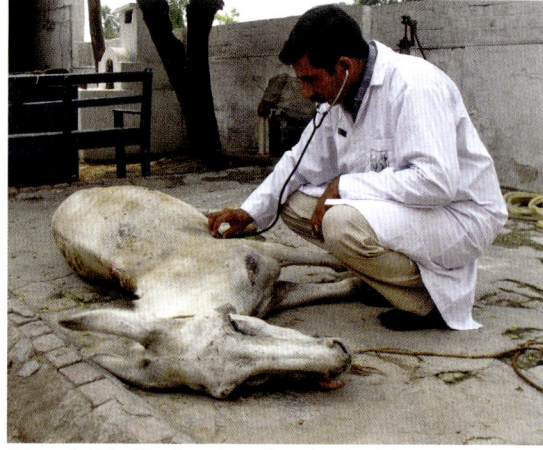

Figure 8.2.3 Check and confirm death of the animal.

Agents that should not be used for euthanasia in equids

- Strychnine
- Hydrogen cyanide
- Nicotine

All of these hypoxic agents are very dangerous to the humans administering them (Jones 1992). Strychnine and hydrogen cyanide both produce violent convulsions before death, and nicotine also produces undesirable stimulation of the central nervous system.

Case study – Euthanasia 8.3

Location Gujranwala, Pakistan

Attending veterinarian Dr Javed Iqbal Gondal

History
Type of work animal was doing: Transportation of goods by carriage or cart in the city area

Number hours per day/days per week the animal worked: 12 hours per day, 6 days per week

Name and age of animal: Rambo, a 22-year-old donkey

It was an extremely hot humid day. The veterinarian encountered Nisar Ahmad and Rambo at the road side. The cart was loaded with heavy goods and the animal was in a terrible condition. Nisar Ahmad was going to the bazaar to unload the goods in a shop; he also had other goods for transportation for the rest of the day. But Rambo was suffering considerably.

Clinical examination findings
Rambo was lame, unable to walk properly and over-loaded; Rambo was not able to work properly (Figure 8.3.1). His owner forced Rambo to work which was very difficult for the animal.

Problems seen:
- Eye problems/poor eye sight
- Very bad lip lesions at both commissures
- Incisor over-bite
- Irregular molars
- Deformed limbs and bowed tendons
- Arthritis of all four fetlock joints
- Thrush in both hind feet
- Severe lameness
- Bronchitis
- Fistulous withers

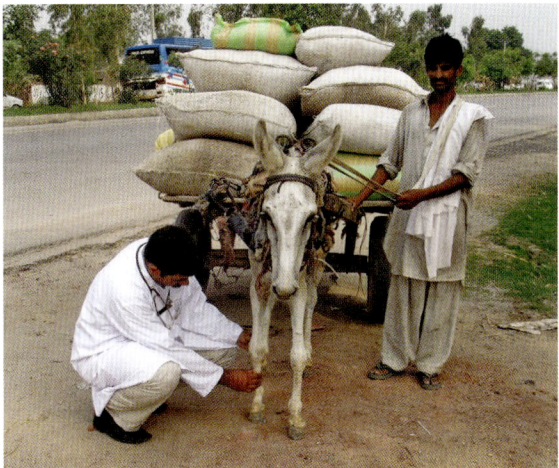

Figure 8.3.1 Initial examination at the roadside.

Diagnosis
Rambo was in considerable suffering and pain, with multiple chronic conditions and an inability to continue working.

Initial treatment
Analgesia was given to Rambo and the owner was asked to meet the veterinarian the next day for further discussion.

Follow-up
The next morning, the veterinarian visited Nisar Ahmad's home and saw Rambo. There was no proper shade or shelter and water for Rambo. Examination showed all of Rambo's welfare needs were compromised including the above list plus multiple galls and severe dehydration.

After a long discussion, the owner was persuaded that Rambo was unfit for work and in severe pain. He agreed to euthanasia (Figure 8.3.2).

8 EUTHANASIA

Procedure for euthanasia
The animal was euthanased by chemical injection using the following procedure:

- Firstly, permission taken from owner and consent form signed
- Animal sedated with xylazine 1.1mg/kg IV
- Administered thiopentone sodium 10mg/kg, slow IV
- Followed by saturated solution of magnesium sulphate
- Confirmed death: absence of breathing, heart beat and corneal reflex

Disposal of carcass
A contract exists with the local municipal committee who collects the carcass and then disposes by proper burial.

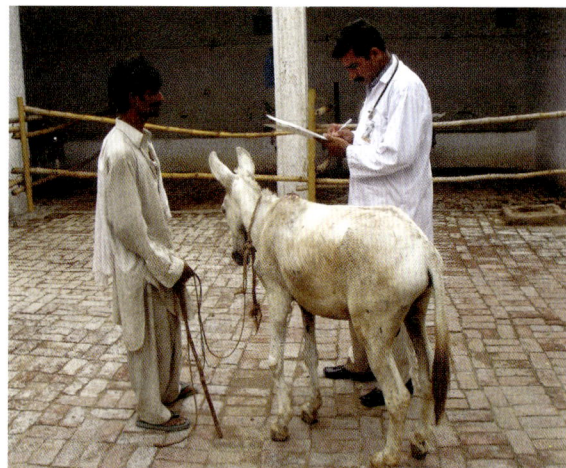

Figure 8.3.2 Consultation with the owner on the decision to euthanase, with written consent obtained.

Discussion
It can be very difficult to persuade poor equine owners to euthanase their animals. Discussion highlighting the income loss, feeding costs and poor welfare of the animal can help to persuade owners. The owner's wife also played a vital role. The couple have since purchased a new animal.

References

8.4

Abass, B.T., Weaver, B.M.Q., Staddon, G.E., Waterman, A.W. (1994) Pharmacokinetics of thiopentone in the horse. *J. vet. Pharmacol. Therap.* 17, 331–338.

AVMA (2007) AVMA guidelines on euthanasia. (Online) Available at http://www.avma.org/issues/animal_welfare/euthanasia.pdf (accessed 13 December 2012).

Knottenbelt, D.C. (1995) Euthanasia of the horse – alternatives to the bullet. *In Practice.* 17, 462–464.

Knottenbelt, D.C. (2006) Equine formulary. Saunders Elsevier Ltd. pp. 311–320.

Jones, R.S. (1992) Euthanasia in horses. *Equine vet. Educ.* 4 (3), 154–157.

Jones, R.S., Knottenbelt, D.C. (2001) Disagree with use of muscle relaxant before euthanasia. (letter) *J. Am. Vet. Med. Assoc.* 218 (12), 1884.

Muir, W.W., Scicluna, C. (1998) Anaesthesia and anaesthetic techniques in horses. *Equine vet Educ.* 10 (1), 33–41.

Further reading

UC Davis. Emergency Euthanasia of Horses. (online) Available at http://www.vetmed.ucdavis.edu/vetext/animalwelfare/euthanasia/emergEuth_horses2-2.pdf (accessed 13 December 2012).

Ophthalmology

9

Introduction	9.1
Equine vision and blindness	9.2
Anatomy of the eye and clinical significance of these structures	9.3
Ophthalmic examination and diagnostic tools	9.4
Ocular therapeutics – Preparation, administration and principles	9.5
Common eye diseases	9.6
Case study – Ophthalmic habronemiasis	9.7
References	9.8

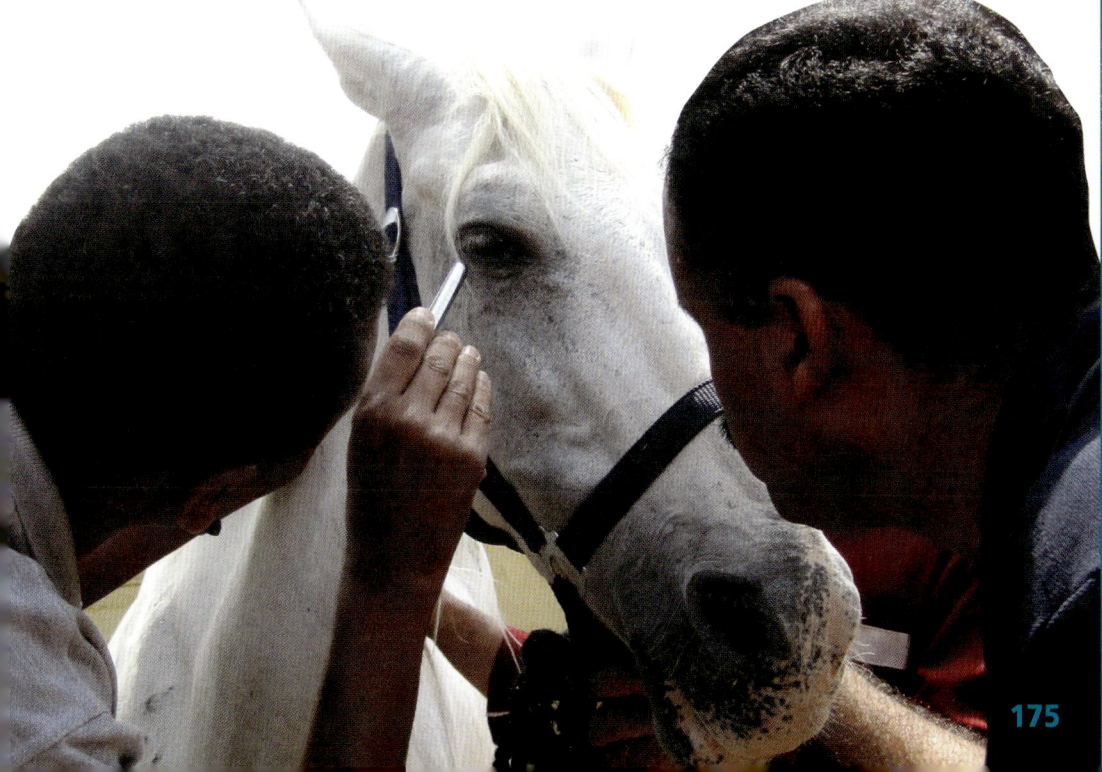

9.1 Introduction

Eye problems are commonly encountered in the working equid population, and in most cases they are preventable. Most eye problems begin as a slight discharge caused by irritation from dust, flies or poorly fitting blinkers. However, due to the intense inflammatory reaction of equine eyes, the initial problem can quickly progress to scarring and blindness.

It is very important to understand how the eye functions and the importance of good husbandry. Advising the owner on early recognition of ocular changes and good eye management is an important responsibility as a working equine veterinarian. Prevention is better than cure.

9.2 Equine vision and blindness

How do equids see the world?

Equine eyes are designed to detect motion and act as an 'early-warning system' for predators. Equids have a wide range of vision, greater than 350 degrees (Hanggi and Ingersoll 2012) due to the positioning of the eyes on the sides of the head (Figure 9.2.1) with only two 'blind' spots; right in front of the head and right behind the tail. This allows them to see approaching predators even when their heads are lowered for grazing, initiating the 'flight' response if necessary (see Section 2.2 *Behaviour*).

The majority of the equine retina is comprised of rods with no area having only cones. This means that they are able to detect movement well, especially in low-level lighting (Saslow 2002).

There is limited information available on equine vision, evaluation of vision loss, or correction of vision defects.

Do equids have colour vision?

Reports state limited colour vision in horses (Saslow 2002); some studies found an ability for horses to distinguish red, blue, yellow and green from grey, but the number of animals in the studies was very small (Hanggi and Ingersoll 2007).

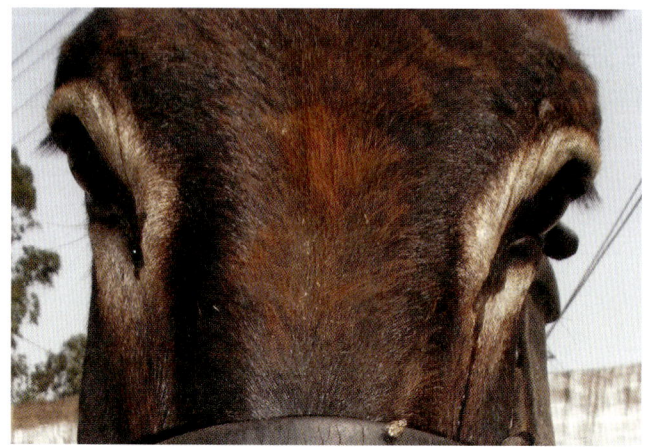

Figure 9.2.1 The equine eyes are positioned on the sides of the head to allow a wide range of vision.

ANATOMY OF THE EYE AND CLINICAL SIGNIFICANCE OF THESE STRUCTURES 9.2

> Question: *Which of the Five Freedoms is compromised in a blind animal?*
> Answer: Potentially all!

Blindness

Signs of blindness

- Bumping into objects
- High-stepping gait
- Reluctance to move forwards or turn
- Difficult to lead
- Fear/nervousness
- Startled easily

Blindness due to chronic injury vs. sudden onset

> **In working equids, it is rare to find blindness without any sign of chronic eye damage.**

As stated earlier, most cases of vision loss in working equids will be due to chronic eye irritation leading to uveitis, corneal scarring and cataracts. Sudden onset blindness will most likely occur from damage to the optic nerve or retina from trauma such as head injuries or acute blood loss.

> **In true acute blindness, the pupil will be dilated, whereas blindness due to chronic irritation will normally have signs of pupil constriction, chronic uveitis, keratitis or injury.**

In the same way that humans adapt, working equids may not show overt signs of blindness if kept in familiar conditions. However, once a routine is changed, the owner may notice something is wrong, and punish the animal for not going forwards. It is the responsibility of a veterinarian to diagnose blindness and inform the owner on ways to manage this. The animal may suffer unnecessary harsh treatment from the owner if a visual impairment is not diagnosed and treated. At the very least the animal will experience fear and distress if it cannot see properly from both eyes.

9.3 Anatomy of the eye and clinical significance of these structures

Orbit

The equid has a complete bony orbit. If the orbit is fractured concurrent palpation of both orbits will reveal crepitus.

Globe (eyeball)

Look at the size of the eyeball and compare to the other eye. The angle of the eyelashes and protrusion of the third eyelid often indicates an abnormal globe size, especially when the other eye is normal. A smaller globe (usually resulting from injury or chronic disease) should be differentiated from exophthalmos and enophthalmos.

> **Enophthalmos** The normal-sized globe recedes into the orbit, usually as a result of pain (Firshman *et al.* 2003).
>
> **Exophthalmos** The normal-sized globe is pushed forwards, usually due to retrobulbar disease, e.g. abscess/tumour in the orbit behind the globe (Naylor *et al.* 2010).

Eyelids

- The upper eyelids are used more in blinking than the lower, therefore any damage to the upper eyelids is extremely serious. To restore function very careful reconstruction, using good anatomical knowledge, must be carried out.

- Assess symmetry by comparing with the other eye, look out for swelling, tumours (Figure 9.3.1), wounds, etc.

- Eyelids must also be carefully inspected for signs of distichia (inappropriately placed eyelashes which could cause corneal ulceration) and foreign bodies.

- The orbicularis oculi muscle produces a strong closure of the eye and if stimulated may cause blepharospasm (an involuntary, forced closure of the eye) making examination impossible. The auriculopalpebral nerve block (see later in this chapter) can be used to stop blinking and make examination easier.

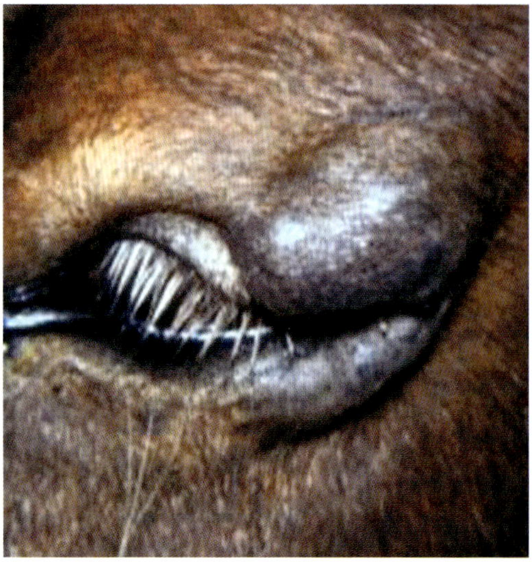

Figure 9.3.1 Appearance of a tumour involving the equine eyelids.

> Remember the auriculopalpebral nerve block is a motor function block and will not provide pain relief.

▌ The eyelids have a large blood supply. Surgical treatment of eyelid damage must be attempted **very carefully** as even a slight misalignment of wound edges can cause painful scarring, resulting in dysfunction of the eyelid and the inability for the eyelids to close, leading to dry eye and keratitis/uveitis and subsequent blindness.

Nictitating membrane (third eyelid)

Gently press the upper eyelid onto the globe to cause eversion of the third eyelid (Herring 2003). It can be assessed for tumours, or granulation tissue from *Habronema* infection (see later in this chapter). The ventral fornix can be inspected for foreign bodies by pulling the third eyelid out gently with soft-end forceps and looking into the space.

Lacrimal system

The nasolacrimal duct runs from a small hole in the medial corner of the eye and exits from the nose. It is this duct which allows fluorescein dye solution to exit from the nose when placed in the eye to examine for corneal ulceration (see Section 9.4). Dye should pass within a minute, but allow up to 5 minutes (Ramsey 2003). Blockage of the puncta, either from dirt, dust, *Habronema* infection or swellings, causes tears to build up and watering of the eye which results in further dust accumulation potentially leading to conjunctivitis and even more severe ocular pathology.

> The nasolacrimal duct can be catheterised and slowly flushed with warm saline. This is a good way to ensure a clear passage exists between the eyes and nose.

The nasolacrimal duct can also be used for medicating the eye, or flushing it, when the animal is head-shy; however, after repeated days of treatment the animal can become adverse to catheterisation.

Conjunctiva

These are the mucous membranes on the inside of the eyelids. Normally they are a pale pink colour and should be smooth and moist. They can be assessed for swelling, foreign bodies or inflammation; they are a place to assess mucous membrane colour.

Cornea

The cornea is a very thin epithelial layer over the front of the eyeball. It can be easily damaged by dust, flies and trauma, causing ulceration. Once the cornea is ulcerated, the return to full vision (if at all) is only possible if acted upon quickly. Equids have intense inflammatory reactions in the eye and scarring occurs quickly which permanently affects the vision.

> The normal cornea will have no blood vessels and will be transparent.

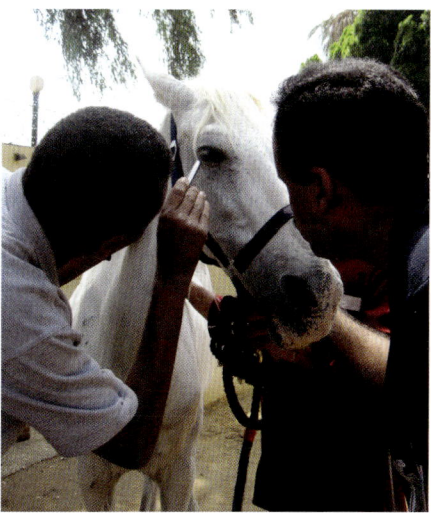

Figure 9.3.2 Examination of the eye with a pen torch.

9 OPHTHALMOLOGY

Any disruption to the cornea will cause opacity which results in various colour changes to the eye (see Table 9.3.1).

Using a pen torch correctly (see detailed examination of the eye later in this chapter and Figure 9.3.2) will help differentiate between corneal opacities and a generalised problem within the globe, such as pus/blood/oedema in the anterior chamber.

Colour of the cornea	Potential cause	Photograph to illustrate
Blue/opaque	Corneal oedema: **Focal** Injury from external source, e.g. a stick, or directly around a corneal ulcer **Diffuse** More widespread intraocular inflammation, glaucoma	
Red	Corneal vascularisation: **Focal** Superficial injury. Blood vessels will grow from the limbal area (edge of the eye) towards an injured area of cornea, bringing cells and nutrients to assist healing. This takes time and, if blood vessels are present, it indicates that the corneal injury has not recently occurred. **Diffuse inflammation** With more widespread inflammation, blood and superficial blood vessels may be seen across the cornea. These can be circumferential and an indicator of widespread diffuse inflammation.	
White	Corneal scarring from an old injury. If a scar is present there will be no active inflammation in the eye. Provided it is small or out of the field of vision, it may have no impact on sight. However, if extensive and across the field of vision it can extensively limit sight.	
Other	Pus (yellow) from intraocular bacterial infection, or other colours due to corneal pigmentation, neoplasia	

(Dwyer 2012)

Table 9.3.1 Corneal colour changes and potential causes.

ANATOMY OF THE EYE AND CLINICAL SIGNIFICANCE OF THESE STRUCTURES 9.3

Anterior chamber

In a healthy eye the anterior chamber is filled with a clear fluid called aqueous humour. Abnormal contents (such as pus or blood from haemorrhage) can be seen in the ventral portion of the anterior chamber often obscuring the iris in this region. If there is severe damage the entire anterior chamber can fill with inflammatory exudate or pus and the whole eye looks a different colour. (This must be differentiated from problems isolated to the cornea).

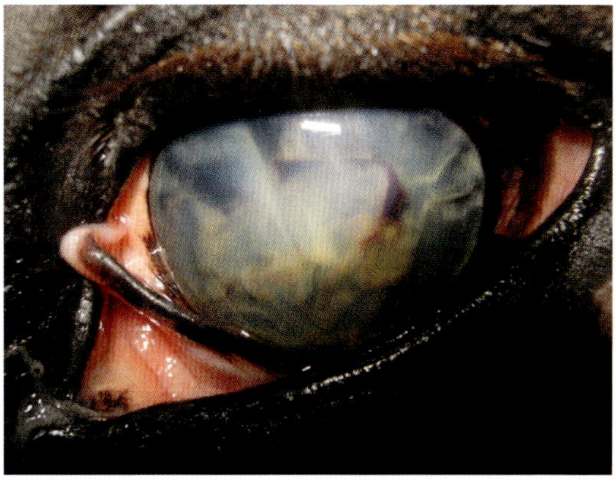

Appearance of the anterior chamber:

- **Yellow/white** Diffuse inflammation, fibrin or infection (Figure 9.3.3) Do not drain!
- **Red** Haemorrhage or settling of red blood cells from an earlier bleed
- **Black/brown** Pupil distortion, iris adhesion, or neoplasia
- **Blue** Diffuse oedema

Figure 9.3.3 Inflammatory changes in the anterior chamber, the posterior structures of the eye can no longer be seen.

Iris

Usually brown coloured in most equids (Figure 9.3.4) but can be blue or white ('wall eye') in some animals (Figure 9.3.5); these are more common in colour dilute equids such as appaloosas, piebalds and skewbalds.

In equids, the iris has proliferative, well vascularised extensions of the iris that look like black cystic masses along the edge of the iris. These are not pathological; they are known as 'corpora nigra' (Figure 9.3.5) and are a variation of normal.

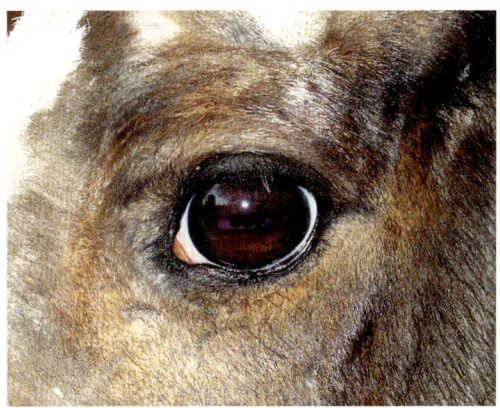

Figure 9.3.4 A brown-coloured iris.

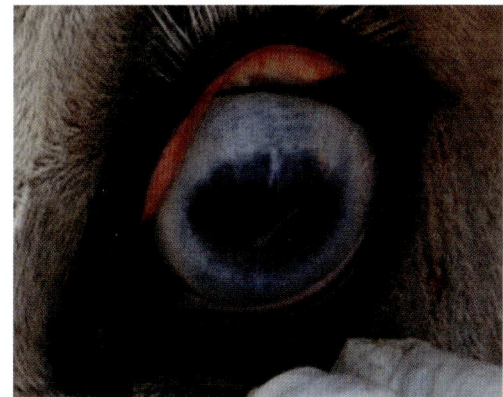

Figure 9.3.5 A blue-coloured iris or 'wall' eye.

181

9 OPHTHALMOLOGY

Pupil

The pupil is the black space in the middle of the eye. The pupillary light reflex/response (PLR) – a reduction in pupil size when light is shone on the eye – indicates whether the nerve pathways (retina, cranial nerves II and III) are working correctly, see Section 9.4 (Dwyer 2012). The equine pupil reduces down to a thin horizontal gap, see Figure 9.3.4 (not round as in humans). As light is shone in one eye there is a consensual response in the opposite eye where the pupil also constricts slightly.

The pupil can look distorted if there is neoplasia or scarring of the ciliary body preventing normal movement of the iris. During the inflammatory processes which occur with intraocular disease, adhesions can form between the iris and other structures; these are known as synechiae and are permanent. The normal oval shape of the iris will be distorted and this area will be unable to move, which can be easily assessed by the PLR.

Lens

The lens needs to be clear for the animal to see. A cloudy lens could either be a cataract or nuclear sclerosis which is a hardening of the lens in old animals where the fundus is still visible. Alternatively, lens luxation can occur secondary to trauma or uveitis (see detailed eye examination later). Any condition involving the lens requires surgery with specialist ophthalmological equipment, personnel and facilities; thus it is not suitable for field conditions. Common variations of normal may be seen, such as an 'onion ring' appearance which is of no concern.

Figure 9.3.6 shows a horse with anterior lens luxation in the left eye; this is not the normal position of the lens. There are also corneal striae on the corneal surface – this could be an indication of glaucoma.

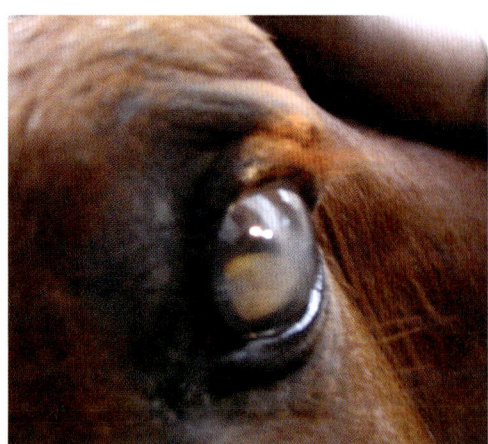

Figure 9.3.6 Anterior lens luxation in the eye of a horse.

Fundus (retina and optic nerve)

> The structures at the back of the eye (fundus) can only be viewed with an ophthalmoscope and good pupil dilation.

There is a large variation in what is considered normal when examining an equine retina; both eyes should always be checked and this can provide a useful comparison, unless the pathology is bilateral. Refer to ophthalmic texts for further information on this, as well as Section 9.4 of this chapter.

Retina This contains neurosensory epithelium and is responsible for vision. It contains photoreceptors (rods and cones) which turn the light that reaches the back of the eye (fundus) into electrical impulses.

- **The tapetal fundus** is located dorsally. It is hyper-reflective and improves night vision. It can be green, yellow, blue or red.

  Note: In colour dilute horses it can be absent and the underlying vessels will be visible in a tree-like pattern.

- **The non-tapetal fundus** is located ventrally. It is usually brown/black in colour due to pigmented cells within the retina.

  Note: In colour dilute horses there can be none of this pigmentation so the underlying vessels will be visible in a tree-like pattern.

- **The optic disc** is normally circular in shape and salmon pink with many blood vessels extending out from it. It is situated just below the junction of the tapetal and non-tapetal fundus. The disc is where the optic nerve enters/leaves the retina and is also the entry point for many of the blood vessels which supply the retina and vitreous humour.

Ophthalmic examination and diagnostic tools

Examine the eye in a routine manner so nothing is missed. The early signs of ocular disease can be very subtle so a thorough examination is vital. It is extremely important to spend time with the owners of working equids stressing the importance of referring any eye problem to a trained health professional at an early stage in order to prevent serious complications arising, as these may end up threatening the vision of the animal (Dwyer 2012). Ensure that all foals, as well as older animals, have an eye examination. General aspects of an ophthalmic examination can be incorporated into all general clinical examinations to pick up any early symptoms of eye disease before they progress into serious eye problems (Figure 9.4.1).

Take a good 'eye' history

- Does the animal have problems seeing things? If so, for how long has it done so?
- Is the problem worse in one eye, or present in both?
- Is there a previous history of eye problems?
- Has there been any medication given previously?
- Are there any signs of pain in the eye?
- Are there signs of ocular discharge?
- Are there signs of upper airway respiratory disease?
- Is the problem getting worse, better, or staying the same?
- Are any other animals affected?

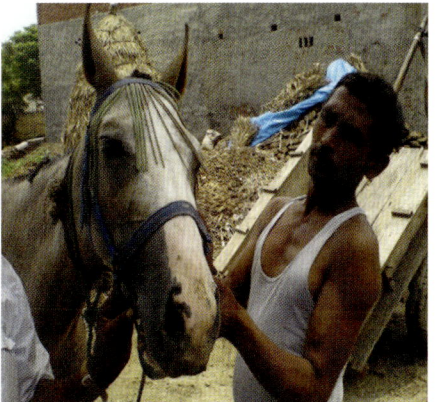

Figure 9.4.1 Take a full history and perform a clinical examination.

9 OPHTHALMOLOGY

Signs of ocular disease

Signs of an eye problem are closely associated with ocular pain (see Chapter 3 *Pain*).

- Epiphora (excessive tearing) (See Figure 9.4.2)
- Blepharospasm (blinking)
- Blepharoedema (swollen eyelids/conjunctivae)
- Enophthalmos (normal-sized globe that is retracted into the orbit)
- Third eyelid prolapse
- Change in eye colour/cloudiness to the cornea
- Photophobia (sensitivity to light)
- Miosis (constricted pupil as a result of ciliary body spasticity)
- Reluctance to allow examination (head shy)
- Depression and anorexia

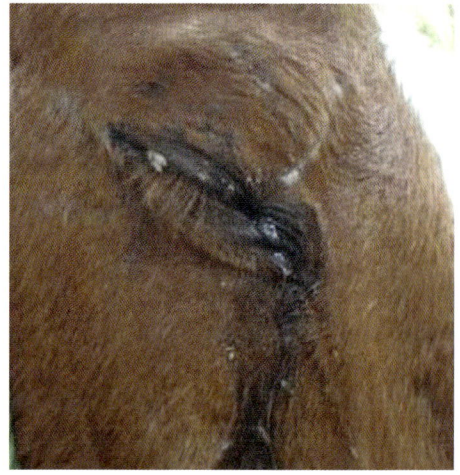

Figure 9.4.2 Epiphora (excessive tearing) and blepharospasm.

Initial examination of the eye in good light

For all examinations of the eyes ensure there is a competent handler, or sedate the animal if it is in distress or severe pain. Keep the handler on the opposite side of the head to the examiner so that there is space to view the eye easily.

> **Always examine both eyes.**

Ocular discharge: Any amount is significant.

- **Colour** Clear indicates viral infection or allergy, whereas yellow/green suggests bacterial infection.
- **Consistency** Watery indicates ongoing/acute condition, whereas dry/crusting indicates chronicity.
- **Amount** Viral infections usually produce small amounts compared to the 'streaming' eyes associated with allergy or the presence of a foreign body.
- **Lacrimal duct obstruction** Suspect with signs of *Habronema* infection.

Always have an examination plan and check in a systemic way for any abnormalities to focus on when doing the detailed ophthalmic examination (Figure 9.4.3).

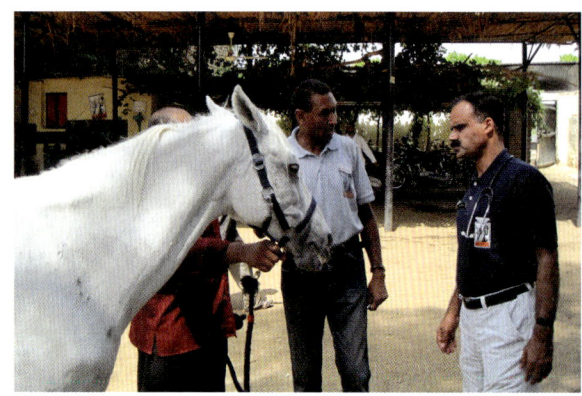

Figure 9.4.3 Initial examination from a distance.

OPHTHALMIC EXAMINATION AND DIAGNOSTIC TOOLS 9.4

Detailed eye examination

Equipment required: Dark area, pen torch, ophthalmoscope (if available, although an examination can be achieved with a pen torch alone)

A dark area and a quiet, calm animal are the two factors standing between a detailed examination and an examination where nothing useful is discovered. It is very important to have a competent handler. If there is not a trained equine handler available, select a competent person from the local community – this may not be the animal's owner, and often it is best if not, as the owner will want to observe and discuss the examination rather than staying on the opposite side of the head and concentrating on calming the animal.

Table 9.4.1 lists the anatomical structures of the eye and the abnormalities to look out for in the examination.

Structure	Abnormalities to look for
Globe	Exophthalmos/enophthalmos
Eyelids	Wounds, swellings
Conjunctiva	Colour, swelling, foreign bodies
Third eyelid	Protrusion, swellings, granulation tissue, foreign body trapped underneath the third eyelid
Cornea	Opacity, ulcers, vascularisation, oedema, rupture
Anterior chamber or 'aqueous humour'	Blood (hyphaema), pus (hypopyon), foreign bodies, 'aqueous flare' (mild greyish appearance of aqueous humour)
Iris	Size, symmetry, shape, colour changes, swellings, synechiae (adherence to back of cornea or front of lens), pupillary light response
Lens	Cloudiness, cataracts
Vision	*See vision tests below.*

Table 9.4.1 Anatomical structures visible in normal light and associated abnormalities.

> **Acute eye conditions will be very painful.**

It is likely that even a chronic condition will have left the animal head-shy at some point in the early, painful stages. For this reason consider local anaesthesia (topical or via nerve blocks, see below) or even sedation to assist in the examination, especially if examination of the eye is not possible or a foreign body needs to be removed.

When out in the field, a dark area can be created if the animal allows a blanket to be placed over both the examiner's and the animals' head. However, this can be very dangerous for both parties so only attempt if the animal is known and fear and distress can be minimised. Consider sedation.

9 OPHTHALMOLOGY

Ophthalmic reflex testing

Pupillary light reflex (PLR)

- This is the reduction of pupil size in response to a light source.
- It tests the functionality of the optic nerve – cranial nerve (CN) II, the retina (sensory arm of the reflex) and the parasympathetic portion of the oculomotor nerve – CN III (motor arm of the reflex resulting in iris constriction).

> - This test needs to be done in a dark area so that the pupils are dilated in response to decreased light.

- Shine the pen torch in the eye and observe constriction of the pupils. This should occur in both eyes since the neuronal pathways cross over. When a light is shone in one eye, ensure that the pupil in the other eye constricts as well – the 'consensual reflex'. (The opposite eye will constrict less than the one with the light shining in it.)
- This reflex shows that the retina and the nerves to and from the eye are working. However, it does not necessarily indicate that the eye is visual as it is a subcortical reflex, and, therefore, does not involve the brain cortex which is required for vision.
- If the pupil is obscured by pathology in one eye, the PLR can still be tested by shining a light in the affected eye and looking for constriction in the other normal eye – i.e. checking the consensual reflex (Dwyer 2012).

Dazzle response

- A bright light is suddenly shone in the eye and the animal will partially close the eyelids to retract the globe.
- Loss of this subcortical reflex could be due to damage in any of the following areas: retina, rostral colliculus, supraoptic hypothalamic nuclei, or CN II, CN VII, and the orbicularis oculi muscle controlling closure of the eyelids (Dwyer 2012).

Palpebral blink reflex

- This tests the functionality of the trigeminal nerve (CN V) and the facial nerve (CN VII).
- Touching a clean cotton bud onto the skin next to the medial canthus should cause a blink reaction (eyelids close). Any area of the immediate peri-ocular skin can be touched for this test, but do not touch the eye itself as this could scratch the cornea.
- If there has been damage to either the CN V or VII there will be no blink reflex (Dwyer 2012).

Menace response

- This test produces a blink or head withdrawal response by the animal in reaction to a threatening movement towards the eye.
- It assesses vision (retina), the function of the oculomotor nerve (CN III), which is responsible for eye movement, and CN VII.

> - In a neonate the menace response may be absent until 1–2 months of age.

- This test is done by standing at the side of the animal and moving a hand quickly towards the eye. Be careful not to create air currents when doing this, as the animal will blink from the sensation of air moving near its face rather than because it can visualise the 'menace' threat.

- If there is no response this may indicate damage to CN III, CN VII, the retina or the visual cortex.

Corneal response

- Touching the cornea will result in closure of the eyelids.
- This assesses CN V and VII. Damage to these nerves (or other pathologies) will result in inability of the eyelids to close, preventing the blink response.

> Take care with this test. Ensure that anything used to touch the cornea is clean and preferably sterile (a sterile sampling swab is a ideal). Ensure the animal is calm and well handled so as not to cause any iatrogenic injury to the cornea.

Diagnostic tests

Intraocular Pressure (IOP)

- IOP should be the same over all areas of the globe; it measures the hydrostatic aqueous pressure. Reported normal values in horses give a range of 17–28 mmHg.

- IOP can be raised due to inflammation in the eye and is commonly associated with glaucoma and chronic uveitis. Although a tonometer is the tool of choice, it is possible to make an estimate of increased pressure by gently palpating both globes through the eyelids at the same time, and making a comparison. Knowledge of whether IOP is raised can help differentiate exophthalmos (see above) from an enlarged globe due to glaucoma. Never place digital pressure on the globe unless it is through the eyelids.

- Studies have shown that IOP is reduced in horses sedated with xylazine and detomidine (Holve 2012) so bear this in mind when assessing and interpreting IOP in sedated equids. The study by Holve (2012) also suggested an initial increase in IOP after application of topical anaesthesia (proparacaine 2% ophthalmic solution).

> Remember that the height of the head (and therefore the eyes) relative to the height of the heart can affect IOP. Recommendations are to keep the head up for 10 minutes prior to measuring the IOP (Holve 2012).

Fluorescein test

- Fluorescein is an orange dye (in drops or strip form) used to diagnose corneal ulceration.
- Place in the eye and wait 2 minutes. (It can also be done by placing strip/drops in a syringe with 2 ml sterile saline and squirting gently into the eye, as for local anaesthesia below.)
- If a corneal ulcer is present, it will stain bright green (positive) due to the alkaline environment (Brooks 2012b) as shown in Figure 9.4.4.

- Fluorescein is a good tool to use to measure the healing progress of an ulcer. Draw diagrams of the ulcer in the clinical notes with mm measurements and assess the decrease in size over time.
- It can also be used to test the patency of the nasolacrimal duct – the dye should appear around the nose after a few minutes if the duct is clear; allow up to 5 minutes (Ramsey 2003).
- If the ulcer is very deep, a crater will form which will stain. However, if the base of this crater does not take up stain this indicates that the cornea has been eroded to the level of descemet's membrane – the final layer of the cornea. It is extremely important to recognise this; it very dangerous as it indicates that the cornea is close to perforation. Intensive treatment is required.

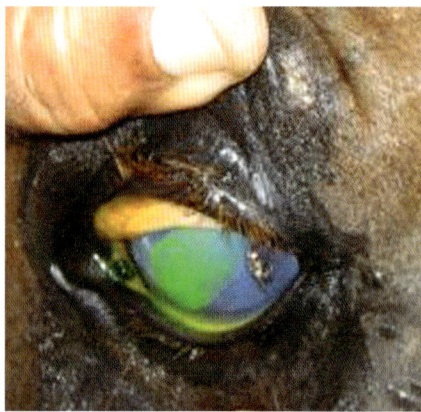

Figure 9.4.4 A positive fluorescein test result showing a superficial ulcer with no obvious crater.

> **Application of fluorescein dye should be a routine part of all ophthalmic examinations in order to detect early corneal ulcers (Brooks 2012b).**

Rose Bengal stain

- This is a red dye used to detect defects in the surface epithelium and defects in the mucin layer of the tear film (Brooks 2012b).
- It may also indicate fungal infections or inadequate tear film (Brooks 2003, Dwyer 2012).
- There are varying reports on whether this is an irritant for the eye (Brooks 2012b).
- Place Rose Bengal in the eye after the fluorescein test.
- It is an important test to use in cases on non-healing ulcers (Brooks 2012b).

Schirmer Tear test

- This measures reflex tear production: the pre-corneal tear film.
- Application of topical anaesthetic (1% tropicamide) to the eye, prior to testing, significantly reduces tear production (Ghaffari *et al.* 2009).
- Test strips can be purchased – follow the instructions on the packet for application, length of time to be left in place (usually 60 seconds) and interpretation of reading.

> **Take care in interpretation as there are reported differences over the day, season, gender and sides! (Piccione *et al.* 2008, Beech *et al.* 2003).**

- Values from 10 mm to over 35 mm have been reported as normal (Beech *et al.* 2003, Brooks 2012b). Lower values, less than 10 mm, indicate a reduced tear production, and very low values, less than 5 mm, indicate keratoconjunctivitis sicca (KCS) (Brooks 2012b).

Differentiating corneal injury from generalised intraocular conditions

If an ophthalmoscope is not available it is still possible to differentiate corneal injury from generalised intraocular conditions.

'How do I tell the difference between a focal problem with the cornea (e.g. corneal ulceration) and generalised inflammatory conditions of the eye such as uveitis – especially since both can present with similar signs of disease?'

Stand at the side of the animal in a dark area and shine the pen torch *through* the eye from the other side. Figure 9.4.5 shows the aspect to view the eye. By examining the eye from this direction it is possible to see whether the whole eye is cloudy (suspect intraocular disease), or whether it is just the cornea/anterior chamber affected. Use of fluorescein dye can help diagnose corneal ulceration if this is suspected (see below).

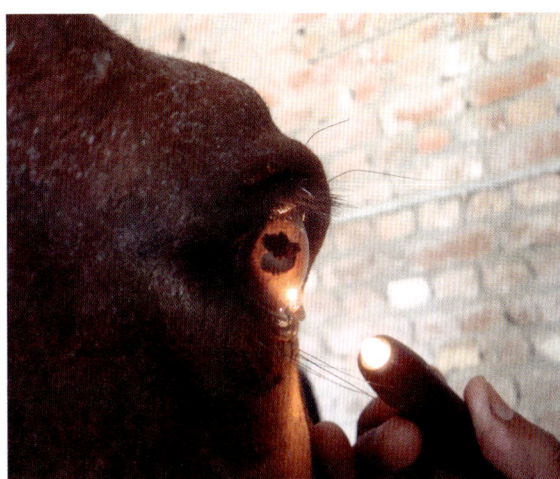

Figure 9.4.5 Angle of view to differentiate corneal conditions from more generalised inflammatory conditions. The corpora nigra can clearly be seen in this photograph.

In very severe corneal injury, a full-thickness injury to the cornea can occur and in these cases aqueous humour can be seen leaking from the defect, or part of the iris may be seen prolapsing through the defect. This is a very serious condition that requires emergency surgery with specialised ophthalmic surgical equipment which will be neither available nor appropriate for the field situation.

> A pen torch and a lot of practice looking at normal eyes will help make this differentiation.

Ophthalmoscopy

An ophthalmoscope is used to examine the fundus (retina, choroid, sclera and optic nerve). Alternatively, use a diopter lens to conduct *indirect ophthalmoscopy* in which the whole fundus is seen at once. Either way, a dilated pupil will enable visualisation of a much bigger area of the fundus than a constricted one. Atropine drops (0.2 ml 1%) will result in a dilated pupil after 15–20 minutes, and are helpful when attempting ophthalmoscopy.

Indirect ophthalmoscopy

Indirect ophthalmoscopy uses a focal light source (pen torch or transilluminator) and a separate diopter lens (condensing lens) to scan the whole retina. This is done by standing about an arm's length away from the eye and directing the light source into the diopter lens which is held next to the eye. Different magnifications depend on the lens type so identify the lens type in use. A reverse image is provided this way, hence the tapetum (coloured part) appears in the ventral portion of the eye. Remember also that any medial lesion will appear in the lateral section of the fundus. The advantage of this method is that it allows visualisation of more of the fundus

9 OPHTHALMOLOGY

at once, for a more rapid examination. A dark environment is essential for this examination (Brooks 2012a).

Direct ophthalmoscopy

This is done with an ophthalmoscope, examining the eye up close to the animal. The disadvantage of this is that it is slower as only a small portion of the fundus can be seen at any one time. It is especially difficult/dangerous in nervous animals as the examiner's face is close to the eye. The advantage is that ophthalmoscopes are portable and simple to use, and the image is true (i.e. not reversed as with indirect ophthalmoscopy). There are many different types of ophthalmoscope. Ophthalmoscopy is not difficult but it does take practice. Here are some tips on its use:

> **Distant direct ophthalmology** This can be done as an initial quick scan for abnormalities.
>
> **Close direct ophthalmology** This can be used to examine all aspects of the eye, and is essential to full evaluation of the retina and origin of optic nerve (Bedford 1985, Brooks 2012a).

- Make sure the instrument is working. Ensure the batteries are charged.
- Test the settings. Ensure the light source is:
  - **White** Ignore the red; blue can be used to look at ulcers (Brooks 2012b).
  - **Bright** Have the light at maximum force rather than dimming function.
  - **Circular** Ignore the slits/crosses, turn the dial to a circle.

> Get close. The closer to the animal's eye, the larger the field of vision.

- Remember human safety. Rest a hand on the head of the animal while examining the eyes.
- Observe the fundus with the setting on 0 to 3 diopters. (This number represents focal length; the negative numbers are usually in red.) The setting can be changed to bring abnormalities into focus. Beginning with the magnifying lens (from +30D), and gradually reducing the strength through to the reducing lens (to -30D), start from the outside surface of the eye and finish by viewing the retina (Brooks 2012a). Compare with the other eye. There is large variation of 'normal' in the equine eye. Note the reflectivity of the retina and the 'Stars of Winslow' (small dots in the tapetal fundus that are end-on normal blood vessels supplying the retina) which are scattered over the tapetum; do not mistake these for abnormalities. Look at the size, shape and position of the optic nerve papilla (disc).

> Ensure that the animal's pupil is well dilated.

- The fundus is examined through the pupil and, if the pupil is miotic, visualisation is not possible. Having the animal in a darkened room will achieve this, although occasionally it is helpful to use a short-acting mydriatic to dilate the pupil (e.g. tropicamide).

> A dark environment is essential for the best examination and visualisation.

Vision testing

The menace response is one way to test vision (see earlier in this chapter). Alternatively, conduct obstacle tests using locally available materials which will not cause harm to the animal if it knocks into them (Dwyer 2012). A good way for a worried owner to test an animal's vision is to change the routine slightly (e.g. put the animal in a different stall/stable, take a right turn instead of a left in the brick kiln or market, anything that will reveal a vision defect being covered up by the animal remembering its routine).

> Careful observation of behaviour may reveal blindness.

By blindfolding each eye in turn, it is possible to assess sight in both sides and detect if there are unilateral defects in vision (Dwyer 2012).

Remember there are differing levels of vision defects. Many working equids have a white plaque over the front of the cornea, 'corneal scarring', from an old corneal ulcer or eye injury. This gives the appearance of looking through frosted glass; the animal can see shadows but not defined shapes. This could have an effect on the fear or distress that the animal experiences; the owners' actions may be unnecessarily harsh if they do not realise their animal cannot see well.

> A veterinarian has a responsibility always to point out suspected vision defects to the owner, however slight, and ensure that the animal is managed appropriately.

Chemical restraint

Equids have fast reflexes and strong ocular muscles, the combination of which makes them averse to examination of the eye, even more so if the eye is painful. The eye has many sensitive nerves (and therefore can be extremely painful when injured) and a strong orbicularis oculi muscle producing the blink response and blepharospasm. If necessary, a combination of intravenous sedation and local anaesthesia can be used to facilitate examination and avoid unnecessary pressure when handling an injured globe.

Complete desensitisation of the eye (for painful procedures) will require blocking the supraorbital, lacrimal, zygomatic and infratrochlear nerves. However, topical anaesthetic will still need to be applied to the surface of the globe, in an ocular preparation.

> For ophthalmological examination the supraorbital block alone will be sufficient as this will inhibit blepharospasm and most of the blinking that obstructs examination *(see later in this chapter for details of these nerve blocks)*.

- **Sedate** Administer an alpha2-adrenergic agonist (e.g. xylazine/detomidine), ideally with an opioid (e.g. butorphanol) IV (see Chapter 5 or other equine formulary texts for dose rates).
- **Topical anaesthesia** This anaesthetises the cornea, facilitating examination, foreign body removal and washing; and makes the animal more comfortable. Examples include proxymetacaine or topical 4% lignocaine *without* adrenaline. Place 0.2–0.3 ml into a syringe (without the needle) and apply gently from a few centimetres. Analgesia occurs after 3–4 minutes and lasts about 20 minutes. This is not a long-term solution for analgesia. Topical anaesthetic has toxic effect on corneal epithelial cells and is short acting. So, while it may temporarily relieve an animal's pain, it will also impede healing. Therefore, although

9 OPHTHALMOLOGY

useful in the short term for examination and essential veterinary procedures, it is not suitable for long-term use, and alternative analgesics should be provided.

- **Nerve blocks** Know the anatomical landmarks. 2% Mepivicaine hydrochloride can be used (Pollock *et al.* 1998).

> **Remember, if sedation is used the head will lower towards the ground.**

In order to comfortably conduct a thorough examination, the animal's head will need to be held up to the examiner's head height. If the handler is holding the head up he/she will tire, so ensure either that there is a second handler to take over or make a 'head-rest' out of suitable local objects. Ensure that the person holding up the head is not constricting the airways at the throat and neck.

Local anaesthesia for examination or treatment of the eye

A thorough examination of the eye and eyelids is difficult without the use of local anaesthesia, (often together with sedation). Complete desensitisation of the eye muscles and skin requires blocking the supraorbital, lacrimal, zygomatic and infratrochlear nerves, however the supraorbital block alone will often be enough for a thorough examination.

> **Note: With all of these nerve blocks the surface of the eye is not desensitised, so ensure topical local ocular anaesthetic is applied if this is required.**

Auriculopalpebral nerve block

This does not provide analgesia.

This block will prevent blinking as it blocks the motor function of the upper eyelid. The nerve runs over the highest point of the zygomatic arch; moistening the area with surgical spirit will make the nerve easily palpable.

- First, without the syringe attached, insert the 22–23G needle as the animal will react and move the head.
- Inject 2 ml local anaesthetic.
- Always use topical local anaesthesia on the cornea too, for the sensory block.

Supraorbital (frontal) nerve block

The supraorbital nerve emerges through the supraorbital foramen, located 5–7 cm dorsally to the medial canthus of the eye. It provides sensory innervation to the middle part (2/3rds) of the upper eyelid only. If the whole upper eyelid needs to be blocked do the frontal block first, then, once the middle is numb, inject local to the lateral areas via local anaesthetic infusion.

- Find the supraorbital foramen by palpation of the bony orbit over the top of the eye.
- Inject 3–4 ml local anaesthetic into the foramen itself, or along the dorsal orbital rim.
- Be careful not to inject into any of the blood vessels.
- Place the needle first, before attaching the syringe, and draw back before injecting.

OCULAR THERAPEUTICS – PREPARATIONS, ADMINISTRATION AND PRINCIPLES **9.5**

Lacrimal, Zygomatic and Infratrochlear block

- Precise location of these nerves is difficult.
- Infiltration of 2–3 ml at each site of the four corners of a diamond positioned around the eye (ring block) will achieve complete desensitisation of the eye and eyelids (Pollock *et al.* 1998).
- This is very useful for examining and suturing injuries to the eye, or for enucleations.
- Again, remember to place the needle first before attaching the syringe.

Enucleations

The technique for enucleation is outside the scope of this text. Refer to a recent surgical text for the exact procedure.

Ocular therapeutics – Preparations, administration and principles 9.5

The challenge with ocular therapy is getting the right drug to the right place for an extended period of time so that effective therapeutic levels are reached. Ideally, any topical application of drops/ointments should occur at least four times daily. However, as time goes by, equids often become more resistant to intraocular medication and examination. It is the responsibility of the prescribing clinician to help owners understand the importance of continuing treatment, and to instruct them on the correct handling methods which will allow them to do this.

Routes of drug administration

There are four main routes for drug administration in ocular treatments:

- Systemic (e.g. IV NSAID therapy)
- Topical (e.g. eye drops/creams)
- Lavage (e.g. nasolacrimal or subpalpebral)
- Subconjunctival injections

The first three are the recommended routes, as subconjunctival injections are not well tolerated in equids; the level of restraint required would cause excessive fear and distress.

Systemic

This is the route of choice for conditions affecting the fundus (as topical treatment will not reach this) and to provide analgesia and anti-inflammatory medication in addition to topical treatments, for example in corneal ulceration, eyelid wounds/swellings. Although topical NSAIDs are the drug of choice for conditions such as corneal ulceration, these may be unavailable locally. Systemic NSAIDs will improve the general comfort of the animal.

Topical

This is the most well-known route (Matthews 2009) and theoretically the easiest for owners to use. It is used successfully to treat eyelids, conjunctival, corneal, anterior chamber pathology and adnexal disease.

Depending on the drugs and the formulation, some drugs (e.g. chloramphenicol) penetrate the intact conjunctival and corneal epithelium, resulting in therapeutic levels in the corneal stroma and anterior chamber, but topically drugs do not reach the posterior chamber.

> **Disadvantages of topical medication include the reluctance of the animal to co-operate after the first days of treatment, or the owner giving up or not actually succeeding in getting drops into the eye.**

Additionally, if several different types of eye drops are being provided, 15 minutes needs to be left between each different drug to avoid too large a volume of fluid added to the eye, resulting in the medication overflowing.

One easy method of applying eye drops is via a syringe with a cut-off 22G needle (for veterinarians), or through a plastic intra-mammary syringe (for owners, to avoid unnecessary damage to the eye if the animal moves its head). This allows for greater control over placing the medication and it is not necessary to be as close to the eye so, theoretically, it will be better tolerated. Any topical application should be applied slowly and gently as the animal will react strongly to anything squirted into the eye.

> **As well as the pharmacokinetics of the drug administered, the preparation type effects the penetration and drug availability.**

Solutions These have a high bioavailability which means that therapeutic concentrations are easily achieved. However, they have a short ocular contact time. As a general rule, solutions should be applied at least every 4 hours and, ideally, in the acute/initial stages of treatment, every 1–2 hours. If two or more solutions are being used, 15 minutes should be left between applications to avoid dilution, washing out or reactions. Failure to do so is a common cause of therapeutic failure.

Ointments On application, these melt into the tear film, aided by blinking. These preparations have relatively poor availability but much longer retention. Therefore they should be instilled every 6–8 hours. Although their availability is not as good as that of solutions, if an owner is not able to administer solutions at the correct frequency, then an ointment may be a better option.

Lavage

This method is useful since it allows application of eye preparations over a period of time without direct contact with the eyes, and once in place can theoretically be taught to owners.

OCULAR THERAPEUTICS – PREPARATIONS, ADMINISTRATION AND PRINCIPLES 9.5

> The disadvantage is that the lavage system needs to be checked daily which is difficult in a field situation, and medications must be infused slowly as the animal will react strongly and start to resent the treatment.

The two main types of ocular catheterisation are via the nasolacrimal duct or a subpalpebral lavage.

Nasolacrimal lavage

This is a good method for flushing out larvae from *Habronema* infection, and in some cases can be used to administer eye drops if the animal is head shy.

Where are the nasolacrimal puncta?

There are species differences here:

- **Horses** The nasolacrimal opening is found ventromedially, very near the junction between the pigmented and non-pigmented mucosa (see arrow, Figure 9.5.1).
- **Donkeys** The puncta are found dorso-laterally and are often harder to find; evert the upper part of the nostril.

Insert a 16–18G catheter (or a very small urinary catheter) gently into the nasal punctum (Figure 9.5.2); this does not have to be inserted all the way. First applying local anaesthetic onto the catheter, and around the punctum, will allow its passage more easily. Gently slide the catheter up towards the eye for a small distance; *do not force* it which will risk puncture of the nasolacrimal duct. Slowly flush warm sterile saline gently through the catheter to encourage patency.

> Always flush gently and be very cautious if resistance is encountered to avoid inadvertently rupturing the nasolacrimal duct.

The catheter can be left in place to administer long-term or frequent ocular treatment (Barnett et al. 1995).

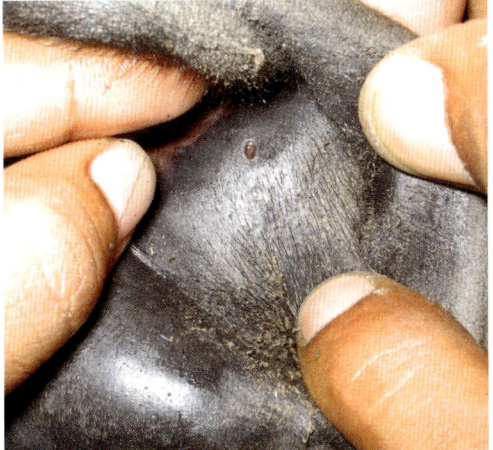

Figure 9.5.1 Position of the nasolacrimal punctum in the horse.

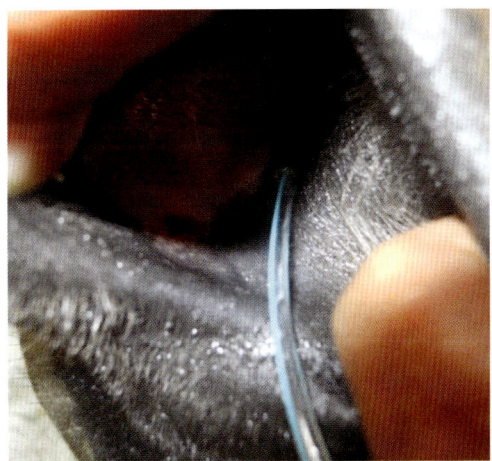

Figure 9.5.2 Flushing tube inserted into the nasal punctum.

9 OPHTHALMOLOGY

Subpalpebral lavage

Subpalpebral lavage involves inserting a length of pliable polyethylene tubing through the upper eyelid through which medication can be delivered. Details of this technique are included in many equine veterinary reference texts. It allows medication of the eye, over a number of days, with multiple preparations. This technique should not be used unless the practitioner is confident of how to place the sub-palpebral lavage system and is able to ensure follow-up involving daily visits to the animal. One study by Sweeney and Russell (1997) reported minor complications in 34% of cases and severe complications in 24% of cases. Minor complications were mild eyelid swelling, tearing of tubing and losing the cap; severe complications were removal of the system by the animal, eyelid infections, losing the footplate in the eye and ulceration of the cornea.

Therapeutic preparations for treatment of common ocular diseases

- **Mydriatics** Atropine/tropicamide. This causes mydriasis or 'dilation' of the pupil, allowing easier visualisation of the fundus. It is also an essential part of treatment for recurrent uveitis (see later in this chapter).

> **Caution:** Atropine reduces gastrointestinal motility in equids so should only be used to effect, and animals on this treatment should be carefully monitored for colic.

Pupil miosis is a natural reaction to bright light which protects the retina by limiting the amount of light passing to it. If the pupil is chemically dilated this protective reflex is inhibited, therefore the animal must be kept in a darkened environment so harmful bright light does not damage the retina and cause discomfort.

> **Caution:** Prolonged mydriasis has been reported in horses after a single dose of atropine, with effects for up to 14 days in one study (Davis *et al.* 2003) and more prolonged effects in Arabian horses.

- **Miotics** e.g. Pilocarpine. These constrict a dilated pupil, for example if an animal is uncomfortable after atropine administration. Often in chronic uveitis, synechiae form where the iris is stuck to the lens. Alternative administration of atropine and pilocarpine at 3-hour intervals is the treatment of choice to attempt to break down these synechiae.

- **Antibiotics** Gentamicin or chloramphenicol, in drop or ointment form, are commonly used preparations for treatment of conjunctivitis, keratitis and recurrent uveitis and wounds in the eye area. These need to be applied every 4–6 hours. Refer to Matthews (2009).

- **Corticosteroid anti-inflammatory drugs** Prednisolone or dexamethasone (topical applications). These are the drug of choice for uveitis and allergic conjunctivitis, however do not use if any infection is suspected, e.g. bacterial, viral or mycotic, as this will delay healing and may cause a sudden deterioration. Do not use systemically for eye conditions.

> Never use corticosteroid preparations in the presence of corneal ulceration as this will severely damage the eye and cause irreversible blindness.

- **Non-steroidal anti-inflammatory drugs (NSAIDs)** Diclofenac drops (topical), phenylbutazone or flunixin meglumine administered IV (systemic).

> Systemic NSAIDs should be considered in all painful eye conditions (see Chapter 4).

Diclofenac drops are also very effective in reducing eye pain; however, the drug itself has been legally banned in many countries due to environmental concerns (Oaks *et al.* 2004).

- **Serum** This can be easily collected and then separated (leave a blood sample to settle in a plain tube). It contains naturally occurring anti-proteinases and anti-collagenases which inhibit corneal autolysis. It is also thought to contain anti-inflammatory agents which may reduce ocular inflammation and can be an adjunct to the treatment of corneal ulceration (Brooks 2010a). This is now considered better than EDTA.

> Remember that any unused serum must be kept cool and clean and discarded after 3 days if not used.

- **EDTA 2%** Anti-collagenase used as an adjunct to the treatment of severe or 'melting' corneal ulcers (Brooks 2012b) to stop autolysis of corneal tissue. This drug is easily acquired by mixing other topical treatments in an EDTA tube before applying to the eye. This is painful when added to the eye so the animal may resent administration.

Common eye diseases 9.6

> With all conditions of the eye ensure adequate pain relief.

Conditions of the eyelids

Entropion

This is inversion of the margin of the lower eyelids, more frequent in foals and either primary (congenital) or secondary to malnutrition, dehydration, septicaemia or uveitis. In equids this is usually *secondary* to another problem rather than primary congenital entropion found in other species. Diagnose and treat the underlying cause.

Clinical signs

- Eye irritation – a few days after birth with congenital entropion, or following another primary inciting cause if entropion is secondary
- Excessive lacrimation
- Blepharospasm
- Photophobia
- A potential sequela is corneal ulceration.

9 OPHTHALMOLOGY

Diagnosis

A history of the systemic conditions and clinical signs described. Observation of corneal ulceration due to eyelashes rubbing on the cornea (fluorescein staining is an essential part of diagnosis see Section 9.4. of this chapter). Close examination of the eye will reveal inverted margins of the lower eyelid.

Treatment

Manual eversion of the lower eyelid is often possible and topical antibiotic treatment is recommended for secondary ocular infection, especially in the case of corneal ulceration and conjunctivitis.

> **Always treat the underlying cause as most cases resolve spontaneously when this is done, e.g. correct hydration status.**

If congenital primary entropion is suspected, use a temporary vertical mattress suture to pull out the skin slightly (Brooks 2002). This is easier, less painful and more successful than saline/tetracycline/penicillin injections into the lower eyelids which should not be done.

Eyelid swelling (blepharoedema)

Injuries, orbital fractures and bites/stings are common in working equids. The eyelids are very vascular and bleed profusely when injured although this excellent blood supply also helps in the healing process. Eyelids swell quickly in response to allergic reactions or other injury, including systemic illness.

Wounds should only be cleaned with clean water, mild saline solutions or 0.2% saline dilution of povidone iodine (1:50). Use of irritant solutions such as chlorhexidine/cetrimide or surgical spirit will cause severe corneal inflammation and damage. Use only antibiotic creams or ointments designed for ocular use.

Diagnosis

> **Remember: Always perform a thorough examination of the eye. If the eyelids are too swollen and painful to do this straight away, treat with anti-inflammatory drugs and antibiotics (if required) and reassess at a later stage (Millichamp 1992).**

Palpation will reveal warm oedematous eyelids (Figure 9.6.1) and possible orbital fracture, as well as obtaining an accurate history of recent trauma.

> **Remember in any case of trauma near the eye that there is potential for the globe to be injured due to the prominent position of the equine eye (Brooks and Dan Wolf 1983).**

If systemic disease is suspected, such as African Horse Sickness or hypersensitivity, proceed by diagnosing and treating this condition.

> **Remember that eyelid swelling and conjunctivitis can reflect more serious systemic disease that may be notifiable and contagious e.g. African Horse Sickness.**

Treatment

Systemic treatment is effective due to the aforementioned blood supply. NSAIDs and antibiotics are useful, also cold compresses (e.g. cold water inside a latex glove, or soaked cotton pads placed over the area) can help reduce the swelling. In allergic conditions, corticosteroids such as dexamethasone can inhibit the allergic response and reduce swelling.

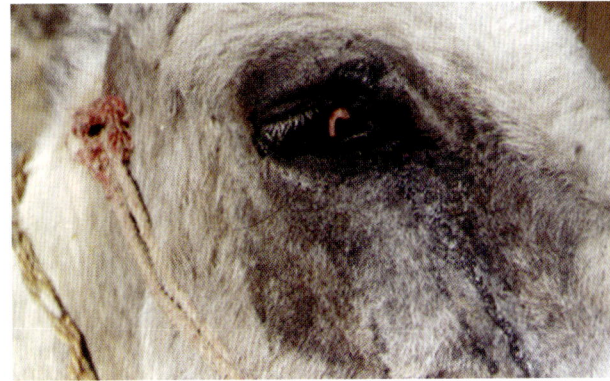

Figure 9.6.1 Upper eyelid swelling and serous discharge.

Eyelid lacerations

These are very common in working equids as they are prone to trauma in their daily work and tend to rub their heads on protruding objects (Figure 9.6.2). Trauma may be secondary to parasites such as lice. Most lacerations heal quite well due to good blood supply; however, assess and treat them very carefully as scarring can be excessive and lead to an inability to close the eye, which can lead to exposure keratitis and corneal ulceration in the future.

> It is important to repair lacerations without delay, removing all dirt and foreign bodies, and ensure restoration of the eyelid margin.

Diagnosis

Standing sedation and local anaesthesia (both motor and sensory nerve blocks, see Section 9.4 of this chapter) are *mandatory* to see the eyelid margins clearly.

Treatment

- When suturing eyelid defects, alignment of the eyelid margin closest to the globe must be exact. Poor alignment leads to corneal ulcers and pain. Wound debridement should be minimal; never cut off skin flaps, unless there is absolutely no doubt that they are necrotic, as this leads to loss of structure and function (Brooks and Dan Wolf 1983) resulting in corneal ulceration and exposure keratitis.

> - The animal must be well sedated and regional/topical anaesthesia should be administered to ensure there is minimal movement and pain during the repair.

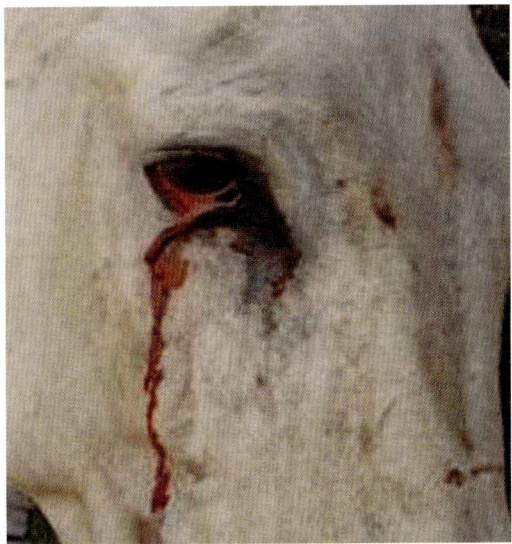

Figure 9.6.2 A lower eyelid laceration.

- Prepare the eyelids using aseptic technique (Section 4.6) as secondary infection is common. Do not use full-eyelid-thickness sutures as this will lead to the suture material rubbing on the cornea, causing ulceration. Start by first aligning the margin of the eyelid closest to the globe to ensure the edges meet exactly which is absolutely critical. Then continue suturing the wound away from the margin edge.

- Use a thin, soft absorbable suture material, such as 4–0, 5–0 or 6–0 catgut or polyglycolic acid (Brooks and Dan Wolf 1983, Millichamp 1992) and cut the ends as close as possible to prevent tags from the knots rubbing on the eyelid. Avoid placing too much tension on the sutures.

- Topical antibiotic eye drops are useful for aftercare but be aware that, if the owner cannot administer these without putting pressure on the injured region, it will be necessary to rely solely on systemic delivery rather than risk wound trauma and infection. Systemic anti-inflammatory drugs should be given for analgesia and to reduce inflammation.

- The area needs to be kept clean, dry and protected by the owner. It may be possible to cover the injured area with a piece of cotton held in place with adhesive tape, although in the field this may be unrealistic. Placing petroleum jelly around the affected area will stop excess discharge/tearing irritating the adjacent skin.

- See surgical texts for more details and diagrams of eyelid repair.

Orbital fracture

The frontal, zygomatic and lacrimal bones are the most commonly injured due to their location (Caron *et al.* 1986).

Clinical signs

- Oedema, swelling, pain, blepharospasm and subconjunctival haemorrhage may result from head trauma.
- Subcutaneous emphysema may be present if the frontal/maxillary sinuses are damaged.
- Palpable disruption of the bony orbital rim occurs if fracture fragments are displaced.
- Globe position may move.
- Nasal discharge may be present.
- Facial asymmetry may be apparent.
- Crepitus can be produced.

Diagnosis

- Diagnosis is normally straightforward due to the history of trauma.

> - **Ensure a complete physical, ocular and neurological examination is performed.**

- Assess the PLR of the injured eye; consensual PLR can be used if extensive trauma obscures the pupil.
- Ensure the cornea is stained with fluorescein dye at the first examination, and all subsequent, as damage can be latent. Fully evaluate the eye movement in all directions.

COMMON EYE DISEASES **9.6**

Treatment

- Cold compress, administer analgesics and anti-inflammatory drugs.
- Systemic antibiotics if an open wound is present. Fractures which extend into the paranasal sinuses should be treated as open fractures due to the normal fungal and bacterial flora present in the sinuses.
- Frequent application of artificial tears to lubricate the eye is essential if there is any impairment to the eyelids.
- Monitor for signs of uveitis secondary to blunt trauma and treat immediately and aggressively if present.
- Observe and treat any developing ophthalmic condition.
- Rapid fibrous fracture callous formation occurs around bone fragments/fracture lines. Surgical repair is usually not practical for working equids. However, satisfactory results can be obtained in some cases with symptomatic care and rest.

Conditions affecting the conjunctiva and cornea

Conjunctivitis: Inflammation of the conjunctiva

Conjunctivitis is a non-specific symptom or response of the eye to injury. The conjunctiva includes the bulbar and palpebral conjunctivae: the mucous membrane covering the sclera and posterior eyelids including the nictitating membrane (third eyelid).

Causes

- **Viral** Seen in association with viral upper respiratory disease (equine influenza, herpes and adenovirus), or other systemic viral disease such as Equine Infectious Anaemia and Equine Viral Arteritis (Brooks 2010b)
- **Irritant** Inflammatory reaction to a foreign body, dust, flies or unsuitable application of eye preparations topically
- **Bacterial** Primary bacterial infections *Moraxella, Streptococcus, Actinobacillus* and *Rhodococcus* spp. (Brooks 2010b), or secondary to viral or irritant conjunctivitis, defined by a mucopurulent (yellow/green) discharge as opposed to the watery, clear discharge of viral and irritant conjunctivitis
- **Foreign bodies** Food or grass seeds in the fornix or under the third eyelid
- **Fungal** Seen with infections caused by *Aspergillus* and *Fusarium* spp.
- **Protozoal** Seen with Equine Protozoal Myeloencephalitis
- **Trauma** Conjunctivitis occuring secondary to trauma
- **Allergic** In response to allergens in the environment
- **Neoplasia** e.g. squamous cell carcinoma, lymphoma and melanoma

> - **Systemic disease** Remember conjunctivitis can be a symptom of systemic disease, e.g. African Horse Sickness and Epizootic Lymphangitis, so always ensure animals are examined for other signs that may indicate this.

9 OPHTHALMOLOGY

Clinical signs

- Hyperaemic (red) conjunctiva, with or without watery/mucopurulent discharge (Figure 9.6.3)
- The type of discharge can often define the causal agent e.g. serous (viral, allergic, environmental) or purulent (bacterial).
- Associated respiratory signs (especially upper respiratory tract) can indicate viral association, which can also be indicated by other animals in the same area showing signs.
- Animal shows discomfort/irritation e.g. rubbing the eye.
- Chemosis (oedema)

Treatment

- Wash the eye area daily with clean water to remove dirt. If it is severely contaminated, apply topical anaesthetic and flush copiously (Brooks 2010b).
- In severe cases of swelling, or where uveitis is suspected, topical corticosteroids can be used to decrease swelling. However, *always use fluorescein first* to check there is no corneal ulceration, especially if a foreign body (FB) is the suspected cause.
- Systemic NSAIDs can be used to provide analgesia and reduce swelling, then check for FB or ulcer the next day, and proceed with topical corticosteroids if there is no ulceration.
- Antibiotic eye ointment (e.g. gentamicin or chloramphenicol) every 4–6 hours for 5 days is recommended if bacterial infection is present. Culture and sensitivity testing can allow changes in initial therapy.
- Fungal and viral infections are treated with appropriately selected medication specific for the causal agent.
- Parasitic causes (habronemiasis and onchocerciasis) are debrided and treated topically and systemically.

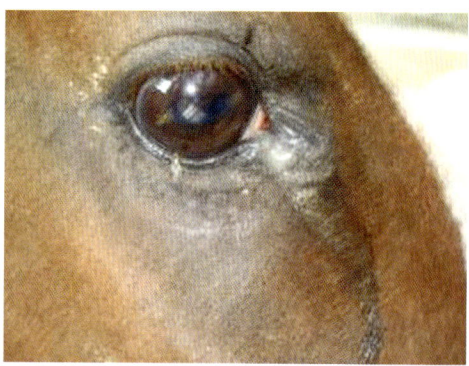

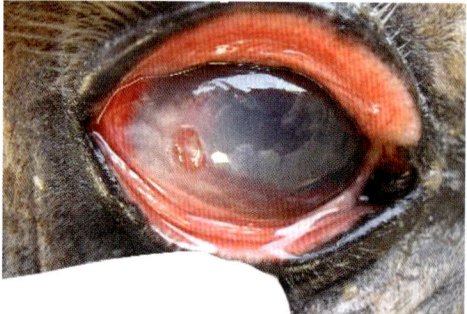

Figure 9.6.3 Mild conjunctivitis (above); note the ocular discharge. Severe conjunctivitis (below) associated with trauma to the eye.

Prognosis

The prognosis is good, if the cornea is not severely damaged.

Corneal ulceration (ulcerative keratitis)

An ulcer is a disruption to the thin corneal epithelium/stroma which covers the front of the eye.

> **Consider every ulcer seriously, with the potential to result in blindness, as the equine cornea is easily inflamed and heals slowly with extensive scarring.**

Furthermore, an infected ulcer can deteriorate rapidly and form 'melting ulcers' where the globe is degraded by infectious and inflammatory processes. To avoid these complications prompt and aggressive treatment is necessary. Consider all ulcers as an emergency and infected unless proven otherwise.

Causes

- **Trauma** Foreign bodies, dust, entropion, rubbing or hitting an object
- **Infection** Bacterial: Primary (*Pseudomonas, Staphylococcus, Streptococcus, Bacillus* spp.), or secondary due to injury or therapy; fungal (*Aspergillus, Fusarium, Penicillium, Phycomycetes* spp.) (Severin 1998)
- **Metabolic** Altered tear production, various corneal disorders
- **Neurogenic** Affecting normal function of the eyelids

Clinical signs

> Pain is pronounced in the acute stages but decreases as scarring occurs.

- Photophobia (light is painful to the eye), blepharospasm (spasm of the eyelids so that they are tightly closed) and increased lacrimation
- Secondary infections and anterior uveitis are common (differentiate from primary uveitis with fluorescein staining to show the ulcer). Assess carefully for signs of secondary reflex uveitis as this will also require aggressive treatment in conjunction with ulcer treatment.
- Corneal oedema is common; it can be localised around the perimeter of the ulcer or can be diffuse across the entire corneal surface.
- Ocular discharge
- The ulcer may be visible with the naked eye without staining and will be seen as a depression in the usually smooth cornea.
- Fluorescein staining will allow better visualisation of the ulcer (Figure 9.6.4). There is uptake of the fluorescein stain by the exposed corneal stroma. Deep ulcers, which extend to descemet's membrane, retain the stain circumferentially as descemet's membrane itself does not take up stain. This is a very serious presentation as only a thin membrane is left and the cornea is almost perforated.
- Note tear production, eyelid position and function, and look for any causes. Carefully examine the cornea, conjunctiva, sclera, and third eyelid for any other pathology or foreign body.
- As healing begins, new blood vessels develop on the cornea and ultimately the cornea heals with grey/white scar tissue.

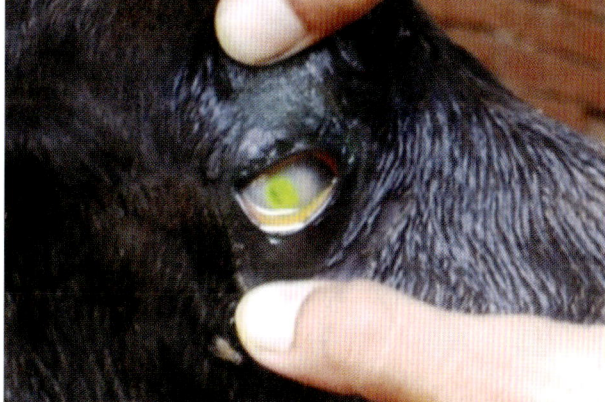

Figure 9.6.4 Corneal ulcers stained with fluorescein dye.

9 OPHTHALMOLOGY

It is crucial to make an accurate note in the clinical records of the ulcer's size, position, depth, amount of corneal oedema and pupil size. This provides a baseline for future examinations and allows monitoring of deterioration or improvement.

Treatment

- Systemic non-steroidal anti-inflammatory drugs are essential to relieve pain and reduce inflammation in the eye, which decreases the likelihood of secondary uveitis (Severin 1998).
- Appropriate topical treatment related to the cause, e.g. if a bacterial cause, apply topical antibiotics e.g. gentamicin drops every 4 hours, or chloramphenicol ointment every 6– 8 hours. (See notes on solution versus ointment eye preparations in Section 9.4 of this chapter.) For fungal agents use miconazole 1% parenterally.
- Apply atropine 1% drops (2 drops every 24–48 hours) if available.

> **Caution: Atropine inhibits gastrointestinal motility, so monitor for colic and use only to effect.**

This will treat miosis (pupil constriction) which results from secondary uveitis.
- Fresh serum has anti-collagenase properties and stimulates growth factors for healing.
- Protect the healing ulcer from further trauma; eyelid/nictitating membrane suturing (be aware that the progress of the ulcer cannot be monitored with this technique).

What is a 'melting ulcer'?

Melting ulcers are characterised by the appearance of a white, stringy ocular discharge due to the breakdown of corneal tissue by autolytic enzymes; the eye is in danger of rupture. This type of ulcer may not be positive to a fluorescein test as the ulceration is so deep in the cornea that descemet's membrane is exposed and this does not take up stain.

> **Note: 'Melting ulcers' carry a guarded prognosis; the globe may perforate due to an untreated corneal ulcer. The eye cannot then be saved.**

Treatment

- Analgesia – systemic anti-inflammatory drugs/analgesics – NSAIDs
- Anti-collagenase therapy is essential – serum (blood collected and left to separate) or EDTA 2% (see ocular therapeutics) should be applied to the eye for at least 48 hours. This is known as 'anti-collagenase therapy' and helps to decrease the production of autolytic enzymes by bacteria and fungi which result in rapid corneal destruction.
- Antimicrobial treatment frequently, e.g. every 2 hours (depending on the preparation) to maintain an effective concentration of the drug in the eye
- Leave 15 minutes between the application of each medication to the eye – to avoid dilution, wash out, or drug reactions (Matthews 1999).
- Mydriatics – atropine 1%
- Owners must be made aware that without this aggressive treatment the globe will rupture, and even with treatment the prognosis is guarded.

COMMON EYE DISEASES 9.6

> Corticosteroids by any route are contra-indicated in the treatment of corneal ulcers as they increase the chance of an ulcer developing into a 'melting ulcer'.

If the cornea is ulcerated, re-examine the eye as often as possible to monitor progress. Ideally, do so daily and stain with fluorescein (and Rose Bengal if available – see Section 9.4 of this chapter), and encourage the owner to continue with intensive treatment. Make an eye bandage to protect ulcerated eyes from light and further damage.

Prognosis Depends on how early the condition is identified and treated. However, in neglected cases, extensive scarring usually results in vision loss.

Intraocular conditions (affecting the iris, ciliary body, choroid, and the aqueous/vitreous humour)

Equine Recurrent Uveitis (ERU, 'moon blindness', 'periodic ophthalmia')

> Uveitis is a common cause of blindness.

Uveitis is inflammation of the uveal tract: the iris, ciliary body and choroid layer of the eye, i.e. inflammation originating from the *inside* of the eye. It can be unilateral or bilateral; taking note of this may help differentiate the initial cause. There are many different causes that are aggravated by specific ocular immune responses. In working equids uveitis most likely occurs as a result of chronic irritation from dust/flies/bacteria or viral respiratory disease. Leptospirosis is an important cause of 'moon blindness'. Uveitis may also occur secondary to Onchocerca infestations (Attenburrow *et al.* 1983).

> As with corneal ulceration, uveitis is serious and needs immediate, intensive treatment to prevent blindness.

If uveitis is not treated aggressively it can initiate immune changes within the eye which can lead to recurrent uveitis (where there are repeated episodes of uveitis that ultimately result in permanent damage, cataract formation and blindness).

> Consider uveitis in any case of acute ocular pain (Matthews 1999).

Clinical signs of active uveitis

- Intense ocular pain
- Blepharospasm – Sedation, topical anaesthesia, and/or an auriculopalebral nerve block to stop the blepharospasm may be needed to allow proper examination of the eye.
- Reddened conjunctiva (conjunctival hyperaemia)
- Aqueous flare (hypopyon) – Inflammatory debris (proteins and cells) in the aqueous humour causes a characteristic flare when examined (Figure 9.6.5). It is usually subtle and best examined in a darkened area.
- Miosis (pupil constriction) – If only one eye is affected, when the animal is placed in a darkened environment there will be a marked asymmetry in pupil sizes (anisocoria) with the affected pupil being much smaller.

- Photophobia – eye pain in response to light (examine in a darkened area)
- Corneal oedema starting at the edge and spreading towards the centre (Figure 9.6.6)
- Thickening/swelling of the iris and hypopyon (pus in the anterior chamber) possible
- Enlarged scleral blood vessels
- Lacrimation (Matthews 1999)

Clinical signs of chronic uveitis

- Corneal changes: diffuse oedema
- Fibrovascular in-growth from the limbus – which can be focal or diffuse
- Synechiae (iris stuck to the lens) (see Figure 9.6.7)
- Distorted pupil shape
- Cataracts with/without lens luxation
- Generalised corneal oedema
- Globe atrophy (Matthews 1999)

Treatment

- Analgesia – Systemic NSAIDs daily, e.g. phenylbutazone or flunixin meglumine. These also give an anti-inflammatory effect.
- Anti-inflammatory drugs – If no corneal ulceration is present (negative fluorescein test), use topical corticosteroid drops, ideally prednisolone acetate 1% frequently according to the formulation (solutions hourly, suspensions every 3–4 hours), or 0.1% dexamethasone (Matthews 1999). If ulceration is present, use topical NSAIDs if available.
- Atropine drops 1–4% administered hourly until pupil dilation is achieved, then as frequently as needed to maintain mydriasis; this is to prevent synechiae formation (Matthews 1999). They can be used alternating every 3 hours with pilocarpine drops (which constrict the pupil) if synechiae are present; the constant dilation/constriction of the pupil will result in the breakdown of adhesions.

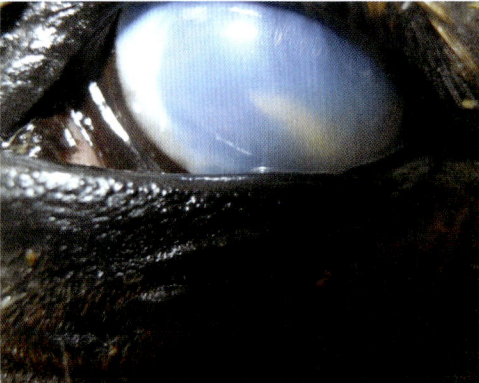

Figure 9.6.5 Aqueous flare seen in the eye of a working equid with uveitis.

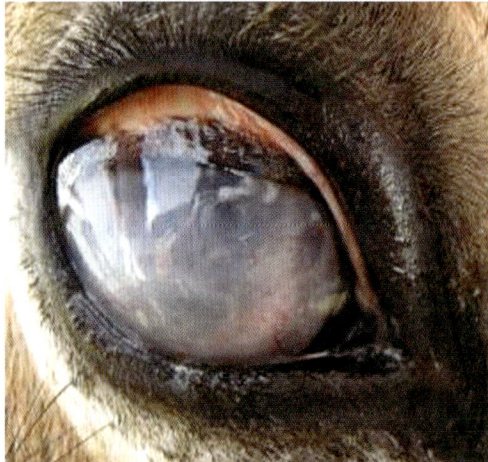

Figure 9.6.6 Marked corneal oedema and corneal vascularisation.

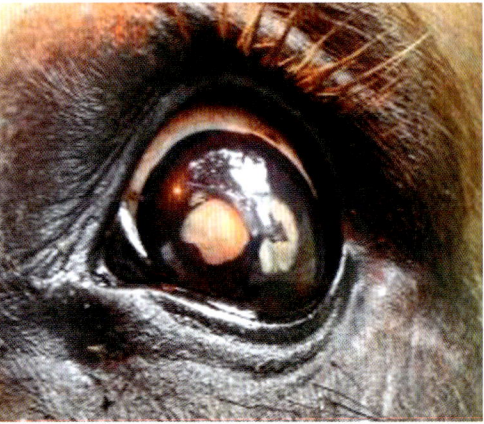

Figure 9.6.7 An eye with chronic uveitis. Note the iris synechia.

> Note: Atropine reduces GI motility and can result in colic, so the minimum effective dose should be given and the animal monitored for signs of colic.

When the pupil is dilated the animal should be kept in a darkened environment as there will be no protection for the retina against bright light.

- Subconjunctival injections of medications such as steroids can be administered under the bulbar conjunctiva (not palpebral); this should only be done if the cornea is healthy and there is absolutely no risk of corneal ulceration. They carry a risk of introducing infection, irritation and pain so caution is advised; good restraint or sedation is required to avoid inadvertent trauma to the globe. They do not substitute topical steroid medication but supplement it. Antibiotics should not be delivered by this route as effective concentrations are not delivered to the eye.
- Good eye care – Clean any discharge regularly, apply petroleum jelly below the eye to prevent staining, keep the animal in a dark environment and feed from the ground.

Prognosis

Fair, if acute condition diagnosed and treated early and aggressively. Poor, when chronic signs are present or uveitis is recurring.

Glaucoma

Glaucoma is associated with elevated intra-ocular pressure (IOP) and is often secondary to recurrent uveitis. Most cases are chronic and insidious in onset. Early signs of glaucoma are subtle and often missed. Although rarely reported in horses, it is a cause of blindness (Pickett and Ryan 1993).

Clinical signs

- Ocular pain is rare.
- Hydrophthalmos (an enlarged globe) is present (differentiate from exophthalmos using IOP – see Section 9.4 of this chapter).
- Dilated, fixed pupil and visual defects/blindness can be suggestive but sight is variable in the horse (Brooks 2002).
- Lacrimation, photophobia, blepharospasm are variably present.
- Corneal changes – oedema can occur: ranging from mild to severe and diffuse.
- Linear white lines/bands of oedema called striae can be seen (Figure 9.6.8).

Diagnosis

Very difficult without a tonometer (to measure IOP). However, glaucoma is suspected with a history of uveitis/vision loss. Use simultaneous digital palpation of the globes, through the eyelids, to detect differences in intra-ocular pressure. Fundic examination with an ophthalmoscope may show changes in the colour/size/shape of the optic nerve in later stages.

Treatment

Options are limited in the field situation:

- Miotics can help but have been known to exacerbate uveitis (Brooks 2002).
- The best thing to do is try to decrease the pressure using systemic NSAIDs and topical treatment of either NSAIDs, if available, or corticosteroids, as long as a fluorescein test is negative.
- If available, use ophthalmic beta-adrenergic antagonists such as timolol maleate (0.5%) every 12 hours and a carbonic anhydrase inhibitor (that reduces the production of aqueous humour, hence lowering IOP) such as dorzolamide every 8–12 hours (Brooks 2002). These medications work to reduce the volume of aqueous humour present in the globe, thus reducing IOP.

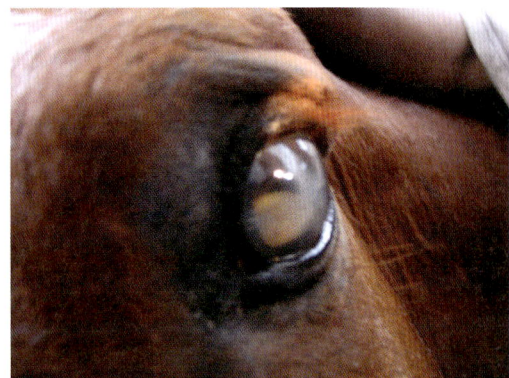

Figure 9.6.8 Glaucoma – corneal striae evident in this image, see the linear corneal oedema. The lens has luxated and is in the rostro-ventral portion of the globe.

Prognosis

Generally poor in the field situation; the disease is difficult to manage, usually leading to blindness.

Disease of the lens

Cataracts

'Cataract' means increased density or opacity of the lens reducing the transmission of light to the retina. Cataracts can be focal or diffuse, unilateral or bilateral, congenital or acquired.

Causes

- **Congenital/developmental** result from disrupted evolution/development of the lens in-utero and in development/growth after birth.
- **Acquired/secondary** result from ocular insult (trauma) or disease; this includes ocular (ERU) and systemic disease, in addition to well documented external factors such as UV light, ionising radiation and toxin ingestion.
- **Senile cataracts** are seen in aged horses (> 20 years old) (Brooks 2002).

Clinical signs

- Lens opacity is observed as greyness or 'bubbles'/'cracks' in the lens. Progresses to white or grey density which prevents light being reflected from the retina, so structures behind the lens cannot be seen (Figure 9.6.9).
- Normal PLR unless associated with adhesions between iris and lens
- Progressive loss of vision leading to total blindness in diffuse disease
- Small focal cataracts which are out of the field of vision may not cause any visual impairment – however, these are usually not visible to the naked eye.

Treatment

▌ Treat associated/underlying conditions (uveitis, pain etc.) if present. However, once a cataract has formed it is irreversible with medical treatment.

▌ Surgery, the only curative treatment, requires an ophthalmologist and specialist equipment thus is not suitable in field conditions.

In cases of extensive bilateral cataract formation with poor vision the safety of both the animal and the owner must be considered in the management plan.

For more information refer to the article by Matthews (2004) on the lens and cataracts.

Lens luxation

This is usually secondary to uveitis, trauma, cataracts or glaucoma (Brooks 2002) and treatment involves correction of the underlying disease process; it can be congenital. Lens removal is not usually attempted in equids (compared to other species where spontaneous luxation can occur) as damage to the rest of the eye is usually so pronounced that the vision will never return to normal. Diagnosis is difficult as there is usually a lot of inflammation. Uveitis is commonly seen.

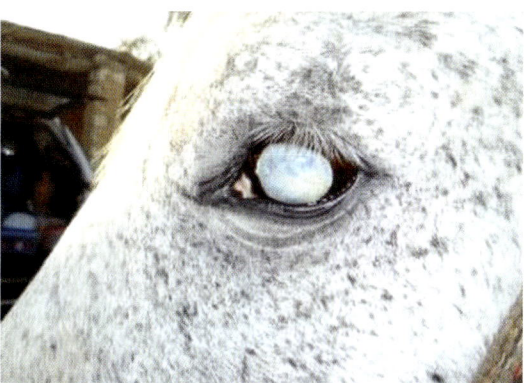

Figure 9.6.9 This horse had very little vision in this eye and the other eye was equally affected.

Figure 9.6.8 shows a horse with lens luxation – the lens can be seen in an abnormal location in the rostro-ventral globe in this image. This eye also shows corneal striae, the 'lines' of corneal oedema.

Diseases of the retina and optic nerve

Definitive diagnosis of these conditions is impossible without an ophthalmoscope. Make an informed decision by linking the history with clinical signs and thinking about the anatomy. This is important in terms of prognosis. If there is access to an ophthalmoscope diagnosis of abnormalities becomes easier once plenty of normal animals have been examined.

> Any presentation of a blind/poorly sighted animal with a normal looking anterior eye on visual/pen-torch examination should have retinal/optic disc disease as a differential diagnosis.

Retinal disease

Retinal disease can occur for a number of reasons. However, in working equids it is most likely to be associated with inflammatory episodes, for example acquired retinal detachment secondary to chronic uveitis. Conditions seen may be retinopathies such as chorioretinitis, or retinal detachment (Brooks 2002). Retinal detachment may be uni- or bilateral, partial or complete, and may be subsequent to ERU, trauma or tumours.

9 OPHTHALMOLOGY

Clinical signs

- The visible portion of the eye can appear normal although, if retinal detachment has occurred, there is evidence of inflammation (oedema, uveitis) in the anterior segment.
- Blindness (may be acute with retinal detachment), poor night vision
- Dilated pupils or poor/slow PLR
- Poor performance on vision tests
- Fundic examination may show poorly pigmented non-tapetum, decreased size of blood vessels or avascularity around the optic disc and a hyporeflective tapetum. (Looking at many normal animals will help diagnosis of abnormal cases.)

Treatment

Systemic NSAIDs, e.g. phenylbutazone or flunixin meglumine in cases of chorioretinitis

> **Remember: Any topical treatment will not reach the back of the eye (the retina).**

Treatment is limited and, in the majority of retinal pathological processes, the prognosis is poor.

Optic nerve disease

Damage to the optic nerve can be unilateral or bilateral, and should be considered with all cases of blindness presenting with fixed, dilated pupil(s). The history will also help determine possible optic nerve damage.

Causes

- Head trauma (rearing over backwards, accidents)
- Profuse bleed somewhere else in the body (e.g. haemorrhage after castration)
- Systemic inflammatory disease such as septicaemia
- Guttural pouch disease affecting carotid arteries such as mycosis
- Sequalae to spheno-palatine sinus infections (Barnett *et al.* 2008)
- Neoplasia

> *Why do the above causes, especially profuse haemorrhage for any reason, lead to blindness? The answer is hypoxia.*

Diagnosis

- History of trauma, surgery or haemorrhage and presenting signs – e.g. sudden-onset blindness
- Slow or absent PLR (Brooks 2002, Barnett *et al.* 2008)
- Dilated pupils unresponsive to light
- Ophthalmoscopy may show changes to the optic disc, e.g. oedema, or decreased blood supply/avascularity of the optic disc.

Treatment

- If trauma is suspected: High doses of systemic corticosteroids (10-20 mg dexamethasone IV or IM daily) should be used for a strong, fast onset anti-inflammatory response.
- Attempt corticosteroid use even if injury happened a few days ago, however treatment is even less likely to work in this case.
- Treat underlying causes (e.g. sinusitis).

> The prognosis for return of vision is usually poor with damage to the retina or optic nerve due to the irreversible nature of most changes.

Parasitic conditions affecting the eyes of working equids

Habronemiasis

See Section 17.5 for more information on habronemiasis.

Habronema infection commonly involves the conjunctiva, eyelids (including the third eyelid) and nasolacrimal system (Rebhun 1996), as well as the skin of the ventrum, genitalia and legs (Down et al. 2009, Paterson 2009).

Owner communication is important in the control of this disease, because the flies that transmit the infected larvae (house and stable flies – *Musca domestica* and *Stomoxys calcitrans*) are attracted to the ocular discharge, dust etc. around the eyes.

> Habronemiasis is a common result of neglecting to clean the eyes daily which can have serious welfare consequences including blindness. It can be easily avoided through owner education.

Cause

Intense granulomatous reaction to the larvae of the nematodes *Habronema muscae, H. majus* and *Draschia megastoma* that migrate into the conjunctiva and nasolacrimal system

Clinical signs

- Ulcerated nodules around the area of the medial canthus/third eyelid
- Often with secondary corneal abrasions – use fluorescein dye to check.
- Eyelids – granulomatous or ulcerative lesions (Rebhun 1996)
- Nodules are often seen extending down over the nasolacrimal duct (Figure 9.6.10), so examine carefully.
- Diagnose by demonstrating larvae in the exudate.
- Lesions may coincide with peak fly season.

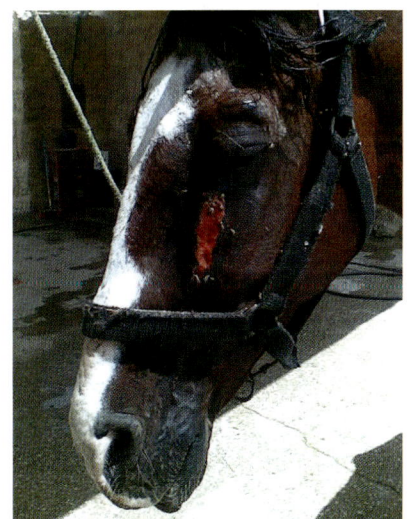

Figure 9.6.10 A horse showing signs of ocular habronemiasis with a lesion extending down over the face below the left medial canthus.

9 OPHTHALMOLOGY

Treatment

- Systemic ivermectin (0.2 mg/kg, orally). Remember larvae die gradually and further signs of disease may continue to be seen after treatment.
- Control of flies to prevent re-infection
- Debridement of calcareous plaques and nodules (Rebhun 1996)
- Topical antibiotics for secondary infection if required
- Topical or systemic corticosteroid anti-inflammatory drugs (if no corneal abrasions or ulceration are present)
- Nasolacrimal lavage with sterile saline to remove larvae and debris (Figure 9.6.11)

Prevention

> **Wound management and fly control are essential to prevent the deposition of infected larvae by flies when feeding on the exudate from open wounds (Pusterla *et al.* 2003).**

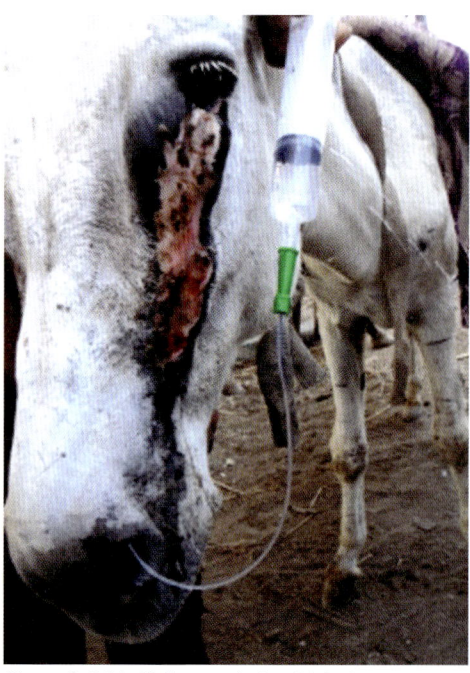

Figure 9.6.11 Habronemiasis with lesions overlying the nasolacrimal duct; the duct has been catheterised for flushing from the nasal puncta.

Prognosis

Good if the cornea is not severely damaged and re-infestation is prevented; healing of corneal lesions is reported at between 5 and 18 days (Pusterla *et al.* 2003).

Onchocerciasis

See also Section 17.5.

Cause

Microfilariae of the nematode *Onchocerca cervicalis* are spread between animals by the female biting midges culicoides spp. (Moore *et al.* 1983). The adults tend to collect in the ligamentum nuchae, whilst microfilariae reside in the dermis (Marques and Scroferneker 2004). Ocular onchocerciasis is the result of aberrant migration and invasion of the eye (Attenburrow *et al.* 1983); it is seen in approximately 50% of cases with cutaneous onchocerciasis (Moore *et al.* 1983).

Clinical signs

- Conjunctival and corneal hyperaeamia and chemosis (inflammation – keratitis) leading to uveitis (Attenburrow *et al.* 1983)
- May get loss of pigment and inflammation at the junction between the cornea and bulbar conjunctiva – depigmentation of the lateral limbus
- Small nodules and corneal opacities on the cornea

- Photophobia
- Epiphora (Moore *et al.* 1983)
- Can result in retinal inflammation and lead to blindness
- Severe cases develop corneal opacity.
- Microfilariae are rarely identified. (Conversely microfilariae have been identified in clinically normal horses: Moore *et al.* 1983.)

Diagnosis – from ocular lesions, and possibly identification of microfilariae

Treatment

- This depends on the stage of disease (acute or chronic) and the presenting ocular signs. After ensuring that there is no corneal ulceration (fluorescein test), administer topical corticosteroids and systemic NSAIDs – for anti-inflammatory and analgesic effects. Start this treatment 2 days prior to parasiticide treatment (e.g. ivermectin) and continue for a few days after it to minimise the inflammatory process sparked by the killed parasites.
- Dead microfilariae stimulate greater immune reaction and damage than live ones, hence use NSAIDs before and during anthelmintic treatment.
- Systemic ivermectin (0.2–0.5 mg/kg PO or SC) 2–3 days *after* NSAIDs are started

Prevention

> **Educate owners as to the importance of midge control to reduce infection rates and transmission.**

This may include stabling during the peak biting times (just before sunset) and insecticide treated shelters (Moore *et al.* 1983).

Prognosis

Good for conjunctivitis. Corneal lesions and uveitis may be chronic or recurrent.

Thalaziasis

Cause

The eye worm *(Thelazia spp.)* is common in horses and cattle. *Thelazia lacrymalis* is commonly found in equids.

Life cycle and transmission

- The face fly (*Musca autumnalis*) is a vector for *Thelazia* spp. (Moore *et al.* 1983). It feeds on lacrimal secretions on the host's face. Infective larvae pass from the fly to the host during feeding and commonly invade superficial structures such as the cornea, conjunctival sac and bulbar aspect of the third eyelid, or more deeply into the conjunctiva, lacrimal gland and duct (Moore *et al.* 1983).

Clinical signs

- May be asymptomatic

- Epiphora, photophobia, and blepharospasm
- Conjunctivitis – The larvae cause local irritation and inflammation, resulting in mild to severe conjunctivitis.
- Keratitis (Moore *et al.* 1983)
- Uveitis/corneal ulceration – The conjunctivitis can lead to more severe conditions such as uveitis and ulceration.
- Inflammation and potential obstruction of the lacrimal duct

Diagnosis

- Identification of the adult worm on the cornea or in the conjunctival sacs

Treatment

- The larvae can be mechanically removed from the surface of the eye: after applying topical local anaesthetic, tweezers can be used to carefully remove the larvae.
- Flushing of the nasolacrimal duct and conjunctival fornices may remove some parasites (Moore *et al.* 1983).
- Concurrent use of topical antibiotics, and systemic or topical NSAIDs. If no corneal ulceration is present topical steroids can also be useful to minimise inflammation.
- Ivermectin is largely ineffective. Fenbendazole at a dose rate of 7.5–10 mg/kg given daily for 5 days has been effective in killing adult worms (Wescott 1987).

Prevention

- Fly control

Setaria (intraocular filariasis)

Setaria spp. are commonly found in the peritoneal cavity of equids where they are non-pathogenic and do no harm. Occasionally aberrant migration occurs and larvae migrate into the anterior chamber resulting in marked ocular pathology. The infective microfilariae are transmitted by blood-sucking insects such as mosquitoes (Moore *et al.* 1983).

Clinical signs

- Larvae may be visible wriggling around the anterior chamber (Figure 9.6.12).
- Ocular pain, epiphora, photophobia, miosis, hypopyon, aqueous flare and corneal oedema
- Signs of intra-ocular irritation (uveitis) which can lead to corneal opacity and blindness

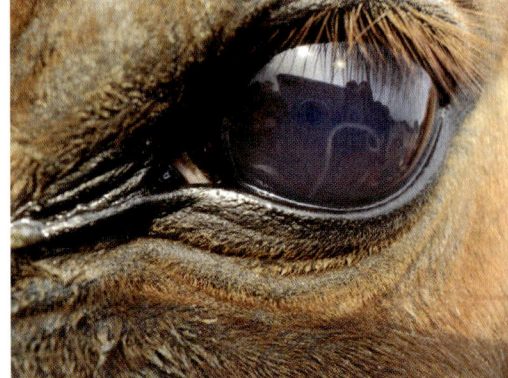

Figure 9.6.12 Aberrant migration of Setaria spp.; worm visible in the anterior chamber.

Treatment

- Systemic ivermectin is reported as over 80% effective in treatment at a dose rate of 0.2–0.5 mg/kg, although medical treatment will not remove dead intraocular parasites.
- Anti-inflammatory treatment – systemic and topical
- Treatment of concurrent ocular disease, e.g. uveitis
- Surgical removal can be curative but involves making an incision and removing the parasite from the aqueous humour. See details below and refer to the paper by Marzok and Desouky (2009) for more details.
- *S. equina* and *S. digitata* have been identified in equid eyes (Marzok and Desouky 2009, Moore *et al.* 1983, Shukla *et al.* 2010).

Surgical removal

It is absolutely essential to provide antibiotic cover topically after the procedure (e.g. gentamicin eye drops). This should not be an ointment as a full-thickness corneal lesion will result from the procedure. Systemic and (topical) NSAIDs are also essential (e.g. phenylbutazone or flunixin meglumine systemically, and diclofenac sodium eye drops) to minimise inflammation, uveitis, and provide pain relief. The procedure must be carried out aseptically to avoid secondary bacterial infection.

- Sedate the animal (e.g. xylazine and butorphanol), perform local nerve blocks (auriculopalpebral and retrobulbar) and apply topical corneal anaesthesia (lignocaine hydrochloride).
- With good restraint and a sterile scalpel, make a small sharp nick (3 mm) on the cornea at the dorsolateral-corneosceleral junction of the affected eye (at the 1 o'clock position: Shukla *et al.* 2010). This will open the anterior chamber and the worm will come out along with forceful oozing of aqueous humour from the eye. Lavage the anterior chamber with sterile saline to flush out stubborn larvae.
- Replace humour with sterile isotonic solution, if required. However, it should refill the anterior chamber within hours.
- Ensure good topical antibiotic cover is provided and analgesics to minimise pain (see above).
- Recovery takes 1–2 weeks after the procedure and careful monitoring is needed for this time to ensure than any complications are identified without delay.
- 10% formalin can be used to preserve worms for transport to a laboratory for morphological identification.

Prevention

- **Mosquito control** Fly repellents, fly masks/fringes/rugs, keeping equids away from standing water, stabling equids at dawn and dusk
- Proximity to other animals that attract flies, such as water buffalo, may also be a risk factor (Shukla *et al.* 2010).

9 OPHTHALMOLOGY

Miscellaneous conditions which can present as eye problems

Tumours

The most common ocular tumour seen in equids are squamous cell carcinomas (SCC) see Figure 9.6.13 (Kaps *et al.* 2005). The next most common are sarcoids (Dugan 1992), followed by small numbers of melanomas, papillomas, and schwannomas/neurofibromas (nerve sheath tumours) (Dugan 1992, Moore *et al.* 2000).

Differential diagnosis

May include habronemiasis (see earlier). Intraocular melanomas are reported in grey-coloured adult horses (Moore *et al.* 2000) with an average reported age of 9 years. SCC are reported as more common in horses with non-pigmented eyes (e.g. Albinos) with an average age of 8–10 years (King *et al.* 1991).

Diagnosis

This can be by fine-needle aspirate or excisional biopsy which treats (by removal) and diagnoses at the same time (Dugan 1992).

Treatment

This will depend on the size, location, nature of the tumour, available treatment and patient considerations of working equids and their owners. Reported treatments are: surgical removal, cryotherapy, hyperthermia, irradiation, chemotherapy, immunotherapy, radiotherapy, laser treatment, and enucleation (Dugan 1992). In severe, invasive cases and moderate cases with poor prognosis, enucleation may be considered in working equids.

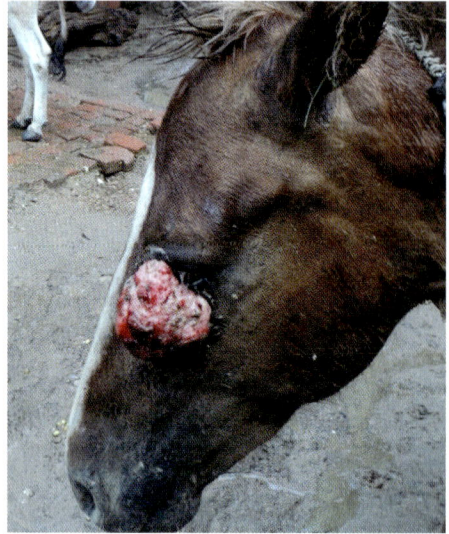

Figure 9.6.13 An ocular squamous cell carcinoma in a working equid.

Recurrence

This may be around 50% after surgical excision (Schwink 1987).

Prognosis

This will depend on the size, location, presence of metastases (check regional lymph nodes and salivary glands) and rate of recurrence after therapy.

See Section 15.3 for more information on tumours of the equine skin.

Lacrimal histoplasmosis

- **Caused** by the fungus *Histoplasma farciminosum* and reported as more common in donkeys. It is described in more detail in Section 15.3 under *Epizootic Lymphangitis* (with photographs).
- **Clinical signs** of the ocular form of the disease are conjunctivitis, signs of eye pain, blepharospasm, ocular discharge, and inflammation extending to the eyelids and around

CASE STUDY – OPHTHALMIC HABRONEMIASIS 9.7

the tear duct (Heragy 2002, Powell *et al.* 2006). Secondary bacterial infection leads to a purulent unilateral nasal discharge from the affected nostril, and a characteristic area of dermatitis from the canthus of the eye spreading towards the nostrils which must be differentiated from habronemiasis (see above).

- **Treatment** Local and systemic anti-fungal drugs, antibiotics if secondary bacterial infection, flushing nasolacrimal ducts; surgical excision may be considered (Heragy 2002).

Tooth root abscess

A large bony swelling below the eye may be a tooth root abscess, as the roots of the maxillary cheek teeth are embedded in the maxillary sinus. Check the cheek teeth for cracks, poor alignment or a foul smell (see Chapter 10).

Trauma

Blunt trauma to the face can cause a bone fracture or chip (sequestrum). Small infected sequestrae may be surgically removed under standing sedation and local anaesthetic (Chapter 7).

Case study – Ophthalmic habronemiasis 9.7

Location Jordan

Attending veterinarian Dr Murad Farajat

History
A 7-year-old bay local-breed stallion presented with a history of extended exudative nodules over the nasolacrimal duct. The horse first presented with a skin lesion around the medial canthus of the left eye. This lesion was first noticed by the owner 3 weeks previously; he had done nothing until it became worse when he decided to bring the horse to the veterinary clinic. The horse was last de-wormed one year previously. The owner had no other horses.

Clinical findings
The horse was showing signs of pain including blepharospasm, reluctance to allow examination, discomfort and rubbing. An ulcerative lesion, present around the medial canthus of the left eye, extended down over the nasolacrimal duct. The lesion had bloody and slightly purulent discharge, no corneal ulceration was present; flies were attracted to the discharge (see Figure 9.7.1). A thorough ocular examination was performed in good light, then, using a pen torch, in a dark place. Pupillary light reflex (PLR), a fluorescein test, menace response and vision testing were completed. The diagnostic procedures were performed with standing sedation: butorphanol tartrate IV and romifidine hydrochloride IV. The PLR was present and normal which indicated that there was no problem with the oculomotor nerve nor within the brain itself. The horse responded normally to the menace response. The fluorescein test was negative indicating no ulcer.

9 OPHTHALMOLOGY

Diagnosis
The diagnosis of ocular habronemiasis was made on the basis of history, clinical signs and location of the lesion.

Treatment
Treatment aimed to decrease the lesion size, reduce inflammation, reduce pain, and prevent recurrence. The treatment was performed initially by using systemic ivermectin orally, primarily to kill adult nematodes in the stomach. Further treatment included topical antibiotic for secondary infection, and nasolacrimal lavage by nasolacrimal catheter flushing daily with sterile saline to remove larvae and debris (Figure 9.7.2). Topical ivermectin (systemic ivermectin paste used as topical ointment) was applied to the extended skin nodules, flunixin meglumine was given as pain relief/anti-inflammatory administrated daily IV, as were diclofenac sodium eye drops to reduce eye pain every 6 hours and gentamicin eye drops every 6 hours. Other therapies included debridement of the wound, wound dressing and application of fly repellent daily.

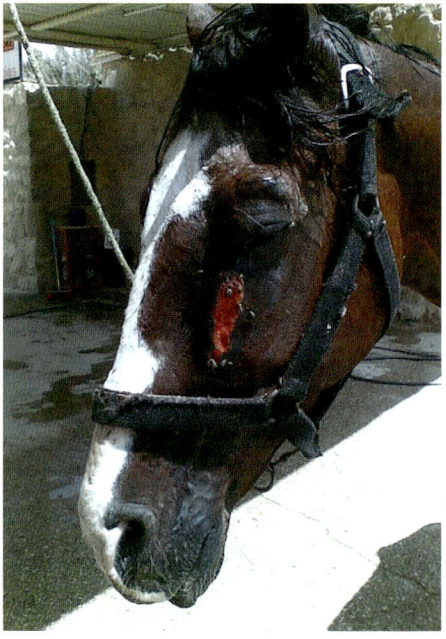

Figure 9.7.1 *Cutaneous lesion of habronemiasis overlying the nasolacrimal duct.*

Outcome
In general, the prognosis was good and, after 7 days of treatment, the lesion around the medial canthus of the eye showed progressive healing and the horse was responding well to treatment and follow-up. After 4 weeks the extended lesion was healed. Follow-up was carried out at the owner's home. The eye was washed daily by the owner with a clean, wet cloth to remove the dust and dirt that can cause further complications; this was also an opportunity for the owner to look at the eye carefully. The use of fly repellents and eye fringes, as well as appropriate de-worming, was recommended to reduce the incidence of habronemiasis. Proper removal and disposal of manure is essential for the reduction of incidence and prevention of recurrence of habronemiasis as manure provides a suitable environment for the intermediate host, maggots of the flies *Musca* and *Stomoxys*, to develop (Watson and Friedman 2007).

Discussion
In this report, a case of ophthalmic habronemiasis has been described. Many of the previous findings and treatments for habronemiasis that have been reported suggest that the probability is high for habronemiasis lesions to be resolved spontaneously following the end of fly season. Lesions usually appear during hot and warm weather, probably related to high fly activity, and regress in wintertime (Higgins and Snyder 2005). The disease is sporadic. Some lesions may become chronic

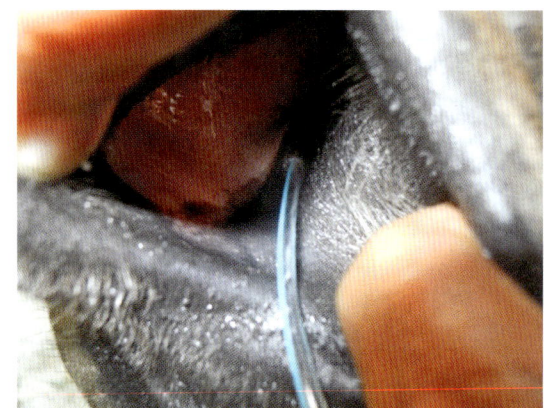

Figure 9.7.2 *Tubing inserted into the nasolacrimal duct (at the nasal end) for flushing.*

and will not heal easily, and persistent ocular irritation may be seen even during the seasons without flies. Some reports recommended surgical intervention initially (Down *et al.* 2009). However, this case responded well to intensive medical care and surgical intervention should be reserved for cases where it is needed later.

The use of topical ivermectin using oral or topical ivermectin in the form of an aqueous cream base has been reported as being effective. Also an ophthalmic form of oral ivermectin made of 50% injectable ivermectin with artificial tears has been reported by Pascoe and Knottenbelt (1999).

In this case, diagnosis was based on history, clinical signs and location of lesions. Some other reports recommend that histopathological examination of biopsies is currently the method of choice for confirming the diagnosis (Rebhun 1996). Many treatments for ophthalmic habronemiasis have been reported. All the reports state that ivermectin was used to kill the larvae and adult worms in the stomach (Pusterla et al. 2003). In our report, ivermectin was used topically in combination with systemic ivermectin. Surgical intervention has been described for some cases in other reports, mainly for the condition related to persistence of degenerated larvae in the lesion.

References

Attenburrow, D.P., Donnelly, J.J., Soulsby, E.J.L. (1983) Periodic ophthalmia (recurrent uveitis) of horses: an evaluation of the aetiological role of microfilariae of *Onchocerca cervicalis* and the clinical management of the condition. *Equine Vet. J.* 15 (S2), 48–56.

Barnett, K.C., Blunden, A.S., Dyson, S.J., Whitwell, K.E., Carson, D., Murray, R. (2008) Blindness, optic atrophy and sinusitis in the horse. *Vet. Ophthal.* 11 (S1), 20–26.

Bedford, P. (1985) Ocular disease of the horse. *In Practice.* 153–157.

Beech, J., Zappala, R.A., Smith, G., Lindborg, S. (2003) Schirmer tear test results in normal horses and ponies: effect of age, season, environment, sex, time of day and placement of strips. *Vet. Ophthal.* 6 (3), 251–254.

Brooks, D.E., Dan Wolf, E. (1983) Ocular trauma in the horse. *Equine Vet. J.* 15 (S2), 141–146.

Brooks, D.E. (2002) Equine Ophthalmology. Proceedings of the 48th Convention of the American Association of Equine Practitioners, Orlando, Florida. pp. 300–313.

Brooks, D.E., Andrew, S.E., Denis, H.M., Strubbe, D.T., Biros, D.J., Cutler, T.J., Samuelson, D.A., Gelatt, K.N. (2003) Rose bengal positive epithelial microerosions as a manifestation of equine keratomycosis. *Vet. Ophthal.* 3, 83–86.

Brooks, D. (2010a) Catastrophic Ocular Surface Failure in the Horse. Proceedings of the 56th Convention of the American Association of Equine Practitioners, Baltimore, Maryland, USA. pp. 68–117.

Brooks, D.E. (2012a) How to get the most from your ophthalmoscope. Proceedings of the 51st British Equine Veterinary Association congress, Birmingham, UK. pp. 42–43.

Brooks, D.E. (2012b) Determining the significance of abnormalities of the outer eye and cornea. Proceedings of the 51st British Equine Veterinary Association congress, Birmingham, UK. pp. 46–47.

Caron, J.P., Barber, S.M., Bailey, J.V., Fretz, P.B., Pharr, J.W. (1986) Periorbital skull fractures in five horses. *J. Am. Vet. Med. Assoc.* Feb 1;188 (3), 280–284.

Davis, J.L., Stewart, T., Brazik, E., Gilger, B.C. (2003) The effect of topical administration of atropine sulfate on the normal equine pupil: influence of age, breed and gender. *Vet. Ophthal.* 6 (4), 329–332.

Down, S.S., Hughes, I., Henson, F.M.D. (2009) Cutaneous habronemiasis in a 9 year old Arab gelding in the United Kingdom. *Equine vet. Educ.* 21 (1), 4–8.

Dugan, S.J. (1992) Ocular neoplasia. *Vet. Clin. N. Am. – Equine.* 8 (3), 609–626.

Dwyer, A.E. (2012) Ophthalmology in equine ambulatory practice. *Vet. Clin. N. Am. – Equine.* 28, 155–174.

Firshman, A.M., Hayden, D.W., Valberg, S.J., McKenzie, E.C. (2003) Horner's syndrome associated with fungal mediastinitis in a horse. *Equine vet. Educ.* 15 (2), 82–85.

Ghaffari, M.S., Sabzevari, A., Radmehr, B. (2009) Effect of topical 1% tropicamide on Schirmer tear test results in clinically normal horses. *Vet. Ophthal.* 12 (6), 369–371.

Hanggi, E.B., Ingersoll, J.F. (2012) Lateral vision in horses: A behavioural investigation. *Behav. Process.* 91 (1), 70–76.

Heragy, A.M. (2003) Lacrimal Histoplasmosis in the working donkeys of Luxor villages. 4th International Colloquium on Working Equines, Syria.

Herring, I.P. (2003) Examination of the eye. In: Robinson, N.E. Ed. 2003. Current therapy in equine medicine 5. Elsevier USA. p. 452.

Higgins, A.J., Snyder, J.R. (2005) The Equine Manual, 2nd Edition, A Saunders Ltd.

Holve, D.L. (2012) Effect of sedation with detomidine on intraocular pressure with and without topical anaesthesia in clinically normal horses. *J. Am. Vet. Med. Assoc.* 240, 308–311.

Kaps, S., Richter, M., Philipp, M., Bart, M., Eule, C., Spiess, B.M. (2005) Primary invasive ocular squamous cell carcinoma in a horse. *Vet. Ophthal.* 8 (3), 193–197.

King, T.C., Priehs, D.R., Gum, G.G., Miller, T.R. (1991) Therapeutic management of ocular squamous cell carcinoma in the horse: 43 cases (1979-1989). *Equine Vet. J.* 23 (6) 449–452.

Matthews, A. (1999) Equine recurrent uveitis - an update. *In Practice.* 21 (7), 370–376.

Matthews, A.G. (2009) Ophthalmic antimicrobial therapy in the horse. *Equine vet. Educ.* 21 (5), 271–280.

Marques, S.M.T., Scroferneker, M.L. (2004) Onchocerca cervicalis in horses from Southern Brazil. *Trop. Anim. Health Pro.* 36 (7), 633–636.

Marzok., M., Desouky, A. (2009) Ocular infection of donkeys (Equs asinus) with setaria equina. *Trop. Anim. Health Pro.* 41 (6), 859–863.

Millichamp, N.J. (1992) Ocular trauma. *Vet. Clin. N. Am. – Equine.* 8 (3), 521–536.

REFERENCES 9.8

Moore, C.P., Collins, B.K., Linton, L.L., Collier, L.L. (2000) Conjunctival malignant melanoma in a horse. *Vet. Ophthal.* 3, 201–206.

Moore, C.P., Sarazan, R.D., Whitley, R.D. (1983) Equine ocular parasites: a review. *Equine Vet. J.* 15 (S2), 76–85.

Naylor, R.J., Dunkel, B., Dyson, S., Paz-Penuelas, M.P., Dobson, J. (2010) A retrobulbar meningioma as a cause of unilateral exophthalmos and blindness in a horse. *Equine vet. Educ.* 22 (10), 503–510.

Oaks, J.L., Gilbert, M., Virani, M.Z., Watson, R.T., Meteyer, C.U., Rideout, B.A., Shivaprasad, H.L., Ahmed, S., Chaudhry, M.J.I., Arshad, M., Mahmood, S. Ali, A., Khan, A.A. (2004) Diclofenac residues as the cause of vulture population decline in Pakistan. *Nature.* 427, 630–633.

Pascoe, R.R.R., Knottenbelt, D.C. (1999) Manual of Equine Dermatology. W.B.Saunders. pp. 139–141.

Paterson, S. (2009) Cutaneous Habronemiasis. *Equine vet. Educ.* 21 (1), 4–8.

Piccione, G., Giannetto, C., Fazio, F., Giudine, E. (2008) Daily rhythm of tear production in normal horse. *Vet. Ophthal.* 11 (S1), 57–60.

Pickett, J.P., Ryan, J. (1993) Equine glaucoma: a retrospective study of 11 cases from 1988 to 1993. *Vet. Med.* 756–763.

Pollock, P.J., Russell, T., Hughes, T.K., Archer, M.R., and Perkins, J.D. (1998) Transpalpebral eye enucleation in 40 standing horses. *Vet. Surg.* 37 (3), 306–309.

Powell, R.K., Bell, N.J., Abreha, T., Asmamaw, K., Bekelle, H., Dawit, T., Itsay, K., Feseha, G.A. (2006) Cutaneous histoplasmosis in 13 Ethiopian donkeys. *Vet. Record.* 158, 836–837.

Pusterla, N., Watson, J.L. Wilson, W.D., Affolter, V.K., Spier, S.J. (2003) Cutaneous and ocular habronemiasis in horses: 63 cases (1988-2002). *J. Am. Vet. Med. Assoc.* 222, 978–982.

Ramsey, D.T. (2003) Abnormal ocular discharge. In: Robinson, N.E. Ed. 2003. Current therapy in equine medicine 5. Elsevier USA. p. 491.

Rebhun, W.C. (1996) Observations on habronemiasis in horses. *Equine vet. Educ.* 8 (4), 188–191.

Saslow, C.A. (2002) Understanding the perceptual world of horses. *Appl. Anim. Behav. Sci.* 78, 209–224.

Schwink, K. (1987) Factors influencing morbidity and outcome of equine ocular squamous cell carcinoma. *Equine vet J.* 19 (3) 198–200.

Shukla, A., Tiwari, R., Kumar, S., Banerjee, P.S. (2010) Identification of species and sex of worm present in anterior chamber in equine eye. Poster. Proceedings of the 6th International Colloquium on Working Equids. New Delhi, India. pp. 214–218.

Sweeney, C.R., Russell, G.E. (1997) Complications associated with use of a one-hole subpalpebral lavage system in horses: 150 cases (1977-1996). 211 (10), 1271–1274.

Watson, J., Friedman, R. (2007) Intestinal Parasites in Horses. A Publication of the center for the equine health, UC Davis School for Veterinary Medicine. 25, 4. (online) Available at: http://www.vetmed.ucdavis.edu/ceh/docs/horsereport/pubs-HR25-4-bkm-sec.pdf (accessed May 2011).

Wescott, R.B. (1987) Anthelmintics in horses. *Int. J. Parasit.* 17 (2), 503–510.

Further reading

Barnett, K.C., Crispin, S.M., Lavach, J.D., Matthews, A.G. (1995) Color atlas and text of equine ophthalmology. Mosby-Wolfe. Times Mirror International Publishers Ltd. London. pp. 51–52.

Brooks, D.E. (2010b) Equine conjunctival diseases: a commentary. *Equine vet. Educ.* 22 (8), 382–386.

Matthews, A. (2004) The lens and cataracts. *Vet. Clin. N. Am. – Equine.* 20, 393–415.

The teeth – Ageing and a practical approach to dentistry

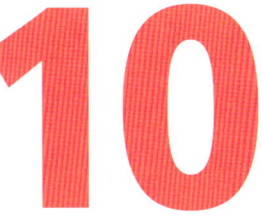

Introduction	**10.1**
Review of the anatomy and physiology of equine teeth	**10.2**
Ageing of equids using the incisors	**10.3**
Complete oral examination	**10.4**
Dental equipment	**10.5**
Common problems due to mastication and wear	**10.6**
Other dental abnormalities seen in working equids	**10.7**
Treating dental conditions in the field	**10.8**
Case study – Fracture of an incisor tooth	**10.9**
References	**10.10**

10.1 Introduction

Equine teeth are constantly erupting throughout the animal's life. Unlike carnivores, whose jaws move in an up-and-down 'biting' motion for catching prey, equine jaws move in a lateral motion, simultaneously grinding the food and wearing down the teeth. However, many things prevent even wear of the teeth, causing discomfort and preventing proper digestion of food. Pain in the mouth, caused by ulceration or pressure from the bit, can result in behavioural changes.

Definition of words used in dentistry

Occlusal surface The surface of the tooth in contact with the food (and other teeth). This is large in size in cheek teeth and thin in incisors.

Lingual surface Tongue-side (medial aspect)

Buccal surface Cheek-side (lateral aspect)

Mandibular Bottom of the mouth (teeth inserted into the mandible bone)

Maxillary Top of the mouth (teeth inserted into the maxilla bone)

Rostral Towards the front of the mouth (nose end)

Caudal Towards the back of the mouth

Arcade Describing the teeth on half or one side of either the upper or lower jaw

Apex or Apical point The surface of the tooth which has contact with the gum

Dental charts

It is good to get into the habit of numbering the teeth from 1 to 11 on each quarter (upper right, upper left, lower left, lower right) for ease of identifying teeth and tooth problems and for case records. See Section 10.4 of this chapter for more information on the **Modified Triadan system** of numbering teeth (Dixon and Dacre 2005). Record charts make dentistry more interesting and meaningful, and is necessary if an animal has severe dental problems and requires regular treatment. It means that areas of known pathology are recorded so can be rechecked regularly, any changes can be tracked and different people can follow up the same case.

> **It is important to involve the owner and help compliance with treatment by good owner management.**

Review of the anatomy and physiology of equine teeth 10.2

Like other domestic animals, equids have temporary or 'deciduous' teeth which are lost at a young age and replaced by permanent teeth, apart from the 4th, 5th and 6th molar cheek teeth which erupt only as permanent teeth.

Dental anatomy in the equid

- **Incisors** The six teeth at the front of the mouth. These are used to 'cut' grass when grazing, and help in estimating the age of equids, as described in Section 10.3 (see Figure 10.2.1).

- **Canines** These teeth are sometimes present between the incisors and premolars. They erupt between 4 and 6 years of age and are uncommon in females (Figure 10.2.2).

- **Wolf teeth** Only present in some animals, these teeth are vestigial premolars that sit right against the first premolar (further back in the mouth compared to canines); they have a greater significance in animals which have a bit placed in their mouth as they may cause interference.

- **Premolars** Cheek teeth (CT) 1, 2 and 3. These teeth erupt within the first 2 weeks of life as deciduous teeth which fall out and are replaced with permanent forms appearing from 2.5 years of age (Figure 10.2.3).

- **Molars** CT 4, 5 and 6. These are permanent teeth only, with CT 4 being the oldest tooth in any equine mouth.

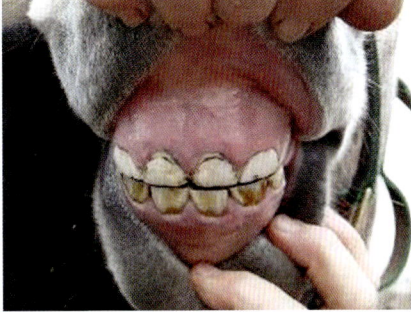

Figure 10.2.1 Deciduous incisor teeth.

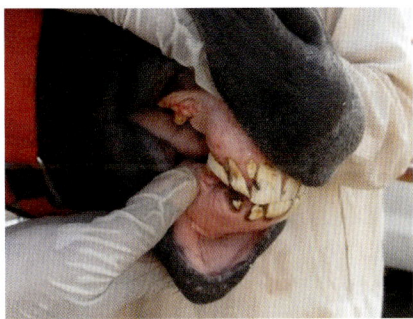

Figure 10.2.2 Canine tooth visible in upper jaw between the incisors and the corner of the mouth.

Combined premolars and molars act as a single unit for food breakdown as they are so close together they effectively form one long occlusal surface (see Figure 10.2.3). There is an angulation in the occlusal surfaces between the mandibular and maxillary cheek teeth in the lateromedial (buccolingual) direction, with the maxillary teeth being longer on the lateral (buccal) aspect, and the mandibular teeth longer on the lingual (medial) aspect (Brown *et al.* 2008).

> Most of the dental work relevant to working equids will focus on the cheek teeth (molars and premolars).

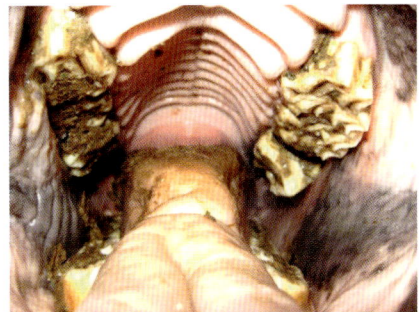

Figure 10.2.3 Molar arcades seen from the cranial view. Note: Packing of food material in teeth and dental caps on 3rd premolars bilaterally.

10 THE TEETH – AGEING AND PRACTICAL APPROACH TO DENTISTRY

Structure of the teeth

Enamel forms the outer covering, it is very hard and has no ability to repair itself.

Dentine makes up the bulk of the tooth, with secondary dentine laid down constantly over the animal's life thus preventing exposure of the pulp as the tooth wears down whilst chewing.

Pulp is the substance with the inner cavity of the tooth containing vascular tissue and nerves.

Cement is the white, hard layer seen at the occlusal surface.

Occlusal surface is the erupting surface of the tooth, seen when examining the teeth.

Figures 10.2.4, 10.2.5 and 10.2.6 illustrate the appearance of occlusal surface of the incisor teeth. It is possible to distinguish the different layers of enamel, dentine and cement. The appearance changes over the animal's life as the teeth wear down. These changes are used to estimate the age of equids. See equine dental texts such as Easley *et al.* (2011) for more detailed descriptions of dental anatomy.

Donkeys

Research into the dental anatomy of donkeys shows general similarities to that of horses (du Toit *et al.* 2008b). Differences in the timing of appearance/disappearance of occlusal surface structures used in ageing are explained in the next section (Section 10.3).

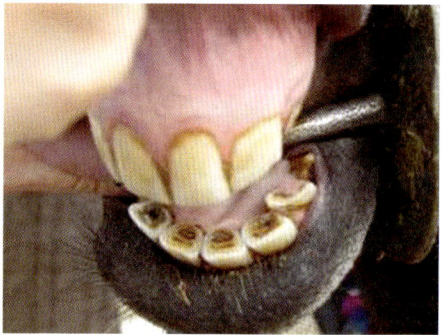

Figure 10.2.4 Occlusal surface of a 3 to 4-year-old equid showing the linear dental stars (buccal side) and infundibula cups (lingual side).

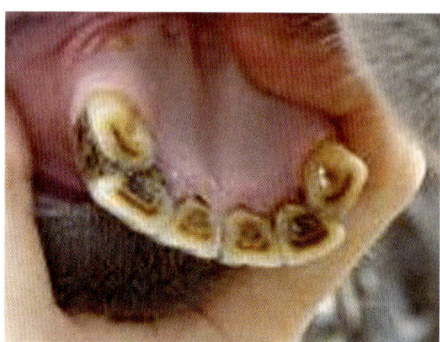

Figure 10.2.5 A 10 to 15-year-old equid, the dental star (secondary and tertiary dentine) is seen as a more oval shape on the labial side of the teeth; the cups are beginning to disappear.

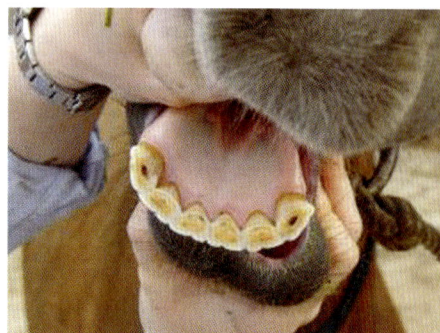

Figure 10.2.6 An equid over 16 years old; the stars have disappeared and the pulp cavity (mark) has been occluded by secondary dentine.

Ageing of equids using the incisors   10.3

The eruption of deciduous and permanent incisors can be used to estimate, fairly accurately, a horse's age until it is 5 years old but, after that, ageing by teeth becomes less reliable. For donkeys, remember that the eruption times of the incisor teeth have been reported as up to one year later than that of horses (Muylle *et al.* 1999). The presence of hooks and Galvayne's groove are unreliable in ageing donkeys (see also Section 1.4).

The information below details how an equid's age can be estimated, but always warn the owner that this is an estimate and, once an animal is over 6 or 7 years old, it is increasingly difficult to give a reliable age.

Ageing in the first 5 years – Incisor eruption

Incisor teeth are either deciduous or permanent. It is important to be able to distinguish the difference in order to estimate the age of an equid.

Deciduous teeth are whiter in colour and more rounded at the apex (Figure 10.3.1).

Permanent teeth are squarer in shape at the gum margin and yellower in colour (Figure 10.3.2).

Table 10.3.1 shows the reported eruption age for incisor teeth of horses and donkeys.

Teeth	Age of deciduous teeth eruption		Age of permanent teeth eruption	
	Horse	Donkey	Horse	Donkey
Central incisors	0–1 week	0–2 weeks	2.5 years	3–3.5 years
Middle incisors	4–6 weeks	8 weeks	3.5 years	4 years
Corner incisors	6–9 months	12 months	4.5 years	5–5.5 years

Table 10.3.1 Incisor eruption timing for horses (Tremaine 2012) and donkeys (Muylle et al. 1999).

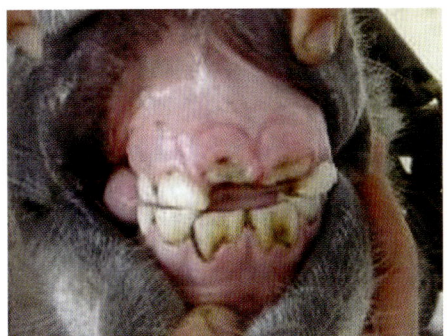

Figure 10.3.1 Erupting incisors. It is important not to confuse these with an injury or as being the chipped or missing teeth of a much older animal. Note that the shape of the gum line for deciduous incisors is rounded.

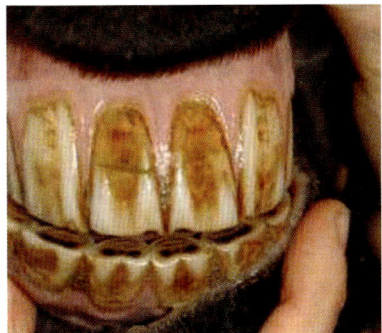

Figure 10.3.2 Permanent incisors: more yellow in colour and squarer at the gum line (apex).

10 THE TEETH – AGEING AND PRACTICAL APPROACH TO DENTISTRY

Dental stars are reported to appear in donkeys at an earlier age than in horses (Muylle *et al.* 1999), with appearance of the dental star in the central incisors at 3.5–4 years old, the middle incisors at 4–4.5 years old and the corner incisors at 5.5–7 years old. Reported appearance of stars in horses does not occur until after 5 years old (Muylle *et al.* 1996).

Ageing between 5 and 15 years – Occlusal surface and angle of incisors

As the animal increases in age, the shape of the occlusal surface changes from oval to a binomial or triangular shape; the incisor slope angle becomes greater when viewed from the side (Figures 10.3.3 and 10.3.4).

Structures of the occlusal surface of incisor teeth change as the animal ages (see also Section 10.2 of this chapter).

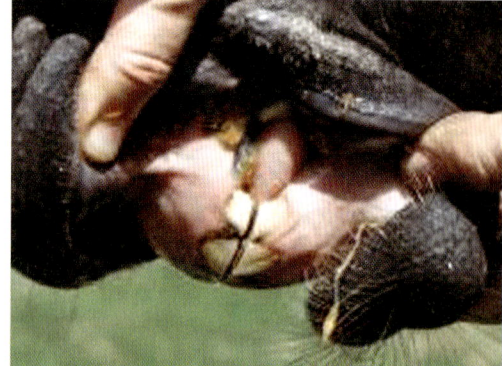

Figure 10.3.3 Lateral (side) view of deciduous incisor teeth, showing steep occlusion angle.

- **Infundibular 'cup'** This funnel-shaped structure appears as a round, white circle when the permanent tooth erupts, becoming blacker (filled with food) and smaller (getting towards the funnel base) as the tooth grows. In horses, it is reported to disappear from the central incisors by 7 years old, middle incisors by 7 to 10 years old and in the corner incisors by 10 to 14 years old, leaving a 'mark' (Muylle *et al.* 1996). In donkeys, the cup disappears from the central incisors by 11 years old, indicating a later date for loss of this structure than in horses (Muylle *et al.* 1999).

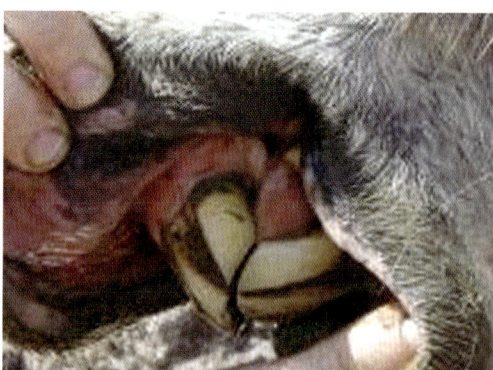

Figure 10.3.4 Lateral view of permanent incisor teeth, showing a more acute occlusion angle.

- **Enamel spot or 'mark'** A small ring of infundibular enamel which is left once the cup has disappeared. It is found on the lingual aspect of the incisors.

- **Dentine 'star'** (See Figure 10.3.5) Reported to appear in horses in the central incisors from 5 years old, middle incisors from 6 and corner incisors from 7 or 8 years old (Muylle *et al.* 1996). The reported age of appearance of the dental star in donkeys is younger than that reported for horses, with appearance of the dental star in central incisors at 3.5–4 years old, the middle incisors at 4–4.5 years old and the corner incisors at 5.5–7

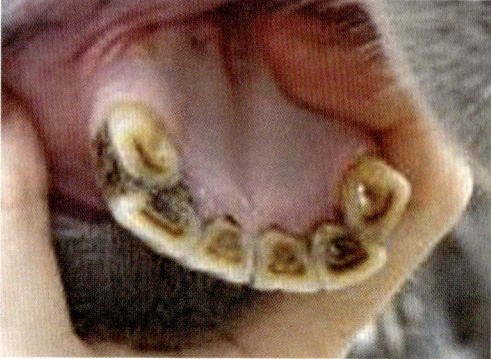

Figure 10.3.5 The 'star' is seen as the darker line on the buccal side of the incisor teeth; the 'mark' is seen as the ring-like structure on the lingual side of the teeth.

AGEING OF EQUIDS USING THE INCISORS 10.3

years old (Muylle *et al.* 1999). At around 7–8 years, secondary dentine starts to deposit in the pulp cavity, becoming larger and changing position on the occlusal surface with age.

After 15 years of age, the appearance of the biting surface does not alter greatly.

Ageing between 10 and 30 years – Upper lateral (corner) incisors

- **Galvayne's groove** This is a dark vertical line which appears on the upper corner incisor teeth (Figure 10.3.6). Historically it was considered to appear at the gum line after 10 years of age in horses, to be half way down the tooth at 15 years, and reach the occlusal surface at 20 years of age.

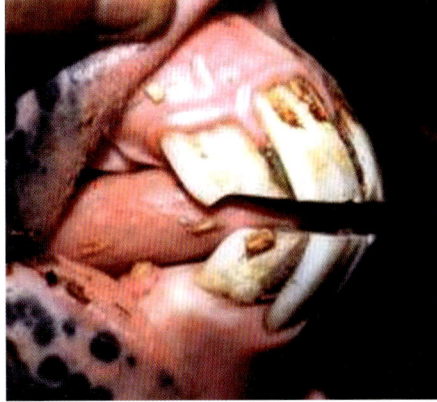

Figure 10.3.6 Galvayne's groove present on the corner incisor.

> Galvayne's groove is now considered to be an unreliable indicator of age, due to differing ages of appearance, growth and bilateral asymmetry (Muylle *et al.* 1996).

Therefore, Galvayne's groove should not be used alone to age an animal, but may add to the overall impression.

- **Donkeys** Galvayne's groove has been reported as present in some animals over 12 years old, but is too inconsistent in presence and growth to be useful as an estimator of age (Muylle *et al.* 1999).

- **Hooks on the upper corner incisors** Historically this was reported to appear at 7 years old, disappear then reappear at 11 years old (due to uneven wear of incisors). However, recent reports dispute the reliability of this, and state that hooks can appear at any time from 5 years old in some horses and can be unilateral (Muylle *et al.* 1996). Again, in **donkeys**, hooks are reported to appear from 6 years of age and can be present at any age after this, with no consistent and reliable age category (Muylle *et al.* 1999).

> Presence of a hook is, therefore, not a reliable indicator to use to estimate the age of equids.

Ageing the donkey

As stated above, the eruption times of incisor teeth are generally a little later than in the horse, and the corner incisors may not be in wear until 9 or 10 years old (5 or 6 years in the horse). The following differences have also been noticed:

- Cups in the teeth of some donkeys may not disappear until 20 years old, whereas they are gone in most horses by 14 years.
- Dental stars appear earlier on permanent incisors.
- Galvayne's groove does not appear in all donkeys.
- Hooks on the corner incisors are not reliable in donkeys.

10.4 Complete oral examination

If oral disease or pain is suspected, attempt to do a complete visual and manual examination to assess the mouth and dentition and ensure all findings are communicated to the owner.

History and clinical signs of dental disease

As usual, carry out a thorough clinical examination to assess all body systems, see Chapter 1.

> Remember, many illnesses can result in a thin animal (Figure 10.4.1) that is not eating, with associated behaviour changes.

When a problem in the mouth is suspected, take a detailed history, looking out for **clinical signs of dental disease** (Tremaine and Casey 2012).

- Reluctance to eat? It can be very useful to watch the animal eat if the owner reports problems associated with this.
- Quidding (oral dysphagia: dropping of balls of food from the mouth), or does the animal only chew on one side of the mouth?
- Hypersalivation?
- Halitosis (bad-smelling breath)?
- Food packing? Food can collect in the cheeks of equids with dental pathology or pain. This can be easily identified when the mouth is opened, and sometimes even palpated through the cheeks.
- Dropping food from the mouth whilst eating?
- Slowness in prehending and eating food?
- Inappetance?
- Faecal consistency changed?
- Weight loss?
- Nasal discharge (may be unilateral)?
- Pain or bahavioural changes when opening the mouth to put in the bit?
- Changes in behaviour when working, or in general?
- Problems with the bit in ridden/driven animals? Head shaking, abnormal head carriage and/or reluctance to accept the bit?
- Intermittent colic signs?
- Facial swellings/asymmetry/discharging sinus tracts?

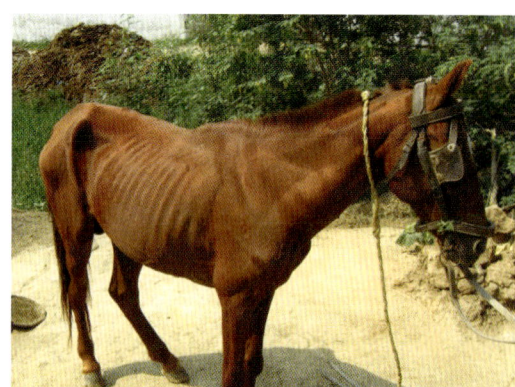

Figure 10.4.1 A thin horse can be the consequence of many diseases, including dental.

> Excessive salivation can be associated with the dumb form of rabies (Section 16.1), especially in donkeys – a good reason always to wear gloves when examining the mouth!

COMPLETE ORAL EXAMINATION 10.4

Having considered all these signs, remember equids are 'flight' animals and are very good at concealing mouth/tooth problems and pain. Ask the owner about any symptoms which could indicate a dental problem. Open the mouth of every animal to look for signs of dental disease. Do a thorough oral examination if dental disease is suspected.

Extra-oral examination

Before opening the mouth, carefully observe the head and neck area for the following signs:

- **Discharge** Nasal and/or ocular
- **Asymmetry** Muscle wasting or swelling of the face
- **Swellings** of the submandibular lymph nodes: unilateral or bilateral
- **Pain** on palpation of the structures on the outside of the face surrounding the oral cavity
- **Buccal retraction** Retract the cheek at the sides of the mouth to visualise the evenness of the cheek teeth and do a preliminary check of the upper arcade for lateral points or injury to the buccal cheek surface.
- **Lateral excursion test** Gently move the mandible laterally in each direction to assess the range of lateral movement. The mandible should move an equal distance to both sides. Note any pain on excursion (Pascoe 2010).

Initial examination will give an indication of the nature of the animal and inform the amount of sedation and restraint needed to continue with a full examination of the mouth (Tremaine and Casey 2012). Figure 10.4.2 shows an initial examination without a speculum.

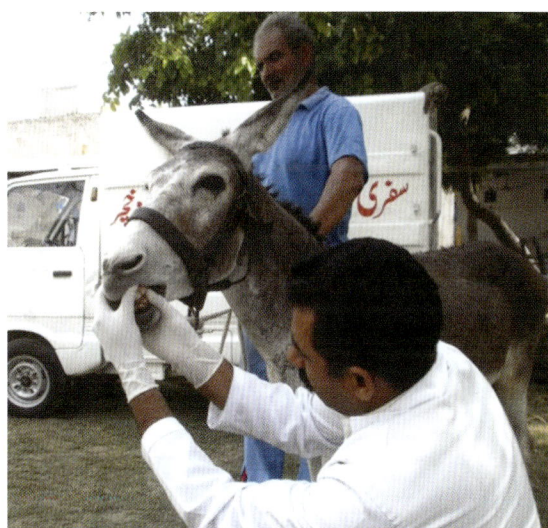

> **Note:** Always take care when examining near the mouth, and do not put a hand in the mouth without a dental speculum (gag) in place.

Studies have shown that horses should utilise both sides of the mouth equally; unilateral favouring may indicate, pain, pathology and shear mouth (Pascoe 2010).

Figure 10.4.2 Preliminary examination of the mouth without a dental speculum.

> Just as a clinician would observe a lame horse walking, it is good to watch an animal with a history of mouth/dental problems eating in order better to identify the potential problem.

10 THE TEETH – AGEING AND PRACTICAL APPROACH TO DENTISTRY

Examination of mouth with a dental speculum

Placement of the speculum

Sedation If the animal is fractious or in pain, ensure adequate sedation before placing the speculum on the head. An animal fitted with a metal speculum can cause injury to people handling or treating so, if in doubt, sedate the animal (Tremaine and Casey 2012).

> **Accurate placement is absolutely essential to do a good oral examination which is safe and allows effective manual and visual assessment.**

The size of the speculum needs to fit the animal well, so a different size would be needed for large horses compared with smaller donkeys; smaller 'pony' plates are available for donkeys.

It is no longer acceptable practice to pull the tongue out for dental examination and rasping (as was done in the past). A full examination and rasping is only possible with the use of a specialised equine speculum, e.g. the Hausmann, which is safer than side-placing gags.

When positioning a Haussmann gag, ensure the **strap over the head is sitting directly behind the ears,** not further down the neck because, if it moves forward, the mouth-pieces could come away from the teeth and the animal will close its mouth, most likely on the clinician's arm!

Examine with hands first (speculum in place)

Before washing out the mouth, always feel for food impaction (Pascoe 2010). Next, wash out the mouth using a large syringe and copious water. Inspect the mouth both manually and visually, using a bright light source.

> **Palpate the entire oral cavity – feeling the buccal, occlusal and lingual surfaces of all arcades.**

Any deviation or asymmetry in cheek teeth should be noted and each tooth should be grasped between the thumb and forefinger and checked for instability, movement or a pain reaction (see the following section on loose teeth). Feel for sharp edges, hooks or spikes, or other major pathology such as fractured/missing teeth and lesions/swellings on the soft tissues.

Visual examination (speculum in place)

Using a bright light source (head torch or pen torch – Figure 10.4.3) examine the soft tissues for evidence of ulceration (due to sharp buccal/lingual ridges), bit trauma or other wounds, swellings or tumours. The commissures of the lips and the inside of the cheeks are common areas for injury. Evaluate all three surfaces of the teeth on each arcade. If there is food impaction re-flush, or examine carefully with a probe to evaluate for diastemata. Use a mirror with a long handle (purchased or made locally) to see the buccal sides of the teeth and gums more easily (Pascoe 2010).

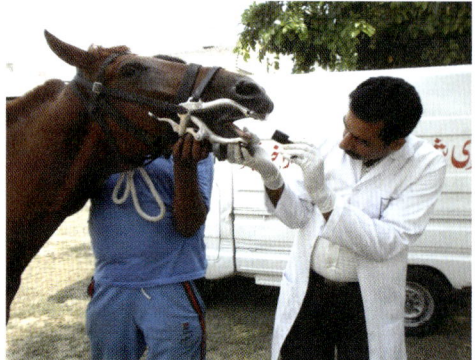

Figure 10.4.3 Examination of the mouth with a dental speculum fitted, using a pen torch to visualise inside the mouth.

Inspect the gums and tongue for injury or ulcers. The upper and lower interdental spaces (where a bit sits in the mouth – between the incisors and first cheek teeth) should be observed (and palpated), checking for bone irregularities, mucosal ulcers/thickenings or trauma from bitting. The tongue should be checked for function as it can be easily injured by harsh bits or tongue ties, as can the lip commissures which are more easily visible.

> The combination of oral and manual examination will indicate whether the animal is experiencing any pain or discomfort when eating or working.

Dental equipment 10.5

The equipment described below is a comprehensive list of equine dental tools. Although not all of these may be available or necessary, they have been included here for information.

Depending on the confidence of the clinician and the frequency of dental work conducted in the field, some of the equipment described below may be required. Ideally, aim to have a full-mouth dental speculum, e.g. Hausmann's, a bright light source (head torches are preferable to leave hands free for examination), a set of dental rasps and flushing equipment for dentistry (large syringe and bucket to collect the dirty water and dispose of somewhere away from the examination site). Local alternatives may actually be a potential source of equipment – provided that it is safe to use and does not cause any welfare problems or risks to the animal.

Dental records

> Ensure that all findings are recorded.

A Modified Triadan system for dental nomenclature can be used (Dixon and Dacre 2005) with the teeth of the upper right arcade numbered from 101 to 111, the upper left numbered from 201 to 211, the lower left numbered from 301 to 311, and the lower right numbered from 401 to 411.

Examination equipment

Speculum or gag

- The Hausmann's is most commonly used – it is a safe oral speculum; however, there is a range of gags available.

  > - A speculum is essential for complete oral examination (Tremaine and Casey 2012).

- A speculum avoids damage to the tongue, which is very common if the tongue is pulled aside to examine and rasp teeth.

Light source
- This is essential for viewing the oral cavity, especially the caudal part.
- Head torches are preferable as they leave both hands free (Tremaine and Casey 2012); cheap versions are widely available.
- LED lights are better as they don't produce heat and have good battery life.

Dental syringe, mouthwash and bucket
- These are all readily available.
- Use chlorhexidine gluconate (< 0.1% concentration) ideally, or salt water, for flushing (very dilute povidone-iodine can be used, but it tastes unpleasant).

> - **Keep the animal's head down so that water falls out of the mouth and is not aspirated (Tremaine and Casey 2012).**

- Collect the water falling from the mouth in a bucket so as not to flood the work area.

Dental mirror
- This allows a good view of the caudal oral cavity and all three sides of cheek teeth (to diagnose diastemata, etc.).
- Strong, rigid mirrors are best as they can move soft tissues, such as the tongue, out of the way to allow better visualisation of the teeth (Tremaine and Casey 2012).
- Mirror fogging can be a problem particularly in cold weather; warming the mirror before use (e.g. placing in some warm water) can reduce this (Pascoe 2010).
- **The** ideal size is 5 cm diameter and angled for ease of use.
- Care: They are fragile and can be broken!

Probes and picks
- Useful to investigate the condition of the occlusal surfaces or the depth of pockets between teeth
- Can identify sharp points and loose fragments (Tremaine and Casey 2012)
- Can be used to clean out diastemata
- A range of shapes and sizes available depending on your requirements (see further dental texts for more information)

Head stand
- Holding the animal's head at head height will make examination easier.
- A sedated equid's head can become very heavy for the handler to hold for the length of a full dental examination.
- Specially made equine head supports are available, but it is possible to improvise with items in the local environment to provide a comfortable support for the animal.

> - **ENSURE that the support does not constrict the airway (throat) of the animal.**

Manual instruments
Dental rasping blades

- A large range of dental rasps are available to deal with the teeth in different parts of the mouth. However, most things can be done with three or four (a minimum of one straight and one angled).
- There are many different types; the angle and blade on the head is more important than the handle type which is usually a question of personal preference.
- Blades can be set in the handle head so the cut is on push or pull; again, this is personal preference.

The following blades are the most commonly used:

- **Tungsten chip blades** Rough chips of tungsten carbide bound on to a solid steel backing plate. These can be quite aggressive if not used correctly. They cut in both directions and are cheaper, but they blunt and corrode quickly. Studies show that they cut deep grooves into the surface of the teeth and damage cement and enamel (Kempson *et al.* 2003).
- **Solid tungsten blades** Serrations are cut into the blade surface by a machine, and there are many different degrees of blade coarseness available. However, the coarse blades are often too aggressive and blunt easily so most dentists prefer a medium/fine cut. They cut in one direction only and can be re-sharpened. They are medium price but better wearing, and are a good option if available. Studies show these blades leave a smooth surface to the teeth post-rasping (Kempson *et al.* 2003).
- **Diamond coated** Diamond bonded onto steel. Cut in both directions. These are durable, but expensive and can corrode.

> - Take care: It is easy to over-rasp with this type! (Tremaine and Price 2012)

Rasp design

There are many different types of rasp handles/heads which can accept different blades, with variations in the style and shaft necessary to fit different parts of the mouth (Tremaine and Price 2012). There is not one rasp that can do everything so ideally have a selection.

Straight blades

- Short straight
  - Used for rostral cheek teeth in both upper and lower arcades
  - Set to cut on the pull as this is easier and less likely to damage soft tissues
- Long straight
  - Used on middle-caudal part of the upper and lower arcades
  - Ensure blade set to cut on the pull stroke

Angled blades (for use on the upper arcade only; the angle makes rasping of uppers easier)

- Short open-angled
  - Rostral upper arcades
  - Blade usually set to cut on the push stroke
  - Cannot rasp rostral hooks on 06s

10 THE TEETH – AGEING AND PRACTICAL APPROACH TO DENTISTRY

▌ Medium open-angled
- Middle-caudal upper arcade
- Blade set to cut on the pull stroke

▌ Up-angled rasp
- Used for upper 10 and 11, especially the caudal aspect where hooks are hard to reach
- Set to cut on the pull stroke as soft tissues are easily damaged in this area

▌ Short offset rasps (down-angled)
- Used to address rostral hooks on upper and lower 06s and round them off
- More useful than other angled rasps
- Blade set on the push or pull stroke

> **Use of any type of tooth-cutting instrument is contra-indicated.**

Motorised equipment

▌ A variety of motorised rasps are available, with varying sources of power-switches, blade movement (disc, axial) and power sourcing.

▌ Motorised rasps can offer greater precision than manual instruments, and can be good for long overgrowths. However, proper training is required to operate them because, if used incorrectly, they can result in a serious amount of damage.

▌ They can be very dangerous in inexperienced hands due to the possibility of excessive reductions of teeth, soft tissue trauma and thermal trauma. However, these dangers can be minimised with good training, skill and sedation of the animal, and an efficient cooling system.

▌ The power source may not be reliable when in the field; there are also additional safety concerns.

> ▌ **Cases of severe over-rasping have been seen with improper use of power tools.**

Over-rasping results because it is often difficult to stop the machine in time. This is very distressing for the animal and owner, as the animal has no occlusal surfaces to grind its food with, and is in pain because the sensitive dentine and pulp is all exposed (Lundstrom 2010).

▌ Take care in older animals as motorised equipment may loosen previously functional teeth (Lundstrom 2010).

> **Motorised equipment should NEVER be used without sedation and a dental speculum.**

Table 10.4 shows the advantages and disadvantages of both manual and motorised dental rasping equipment. Consider and be aware of these when deciding on and using dental rasping equipment.

Advantages	Disadvantages
Manual equipment	
Easy to use	May be less precise
Inexpensive	Inefficient on large overgrowths
Less traumatic to soft tissues	Physically demanding for operator
Less likely to require sedation	Causes surface damage to the teeth (enamel and cement)
Motorised Equipment	
More precise	Difficult to use correctly and requires training
Efficient	Expensive
Less soft tissue damage in the caudal mouth (if used correctly)	Traumatic to soft tissues
Less physical effort for the operator	Requires sedation
	Produces dust and heat (which can damage the tooth pulp); always use with a cooling system
	Never to be used without a dental speculum
	Requires efficient, safe power supply which may be difficult in the field
	It is easy to over-rasp
	May loosen previously functional teeth in older animals

Table 10.4 Relative advantages and disadvantages of manual and motorised dental rasping equipment.

10.6 Common problems due to mastication and wear

Due to the infrequent grazing patterns of many working equids, and the diets they consume, there is often evidence of dental problems, especially in older animals (du Toit and Dixon 2012). In a study of 203 working donkeys in Mexico, the prevalence of dental disease was 62% with sharp enamel points in 98% of animals examined (du Toit and Dixon 2012). Dental disease is reported as most prevalent in older donkeys aged 16–20 years (du Toit et al. 2008a).

An equid's teeth depend on *constant lateral movement* for them to wear evenly. If this does not occur, due to disruption of normal grazing/eating behaviours (such as working for many hours per day), then dental problems occur.

Sharp enamel points – buccal (lateral) and lingual (medial) overgrowths

These are a very common abnormality associated with equine teeth worldwide (du Toit and Dixon 2012). The hard points of enamel on the buccal surface of the upper (maxillary) teeth and the lingual side of the lower (mandibular) cheek teeth become very sharp often lacerating the cheeks.

Studies indicate that tight nosebands and head-collars contribute to ulcers and calluses in the mouth (du Toit et al. 2008a) possibly by pressing the cheeks and soft tissues onto the sharp points resulting in trauma and wounds. As well as rasping these sharp points, loosening the noseband could make equids more comfortable.

Besides affecting the ease with which equids can grind food (and hence affecting digestion capabilities and thus the nutritional value of feed), these enamel points can produce painful sores and ulceration of the mucosa lining the cheeks and tongue (Figure 10.6.1) making eating painful, which further exacerbates the problem of overgrown teeth and associated weight loss.

Although focal overgrowths on the first few (rostral) cheek teeth can be visualised, it is necessary to do a thorough examination, with a dental speculum and bright light, to pick up problems at the back of the mouth. Feeling the back of the mouth with a gloved hand can also pick up pathology in hard to see places. It is crucial that the sharp points at the back of the mouth are not missed as these are more likely to result in cheek lesions and pain.

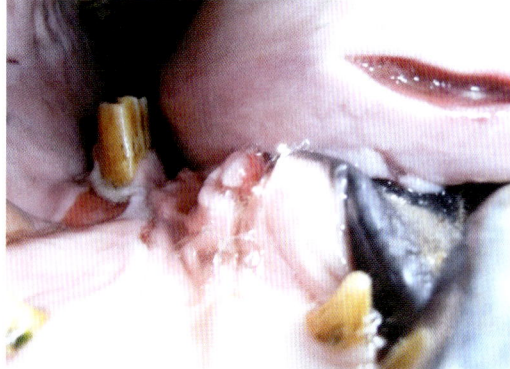

Figure 10.6.1 Laceration of the tongue due to sharp enamel points.

See Section 10.8 of this chapter for treatment and rasping of sharp enamel points (Figure 10.8.1).

Rostral and caudal overgrowths of cheek teeth (hooks)

If the maxillary and mandibular arcades are misaligned or different lengths, uneven wear may produce overgrowths on the front and back (rostral and caudal aspects) of the cheek teeth, in addition to or instead of the lateral overgrowths described above.

COMMON PROBLEMS DUE TO MASTICATION AND WEAR 10.6

> Dental overgrowths cause pain and discomfort when eating and can affect the prehension and biting of food, especially grasses.

Hooks on the rostral aspect of the 1st cheek tooth (06) are easily seen and rasped in a good dental examination; however, hooks on the caudal aspect of the 6th mandibular cheek tooth (11) are often missed (Figure 10.6.2) and it is these which can cause the most pain.

Rasps with solid carbide blades can treat this problem effectively, although it requires patience as it can take a long time. Molar cutters are not recommended since they increase the chance of exposing the sensitive dental pulp (Tremaine and Price 2012).

> For large dental overgrowths, gradually reduce over a number of examinations rather than in one go.

See Section 10.8 of this chapter for more information on treatment.

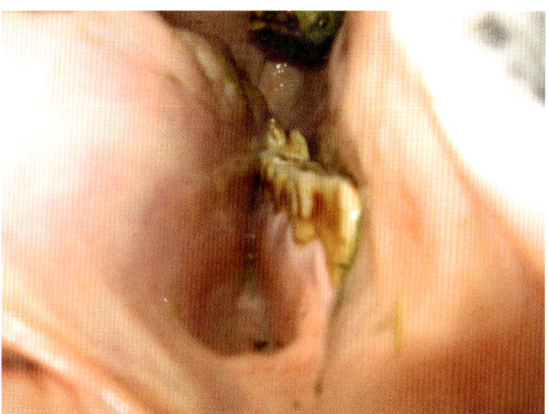

Figure 10.6.2 Caudal hook on tooth 311.

Excessive transverse ridges of the occlusal surfaces (ETRs)

The occlusal surfaces of equine teeth are naturally uneven due to the natural jaw movements and varying rates of wear of the enamel and dentine. This unevenness is related to effective mastication (Tremaine and Price 2012), see Figure 10.6.3.

> There is little current evidence to show that ETRs contribute to equine dental problems; it is *inadvisable to rasp occlusal surfaces* unless they are causing obvious pain.

Occasionally there may be an excessive ridge that protrudes far beyond the level of the others. In this case it may be appropriate to reduce this ridge to the level of the others to allow effective mastication (Tremaine and Price 2012).

It is absolutely essential that the occlusal surfaces have some ridges and roughness as this is the grinding surface that breaks up the food in mastication. If this is rasped smooth, the equid will not be able masticate effectively and this may result in weight loss and quidding (Lundstrom 2010).

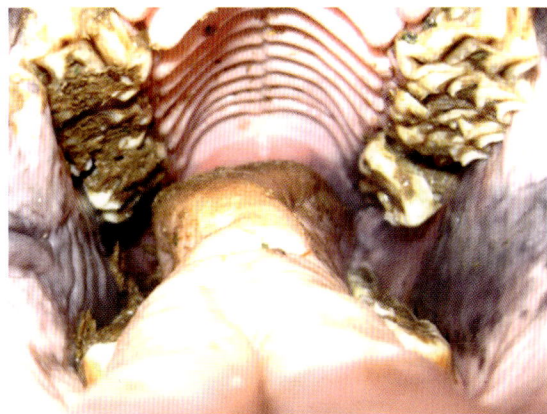

Figure 10.6.3 Transverse ridge pattern seen in these cheek teeth.

Wave mouth

This is when there is a wave-like or undulating appearance to the arcade in a rostro-caudal direction and is especially seen in older horses and donkeys (Dixon and Dacre 2005, du Toit and Dixon 2012). Large focal overgrowths or diastemata may contribute to producing a wave mouth (Dixon and Dacre 2005, Tremaine and Price 2012).

> It is rarely possible to correct such chronic changes (wave mouth) with rasping.

Ideally overgrowths should be treated early on to prevent wave mouth (Dixon and Dacre 2005). Rasp little and often (twice-yearly) to attempt to correct wave mouth.

Step mouth

Focal overgrowths can occur which result in a 'step' in the mouth where one tooth is a lot 'taller' than that the rest of the arcade. This overgrown tooth will stop the other teeth in the arcades coming together in a bite and, therefore, will interfere with the occlusal grinding surface and ultimately may severely disrupt mastication. Severe soft tissue damage can be the result if a tooth overgrows extensively and chewing results in trauma to the opposite gums.

These focal overgrowths commonly occur if a tooth is lost. Equine cheek teeth erupt continuously and are continually worn by the process of mastication. If a cheek tooth is lost the opposite tooth will no longer be worn and will become overgrown. Without any wear this overgrowth will get larger and larger until it causes a serious impact on mastication; it can stop the cheek teeth from meeting, and always results in serious soft tissue injury and pain in the mouth.

> It is really important these overgrowths are treated as they will severely impair mastication (chewing) and will result in severe dental pain.

Furthermore, without treatment they will only get worse. The overgrowths do not need to be rasped right down to the level of the other teeth, but sufficiently to allow normal mastication (du Toit and Dixon 2012). See Section 10.8 for more information on treatment.

Shear mouth

Normally the occlusal surfaces of the cheek teeth sit at a slight angle of 10–30 degrees (Tremaine and Price 2012). If the angle becomes greater than 45 degrees this is termed 'shear mouth' (Dixon and Dacre 2005). If the enamel edges become too long the occlusal surfaces end up sitting at a steeper angle, causing pain, and reduce the occlusal surface available for grinding food.

In extreme circumstances it can altogether stop the animal eating normally. Instead of a side to side movement of the jaw to grind food the eating pattern ends up like a carnivore's with an up-down chewing motion. This is very dangerous for equids and further exacerbates the overgrowth.

> Severe shear mouth leads to quidding and weight loss; further gum and tooth disease can occur due to the large amounts of food which sit in the mouth for long periods as they cannot be chewed.

Severe shear mouth is ideally treated by dental experts with mechanical burring done in stages. With a manual rasp, reduce the buccal and lingual points as normal. This may require frequent (every 3 months) reviews to maintain an adequate functional arcade (du Toit and Dixon 2012).

Smooth mouth

This mostly occurs in older animals (du Toit and Dixon 2012) or where there has been excessive rasping of the teeth, often with a power tool (iatrogenic) (Lundstrom 2010).

> Beware rasping too much off the points in older animals – they may be the only occlusal surface the animal has left for eating!

Smooth mouth cannot be cured and permanent feeding of soft food is required. It is essential that owners are aware of the correct diet for these animals to maintain their daily requirements, especially if they are still working.

Other dental abnormalities seen in working equids 10.7

Retained deciduous crowns ('caps')

The first three cheek teeth (excluding wolf teeth) are the premolars (06, 07, 08) and all have deciduous teeth that grow and fall out before the permanent teeth develop. The last three cheek teeth are the molars (09, 10, 11) and do not have deciduous forms, erupting for the first time as permanent teeth; they are not present in foals.

Around the age of 2–4 years old the crowns of the deciduous cheek teeth can become loose or rotated as the permanent teeth erupt, causing discomfort and trouble eating.

Diagnosis is usually by palpation or visualisation (Figure 10.7.1), or by smell as food becomes caught. An irregularity

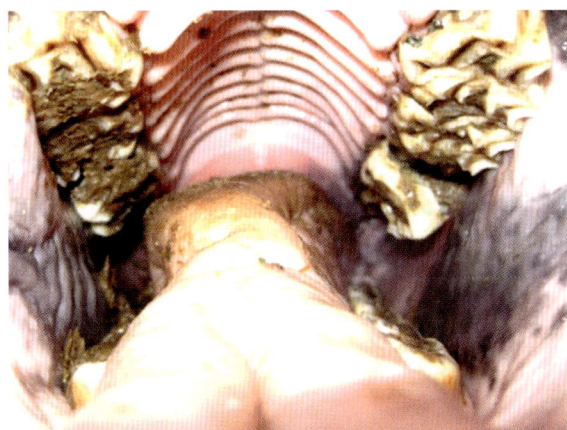

Figure 10.7.1 Dental caps seen on 108 and 208.

or 'rattling' sound may be experienced when rasping – check the animal's age if this is so. In most cases caps will fall off naturally (Figure 10.7.2) and any remaining small pieces should not cause a problem. If small caps are present rasp any sharp hooks left behind, but avoid manual

10 THE TEETH – AGEING AND PRACTICAL APPROACH TO DENTISTRY

removal of caps as this causes other problems if they are not ready to come off. If caps are very loose, and appear to be causing problems, they can be removed carefully using an appropriate instrument (Dixon and Dacre 2005).

Incisors – Uneven, displaced or retained deciduous incisors

Most equids have fairly straight incisors, although sometimes they are crooked, uneven, or have retained temporary teeth behind or between them. A case of polydontia is shown in Figure 10.7.3.

Current thinking is that these conditions rarely cause problems with eating, and incisors should not require rasping or removal unless absolutely necessary (Tremaine and Price 2012).

> Complete incisor removal can have disastrous consequences: these teeth keep the jaw balanced at the temporomandibular joint and allow the animal to prehend food.

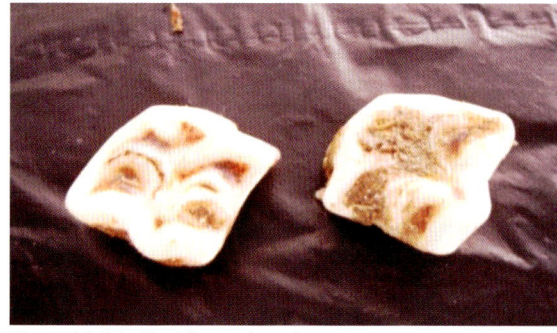

Figure 10.7.2 Deciduous dental caps.

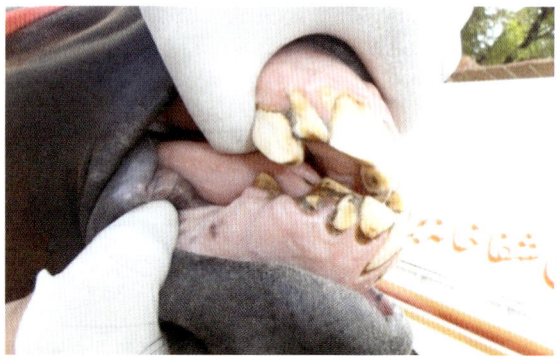

Figure 10.7.3 Polydontia seen in a working horse.

Diastemata

These are abnormal gaps between teeth which occur for a number of reasons, including developmental conditions, periodontal disease, and focal overgrowths which force food down between the teeth, or dental extractions. These gaps allow food material to pack between the teeth causing periodontitis (Casey and Tremaine 2010) with resultant infection. Damage to periodontal ligaments will ultimately result in loose teeth which may fall out.

Studies report that diastemata are the most prevalent dental disorder in donkeys (du Toit and Dixon 2012).

Clinical signs Salivation, pain and a bad smell can indicate diastemata. Thorough inspection with a gag is necessary to identify this.

> Diastemata are usually extremely painful for the animal.

Treatment in the field involves flushing out food from the tooth space using a high-pressure syringe (usually very painful therefore sedation may be required). Use a rasp to reduce the opposite transverse ridge slightly, as this acts to push food further into the diastemata. Be sure to look at the whole mouth and correct any hooks, sharp points, etc. which may be causing the problem. Reducing any overgrowths or sharp edges to improve food flow can minimise food packing. Widening of diastemata is carried out to try to prevent food trapping (du Toit and Dixon 2012). Changes to the diet may also aid in reduction in food trapping (Casey and Tremaine 2010). NSAIDs are recommended for analgesia; antibiotics depend on the individual case.

> There is good current evidence to show that simply flushing out food from the space and treating with antibiotics and anti-inflammatory drugs, along with a diet of larger-sized food particles (i.e. hay and no finely cut roughage such as chaff or short-chopped, hard feed such as alfalfa) (du Toit and Dixon 2012), can be adequate to manage diastemata.

Periodontal (gum) disease

This is inflammation and infection of the gums (alveoli, gingiva, periodontal ligaments and cement); periodontal meaning 'around the teeth'. It is most common in older animals and seen secondary to primary dental disorders such as diastemata and misaligned cheek teeth (Dixon and Dacre 2005, Casey and Tremaine 2010). It is reported as a very painful condition; however, correction of the primary problem may lead to reversal of the periodontitis ((Dixon and Dacre 2005).

Clinical signs can include the generalised signs of dental disease: halitosis, quidding, discomfort with the bit/bridle, behaviour change, nasal discharge (Casey and Tremaine 2010). However, facial and mandibular swelling is not a symptom as any infectious exudate associated with the condition can drain out of the mouth, rather than being trapped in the tooth root, as seen with a tooth root abscess.

If present for a long time, gum problems will lead to loosening and eventual loss of teeth, due to damage/loosening of the periodontal ligaments that hold the teeth in place.

Treatment Early regular attention will avert this problem. However, it may not be possible to reverse severe gum disease once it has passed the superficial stages. Correction of malocclusions/overgrowths and early treatment of diastemata is the key to prevention. In advanced cases, flushing with dilute chlorhexidine and owner management, including feeding practices, may be the only treatment option (Tremaine and Price 2012).

Dental disorders associated with trauma

Trauma is frequently seen in working equids due to road accidents, kicks, falls or biting hard objects. Fractures of the mandible and maxilla bones are common; most have a good prognosis with appropriate therapy. Some dental problems may go undetected until more serious complications develop and, without repair, may result in tooth loss, oestomyelitis, malalignment of the jaws, or functional loss (Moll and Schoonover 2005). Incisors which are missing or damaged in one jaw will affect tooth balance, and opposing overgrowths will need regular attention (Dixon and Dacre 2005). Every attempt should be made to preserve the incisor teeth after trauma (Caldwell 2006).

Such cases may present with painful swellings and trouble eating, with associated lip or tongue trauma (see Section 11.4 *The Gastrointestinal System – Conditions of the mouth and oesophagus*), or more overt trauma (Figure 10.7.4).

> The oral mucosa heals very well due to a good blood supply.

Even though the oral mucosa is exposed to food material and a large number of commensal bacteria, its ability to heal is very good. There is little merit in using topical medications,

10 THE TEETH – AGEING AND PRACTICAL APPROACH TO DENTISTRY

although oral lavage with saline solution or water can temporarily assist in reducing food contamination. Chlorhexidine solutions can be used, but reports state not to exceed 0.2% (Caldewell 2006); dilute povidone iodine (PI) has also been reported for use (Moll and Schoonover 2005), but conflicting reports state PI may affect healing and is best avoided (Caldewell 2006). Similarly, unless wounds are full thickness and require closure to stop food contaminations, suturing of intra-oral injuries is generally not indicated.

If the animal can eat, unilateral fractures are well splinted by the other hemi-mandible and can be treated conservatively with broad-spectrum antibiotics, anti-inflammatory drugs (Caldewell 2006) and feeding only very soft food. Wire can be used for stabilisation in some cases (see surgical texts and references), a mental nerve block (see Section 10.8 of this chapter) is good for suturing broken gums and wiring jaws if necessary. If an injury penetrates the alveolar bone, apical infection and tooth loss can occur.

> **Daily flushing the area aids healing (Moll and Schoonover 2005).**

When the incisor teeth have been involved in a trauma, they may be broken or loose. Fractures of these teeth with no pulp involvement will heal gradually with antibiotics and anti-inflammatory drugs; it is not recommended to remove fragments unless they are 'hanging loose'. Pulp exposure is seen as a gelatinous structure, muddy-red which becomes grey if it has been there for a few days (normally it is pink). Correct any sharp fragments with a rasp, although flattening the incisors too much will lead to problems with jaw alignment.

> **The rasping of incisor teeth is considered painful (Tremaine and Price 2012).**

An example of a dental trauma is presented in the case study in Section 10.9 of this chapter. It involves a working horse which was hit in the mouth by a vehicle on a road, resulting in a fracture of the central left upper incisor (201) (see Figure 10.7.4).

> **Aim to make the animal comfortable and the teeth functional, rather than restore absolute cosmetic appearance.**

Periapical infection, tooth fractures and neoplasia

These can all occur in working equids. Their diagnosis and management is a specialist area for veterinary dentists, often requiring equipment that is out of the scope of a field situation.

Suspect a **tumour** if there is a hard, slow-growing mass on the jaws, or if multiple teeth have been lost over a few months due to resorption of bone and teeth (Dixon and Dacre 2005). Sometimes a benign epulis behind the incisor teeth will cause the same symptoms.

For further information see the references at the end of this chapter.

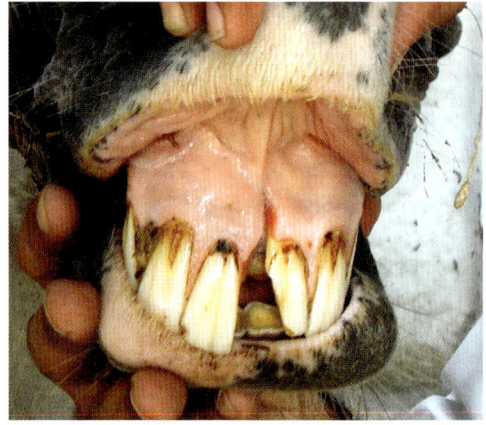

Figure 10.7.4 Fracture of 201 incisor and maxilla in a working horse.

Treating dental conditions in the field

10.8

Health and safety

Although health and safety is important in all veterinary interventions, safety awareness in dentistry is even more important as many procedures involve standing right in front of the animal which is a common place for injury (Pascoe 2010). Also, when a full-mouth dental speculum, such as the Hausmann gag, is used in dental examinations, this heavy piece of equipment can result in injury to bystanders if the animal moves its head suddenly. Therefore, it is crucial always to restrain the animal correctly (consider sedation), and keep one hand on the gag to be aware of its position and avoid injury.

> **Never kneel in front of the animal to look in its mouth as this may result in injury if the animal moves forwards.**

Use of sedatives in equine dental treatment

Any of the sedation techniques (see Section 7.1) can be used to settle the animal if the mouth is painful or the animal is fearful; it should always be considered early on in the procedure for both the clinician's safety and that of the owner/handler and animal. Many working equids will never have worn a dental speculum or had their mouth examined before so, until they become familiar with the process, they may find it distressing.

> **Administering sedation before the animal is very excited or nervous improves the efficacy.**

If a procedure is going to be painful then ensure pain relief is provided **pre-emptively** before the procedure. This improves the efficacy of the analgesia.

Analgesic cover needs to be provided for a suitable period of time. Analgesia, offered by alpha2-agonists and/or butorphanol used for sedation, is very short acting, wearing off before the animal recovers from the sedative effects. Therefore, this should be combined with an NSAID, e.g. phenylbutazone or flunixin meglumine, which will provide analgesic cover for 24 hours (see Section 5.2).

Advantages and disadvantages of using sedation during dental treatment

When considering whether to sedate an animal for a dental examination, consider the behaviour and pain experienced by the animal, as well as the planned examination and treatment, and any increased levels of pain or distress this may cause. Always know the effects of the sedative agent to be used and advise the owner of these effects. Table 10.8.1 on the next page lists the advantages and disadvantages of sedative use for dental interventions.

10 THE TEETH – AGEING AND PRACTICAL APPROACH TO DENTISTRY

Advantages	Disadvantages
Increased safety for the animal, veterinarian and owner/handler	Results in a lowered, heavy head (requires head stand or a person to hold it up)
Improved experience for the animal (decreased pain, fear, distress from the unfamiliar experience of wearing a speculum)	Possibility of an adverse reaction
Enables thorough oral examination and opportunity to do the treatment properly and precisely	Animal may fall, or choke on the water used for flushing the mouth
Provides some pain relief	Potential for increased haemorrhage
Aids the education of client or other health professional.	Requires time for recovery and this needs to be supervised

Table 10.8.1 The advantages and disadvantages of using sedatives for dental interventions in working equids.

Correction of dental problems with rasps

> Rasping (floating, filing) should be done with care and attention – never go too fast as this may result in over-rasping. The objective is just to remove any sharp projections, thus improving dental health and overall mastication.

Enamel points

The jaw curves naturally upwards at the front and back, and is straight in the middle.

The teeth of the upper arcade are slightly wider that those of the lower arcade. This results in a distinct wear pattern whereby:

- the outside edges of the maxillary (upper) cheek teeth develop sharp edges
- the inside edges of the mandibular (lower) cheek teeth develop sharp edges.

These sharp points can cause injury/wounds to the cheeks and the tongue resulting in significant pain when eating and with bitting. It is common for this soft tissue injury to be made significantly worse by **tight nosebands** (du Toit *et al.* 2008a) which press the delicate cheek tissue onto the sharp enamel edges resulting in lacerations and wounds.

Diagnosis

- Signs of dental pain are often present – quidding, resentment of the bit, loss of condition.
- Oral examination – visualise/feel these sharp points.

TREATING DENTAL CONDITIONS IN THE FIELD 10.8

Treatment

▌ Hold the rasp with either one or both hands and carefully remove these sharp enamel points. Aim to rasp **only** these points and do not rasp the entire occlusal surface smooth – i.e. do not place the rasp horizontally on the arcade, but at an angle so only the points are removed (Figure 10.8.1). Equids need this occlusal surface to be ridged to grind their food. If it is smooth they will be unable to masticate (chew) effectively and will lose weight.

▌ Using rasps with angled heads can help rasp these enamel points effectively – an angled rasp is helpful for the rostral cheek teeth of the upper arcade, whereas straight rasps (without angled heads) are useful for the lower cheek teeth and caudal upper cheek teeth.

▌ Only rasp the sharp edges of the tooth (buccal in maxilla and lingual in mandibular arcades) and do not flatten down the occlusal surfaces.

> ▌ Rasp the back molars (11s) on each arcade as these are commonly missed but are often problematic for equids.

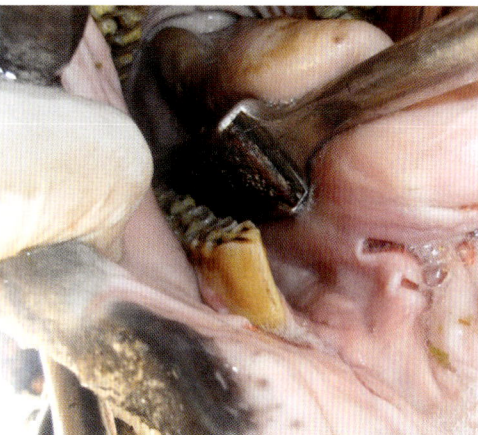

Figure 10.8.1 *Using a manual rasp to file sharp enamel points on the lingual side of the maxillary cheek teeth.*

Complications of rasping – what to avoid

▌ **Avoid over-rasping – particularly in older animals.** The older the animal the slower the eruption of teeth and the less residual tooth crown (that above the gum-line) so, in older animals, it is even more important to avoid excessive rasping – many problems such as wave and shear mouth will never be corrected. Often in older animals rasping is done to prevent soft tissue trauma from overgrown or deformed teeth and to facilitate eating. As a guide, only rasp one-third to half of what is necessary in older animals. Excessive rasping may loosen otherwise functional teeth (Lundstrom 2010).

▌ Common problems of older horses, such as weight loss, reluctance to eat and reluctance to work, may be prevented with even slight amounts of rasping.

▌ Be sure to check the whole mouth, and that any sharp points or hooks at the back of the mouth have been successfully treated. There is no point in correcting the mild enamel points at the front of the mouth if there are large hooks left caudally which are causing much more of a problem.

▌ Be very careful not to injure the mucosa or cause excessive bleeding.

> ▌ Aggressive correction, or rasping at an angle which produces flattening of the occlusal surfaces, can completely remove arcades from occlusion making it impossible for the equid to chew its food (Lundstrom 2010). It doesn't matter how it feels, or looks, but how it works for the animal.

- Excessive rasping can also expose the sensitive parts of the tooth, causing pain and shortening the tooth's life (Dixon and Dacre 2005).

- Always consider **analgesia**. Rasping may be painful for the animal due to the presence of sensory nerves within the dentine (Tremaine and Price 2012).

- If the animal is eating normally, there is no evidence of soft tissue trauma visible in the mouth and no dental pathology that could produce trauma, then do not rasp.

Correcting overgrowths/step mouth

In treatment of focal overgrowths of one tooth (a step) or multiple dental overgrowths (e.g. wave mouth), the correction principles are the same: reduce to a more normal function. Remember, an overgrowth is the symptom not the cause of a problem. Have a good light source and check the opposite arcade.

- Excessive rasping of overgrowths can expose dentine and cause pain (Tremaine and Price 2012). Always stop and check with a good light source.

- It is crucial that during corrective rasping the pulp is not exposed as this will result in severe, potentially permanent damage to the tooth (Dixon and Dacre 2005). It is also extremely painful for the animal as the pulp contains the nerve supply to the tooth. Stop rasping if a pink colour is visible at the centre of the tooth as this indicates that the sensitive pulp has been damaged.

- If an overgrowth is large, ideally it should be gradually reduced over a period of treatments/months, so the pulp is not exposed (Tremaine and Price 2012).

- **Tooth cutters** are generally not advised as they can result in serious side effects including:
  - tooth fracture – Splitting cheek teeth will result in severe dental pain and will permanently damage the teeth. This can lead to severe and long-term pain/infection.
  - exposure of the pulp – If too much tooth is cut the pulp will be exposed. As explained earlier, this can result in permanent damage to the tooth and chronic pain.
  - iatrogenic wounds in the mouth/jaw fracture – from over-zealous molar cutting.

Tooth removal

> **Tooth removal is very rarely indicated in working equids – unless the tooth is loose enough to be easily extracted orally.**

For a cheek tooth to be loose, over 50% of the periodontal ligament attachment must be lost. This damage to the periodontal ligaments commonly occurs through dental disease such as periodontal disease secondary to food packing in a diastema. Once a tooth is lost, this always results in a focal overgrowth (step) in the opposite cheek teeth arcade (Dixon and Dacre 2005). Equine cheek teeth erupt continuously and are continually worn by the process of mastication. If a cheek tooth is lost the opposite tooth will no longer be in wear, resulting in an overgrowth. Without this wear the overgrowth will get larger and larger until it causes a serious impact on mastication. It can stop the cheek teeth from meeting and always results in serious soft tissue injury and pain in the mouth.

Loose teeth can be identified with a thorough oral investigation. Carefully palpate all teeth and test whether any of them wobble with manual pressure. Loose teeth tend to be painful; therefore, if any area of the mouth is painful to this palpation or rasping, look carefully for any evidence of laxity.

> Unless the tooth is extremely loose and can be pulled out with forceps, do not attempt molar removal in the field.

Complications for this surgery are high, and cheek tooth removal is an advanced surgical technique that requires specialist veterinary dental skills, equipment and extensive aftercare. In the context of working equids, suitable facilities are rarely available and the risks of complications, resulting in significant pain, poor welfare and actually making the dental pathology worse, makes tooth extraction impractical and ill-advised. Complications are higher in younger animals (Tremaine and Price 2012).

Complications of tooth removal

- Sequestration – leaving a piece of tooth in the alveolus
- Oro-nasal fistula – damaging the bone separating the oral and nasal cavities
- Super-eruption of opposite tooth – overgrowth of the cheek tooth in the opposite arcade because it is no longer being worn down by the tooth that has fallen out, requiring frequent rasping of the opposing arcade
- Chronic sinusitis and discharging sinus tracts – infection in sinus as a result of incomplete tooth removal or iatrogenic infection

Care after tooth removal

If a cheek tooth is loose and can be easily removed orally – by wobbling until it comes free – it is still important that careful aftercare is provided to ensure rapid healing and to reduce complications.

- Provide soft palatable food (e.g. mashes), not coarse/fibrous hay/straw. This minimises trauma to the healing tooth socket.
- NSAID cover should be provided – for analgesia and anti-inflammatory effects.
- Animals with marked infection may require a course of antibiotics.
- Administer tetanus antitoxin.

> - **AFTER TOOTH REMOVAL** the teeth of that animal will require very regular rasping every 6 to 12 months as a minimum.

Regular care is needed to prevent an overgrowth in the opposite cheek tooth. This will need to be done for the rest of the animal's life. **It is essential that owners are fully aware of this requirement to avoid problems in the future.**

Dental nerve blocks

To aid certain dental procedures, the administration of the following nerve blocks can make the experience less painful for the animal and allow standing dental treatments for minor surgeries

(Lowder 2012). The local anaesthetic (LA) agent of choice is lignocaine, although mepivicaine, bupivicaine and prilocaine can be used (Tremaine 2007) depending on the procedure and length of LA time needed; mepivicaine is shorter-acting than bupivicaine. Know the anatomy well and understand potential complications of the procedure (Lowder 2012). Owners should be aware that recovery time is needed before the animal can eat again or work.

Four nerve blocks are reported: the first two on the list are the most effective (Lowder 2012):

- Maxillary
- Mandibular (inferior alveolar)
- Mental
- Infraorbital

Below are summaries of the different nerve blocks. When planning to carry out one of these blocks, study detailed anatomy and procedures in dental texts or refer to Tremaine (2007). Practice on cadaver specimens will enable the precise location and technique to be mastered.

Maxillary nerve block

Caution! This technique runs the risk of arterial puncture. Other side effects include swelling of the face, exophthalmos and Horner's syndrome (Tremaine 2007).

Administer LA around the maxillary foramen. A number of approaches are documented, the most reliable being the approach just ventral to the zygomatic arch, passing in a rostroventral direction until maxilla bone is contacted. This will block sensation to all maxillary cheek teeth. A spinal needle of 7–10 cm in length and 18–19G is recommended (Tremaine 2007).

Mandibular nerve block

Administer LA around the mandibular foramen on the medial side (inside) of the mandible. This nerve has sensory and motor fibres and will block sensation to the mandibular teeth and parts of the gingival mucosa. A very long needle is essential, e.g. a spinal needle of approximately 12 cm for an adult horse (Tremaine 2007). The needle is advanced on the medial side of the mandible close to the bone from the cranial insertion of the masseter muscle towards the medial canthus of the eye until the foramen is encountered; approximately 10 ml of LA can be administered.

Mental nerve block

Administer LA agent around the mental nerve at the mental foramen, ventral to the interdental space on the lateral side (outside) of the mandible. This blocks the lower lip, labial parts of the gingiva and some of the interdental space. If removal of sensation for the incisors and premolars is required, then the LA needs to be administered deeper into the mental foramen canal (Tremaine 2007); a small 23G needle is recommended.

Infraorbital nerve block

Caution! Only perform under heavy sedation or GA due to the reaction if the nerve is hit with the needle (Tremaine 2007).

Administer LA around the infraorbital foramen, found between the end of the facial crest and the nasoincisive notch; this will block sensation to the face around the nostrils, muzzle, and upper lip. By advancing the needle further into the foramen, motor innervation can be blocked to the cheek teeth. A 21G needle is recommended for this procedure.

Case study – Fracture of an incisor tooth

10.9

Location Pakistan

Attending veterinarian Dr Javaid Khan

History
Grey mare, 16 years old, used to transport goods by cart, with a recent history of a road traffic accident when the horse was hit in the muzzle by a moving vehicle.

Clinical findings
The horse was frightened and bleeding from the mouth; the tongue was protruding in and out. There was obvious pain with reluctance to allow examination. Diagnosis was facilitated after sedation (xylazine), and analgesia (flunixin meglumine). Oral examination revealed a fractured incisor 201, there was a broken piece of tooth loosely attached to gum tissue. The fractured line was carefully explored. Upper and lower incisors were examined and were found not to be displaced from the alveoli. There was an obvious gap between the upper central incisors. Neurological examination of the horse was also carried out in order to assess cranial nerves: menace reflex, PLR, palpebral reflexes and facial nerve, all assessments were normal.

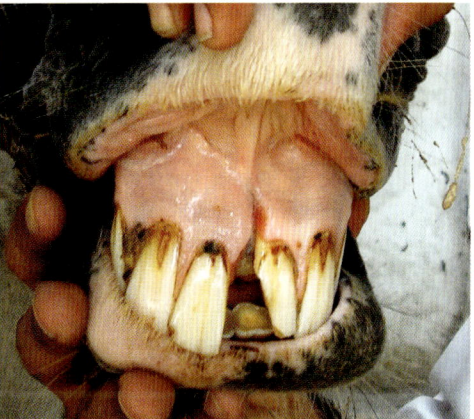

Figure 10.9.1 Fracture of 201 in a working horse.

Treatment
The mouth was rinsed with normal saline. The broken piece of 201 was carefully removed. The injured gum line was coated with a proprietary ointment (Lignocaine 0.6%, Cetylpyridium chloride 0.02%, Menthol 0.06%, Eucalyptol 0.1% and Ethanol 33% v/w) to reduce the pain. Broad-spectrum antibiotic cover was given (procaine penicillin and metronidazole), analgesia was continued (flunixin meglumine) daily.

The owner was advised to check the mouth daily and to remove any food material lodged in the gap between the upper incisor teeth to allow for normal healing. He was also advised to offer soft feed, such as wheat bran with added molasses.

Outcome
The prognosis was good and the horse started eating and drinking soon after initial therapy. Follow-up was encouraging, with no infection noted at the site of gum injury; prehension and mastication were normal. Healing of the injured mucosa was progressive.

Discussion
In this case report, surgical repair was not proposed as the fracture did not involve avulsion of the incisor and the teeth remained embedded in their alveoli. The tooth was not extracted, except for a broken fragment, to avoid future complications (Caldewell 2006).

10.10 References

Brown, S.L., Arkins, S., Shaw, D.J., Dixon, P.M. (2008) Occlusal angles of cheek teeth in normal horses and horses with dental disease. *In Practice*. 162, 807–810.

Caldwell, L.A. (2006) A review of diagnosis, treatment and sequelae of incisor-luxation fractures in horses (from a dentist's viewpoint). Proceedings of the 52nd American Association of Equine Practitioners convention, Texas, USA. 52, 559–564.

Casey, M.B., Tremaine, W.H. (2010) Dental diastemata and periodontal disease secondary to axially rotated maxillary cheek teeth in three horses. *Equine vet. Educ*. 22 (9), 439–44.

Dixon, P.M., Dacre, I. (2005) A review of equine dental disorders. *Vet. J*. 169, 165–187.

du Toit, N., Burden, F.A., Dixon, P.M. (2008a) Clinical dental findings in 203 working donkeys in Mexico. *Vet. J*. 178, 380–386.

du Toit, N., Kempson, S.A., Dixon, P.M. (2008b) Donkey dental anatomy. Part 1. Gross and computed axial tomography examinations. *Vet. J*. 176, 338–344.

du Toit, N., Dixon, P. (2012) Common dental disorders in the donkey. *Equine vet. Educ*. 24 (1), 45–51.

Easley, J., Dixon, P.M., Schumacher, J. (2011) Equine dentistry. 3rd Ed. Saunders, Elsevier Ltd.

Kempson, S.A, Davidson, M.E.B., Dacre, I.T. (2003) The effect of three types of rasps on the occlusal surface of equine cheek teeth: a scanning electron microscopic study. *J. Vet. Dent*. 20 (1), 19–27.

Lowder, M.Q. (2012) Equine dental nerve blocks. *Equine vet. Educ*. 24 (3), 124–125.

Lundstrom, T. (2010) Routine floating – performance or mastication? Proceeding of the 49th British Equine Veterinary Association Congress, Birmingham, UK. pp. 22–23.

Moll, H.D., Schoonover, M.J. (2005) How to repair incisor tooth avulsion fractures in the standing horse. Proceedings of the 51st American Association of Equine Practitioners convention, Washington, USA. 51, 294–296.

Muylle, S., Simeons, P., Lauwers, H. (1996) Ageing horses by an examination of their teeth: an (im)possible task?. *Vet Rec*. 138, 295–301.

Muylle, S., Simeons, P., Lauwers, H., Van Loon, G. (1999) Age determination in mini-shetland ponies and donkeys. *J. Vet. Med*. A. 46, 421–429.

Pascoe, R. (2010) Oral examination in the field. Proceeding of the 49th British Equine Veterinary Association Congress, Birmingham, UK. p. 21.

Tremaine, W.H. (2007) Local analgesic techniques for the equine head. *Equine vet. Educ*. 19 (9), 495–503.

Tremaine, H., Casey, M. (2012a) A modern approach to equine dentistry 1. oral examination. *In Practice*. 34, 2–10.

Tremaine, H. (2012) A modern approach to equine dentistry 3. Imaging. *In Practice*. 34, 114–127.

Tremaine, H., Price, C. (2012) A modern approach to equine dentistry 4. Routine treatments. *In Practice*. 34, 330–347.

The gastrointestinal system

11

Introduction including body condition scoring	**11.1**
Debility and poor body condition – Approach to the thin equid	**11.2**
Diagnostic aids for examination of the GI system	**11.3**
Conditions of the mouth and oesophagus	**11.4**
Colic – A practical approach to diagnosis and treatment	**11.5**
Diarrhoea in adult equids	**11.6**
Conditions affecting the rectum (prolapse and perforation)	**11.7**
Peritonitis	**11.8**
Liver disease	**11.9**
Case study – Impaction colic caused by foreign material consumption	**11.10**
References	**11.11**

11.1 Introduction including body condition scoring

The ability of the working equid to digest and absorb nutrients (and ultimately gain energy to work) depends on a well-functioning gastrointestinal (alimentary) system. It is necessary to consider all aspects of the gastrointestinal tract (GIT), the teeth, mouth, oesophagus, stomach, small and large intestines, caecum and rectum, as disruption to any part of this system can be very debilitating.

Symptoms of a problem with part or all of the GIT include the following:

- Poor body condition
- Dropping food from mouth 'quidding' (see Chapter 10 *The Teeth*)
- Weight loss
- Inappetance
- Colic
- Diarrhoea
- Impaction/constipation
- Rectal prolapse

Taking a 'GIT' history

Ask specific questions regarding the GIT if it is suspected that this is the system affected:

- Eating patterns/appetite altered?
- Dropping food/pain?
- Excessive salivation?
- Weight loss?
- Faecal consistency and colour – diarrhoea/constipation?
- Signs of colic?
- Other animals showing the same signs?
- Type of feed/feeding pattern changed?

Body condition scoring (BCS)

This is an important assessment to make; a lot of information can be gained about the health of the animal and the quality of the husbandry it receives from the owner. It can also be used as a monitoring tool to assess progress in poorly conditioned animals.

> **Body condition score is an estimation of the fat and muscle coverage on the animal's body.**

Procedure

- View the animal from at least two positions in order to assess the body condition.
- Stand approximately 3 metres away from the animal, facing towards its side.
- Stand approximately 3 metres away from the animal, facing towards its tail.

INTRODUCTION INCLUDING BODY CONDITION SCORING 11.1

Horses

A number of BCS systems are described. Carroll and Huntington (1988) described a system with six categories (0 = very poor, 1 = poor, 2 = moderate, 3 = good, 4 = fat, 5 = very fat). The paper describes the body parts to be observed and the conditions for each score. The neck, back, ribs and pelvis are the main indicators.

Henneke *et al.* (1983) used a system of nine categories (1 = poor, 2 = very thin, 3 = thin, 4 = moderately thin, 5 = moderate, 6 = moderately fleshy, 7 = fleshy, 8 = fat, 9 = very fat) and recommend palpating the following body parts: neck withers, back crease, tail head, ribs and behind the shoulder.

Donkeys

Vall *et al.* (2003) reported the use of a body condition scoring system for donkeys with four categories (1 = emaciated, 2 = thin, 3 = average, 4 = good) considering the appearance of the hindquarters, ribs and spine.

When body condition scoring donkeys, consider the following:

- Donkeys have a deceptively large belly.
- Fat pads: these are large uneven lumps which vary in position on the animal (e.g. neck, hindquarters and belly).
- **Do not take these features into account when scoring body condition. Use the other descriptors to decide on a score.**

Repeatability

> The main consideration when choosing a BCS system is to select one that adequately describes each score so that it is repeatable between different observers and the same observer on different occasions. Thus individual animals and groups can accurately be assessed for improvements or deterioration in BCS.

Both Carrol and Huntington (1988) and Vall *et al.* (2003) stated that their systems were repeatable and reproducible.

BCS illustrations

For pictures illustrating BCS refer to the papers mentioned above.

11.2 Debility and poor body condition – Approach to the thin equid

Debilitated equids are commonly presented for treatment (Figure 11.2.1). Conduct a clinical examination to identify the underlying cause(s) and treat appropriately. Remember to obtain a thorough history about the animal's husbandry, nutrition, workload and any previous health problems (see Chapter 1).

> **ENERGY INTAKE < ENERGY OUTPUT = WEIGHT LOSS AND DEBILITY**

When this imbalance is prolonged, body reserves of fat and muscle are used to provide energy, resulting in a thin, weak animal.

Causes of reduced energy intake

- **Insufficient or poor quality** food provided (most common) (Finkler-Schade 2007)
- **Inability to take in** food properly, eg. overgrown teeth, sore mouth
- **Inability to digest** food properly, eg. dehydration, diarrhoea, worms
- **Inability to metabolise** food properly, eg. liver disease

Causes of excessive energy output

- **Overwork** (most common) (Maranhão et al. 2006)
- Concurrent **disease, pain or fever** (Dobromylskyj et al. 2000, Almeida et al. 2008)
- **Cold** environment leading to excessive loss of body heat
- **Lameness** (Weishaupt et al. 2004)

Principles of management of thin equids

1. **Identify underlying cause** Often both health and management issues are involved so it is important to identify all issues and communicate these to the owner. Where possible, a blood smear should be taken to look for signs of anaemia and blood parasites (see Chapter 16).

2. **Communicate with the owner** Discuss improvements which could be made to the energy content of the animal's diet, using locally available feed, to ensure adequate quality and quantity. Be realistic about what the owner can afford. Emphasise that reducing the animal's workload is essential if it is to regain condition.

Feeding sick equids

> **Sick animals have higher energy requirements than healthy ones.**

They may also have a reduced appetite (Dobromylskyj et al. 2000, Almeida et al. 2008) and poorer ability to digest food efficiently. Aim to give small volumes of high quality, digestible food 5–6 times per day.

DEBILITY AND POOR BODY CONDITION – APPROACH TO THE THIN EQUID 11.2

Stimulate the appetite with small meals of green fodder; this acts as an appetite stimulant, improves gastrointestinal function and provides vitamins, minerals, energy and protein. Adding a cup of vegetable oil to each feed increases the energy content.

If eating is painful or difficult, feed (such as grain/cereals) can be soaked in water or cooked to make it easier to eat, and digest. Some sick equids may need to be fed by hand.

A sick animal will not eat well if it is nervous or threatened by a more dominant animal next to it. Feed sick animals separately from healthy ones to prevent bullying and ensure that they receive their share.

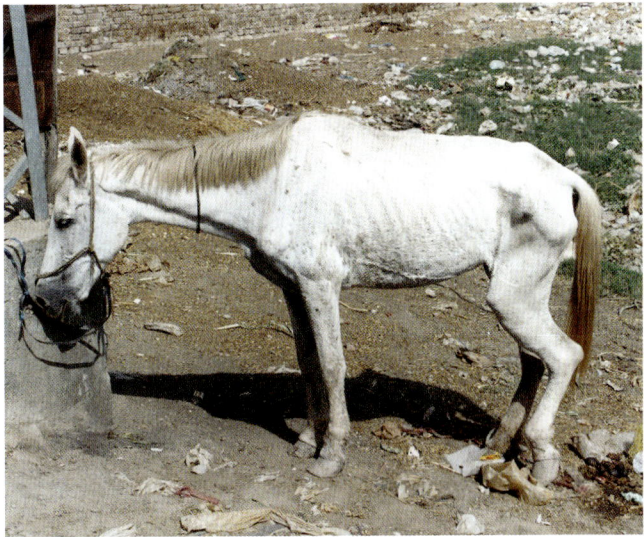

Figure 11.2.1 Weight loss and debility in a working equid.

> Ensure that fresh water is available at all times.

Feeding foals

Foals grow at an extremely fast rate especially in the first 6 months of life; daily weight gains of over 1 kg a day are common in this period (Coleman et al. 1999). Before any milk replacer is offered (Stoneham 2005) it is absolutely essential that all foals have suckled within the first 6 hours of birth so that adequate colostrum is consumed containing a rich mix of antibodies which helps to protect the neonate from disease (Naylor 1979).

> **Foals are very dependent on their mother's milk during the first few weeks of life. It supplies all their needs up to 6 weeks of age (Ousey *et al.* 1997).**

The mare's milk is the main source of nutrition until 4–5 months of age. Foals are born with a monogastric GIT and do not have the capacity to digest fibre in the first few months of life – this develops as the foal grows. Some foals will eat the mare's droppings in the first 2 months of life and this coprophagia is thought to help populate the hindgut with bacteria, provide some nutrients, provide exposure to pheromones for growth and other substances which may increase the gut immunity and maturation of the nervous system (Crowell-Davis and Houpt 1985).

> **Foals suckle very frequently – up to 7 times a day in the first week of life.**

This frequent suckling means it is very important a foal is left with the mare (Carson and Wood-Gush 1983). This is also essential in building the mother-foal relationship which is

11 THE GASTROINTESTINAL SYSTEM

important for good welfare. Owners should be fully educated about this requirement and a mare with a foal should not be worked.

Feeding lactating mares

Lactation places a huge drain on nutrient requirements – especially for energy, water, protein, calcium and phosphorus.

> Reports state lactating mares require 65% more feed than pregnant mares (Boulot *et al.* 1987).

This should be accounted for in the feeding of the mare and her body condition should be carefully monitored. A nutritional deficiency in lactation will not only affect the health of the mare but will also reduce the quality of the milk and, therefore, affect the health of the foal.

11.3 Diagnostic aids for the examination of the gastrointestinal system

As with any diagnostic aids, use of the following has the potential to cause harm or even death to the animal if not done correctly. Rectal examination and abdominocentesis are usually only done in cases of severe colic and so will be found under the *Colic* section (11.5) of this chapter.

Mouth speculum for examining the teeth and oral cavity

See Section 10.4 on teeth and dentistry.

Auscultation

Both left and right sides of the abdomen should be auscultated; about 4–5 minutes is the time required to do this properly in a suspected GIT case.

Normal gut sounds

- 'Rumbling', 'bubbling' and 'splashing' noises can be heard on auscultation of the abdomen.
- Ileocaecal sounds should be heard in the right paralumbar fossa (see Section 1.4 for this location, and Figure 11.3.1) at a rate of 1–3 a minute; this sounds like water flowing down a drainpipe.
- Borborygmi are small intestinal sounds in the ventral abdomen, low-pitched fluid sounds.

Abnormal gut sounds

- Increased 'rumbling, bubbling and splashes' indicate possible spasmodic colic.

- **Absence/decreased** gut sounds are a poor sign (Orsini 2011), indicating ileus associated with possible obstruction or torsion.
- A **'pinging'** sound on percussion indicates gas accumulation. This is significant if there is associated abdominal distension and may indicate an obstruction or impaction.

Repeated auscultation over some hours is vital when monitoring a colic case. A progressive decline in frequency or intensity of gut sounds indicates a poor prognosis, especially if the other clinical signs are also deteriorating.

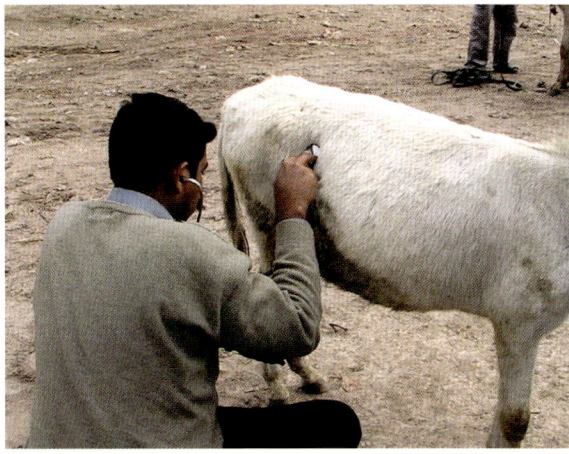

Figure 11.3.1 Auscultation of the right paralumbar fossa.

Anti-spasmodic drugs (e.g. hyoscine-N-butyl bromide/N-butylscopolammonium bromide) can be used for analgesia in various types of colic: spasmodic, tympanic and simple impaction.

Never administer anti-spasmodic drugs in cases of impaction associated with ileus (Bertone 2002).

Faecal examination

It is important to look at an equid's faeces as this can give very useful information about a case and is non-invasive.

Collect the sample of fresh faeces, either on rectal examination, if this is being carried out as a part of the clinical examination, or freshly deposited faeces straight off the ground. Do **not** rectal the animal simply to collect faeces, only if it is part of the clinical examination, e.g. when investigating a colic case. Otherwise wait for the animal to deposit a fresh sample.

Look for the following:
- Pararsites – may be grossly visible.
- In cases of ileus and some cases of colic, faecal output will be reduced.
- In impaction colic and dehydration, the faecal balls will be very small and dry.
- In dental disease, long fibre may be visible in the faeces as this has not been adequately chewed (masticated) as a result of dental pain/pathology.
- In diarrhoea cases, faeces will be loose and watery. Check for any signs of blood or melaena.

The following tests can be carried out:
- Direct observation (see above)
- Smear (see parasitology texts or specialist laboratories)
- Faecal flotation – McMaster (see Chapter 16 *Parasitology*) and Baermanns test for lungworm
- Culture, e.g. bacterial, if suspected Salmonella or clostridium infection (Weese *et al.* 2001)

11 THE GASTROINTESTINAL SYSTEM

Nasogastric intubation

Why is this often done in a case of colic?

Passage of a nasogastric tube can be used to assess whether there is reflux of gastric material.

> **Remember that equids cannot vomit.**

Passage of a stomach tube will release any gastric contents which have built up as a result of this inability to vomit (due to the sharp angle of the oesophagus entering the stomach and the strong oesophageal muscles). Gastric reflux is significant because it indicates an accumulation of fluid in the stomach resulting from an obstruction in the proximal jejunum/duodenum; this obstruction can be a strangulating lesion or a functional obstruction. If the stomach is not decompressed it can rupture leading to peritonitis and fatal endotoxaemia. (See Section 4.1).

Further GIT diagnostics are usually only indicated in severe colic cases – see Section 11.5 of this chapter for further tests.

Glucose absorption test

This test is indicated in suspected malabsorption cases (Mair *et al.* 2006). When weight loss is observed in cases where the equid is consuming sufficient food, malabsorption may be suspected. There may be concurrent diarrhoea and ventral oedema. Rule out more common problems such as parasites, blood protozoa and dental problems before conducting a glucose absorption test. The procedure is as follows:

- Fast the animal for 12 hours (Venner and Ohnesorge 2001).
- Administer 1 g/kg glucose as a 10% (or 20%) solution by stomach tube.
- Collect blood samples in oxalate fluoride tubes at 0 (pre), 30, 60, 90, 120, 150, 180 minutes post glucose administration.

Result

Between 60 and 120 minutes post administration (Mair *et al.* 2006), assess glucose levels:

- In **normal** horses, peak concentrations of glucose of over 85% above the resting level is seen.
- **Partial malabsorption** is seen with results between 15 and 85% above resting blood glucose levels.
- **Complete malabsorption** is seen with levels of glucose less than 15% of the resting blood glucose level.

Differential diagnoses

Inflammatory bowel syndrome, infiltrative bowel disease (neoplastic), infections of the intestinal tract (bacterial, parasitic, fungal), enteritis in foals (Mair *et al.* 2006).

Treatment

Depends on the cause and diagnosis. Nutrition is a major factor; drug therapies include corticosteroids, antibiotics and anthelmintics.

Conditions of the mouth and oesophagus

11.4

Cleft Palate

See Chapter 18.1.

Lampas

Lampas is reported as a swelling of the hard palate just behind the incisor teeth (Pringle 1871).

Cause

It is a **normal physiological adaptation** to a very fibrous diet, commonly seen in working equids fed on poor quality roughage such as straw and husks.

Treatment

Lampas requires no treatment. Explain the cause to owners and try to discourage the use of astringent, blistering agents or surgical removal as these will cause unnecessary pain, suffering and affect normal eating. Even in an equine veterinary textbook of 1871 by Pringle, it is stated that this is a natural process and '*cruel practices – such as firing – should never for a moment be thought of*'. Alterations to the diet and good feeding practices from the start can help prevent, resolve or prevent enlargement of such swellings. If the swelling is large it may make placement of a mouth speculum uncomfortable, so take extra care during dental examination and rasping.

> Remember, lampas is a normal physiological adaptation requiring no treatment.

Oral ulceration

This can be due to a variety of causes: trauma, nutrition, autoimmunity and neoplasia (Tell *et al.* 2008). A high prevalence of traumatic ulcers caused by bits and bridles has been recorded (Tell *et al.* 2008). Infectious causes include '**vesicular stomatitis**', which is a viral disease of equids and a zoonosis and bacterial diseases such as *Pseudomonas*. Additional causes are the ingestion of brittle plant materials, thorns or toxic chemicals (often from drinking from inappropriate water containers), dental disease and oral foreign bodies. Uncommonly, ulcers can occur from kidney disease and associated uraemia, rarely associated with long-term phenylbutazone administration.

Clinical signs

Initially, small vesicles develop into large ulcers over the oral cavity and tongue, sometimes extending into the pharynx and larynx. There may be excessive salivation and inappetance due to pain. In some cases, the tongue may become hard or 'spoon-like', resulting in inability to eat.

Diagnosis

Based on clinical signs and, in the case of toxicity, a history of ingestion of inappropriate substances. Always check the oral cavity using a full mouth speculum (remember, the animal might have pain in opening its mouth) and ensure there are no foreign bodies present. Also check the teeth as ulcers can be secondary to dental disease (see Chapter 10). Caution – Vesicular stomatitis is zoonotic, so wear gloves. Lesions appear on the tongue, gums, lips, teats, prepuce and coronary band (Letchworth et al. 1999); horses are depressed with an increased temperature. If renal disease is suspected from the general examination, biochemistry can confirm this.

Treatment

Treat the underlying cause, e.g. remove the foreign body, treat dental disease and ensure that bits and bridles are well-fitting (Tell et al. 2008). Rinsing the mouth with dilute antiseptic solution daily may be useful to prevent secondary infection (if the animal allows this). Give anti-inflammatory drugs/analgesia if the animal is in pain, and encourage eating by providing soft palatable food.

Trauma to the lips and tongue

> This is common in working equids due to ill-fitting or harsh bits, injuries from wood and wire, and eating inappropriate caustic substances.

Trauma can also be caused by excessive force on the tongue during examination – so be careful.

Clinical signs

Reluctance to eat, often accompanied by blood or excessive saliva dripping from the mouth. Inspection of the bit can reveal dried blood. Often the mouth will be open with the tongue hanging out. There is sometimes swelling under the tongue (sublingual cellulitis).

Diagnosis

Based on history, clinical signs and thorough examination (Hague and Honnas 1998)

Treatment

If fresh wounds are present on the lips and tongue, debride and suture if necessary, preferably with a dissolvable material. Landmarks for the mental nerve block are found in Section 10.8. Lesions of the tongue heal well by secondary intention, often rapidly and without complications. Equids can manage well with even severe tongue defects. Nursing care is important, so give pain relief and soft, palatable foods; administer antibiotics if secondary infection is severe. As with all wounds, ensure that the animal is either vaccinated for tetanus or, if the vaccination history is unknown, give tetanus anti-toxin if available.

Oesophageal obstruction ('Choke')

Oesophageal disorders are uncommon in equids but, among these, the most common presentation is choke.

There are a variety of inflammatory or traumatic forms of choke which cause partial or full blockage of the oesophagus. The most likely scenario with working equids is choke due to eating inappropriate feed which gets lodged in the oesophagus part-way down and presents as an acute condition.

> Always consider choke an emergency (Widman 2008).

Clinical signs

Pain and retching when attempting to swallow, nasal discharge often accompanied by extension of the neck when swallowing often with regurgitation of food through the nostrils. Often a swelling can be seen halfway down the neck due to the impacted food or foreign body. If choke has been present for some time there may be evidence of aspiration pneumonia (dyspnoea, increased lung sounds, pyrexia) from food passing back up the nose and into the trachea.

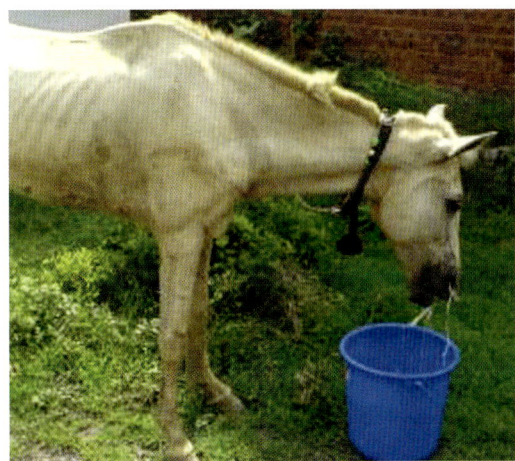

Figure 11.4.1 *Discharge from the nose in a case of choke.*

Diagnosis

Based on the clinical signs, confirmed with passage of a stomach tube which will not pass further when it reaches the level of the blockage

> **Be very careful when passing a nasogastric tube if choke is suspected, to avoid rupturing the oesophagus.**

Treatment

Over the telephone to the owner, tell them to remove food and water.

Most cases of choke resolve spontaneously. It is important to relax the animal (sedation with e.g. xylazine or acepromazine) and provide pain relief. Oxytocin (0.11–0.22 IU/kg IV, administered once only) can help oesophageal relaxation (unless the animal is pregnant) if the obstruction is in the top third of the oesophagus.

If none of the above is effective then **lavage** can be performed.

Insert the stomach tube to the level of the impaction and lavage with warm water to encourage lubrication and mass breakdown. Lavage *slowly and gently* and keep the head as low as possible to avoid causing aspiration pneumonia (see complications of nasogastric tube insertion in Section 4.1). Placing 20–50 ml of local anaesthetic down the tube promotes oesophageal relaxation and helps with the animal's discomfort. Lavage may need to be repeated over a few hours.

Ensure that only soft food is fed for a few days after the obstruction has been cleared and provide pain relief if the obstruction was severe and required a lavage to remove it, as the animal will continue to suffer discomfort when swallowing.

After every choke case check the teeth and carefully discuss diet with the owner as this may reveal a predisposing cause that can be avoided in the future. For example, choke can be caused by feeding very dry food which swells in the oesophagus; this can be easily avoided by ensuring that soaked feed is given.

11.5 Colic – A practical approach to diagnosis and treatment

'Colic' is a general term meaning abdominal pain. There are a large number of known causes of colic in equids, so a thorough work-up is necessary.

> Colic is a symptom, not a diagnosis!

This section covers colic due to gastrointestinal (GI) disturbances, although there are a number of other causes – see relevant sections.

> Colic can be fatal and is one of the most frequent causes of mortality in horses (Nolen-Walston *et al.* 2007).

However, 80% of colic cases resolve spontaneously or with simple medical treatment, with a further 10% requiring intensive medical treatment (Orsini 2011). It is the remaining 10% that are fatal without surgical intervention; humane euthanasia may be considered in these cases when surgical intervention is not possible or appropriate. To determine whether a colic case is mild or serious conduct a thorough clinical examination and monitor the response to treatment closely.

> Do not delay in the response to a colic case.

What might be happening internally when colic signs are observed?

- **Inflammation of the stomach or intestinal walls** This could be due to parasitic worm damage, sand ingestion, bacterial infection or ingested foreign bodies (e.g. plastic bags). It can lead to altered motility and diarrhoea.

- **Stretching of the intestinal wall** This is due to distension with gas (tympany) or food material (grain overload, or colonic impaction).

- **Altered intestinal motility** Peristaltic movements may be abnormally increased (spasm), decreased or absent (ileus). Changes in motility may be caused by dehydration, dietary changes, parasitic worms, toxins, or obstruction from inappropriate ingested materials. They often lead either to diarrhoea or to constipation.

- **Loss of blood supply to an area of intestine (ischemia)** This is caused by intestinal torsion, strangulation, intussusception or total blockage. It leads to the release of toxins into the blood, inflammation and severe pain followed by necrosis and death of the affected section of intestine.

In many cases, the underlying cause of the colic will result in a combination of the above effects on intestinal walls. The first three categories listed often recover spontaneously or with medical treatment alone. Those in the fourth category can develop from one of the other three, or may have no obvious cause. Medical treatment does not relieve the symptoms, in this last category, which progress rapidly over a few hours and are fatal without surgical intervention; euthanasia is recommended in these cases to relieve pain and suffering.

COLIC – A PRACTICAL APPROACH TO DIAGNOSIS AND TREATMENT 11.5

The approach to a colic case

History

The following questions are important:
- When did the colic signs start?
- Has the animal had colic before? If so, when was the last time?
- When did it last pass faeces? How much? What consistency?
- Does it have diarrhoea?
- When was the last de-worming treatment?
- When did the animal last eat? What does it eat? Has the diet changed recently?
- When did it last drink and how much?
- When did it last pass urine?
- Is the animal pregnant?
- History of teeth problems/quidding? (See Chapter 10 *Teeth*.)

> **Dehydration is a common cause of colic in working equids.**

Around 100 L of fluid passes daily through the GIT of an adult horse and is partly responsible for keeping ingesta moving through the system.

Urine retention is an extremely rare cause of colic; it is more likely that colic signs are due to dehydration.

> **Never give diuretics in cases of colic – they will make the animal more dehydrated.**

When the animal is rehydrated and given pain relief it will urinate without the need for diuretics or catheterisation (see Section 13.1).

Always examine the teeth as dental problems are a common cause of colic in working equids.

Clinical signs

It is important first to observe the animal at a distance to ascertain physical signs of colic.

- **Horses** show varying symptoms, some of which can be very dramatic and can potentially harm the animal or people in the vicinity. Lying down 'flat out', rolling and kicking are common. Milder signs include sweating, pawing at the ground and frequent looking back at the abdomen (Figures 11.5.1). (See Chapter 2 for further behavioural signs of abdominal pain.) Some animals may strain as though attempting to pass faeces, whilst others are just subdued with dehydration and decreased appetite. Try to perform a thorough clinical examination *before* giving any drugs, as these may quickly hide the clinical signs and make diagnosis more difficult.

- **Donkeys** often show more subtle pain symptoms which may be overlooked (Figure 11.5.2). They must be examined thoroughly in order to assess the severity of colic as behavioural signs of pain may be different from those shown by horses. Dullness and depression are signs of colic as well as subtle changes in behaviour.

11 THE GASTROINTESTINAL SYSTEM

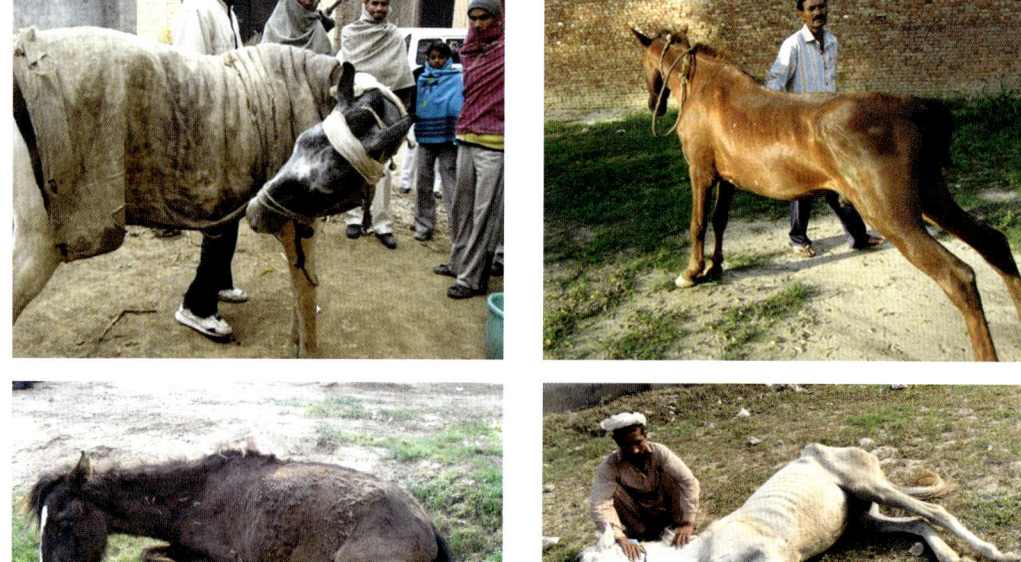

Figure 11.5.1 Colic signs in horses: flank-watching (top left), stretching (top right), sitting down (bottom left) and lying flat out on the ground (bottom right).

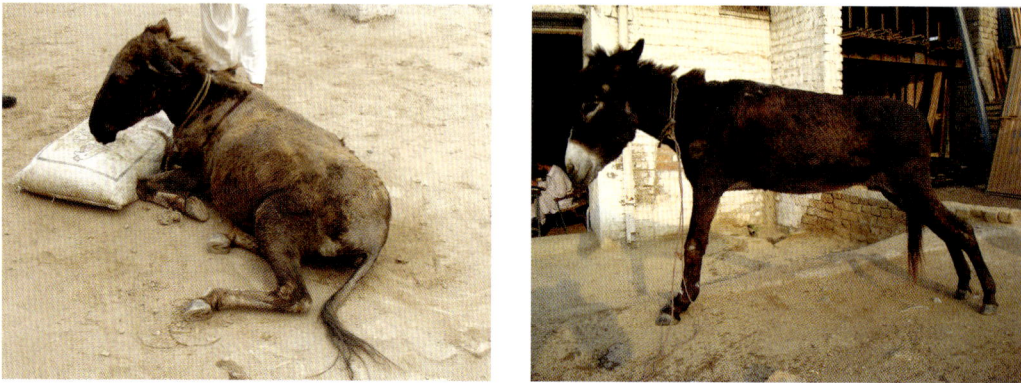

Figure 11.5.2 Colic signs in the donkey may appear more subtle than in the horse, including sitting down and stretching out.

Clinical examination

A thorough clinical examination should take place, including the length of the GI tract that is either physically palpable (mouth, oesophagus, abdomen, rectum), or via auscultation and percussion (all four quadrants of the abdomen). Auscultation of the abdomen, and knowledge of what normal gut sounds are, will be the first step in the colic diagnosis as, even with mild/inapparent clinical colic signs, changes in gut motility can be detected. Heart rate, respiratory rate, mucous membrane colour (pale/anaemic, icteric/jaundice, purple/toxic), capillary refill time, pulse quality and hydration status should all be assessed.

> Other conditions can be mistaken for colic in equids, especially if the signs are mild.

In equids exhibiting colic signs, check also for laminitis, rhabdomyolysis, tetanus or even foaling.

Other diagnostic procedures

These include the following:
- Nasogastric intubation
- Rectal examination
- Abdominocentesis (peritoneal fluid sampling)
- Blood sampling

Nasogastric intubation

This procedure should be carried out in all equids suspected of colic, if there is a suitably trained and competent veterinarian to carry out the procedure, a suitable nasogastric tube, a calm (possibly sedated) animal and a competent handler. Passing the tube will help with diagnosis of an obstruction in the pharynx or oesophagus, it will release air and gas from the stomach and, in severe colic cases, fluid accumulated in the stomach can be released or siphoned off. This procedure will ease the pain and suffering caused by a distended stomach as well as aiding in diagnosis and treatment of the case. The same technique can be used to pass fluid into the animal if required as part of the treatment regime. For details of the full technique refer to Section 4.2.

Rectal examination

Why do a rectal examination in a case of colic?

- Rectal examinations give us an insight into what is happening internally so that we can refine or confirm our diagnosis or gain a better indication of prognosis. Although frequently carried out for colic cases, rectal examination is also performed to confirm pregnancy or to assess for tumours or other abnormalities in animals with a history of chronic weight loss or diarrhoea. Rectal examination is not generally well tolerated by mules; it is most commonly used in horses; it can also be safely carried out in donkeys. Do not attempt in mares known to be heavily pregnant as it is difficult to palpate structures other than the foal.

> Only the caudal third of the abdomen can be palpated, so abnormalities higher up in the digestive system (small intestine or stomach) will not be detected.

11 THE GASTROINTESTINAL SYSTEM

When is the best time to do a rectal examination? And what if it seems too dangerous?

- A rectal examination should be done as soon as possible in cases of **severe colic** (see Table 11.5.2 on page 271 for other external indictors of whether colic is severe) to get an early diagnosis and prognosis. It is important that the severity of the colic is determined as early as possible so that cases with a poor prognosis (gut torsion, rupture, etc.) can be euthanased quickly to prevent further suffering.

- In many cases of severe colic the animal may harm the clinician while the rectal examination is being carried out, for example if it is rolling on the ground or kicking out. An early attempt at a rectal examination in this case could also damage the sensitive rectal mucosa so calm the animal first with analgesia (NSAIDs such as flunixin meglumine) and sedate with an alpha2-agonist sedative drug (xylazine or detomidine), then attempt the examination after 10–20 minutes. Weigh up the potential harm caused by the hypotensive effects of sedation compared to the harm the animal will do to itself, or those present, if it is not sedated. Alternatively, leave out a rectal examination altogether if the potential harm is going to outweigh the benefit to the animal, and use other information you can gather (mucous membrane colour, heart rate, history, response to analgesia etc.) to make an informed decision about the prognosis.

- In cases of **mild to moderate colic** a rectal examination may be performed at a later stage of treatment than it can in severe cases. This would be appropriate if there is no response to fluid or analgesic therapy after several administrations, no faeces have been passed after 48 hours despite settling of clinical signs, or the colic signs are recurring.

> **Blood on an equine rectal glove is a bad sign. Do not use the same force as when conducting a rectal examination on a bovine animal.**

What if there is blood on the glove after examination?

- The rectal wall of the horse is extremely sensitive and damage is often indicated by the presence of blood on the rectal glove. Any amount of blood is serious and the depth of the rectal tear will determine the consequences. Refer to Section 11.7 of this chapter (*Rectal perforation*) for guidance on what to do if a rectal tear is suspected.

- The seriousness of a rectal tear and associated peritonitis reiterates the importance of using good restraint, patience and good technique when doing a rectal examination. Peritonitis is a very painful, unnecessary and fatal consequence of poor rectal technique.

How to perform a good, safe rectal examination?

A good knowledge of the internal anatomy is essential for conducting a rectal examination. Without this knowledge a rectal examination cannot be justified.

Observe the following technique:

1. **Excellent restraint and lots of lubrication** are vitally important. Stand beside the animal and insert an arm slowly and gently into the rectum. If the animal is straining, do not push against it as this may damage the rectal wall.

2. **Pull the faeces out slowly** and observe consistency (e.g. dry and hard) or whether it contains blood, sand or mucus. Removal of faeces gives better access to the rectum.

3. **Gently palpate the internal organs** with a flat hand.

   a. **Rectal mucosa** should be smooth. Roughening or thickening of the rectal wall is abnormal.

   b. **Small colon (left side)** is detected by palpation of small faecal balls within the lumen and is relatively mobile. Distension or impaction of this is abnormal.

   c. **Pelvic flexure** is normally in the ventral part of the abdomen, left of the midline. Impaction is common due to the sharp bend in the colon at this point and the natural reduction in luminal diameter there. If impacted, it will feel distended and 'doughy' on palpation and, when gently pressed, a small indent will remain. When impacted, the pelvic flexure may be displaced from its normal position; it may be the first thing palpated on entering the rectum.

   d. **Caecum** This sits in the right-hand side of the abdomen, internal to the right paralumbar fossa. The ventral band is felt running top to bottom of the caecum from right to left, in a diagonal direction. Distension of the caecum with gas or ingesta changes the direction of this band, and tight bands are pathognomonic. If it is possible to palpate the bottom part of the caecum it is distended.

   e. **Large colon** Distension and bands (similar to the caecum) are abnormal.

   f. **Small intestine** This cannot usually be palpated. If it is palpable in the middle part of the abdomen (usually because it is distended with gas), it could indicate a problem higher up the tract, such as a small intestinal obstruction, strangulation or torsion. When distended it feels like a tight balloon or rubber rings.

   g. **Spleen** This is close to the left abdominal wall near the level of the last rib. It should feel very close to the abdominal wall and is firm to palpate with a sharp caudal edge. Always check the dorsal margin of the spleen and feel along the nephrosplenic ligament which joins to the left kidney on the dorsal aspect of the left abdominal wall because the large colon can displace and lodge here. This is known as nephrosplenic entrapment.

   h. **Peritoneum** This is the final structure examined. Be very gentle so as not to rupture the large intestine. It should be smooth. Nodules, roughening and fibrous tags indicate possible peritonitis.

   i. **Other** Occasionally other abnormalities such as tumours, uterine torsion or adhesions can be found. These are useful findings to aid diagnosis especially if associated with chronic weight loss or diarrhoea.

Abdominocentesis/paracentesis/peritoneal tap

What information can abdominal fluid provide, and when should it be sampled?

- Examination of the colour and viscosity of abdominal fluid (see Table 11.5.1 on the next page) is useful in determining the prognosis for suspected peritonitis cases and can also be used to give more information about the cause of colic. It should be done if clinical signs are **severe or worsening over time** to give a possible indication of whether torsion or rupture has occurred.

> Sterile technique is extremely important; do not introduce infection into the abdomen.

11 THE GASTROINTESTINAL SYSTEM

1. **Restrain the animal (sedate if necessary)** and clip and disinfect the abdominal midline thoroughly. Find the umbilicus; the ideal place for needle insertion is 2–3 fingers' width from the umbilicus back towards the tail end of the animal at the most dependant point of the abdomen.
2. **Stand next to the animal at the elbow, facing the rear.** It is easier to move the arm, rather than the whole body, out of the way if the animal kicks.
3. **Using a sterile 18G, 1.5-inch needle**, insert it sharply and quickly through the skin and muscle and then slowly advance it into the peritoneal space. Once it is inserted move it around gently until fluid appears at the hub. Collect a sample in a sterile tube. **Normal peritoneal fluid** is yellow/straw coloured and clear enough to read the text of a newspaper through the vial.
4. **If not successful** repeat more caudally.
5. **Refractometry** Put a drop of peritoneal fluid onto the refractometer and read the total protein concentration (opposite scale to the USG). This is a simple and useful tool which can provide useful information (see table below).

Colour	Possible condition	Total protein (TP) (g/dL)
Yellow/straw, clear	Normal	< 2.0
Streaked with fresh blood	Hit a blood vessel in the skin or muscle on the way through the abdominal wall (blood free in abdomen with be defibrinated and will not clot)	
Yellow/straw/amber, opaque	Impaction, obstruction, peritonitis, early gut compromise	< 3.0
Red/brown, serous	Possible strangulation, early torsion. Dark blood that clots is from the spleen.	2.5–6.0
Brown/black/green-tinged	Bowel necrosis/rupture, torsion, peritonitis, severe gut compromise (turbid and cells settle out)	5.0–6.5
Green/fibrous	Intestinal contents/penetrated gut with needle (with sediment)	Variable

Table 11.5.1 Findings when examining peritoneal fluid.

Normal peritoneal fluid

- Approximately 5–10 mls in drips over 4–5 minutes
- Clear (low turbidity) pale yellow fluid, low cellularity
- Can use a refractometer to measure TP, < 2 g/dl is reported as within normal limits.
- Look at the cells under a microscope for WBC count, for adult horses < 10×10^9/l has been reported as the maximum limit of the normal range, for foals a count > 1.5×10^9/l should be should be considered abnormal (Grindem *et al.* 1990).

COLIC – A PRACTICAL APPROACH TO DIAGNOSIS AND TREATMENT 11.5

Guidelines for making informed decisions in the management of colic cases

Colic, especially if severe, is an emergency.

Stay with the animal to monitor the response to treatment, and follow up over the following days until the animal is passing faeces and behaving normally again.

Table 11.5.2 is included to help determine how severe a colic case is, the possible cause, and what actions should be taken after the initial examination. Use this as a guide only and treat each case individually based on clinical findings. It is impossible to classify every case into a table with specific guidelines for approach to management.

Clinical sign	Mild/moderate colic	Severe colic
Pain	Mild/moderate	Severe
Sweating	Absent/mild	Severe
Mucous membranes	Normal or mild congestion	Severe congestion, purple, grey, 'toxic line' at the base (gum line) of the teeth
Capillary refill time	Normal	> 3 seconds
Pulse quality	Normal	Weak
Heart rate, beats per minute (bpm)	< 70 bpm	> 70 bpm and rising
Gut sounds	Normal or increased	Decreased or absent
Faeces	Present	Absent or small dry faecal balls
Hydration	Normal or mildly dehydrated	Severely dehydrated
Gastric reflux*	None or very little	Large volume
Rectal examination*	Normal, impaction, mild tympany	Displacement, severe tympany, loops of small intestine, foreign body
Paracentesis*	Normal	Abnormal
Response to analgesia	Good response within 30 minutes to an hour. Symptoms do not recur if underlying cause is treated.	Poor/slight response after an hour. Symptoms recur quickly within hours and often appear worse than before.

Those diagnostic aids marked with an asterisk (*) are normally only done if other clinical signs are severe. If mild colic is suspected treat and reassess 1–2 hours later.

Table 11.5.2 Interpreting clinical signs in colic cases.

11 THE GASTROINTESTINAL SYSTEM

Diagnosis

Mild to moderate clinical signs with increased gut sounds

This usually indicates spasmodic colic or intestinal wall inflammation due to intestinal worm damage or diet.

Treat with NSAIDs and rehydrate. Anti-spasmodic drugs (hyoscine) are good if available although never use them if gut sounds are decreased. Give anthelmintic treatment only when the animal has recovered; giving this while the animal still has clinical signs can greatly increase the colic symptoms.

Remember, flunixin meglumine is a very potent visceral analgesic and will mask early signs of deterioration and the development of endotoxaemia.

> **After analgesia has been given animals should be carefully monitored for signs of further deterioration.**

Mild to moderate clinical signs with decreased/absent gut sounds

This can indicate an impaction or partial obstruction. Rectal examination findings may reveal foreign objects such as plastic bags, rope or cloth in the rectum (see Figure 11.5.3 and the case study in Section 11.9 of this chapter). The pelvic flexure is a common site of impaction due to the narrow lumen at this point; observe its position and consistency noting any abnormalities (see details of rectal examination earlier).

Treatment

Impaction

- Analgesics to control the pain (see above)
- If gastric reflux is not present, and there is evidence of gut sounds, give oral fluids by nasogastric tube. 3–6 litres can be given, depending on the size of the animal, and electrolytes can be added. This can be repeated every 2–4 hours; if the impaction is large this may be necessary. Because foreign body impactions are difficult to distinguish from food impactions, laxatives such as mineral oil are often used. However, frequent administration of fluids per nasogastric tube has been shown to be as effective, if not more so. Refer to Section 6.2 on fluid therapy for information on how to make an isotonic solution suitable for nasogastric intubation.
- Food should be withheld and the treatment repeated until the animal starts to pass faeces again.
- Recent research on treatment of large colon impactions shows that oral fluid hourly is the most effective way to treat an impaction. This

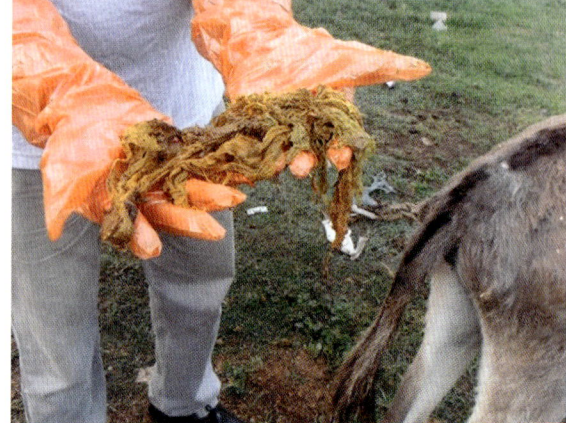

Figure 11.5.3 An example of a foreign body impaction from plastic bags and rope eaten by the donkey.

provides the most rapid resolution and is cheaper, as well as avoiding the complications associated with IV parenteral fluid administration (e.g. thrombophlebitis).

> In the context of working equids the administration of oral fluids, in the case of large colon impactions, is more practical, readily available and safer, so should be considered the treatment of choice.

Refer to the paper *Colic – A Practical Approach to Diagnosis and Treatment* by Hallowell (2008) for more information.

- Once the animal has started to pass faeces, small amounts of a soft laxative diet such as fresh green fodder or crushed concentrates soaked in large amounts of water can be offered 5–6 times daily (little and often) for 3–4 days. Ensure plenty of water is available to drink at all times; this keeps the contents of the intestine soft and reduces the likelihood of recurrence. Warn the owner of the possibility for recurrence, especially if water is withheld or the animal is allowed to eat unsuitable feeds (hard, fibrous or rubbish).

Colonic displacement

Displacement of the left colon dorsally over the nephrosplenic ligament and right dorsal displacement, where the colon rotates around the caecum, are the two most common forms. The cause of these displacements is not known but it is thought to be the result of alterations in gut contents, resulting in an accumulation of gas, or altered motor activity.

- **Nephrosplenic entrapment** The left portion of the colon becomes lodged in the space between the left kidney and the spleen, hooked in place by the underlying nephrosplenic ligament. Once trapped in this position the colon becomes occluded resulting in a partial obstruction. On rectal examination the colon can be felt in this position between the kidney and the spleen in the upper left quadrant.

- **Right dorsal displacement** The large colon rotates 180 degrees around its mesenteric attachment. This can be felt rectally as a gas-distended colon and the pelvic flexure is no longer palpable as this has been displaced more cranially in the abdomen by the rotation.

Treatment regime

- Analgesics to control the pain

- Correct fluid imbalances. Provided that gut sounds are present and there is gastric reflux, this can be administered through nasogastric intubation.

- Withhold food. In mild cases, if food is withheld, the reduction in gut fill allows the colon to shrink and possibly move back to the normal anatomical position. Gentle walking can help this movement.

- Administration of phenylephrine at 20–80 µg/kg dissolved in 500 ml of 0.9% NaCl given slowly over 30 minutes, results in splenic contraction and facilitates the movement of the colon into the normal position. It should only be used if a nephrosplenic entrapment has been definitively diagnosed without doubt. The heart should be carefully monitored for the duration of the infusion and it should be stopped immediately if any arrhythmia is detected. Do not use in cases of myocardial failure.

- In some cases, displacements will not self-correct.

11 THE GASTROINTESTINAL SYSTEM

> In the context of working equids corrective colic surgery is not an option.

If a case is not responsive to analgesia or becomes endotoxaemic (i.e. develops into a more serious disease state) then euthanasia should be advised.

Severe colic signs

Treat initially with pain relief.

It is **very important** to stay for at least an hour and monitor the response to pain relief since these drugs should act within 30 minutes. If it is safe to do so, carry out further diagnostics (rectal examination, abdominocentesis) even if pain relief has worked, as there is still likelihood of a critical condition if severe signs are seen. Further work-up will assist in determining a prognosis. If there is no response, or the animal's condition gets worse over a few hours, the prognosis is hopeless.

Euthanasia should be carried out to alleviate suffering if the prognosis is hopeless.

If the owner does not agree to euthanasia, heavy sedation and pain relief should be given until the animal dies.

Why is colic surgery not advocated in working equids?

Surgical treatment of colic requires a large amount of specialist equipment, strict aseptic conditions, an expert surgeon and excellent facilities and personnel for general anaesthesia and recovery. Post-operative care is intensive, lengthy and the animal always requires at least 4–6 months' rest post-recovery which is normally not possible for a working equid. Colic surgery is therefore logistically impossible in mobile clinic conditions and is not attempted.

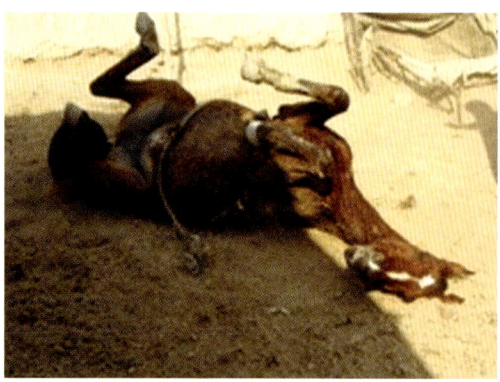

Figure 11.5.4 A horse showing severe abdominal pain.

> Remember harm v. benefit for the animal.

Even with state of the art facilities, 24-hour nursing care, expert equipment and experienced equine surgeons, many colic surgeries result in prolonged suffering and eventual death of the animal, or long-term gastric complications.

Prevention of colic

> The key to a healthy equine gastrointestinal system is the continuous provision of appropriate food and water.

Sometimes colic occurs for no identifiable reason. Good nutrition and feeding practices, free access to clean water, an appropriate living environment, care of dentition, some moderate daily exercise, and management of internal parasites can help prevent many of the common causes of colic.

Risk factors for colic in equids

A number of reviews have been written on the risk factors for colic in equids (see References). Listed risk factors are: age, sex, breed, type of housing, outdoor access to pasture, changes in management practices, activity level of the animal and changes in activity, water supply, control of parasites (use of de-worming products, presence of intestinal parasites particularly tapeworm, and type of de-worming programme), quality and type of food (such as concentrates, feeding of wholegrain corn, changes in feeding practices and types of feed), competence of the person who cares for the animal daily, and medical history such as previous colic episodes or administration of medical treatment (Reeves *et al.* 1996, Proudman and Trees 1999, Gonçalves *et al.* 2002, Proudman 2003). However, many reported risk factors have conflicting reports and weak evidence (Nolen-Walston *et al.* 2007).

Identification of risk factors is important to be able to advise owners on management that will reduce colic incidence (Scantlebury *et al.* 2011).

> **Risk factors for colic related to feeding practices are the most prevalent, especially changes in diet, low levels of forage, and high levels of carbohydrates.**

Anthrax in equids presents as acute colic, with septicaemia and enteritis. Treatment can be attempted, with BID penicillin, if early in the disease course. The disease course is usually 48–96 hours, and is generally fatal. Burn and bury suspect cases that die; do not conduct a post-mortem as this is a zoonotic disease.

Diarrhoea in adult equids 11.6

See Chapter 18 for information about diarrhoea in foals.

Acute diarrhoea (acute colitis)

In most cases, acute diarrhoea results from inflammation of the large colon and caecum.

Clinical signs include depression, abdominal pain, pyrexia and dehydration, which can progress to shock and death. This progression can occur quickly, so rapid identification and correction of fluid deficits must be a first priority (Naylor and Dunkel 2009).

Cause may not always be identified.

Treatment of clinical signs should be implemented without delay. Other treatment should aim to reduce systemic and intestinal inflammation (NSAIDs) and then to promote intestinal mucosal repair (sucralfate). Response to treatment should be monitored.

> Caution! Antibiotic-associated diarrhoea (AAD) has been linked to nearly all antibiotics used in equids (McGorum and Pirie 2010) – so do not use them in treatment of diarrhoea (especially in adult horses) as this may exacerbate the situation.

The **macrolide** group of antibiotics (erythromycin and clindamycin) has been particularly indicated as a cause of AAD (see below) and is therefore contra-indicated in equids (McGorum and Pirie 2010); see Chapter 5 *Medicines*. Antibiotics should be avoided but, if used prudently, should be carefully selected based on diagnostic analysis.

Fluid therapy in diarrhoea

Mucosal inflammation, often found in cases of diarrhoea, can compromise mucosal integrity and function, which in turn can affect the absorption of water and electrolytes. However, in mild to moderate cases of diarrhoea, enteral fluid therapy via a nasogastric tube is still considered an appropriate method of fluid therapy (Naylor and Dunkel 2009). In most cases involving working equids this would be the most appropriate method of rehydration because it is readily available, practical, cheap and avoids the risk of thrombophlebitis associated with venous catheterisation (often increased in diarrhoea cases). See Chapter 6 *Dehydration and fluid therapy* for instruction on how to deliver isotonic enteral therapy.

Salmonella

Cause *Salmonella* spp. of bacteria. Diarrhoea is due to toxin release by the bacteria resulting in increased fluid secretion and inflammation of the intestinal mucosa. Equids of all ages can be affected although younger animals seem more susceptible. This can occur in outbreaks, and stress is often indicated as an underlying factor, e.g. transportation, gastrointestinal disease, changes in feeding patterns, high temperatures and antibiotic therapy (Feary and Hassel 2006). Recovered animals may become chronic carriers, shedding bacteria into the environment and affecting other animals (see *Chronic diarrhoea* below).

Clinical signs Signs of depression, inappetance, pyrexia, and colic are often present a few days before the diarrhoea starts. Profuse watery foul-smelling diarrhoea, possibly bloody, is typical, along with increased systemic parameters and congested mucous membranes. Septicaemia and endotoxaemia are common sequelae, which could lead to complications such as laminitis. Sometimes salmonella can become a chronic condition, reappearing in times of stress and causing chronic poor body condition and failure to thrive.

Diagnosis Should be confirmed by faecal culture but this can be difficult as false negatives are possible. As the bacteria are shed intermittently, a minimum of three samples (ideally five) taken on subsequent days, are recommended to rule out the salmonella infection (Feary and Hassel 2006).

Treatment Correct the fluid deficit via nasogastric tube with oral supplementation. NSAIDs are recommended. The use of antibiotics has been shown in some cases not to reduce shedding of salmonella, and can be detrimental. Indeed, antibiotics have been shown to be associated with the *cause* of some cases (Feary and Hassel 2006). Antibiotics should only be proposed in severe cases of septicaemia and for immune-compromised animals with careful selection of a narrow-spectrum bactericidal agent (Feary and Hassel 2006).

> Remember, salmonella is very contagious to most species, including humans. Appropriate isolation of the animal and owner advice must be given.

Clostridium perfringens

Cause *C. perfringens*

Clinical signs Acute onset depression and shock, with death often occurring before diarrhoea. Intense pain, often unresponsive to analgesia, means that euthanasia is usually indicated; most animals die within 24 to 48 hours of onset. Endotoxaemia is a common finding, and the associated systemic signs of this. Seen in foals in the first few days of life.

Diagnosis Isolation of bacteria in fresh faeces or faecal swabs

Treatment Aggressive fluid therapy can be initiated if *C. perfringens* infection is recognised in the early stages. Foals can be treated with antibiotics (e.g. penicillin and aminoglycoside, plus metronidazole PO/IV 10–15 mg/kg BID). Avoid antibiotic therapy in adult equids as this is reported to induce further diarrhoea (Feary and Hassel 2006).

Chronic diarrhoea

Parasitic enteritis

(See also Chapter 17)

Cause Usually due to the emergence of larval cyathostomes (small strongyles) which damage the walls of the caecum and colon. These cyathostome larvae hypobiose (go into arrested development) in the gut wall at times when external environmental factors are detrimental to their development/life cycle, e.g. cold winters and possibly drought periods. Large strongyles have also been implicated.

Clinical signs Diarrhoea, weight loss, parasitic larvae may be seen in faeces, severe cases may show limb oedema (due to hypoproteinaemia) and increased pulse/respiratory rates. Faecal egg counts will not reveal the true extent of the infection as the hypobiosed larvae are prepatent. Cyathstomiasis has been linked to fatal colitis and is more commonly reported in 1–6 year olds (Feary and Hassel 2006).

Diagnosis Signalment, history, risk factors, faceal and blood analysis, parasitic larvae in faeces

Treatment Due to over-use of de-worming drugs, certain anthelmintics are no longer effective, e.g. benzimidazoles (fenbendazole). Repeated dosing is needed to kill developing larvae; there are no reports of resistance to ivermectin (Feary and Hassel 2006).

> Emergence of resistance of cyathostomes to anthelmintics is a major parasitic control problem and warrants careful monitoring.

Chronic salmonellosis

Clinical signs Soft faeces with intermittent bouts of diarrhoea, persistent weight loss (MacLeay *et al.* 1997). May have fever or poor appetite.

Diagnosis Serial faecal cultures

Treatment As for acute salmonellosis; however, it is usually unsuccessful.

Antibiotic Associated Diarrhoea (AAD)

Clinical signs Diarrhoea starts 2–6 days after antibiotics are first administered.

> Nearly all antibiotics used in horses have been reported to cause diarrhoea; therefore, it is important to use antibiotics responsibly.

It is thought that the antibiotics kill the beneficial gastrointestinal (GI) flora which leads to an overgrowth of *Clostridium difficile* and *C. perfringens* (McGorum and Pirie 2010). Decreased roughage consumption may predispose animals.

Diagnosis By clinical signs and recent antibiotic therapy

Treatment Stop the antibiotic therapy. Give dry forage diet and supportive care. Correct the fluid deficit via nasogastric tube if possible, ideally with isotonic solution (see Chapter 6). NSAIDs may be required to ensure comfort, but use sparingly. Flunixin meglumine is a good choice for its anti-endotoxic properties. Metronidazole 15–25 mg/kg PO 6–8 hours may help in cases of acute toxic enterocolitis (McGorum and Pirie 2010) but, if improvement is not seen, stop the antibiotics.

NSAID toxicity

Cause Phenylbutazone, flunixin meglumine and ketoprofen have been implicated in causing disease. Phenylbutazone is thought to have the highest propensity to cause diarrhoea (MacAllister *et al.* 1993).

Clinical signs Diarrhoea, colic (Hillyer 2004), inappetance, hypoproteinaemia, and dependent oedema

Diagnosis Recent history of NSAID use and clinical signs. Drugs may have been used in the correct doses, or may have been overdosed or used for a prolonged period of time.

Treatment Withdraw the NSAID. Supportive treatment for the diarrhoea: fluids (preferably by nasogastric tube), dry forage diet. Sucralfate 22 mg/kg BID/TID may help.

GI tumours

> This should be considered in older equids with chronic, non-progressive diarrhoea which does not respond to treatment.

The most common form is intestinal lymphosarcoma (Taylor *et al.* 2006), although mesenteric lipomas are also common in older animals.

Clinical signs Persistent weight loss, diarrhoea, colic, and oedema of the ventral abdomen and limbs as, over time, the protein-losing enteropathy leads to hypoproteinaemia. Contrary to other causes of chronic diarrhoea, the animal may or may not have a good appetite or fever.

Diagnosis Clinical signs and a lack of response to therapy. A rectal examination may reveal enlarged mesenteric lymph nodes, or the tumour itself, and a haemogram or abdominal paracentesis may show increased numbers of lymphocytes.

Treatment None available which is curative. Supportive therapy (rest, good quality feed, and pain relief if required) is indicated until the animal is too debilitated to work. These tumours often lead to colic signs, especially if the bowel becomes obstructed or strangulated which is often the case with pedunculated lipomas.

Prognosis Poor – chronic weight loss and debility leads to death or euthanasia. If the animal cannot work and has become anorexic, these are indications that it is suffering and euthanasia should be recommended to the owner. Reported time from the start of signs of the disease to death or euthanasia is less than 2 months (Taylor *et al.* 2006). Make the owner aware of this very poor prognosis to reduce suffering for the animal.

Conditions affecting the rectum (prolapse and perforation) 11.7

Rectal prolapse

Cause This is quite common in some regions and can be due to a variety of reasons, including chronic diarrhoea associated with infection or parasitism, foreign bodies or feed impaction due to poor teeth, dehydration, or following parturition, many of which cause increased straining (tenesmus) (Colahan *et al.* 1999). Other non-gastrointestinal causes can include overloading (the animal strains in the hindquarters to move the load) and prolonged recumbency from other illnesses. A study of 177 donkeys in Ethiopia (Getachew *et al.* 2012) showed over 83% of cases were associated with the presence of *Gasterophilus nasalis*.

A prolapsed rectum is a *symptom* of an underlying problem, not the problem itself!

Treatment This involves not only replacing the prolapse (Figure 11.7.1), but taking a good history and doing a detailed clinical examination to try to identify and treat the underlying cause. Many cases of prolapse are recurring and, unless the underlying cause is rectified, the animal's welfare will be severely compromised with repeated attempts at replacement. Provide analgesia and anti-inflammatory drugs.

How do you replace the prolapse?

- Ensure the animal is adequately restrained. This requires a competent handler, sedation and, ideally, epidural anaesthesia, (details in Section 7.2), particularly if the animal is still straining a lot or distressed.

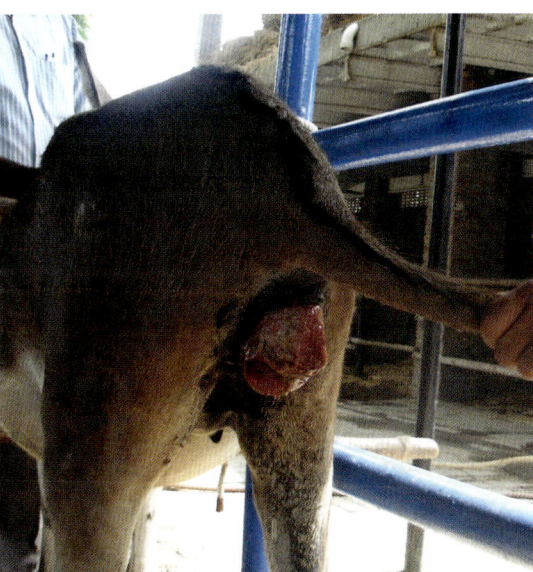

Figure 11.7.1 An example of a case of rectal prolapse in a donkey.

- Tie back the tail and clean any faeces from the tail and perineal area.
- Wash the prolapse gently and remove as much necrotic tissue as possible. Applying table sugar will help decrease any oedema and allow for easier replacement back into the rectum (Myers and Rothenberger 1991).
- Gently push the rectal tissue back into the rectum manually, avoiding excessive pressure which could tear the delicate rectal mucosa; use lubrication to aid the process. If the animal continues to strain and the rectum keeps re-prolapsing, consider sedation, if this has not already been given, or even a caudal epidural (Michou and Leece 2012) if the animal appears to be in a lot of pain. Ensure that a caudal epidural has been administered before suturing the anus.
- Many rectal prolapses can be resolved through manual correction and do not require suturing. If this is not possible then a suture can be placed.

> **Ensure that the animal can pass droppings and that sutures are removed.**

- Using a large needle and thick suture material (cattle vaginal tape is best if available), make a 'purse-string' suture (a single, continuous suture pattern with needle insertion at 4–6 points in a full circle around the rectum). Infuse local anaesthetic into the area first with a 24G needle.
- Gently pull the two ends of the suture so that the rectum closes. Leave a space large enough to insert 2–3 fingers into the hole (so the rectum will not prolapse back through the hole, but that soft faeces and gas can still escape).
- Treat for underlying colic symptoms, pain and infection, if necessary. Pass a nasogastric tube and give liquid paraffin or mineral oil (the same dose as for suspected obstruction in colic – Section 11.5 of this chapter) as this lubricates the faeces to allow for easy passage once the suture is removed. If parasites are suspected to be the underlying cause, **do not give anthelmintics** until the sutures are removed and faeces are passing normally, as this could cause recurrence of the prolapse or colic.

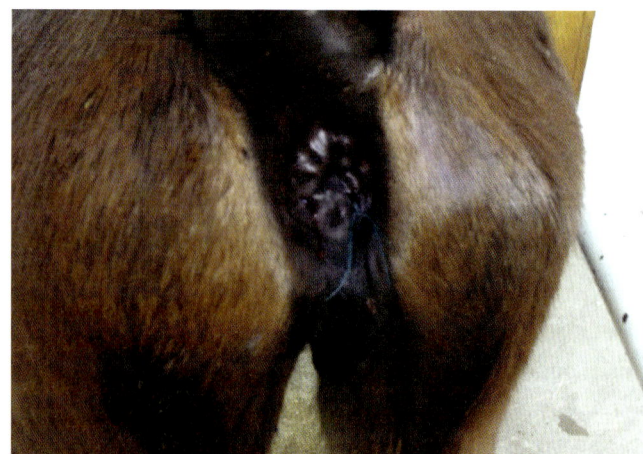

Figure 11.7.2 A replaced rectal prolapse being held in place by sutures.

> **Important:** If the prolapse has been replaced and held in place with sutures, ensure that the sutures are removed after 48 hours (72 at most) (Colahan *et al.* 1999). Leaving in sutures will ultimately lead to the death of the animal, which is far worse than the original prolapse.

CONDITIONS AFFECTING THE RECTUM (PROLAPSE AND PERFORATION) 11.7

- Do not just rely on the owner to take the sutures out – aim to revisit the animal the next day, assess for colic symptoms and pain, and repeat the paraffin or other symptomatic treatment if necessary. If follow-up is not possible, ensure another member of the team or a trusted local health provider is able to revisit. The animal will require several days of soft laxative feed, plenty of water, and a reduced workload for the next week to ensure the prolapse does not recur.

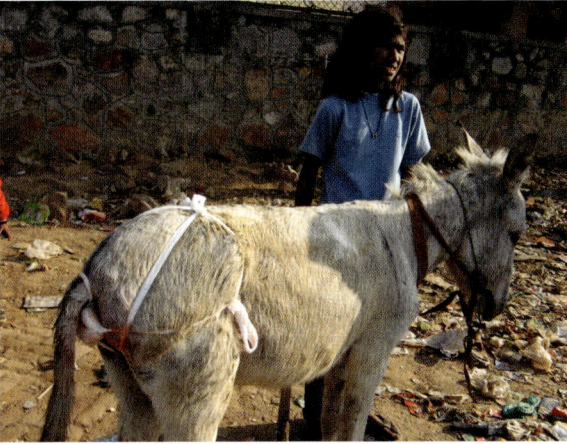

Figure 11.7.3 Bandage preventing recurrence of prolapse.

Always remember to remove the sutures.

A novel treatment in the field, when suturing is not possible or not required (Chittora 2012, personal communication), is to use a bandage pack to keep the prolapse inside after manual replacement (Figure 11.7.3). As before, careful monitoring of the animal is required and analgesia and anti-inflammatory drugs administered. The owner needs to be advised of a soft diet to reduce straining until the symptoms have resolved.

> Prevention: The underlying cause must be found and treated or repeated prolapse may occur.

Rectal tears/perforation

This is a serious condition in equids and can result in fatal peritonitis which requires euthanasia. The rectum consists of three layers. From the lumen side these are: mucosal (lining the rectal lumen), muscularis and serosal layers.

Causes

- Inappropriate rectal examination technique is the most common cause (Watkins *et al.* 1989) possibly due to an unrestrained animal, lack of lubrication and/or excessive force (see rectal examination in Section 11.5 of this chapter).
- Foaling difficulties – excessive straining by the mare, foal hooves tearing the rectal lining, or an explosive delivery
- Inappropriate or violent coitus

Diagnosis

- Suspect if signs of colic or peritonitis are observed, with a history of foaling, coitus or recent rectal examination.
- Abdominocentesis can reveal faecal material or other signs that a complete rectal rupture has occurred.

11 THE GASTROINTESTINAL SYSTEM

- Rectal examination is the only way to determine the size of the tear and whether it is full thickness or involves just the mucosa and/or muscularis layers.
- Rectal tears have been classified from Grades 1 to 4 depending on the depth of the tear: from Grade 1 involving just the mucosa (mildest form) to Grade 4 involving full thickness of the rectal wall leading to contamination of the peritoneal cavity with faeces (which is invariably fatal and calls for immediate euthanasia) (Watkins et al. 1989).

Treatment

- A full-thickness tear (through all three layers – mucosa, muscularis and serosa) will most likely result in fatal peritonitis (Grade 4), and humane euthanasia is recommended early to prevent suffering.
- Semi-thickness or simple mucosal tears may heal themselves if small (Grade 1). However, if the animal is presented with depression/colic/inappetance and a rectal perforation is the cause, the likelihood of healing is reduced.
- If the signs are mild and there is no pyrexia or excessive pain, advise complete rest for 1–2 weeks, feeding very soft food only, with paraffin included 2–3 times daily. Be sure to give pain relief, and antibiotics to avoid secondary infection in the colorectal wall. At the first signs of colic or peritonitis it is advisable to euthanase on humane grounds.
- Good first aid care as soon after the occurrence of the tear can improve the outcome (Watkins et al. 1989). Reduce the straining (consider epidural anaesthesia), remove faecal material and pack the tear with gauze swabs.
- Recommend a soft diet and mineral oil.
- Analgesia and anti-inflammatory drugs should be given.

Prognosis

This is usually poor for all but the most minor type of rectal tear.

Peritonitis

11.8

> Peritonitis is inflammation of the peritoneum that lines the peritoneal cavity.

Equids are much more susceptible to peritonitis than bovine animals.

Peritonitis can be described as:
- primary or secondary
- diffuse or localised
- peracute, acute or chronic
- septic or non-septic.

These descriptions relate to the presentation and underlying cause of peritonitis. Equids most commonly present with secondary peritonitis following damage to the gastrointestinal tract or abdominal wall (Dart and Bischofberger 2011).

Causes Peritonitis is commonly associated with bowel compromise (colic signs), parasitism and abdominal abscesses from infection with *Streptococcus* or *Rhodococcus* bacteria. Injuries which puncture the abdominal wall, rupture of the uterus during foaling, or rectal wall damage during examination, parturition or coitus are frequent causes of acute peritonitis.

Differential diagnoses for peritonitis should include various other causes of colic, as well as myopathies, laminitis, and pleuritis – anything which causes reluctance to move and increased pain, pyrexia and dullness in the animal.

Clinical signs and diagnosis History of trauma, colic or parasitism is extremely suggestive. Diarrhoea, weight loss, and recurrent colic combined with pyrexia are common signs in chronic cases. Systemic signs such as fever and increased heart and respiratory rates are indicative, as is reluctance to move, and ileus in the more critical cases. Severe cases associated with gut rupture show more grave signs of endotoxaemia, septicaemia, depression, acute cardiovascular deterioration, severe abdominal pain, sweating, tachycardia, and red to purple mucous membranes. In severe cases death occurs in 4–24 hours of the rupture.

Rectal exam may reveal 'gritty' peritoneal surfaces or thickening of intestines, as well as possible masses attributing to the peritonitis.

Abdominocentesis This helps achieve a definitive diagnosis (see Section 11.5. of this chapter, on colic).

Treatment Many cases of peritonitis cannot be treated and it is preferable to euthanase the animal. Any type of perforation falls into this category. However, for milder cases, it may be possible to treat symptomatically with fluids, anti-inflammatory drugs and antibiotic therapy; for secondary peritonitis always try to identify and treat the underlying cause (Dart and Bischofberger 2011).

Treatment is long term (> 3 weeks) and may not be ethically justified in working equids, especially if adequate follow-up and nursing care is not possible. Oral trimethoprim-sulphur tablets could be a useful alternative to injectable antibiotics to provide long-term therapy. However, remember the bacteria must be susceptible – if there is no improvement over the course of a week consider euthanasia.

11.9 Liver disease

The liver has an amazing compensatory capacity. In fact 80% of the liver has to be compromised before its functional capacity will start to fail (Pearson 1999).

> Liver disease in working equids is relatively common.

The liver is the major metabolising organ of the body, with large amounts of blood passing through it, so it is a common site for secondary abscessation and pathology after an infection such as strangles, toxicity or an inadequate diet. Many drugs are also metabolised by the liver; it is important to administer the correct drugs in the correct amounts and advise owners of the seriousness of inappropriate drug administration.

Clinical signs of liver disease

Sub-clinical liver disease may be common in equids, but signs are only seen when cases are advanced (Gehlen *et al.* 2010).

Signs are general, variable and often non-specific and many of these common, generalised signs of illness in working equids have any number of underlying causes. It is important to remember the liver during examinations, and take a good history, to be successful in narrowing a case down to a liver problem.

- Depression
- Inappetance
- Weight loss
- Icterus (jaundice)
- Colic
- Neurological signs*: gait abnormalities and motor deficits (rare hepatic myelopathy and encephalopathy – Nout 2011)
- Pruritis and other skin conditions
- Diarrhoea or constipation
- Coagulopathies (dysfunction of blood clotting mechanisms)

*Signs of neurological (central nervous system – CNS) dysfunction can range from mild behavioural changes, which only the owner may notice, to more severe signs such as incoordination, yawning, aimless wandering and dullness.

Acute liver disease

Acute toxicosis is a common cause of sudden onset liver disease – caused by the ingestion/administration of hazardous plants or chemical materials, including drugs, tetanus antitoxin and mycotoxins found in bad feed (Pearson 1999).

> Remember that, due to the compensatory mechanisms of the liver, what seems an acute onset liver problem could also be the sudden inability of the liver to cope with a chronic condition, or liver pathology due to a secondary cause.

Clinical signs Depression, lethargy, anorexia, colic, jaundice (Figure 11.9.1) and possible CNS signs (depression, head pressing, incoordination). The urine may be dark-coloured (high bilirubin). A history of the recent ingestion/administration of harmful substances is suggestive of an acute condition (Pearson 1999).

Diagnosis Usually based on clinical signs and history. A blood test for liver enzyme levels usually shows elevations in plasma or serum total bile acids, serum total bilirubin, AST, ALP, GGT, and bilirubin (see Section 4.5); SDH and GLDH are liver specific. Differential diagnoses include chronic liver failure/abscessation, chronic active hepatitis and other systemic disease causing anorexia/CNS signs/depression.

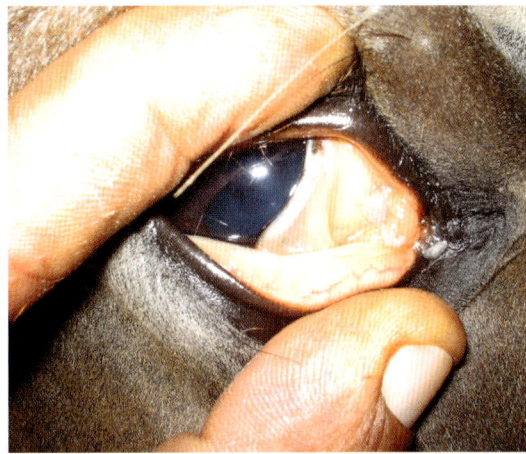

Figure 11.9.1 Yellow-coloured (icteric) mucous membranes of the eye.

Treatment The regime below can be used for any suspected liver disease. The aim of therapy is to be supportive until hepatic compensation and regeneration can occur which may take from weeks to months. Work out a timeline with the owner for indicators of improvement. Rest and appropriate feeding can be ongoing; however, sedation, vitamins and antibiotics are not recommended long term. Monitor the case closely, although euthanasia may be the only option if signs do not improve or deteriorate within the first few days despite initial therapy.

- In the first 24–48 hours, sedation with xylazine or another alpha2-agonist is recommended only if neurological signs result in manic behaviour (Pearson 1999). However, depression is more likely.

> Remember the liver will have to metabolise any drug administered at this time, thus putting extra pressure on it.

- Ensure the animal is kept in a place where minimum harm can come to it from its decreased mental capacity.

- Provide a high-energy, low-protein diet. Aim to boost blood glucose levels without increasing the strain on the liver to break down proteins – a 5% dextrose IV infusion at 2 L/hour may be effective in the short term. Nasogastric intubation of food may be required initially if the animal is anorexic.

- B-complex vitamin administration IM

- Supportive mechanisms such as fluid therapy, pain relief or antibiotics if signs such as dehydration, colic or pyrexia are present. If available, metronidazole is a good antibiotic to use in liver disease as it can penetrate abscessation, otherwise, trimethoprim sulphur or a combination of penicillin/gentamicin is acceptable.

- Rest!

Prognosis For acute conditions, expect a rapid, maintained improvement in signs over 24–48 hours as the toxicity is flushed through the system and the liver returns to functional capacity. A downward trend in liver enzymes is also positive for hepatic function improvement; if possible take a blood sample again after 7–10 days. If blood analysis is not available, expect to see a rapid improvement in the animal's condition, a desire to eat and drink, as well as a substantial reduction in CNS impairment.

Failure/slow improvement, or return to clinical signs once therapy is stopped, is an indication that the damage to the liver is extensive or chronic, and prognosis is not good.

Chronic liver disease/chronic active hepatitis

The causes, diagnosis and treatment are similar to those for acute liver disease; however, a *history of chronic weight loss* is common.

> The most common cause of chronic liver failure is from eating hepatotoxic plants over a sustained period of time, especially those containing pyrrolizidine alkaloids.

Become familiar with any plants in the local area which may contain these compounds; often the owners are aware of them already if they have other livestock. Other potential causes are infectious and immune-mediated (Pearson 1999).

Clinical signs A history of chronic weight loss is the most common differentiating factor between acute and chronic liver disease. Other signs are as above for acute disease (depression, neurological signs), although jaundice may not be as pronounced in the chronic case. If chronic disease has resulted in hypoproteinaemia, oedema may occur in dependent areas such as under the jaw/sternum, and polyuria/polydipsia may have been noticed by the owner. Skin lesions may be visible: photosensitisation/pruritis/dermatitis.

Diagnosis Clinical signs, history and elevations in liver enzymes and bile acids are suggestive. The blood results may not be as pronounced as expected since active liver inflammation may have ceased in the chronic case. Toxicosis from pyrrolizidine alkaloids can only be confirmed by liver biopsy (Pearson 1999) which is not practical. Inspection of grazing areas can aid diagnosis if plants are found containing pyrrolizidine alkaloids.

Treatment As for acute cases: treatment should be supportive and eliminate the cause. Response to treatment can help you to determine prognosis and sometimes to differentiate between acute and chronic conditions.

Prognosis Equids with chronic liver disease have a poor prognosis for survival and, as with acute liver failure, treatment is supportive only in the hope that liver function returns, which rarely happens. Owners should be warned of this before embarking on treatment.

Prevention of liver disease

Ideally, this is the best route. It is vitally important to create awareness in owners and equine health providers of the causes and, therefore, the prevention, of liver disease, especially as subclinical disease may be common and yet undetected until too late.

> Removal and avoidance of toxic plants (pyrrolizidine alkaloids) and correct dosage of drugs are steps that can be taken (Pearson 1999).

Case study – Impaction colic caused by foreign material consumption

11.10

Location Matrouh, Egypt

Attending veterinarian Dr Ahmed Elrwany

History
A 7-year-old female donkey, presented by the owner. The donkey had not defaecated during the last 12 hours. Previous to this, defaecation was less than normal with small balls. The donkey last ate 12 hours previously and did not finish the whole feed. She last drank a small amount of water 12 hours previously. She was not pregnant, had no teeth problems and was last de-wormed a month ago. The owner had noticed colic signs in the donkey (rolling) 6 hours previous to presentation.

Clinical findings
- Dullness
- Rolling on the ground
- No defaecation, no urination
- Anorexic
- Pulse rate 56 beats per minute
- Respiratory rate 25 breaths per minute
- Rectal temperature 37.2°C
- Decreased gut sounds
- Normal mucous membrane

Diagnosis
Made from history and clinical signs, after full clinical examination. Careful rectal examination found that the rectum was completely blocked by foreign material. The donkey was suffering from impaction colic.

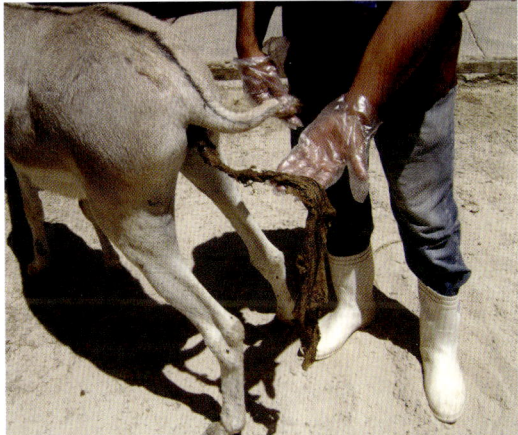

Figure 11.10.1 Foreign material found in the rectum.

Differential diagnosis
Tympanitic or obstructive colic

Treatment
- Immediate pain control – Injection phenylbutazone 2.2 mg/kg IV
- The foreign material could not be brought out of the rectum on the first rectal examination, so oral water and laxatives were given as well as liquid paraffin 1.5 litres administered by nasogastric tube – to soften and lubricate the faeces.
- Further food was withheld, the donkey walked in-hand regularly to stimulate gut motility, and closely monitored.
- After 12 hours, a piece of foreign material appeared at the rectum that was carefully removed; it was a large piece of cloth (Figures 11.10.1 and 11.10.2).

11 THE GASTROINTESTINAL SYSTEM

- Food was withheld a further 12 hours until no other foreign material was passed, only faeces, then small amounts of green fodder was offered 6 times per day for 4 days.
- Normal food was gradually re-introduced.

Prevention
Owner involvement, follow-up plan, good management/husbandry practices and take-home message.

- Feed high-quality hay that is not too mature and hard to digest.
- Feed small meals frequently, instead of large meals once or twice per day.
- Provide plenty of fresh clean water to drink at all times.
- Provide electrolytes to stimulate drinking and replenish any losses.
- Provide preventative care such as appropriate intestinal parasite control and regular dental check-ups.
- Make any changes to the diet, exercise or stabling gradually.
- Observe the donkey daily, looking for any changes in behavior that may indicate ill health.
- Be aware of the average number of piles of faeces that a donkey passes daily and the consistency.

Prognosis
The prognosis was good because, after rectal examination and removing the foreign material, the animal felt comfortable.

Discussion
Colic is a serious welfare issue and may lead to death of the animal. Regular good management/husbandry practices and timely treatment reduces its severity and saves lives. This case of impacted colic was due to foreign material ingestion. The piece of cloth found on rectal examination was twisted with faecal material, totally blocking the rectum; the animal was not defecating and was in constant pain. After rectal examination and removal of these materials the animal was more comfortable and gradually recovered, showing the effectiveness of correct diagnosis and treatment.

Prevention of impaction colic
The following are potential risk factors:

- Dehydration, due to insufficient fresh water availability
- Animals eating straw bedding, plastic bags, rope and cloth – ensure the stabling/grazing area is clean
- Animals grazing on sandy soil may take in sufficient sand to cause impaction of the colon
- A sudden change in management, such as stabling
- A sudden drop in the amount of exercise

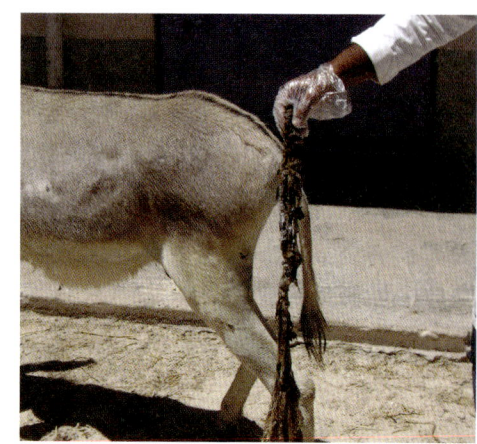

Figure 11.10.2 Foreign material removed from the rectum.

References

Almeida, P.E., Weber, P.S.D., Burton, J.L., Zanella, A.J. (2008) Depressed DHEA and increased sickness response behaviors in lame dairy cows with inflammatory foot lesions. *Domest. anim. Endocrin.* 34, 89–99.

Bertone, J.J. (2002) Clinical field efficacy and safety of N-Butylscopolammonium Bromide in horses. Proceedings of the 48th American Association of Equine Practitioners convention, Florida, USA. 48, 370–374.

Boulot, S., Brun, J.P., Doreau, M., Martin-Rossett, W. (1987) Activites aliminentaires et niveau d'ingestion chez la jument gestante et al.laitainte. *Repro. Nutr. Develop.* 27, 205–206.

Carroll, C.L., Huntington, P.J. (1988) Body condition scoring and weight estimation of horses. *Equine Vet. J.* 20 (1), 41–45.

Carson, K., Wood-Gush, D.G.M. (1983) Behaviour of Thoroughbred foals during nursing. *Equine Vet. J.* 15 (3), 257–262.

Chittora, R. (2012) *Discussion on rectal prolapse in working equids.* [letter] (Personal communication, 21 August 2012).

Colahan, P.T., Mayhew, I.G., Merritt, A.M., Moore, J.N. (1999) Manual of Equine Medicine and Surgery. Mosby, Inc. Missouri. pp. 17–22.

Coleman, R.J., Mathison, G.W., Les Burwash, M.S. (1999) Growth and condition at weaning of extensively managed creep-fed foals. *J. Equine Vet. Sci.* 19 (1), 45–50.

Crowell-Davis, S.L., Houpt, K.A. (1985) Coprophagy by foals: effect of age and possible functions. *Equine Vet J.* 17 (1), 17–19.

Dart, A.J., Bischofberger, A.S. (2011) Peritonitis in the horse: a treatment dilemma. *Equine vet. Educ.* 23 (6), 294–295.

Dobromylskyj, P., Flecknell, P.A., Lascelles, B.D., Livingston, A., Taylor, P., Waterman-Pearson, A. (2000) Pain assessment. In: *Pain management in animals*, Eds: P.A. Flecknell and A. Waterman-Pearson, W. B. Saunders Ltd, London. pp. 53–80.

Feary, D.J., Hassel, D.M. (2006) Enteritis and Colitis in horses. *Vet. Clin. N. Am. – Equine.* 22, 437–479.

Finkler-Schade, C. (2007) Development and nutrition of the foal. *Pferdeheilk.* 23, 569–576.

Gehlen, H., May, A., Venner, M. (2010) Liver disease in horses. *Pferdeheilk.* 26 (5), 668–679.

Getachew, A.M., Innocent, G., Trawford, A.F., Reid, S.W., James, and Love, S. (2012) Gasterophilosis: a major cause of rectal prolapse in working donkeys in Ethiopia. *Trop. Anim. Health. Prod.* 44 (4), 757–762.

Gonçalves, S., Julliand, V., Leblond, A. (2002) Risk factors associated with colic in horses. *Vet. Res.* 33 641–652.

Grindem, C.B., Fairley, N.M., Uhlinger, C.A., Crane, S.A. (1990) Peritoneal fluid values from healthy foals. *Equine Vet. J.* 22 (5), 359–361.

Hague, B.A., Honnas, C.M. (1998) Traumatic dental disease and soft tissue injuries of the oral cavity. *Vet. Clin. N. Am. Equine Pract.* 14 (2), 333–347.

Hallowell, G.D. (2008) Retrospective study assessing efficacy of treatment of large colonic impactions. *Equine Vet. J.* 40 (4), 411–413.

Henneke, D.R., Potter, G.D., Kreider, J.L., Yeates, B.F. (1983) Relationship between condition score, physical measurements and body fat percentage in mares. *Equine Vet. J.* 15 (4) 371–372.

Hillyer, M. (2004) A practical approach to diarrhoea in the adult horse. *In Practice.* 26 (1), 2–11.

Letchworth, G.J., Rodriguez, L.L., Del C. Barrera, J. (1999) Vesicular stomatitis. *Vet. J.* 157, 239–260.

MacAllister, C.G., Morgan, S.J., Borne, A.T., Pollet, R.A. (1993) Comparison of adverse effects of phenylbutazone, flunixin meglumine, and ketoprofen in horses. *J. Am. Vet. Med. A.* 202 (1), 71–77.

MacLeay, J.M., Ames, T.R., Hayden, D.W., Tumas, D.B. (1997) Acquired B lymphocyte deficiency and chronic enterocolitis in a 3-year-old Quarter horse. *Vet. Immunol. Immunopath.* 57. 49–57.

McGorum, B.C., Pirie, R.S. (2010) Antimicrobial associated diarrhoea in the horse. Part 2: Which antimicrobials are associated with AAD in the horse? *Equine vet. Educ.* 22 (1), 43–50.

Mair, T.S., Pearson, G.R., Divers, T.J. (2006) Malabsorption syndromes in the horse. *Equine vet. Educ.* 18 (6) 299–308.

Maranhão, R.P.A., Palhares, M.S., Melo, U.P., Rezende, H.H.C., Braga, C.E., Silva Filho, J.M., Vasconcelos, M.N.F. (2006) Most frequent pathologies of the locomotor system in equids used for wagon traction in Belo Horizonte. *Arq. Bras. Med. vet. Zoo.* 58, 21–27.

Michou and Leece (2012) Sedation and analgesia in the standing horse 2. Local anaesthesia and analgesia techniques. *In Practice.* 34, 578–587.

Myers, J.O., Rothenberger, D.A. (1991) Sugar in the reduction of incarcerated prolapsed bowel. Diseases of the colon and rectum. 34 (5), 416–418.

Naylor, J.M. (1979) Colostral immunity in the calf and the foal. *Vet. Clin. N. Am. Equine Prac.* 1, 169–178.

Naylor, R.J., Dunkel, B. (2009) The treatment of diarrhoea in adult horses. *Equine vet. Educ.* 21 (9), 494–504.

Nolen-Walston, R., Paxson, J., Ramey, D.W. (2007) Evidence-based gastrointestinal medicine in horses: it's not about your gut instincts. *Vet. Clin. N. Am. – Equine.* 23, 243–266.

Nout, Y.S. (2011) Gait deficits in liver disease: hepatic encephalopathy and hepatic myelopathy. *Equine vet. Educ.* 23 (1), 11–13.

Orsini, J.A. (2011) A fresh look at the process of arriving at a clinical prognosis Part 2: colic. *J. Eq. Vet. Sci.* 31 (7), 370–378.

Ousey, J.C., Prani, S., Zimmer, J., Holdstock, N., Rossdale, P.D. (1997) Effects of various feeding regimes on the energy balance of neonates. *Am. J. Vet. Res.* 58, 1243–1251.

Pearson, E.G. (1999) Liver disease in the mature horse. *Equine vet. Educ.* 11 (2), 87–96.

Pringle, R.O. (1871) Purdon's veterinary handbook. The diseases of horses, cattle, sheep, swine, dogs and poultry, their causes, symptoms and treatments. 2nd Ed. William Blackwood and sons, Edinburgh and London. p. 10.

Proudman, C.J. (2003) Diagnosis, treatment, and prevention of tapeworm-associated colic. *J. Eq. Vet. Sci.* 23 (1) 6–9.

Proudman, C.J., Trees, S. (1999) Tapeworms as a cause of intestinal disease in horses. *Parasitology Today*. 15 (4) 156–159.

Reeves, J.R., Salman, Mo. D., Smith, G. (1996) Risk factors for equine acute abdominal disease (colic): Results from a multi-center case-control study. *Prev. Vet. Med*. 26, 285–301.

Scantlebury, C.E., Archer, D.C., Proudman, C.J., Pinchbeck, G.L. (2011) Recurrent colic in the horse: Incidence and risk factors for recurrence in the general population. *Equine Vet. J*. 43 (s39) 81–88.

Stoneham, S.J. (2005) How to feed the sick neonatal foal. In, The 1st BEVA and Waltham nutrition symposia. Eds: Harris, P.A., Mair, T.S., Slater, J.D., and Green, R.E. Equine Veterinary Journal Ltd. Cambridge, England. pp. 33–37.

Taylor, S.D., Pusterla, N., Vaughan, B., Whitcomb, M.B., Wilson, W.D. (2006) Intestinal Neoplasia in Horses. *J. Vet. Intern. Med*. 20, 1429–1436.

Tell, A., Egenvall, A., Lundstrom, T., Wattle, O. (2008) The prevalence of oral ulceration in Swedish horses when ridden with bit and bridle and when unridden. *Vet. J*. 178, 405–410.

Vall, E., Ebangi, A.L., Abakar, O. (2003) A method for estimating body condition score (BCS) in donkeys. *Working animals in agriculture and transport: a collection of some current research and development observations*. 6, 93–102.

Venner, M., Ohnesorge, B. (2001) Glucose and D-xylose absorption test for diagnosis of malabsorption in the horse. *Tierarztl. Prax. G. N*. 29 (4), 256–259.

Watkins, J.P., Taylor, T.S., Schumacher, J., Taylor, J.R., Gillis, J.P. (1989) Rectal tears in the horse: an analysis of 35 cases. *Equine Vet. J*. 21 (3), 186–188.

Weese, J.S., Staempfli, H.R., Prescott, J.F. (2001) A prospective study of the roles of *Clostridium difficile* and enterotoxigenic *Clostridium perfringens* in equine diarrhoea. *Equine Vet. J*. 33 (4), 403–409.

Weishaupt, M.A., Wiestner, T., Hogg, H.P., Jordan, P., Auer, J.A. (2004) Compensatory load redistribution of horses with induced weight-bearing hindlimb lameness trotting on a treadmill. *Equine Vet. J*. 36, 727–733.

Widman, E. (2008) How to deal with the choking horse. *J. Eq. Vet. Sci*. 28 (9) 504.

Further reading

Bezdekova, B. (2012) Esophageal disorders of horses: a review of literature. *Pferdeheilk*. 28 (2), 187–192.

Hague, B.A., Honnas, C.M. (1998) Traumatic dental disease and soft tissue injuries of the oral cavity. *Vet. Clin. N. Am. Equine Pract*. 14 (2), 333–347.

Hillyer, M. (2004) A practical approach to diarrhoea in the adult horse. *In Practice*. 26 (1), 2–11.

National Research Council (2007) Nutrient requirements of horses. 6th Ed. National Academy of Sciences, Washington, USA.

The respiratory system

12

Introduction – The significance of respiratory disease in working equids	**12.1**
Defence mechanisms of the respiratory tract and spread of disease in populations	**12.2**
Examination procedure	**12.3**
Clinical signs of respiratory disease	**12.4**
Disorders of the upper respiratory tract	**12.5**
Viral respiratory disease	**12.6**
Bacterial respiratory disease	**12.7**
Allergic respiratory disease	**12.8**
Parasitic respiratory disease	**12.9**
Epistaxis	**12.10**
Case study – Aspiration pneumonia	**12.11**
References	**12.12**

12.1 Introduction – The significance of respiratory disease in working equids

Respiratory tract problems are **common in working equids** and, even without extensive diagnostic tools such as radiography and endoscopy, it is possible to do a thorough clinical examination and make an informed decision about the most likely cause based on clinical signs.

Respiratory signs can be very **subtle** – often just a small increase in watery discharge from the nose, a slight cough or sneeze, or the animal being described as less vigorous than normal by the owner.

There are many different levels and types of respiratory disease, and secondary bacterial infection is common.

> It is the responsibility of a veterinarian to diagnose the presence or potential for respiratory disease, and explain the implications of this to the owner.

The primary purpose of the respiratory system is to enable **oxygen to enter the body**. Within the alveoli of the lungs, oxygen diffuses into the blood which is then pumped around the body to supply cells with oxygen for **aerobic respiration**. The musculoskeletal system is extremely important to the working equid; effective work is not possible if the blood to the muscles is not well oxygenated (Figure 12.1.1). Therefore, the cost to the animal from respiratory disease is much more than just discomfort and difficulty in breathing (dyspnoea).

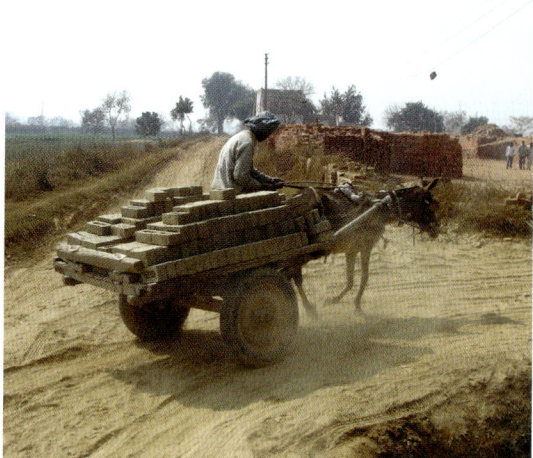

Figure 12.1.1 Any problem with the respiratory system creates an extra burden on a working equid's daily labour.

Defence mechanisms of the respiratory tract and spread of disease in populations

12.2

The working and living conditions of working equids are usually **dusty and polluted** (Figure 12.2.1), often with many animals working or housed together.

> Damaged airway defences and close confinement will increase the rate of transmission of viral and bacterial respiratory infections through the local population.

The respiratory tract has several functions:

- Intake of air for **oxygenation of blood**
- **Thermoregulation** by evaporative cooling
- **Compensatory mechanisms**, e.g. in metabolic acidosis

The respiratory tract does not have a device to scan air quality; all air goes in regardless of quality. Therefore, if an animal is working or living in an area where the air quality is not good (contaminated with dust, smoke and pollution), then the defence mechanisms may become overwhelmed or damaged.

The **mucociliary escalator** protects the respiratory tract by trapping dust particles or pathogens in a mucous layer which is then moved upwards towards the throat by beating cilia (small hairs). It has been shown that the cilia are paralysed in humans who smoke; it is likely that the same effect occurs in equids that are exposed to pollutants.

> Damage caused by dust and pollution leaves the respiratory tract vulnerable to secondary bacterial infection.

Once an infection is established, the pathogens within the respiratory tract will induce an inflammatory response. Subsequently **mucous secretion increases** which can be observed as a nasal discharge. Sneezing and coughing spreads the secretions thus aiding the dissemination of the virus and bacteria to other hosts.

It is essential to implement thorough **disinfection protocols** following the treatment of a respiratory case if an infectious cause is suspected. Disinfect hands, clothes, mouth gags, nasogastric tubes and stables after every respiratory case. Wear gloves when examining and treating cases. Isolate the affected animals from the healthy population.

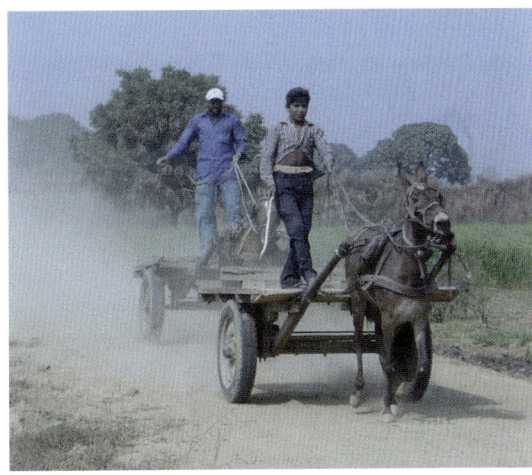

Figure 12.2.1 Dusty working environments increase the risk of respiratory infection in working equids.

Appropriate isolation with no nose-to-nose contact and a separate air space is important to prevent circulation of pathogens. Monitor the remaining population closely for the onset of clinical signs indicating respiratory infection. Treat and isolate any other suspected cases.

> It can often be beneficial to plan isolation facilities in advance. A disused shed or stable could be cleared and prepared.

12.3 Examination procedure

As always, it is important to conduct a thorough clinical examination, even if the animal presents with an obvious breathing problem. Many respiratory diseases result in systemic signs, and also many 'coughs', which may worry the owner, can reflect environmental conditions or secondary bacterial infection, rather than being the primary cause.

Overall assessment of the respiratory case

Taking a good history. Ask the owner:
- What signs/symptoms has he noticed?
- How long have the signs been present?
- Have the signs been more common at a particular time of day or during a particular activity?
- Are they getting better, worse or staying the same?
- How old is the animal?
- Are there other animals in the area showing similar signs?
- Have any animals been brought in recently or has anyone been to an equine fair?
- Has the animal been treated by anyone else recently (e.g. drenched)?

Detailed examination of the respiratory system

> Look at the body and coat condition and hydration status in conjunction with the clinical parameters of temperature, heart rate and respiratory rate.

- **Head and neck** Examine the head and neck for signs of asymmetry. Look for swelling of lymph nodes, especially in the submandibular area, as this may indicate strangles. Asymmetry of the face could indicate sinus problems or tumours.
- **Mucous membranes** Check the colour (cyanosis, a blue colour, may indicate poor perfusion) and for any haemorrhage.

- **Nostrils** Feel the air flow to ensure that it is equal on both sides. Listen for abnormal sounds/smell coming from a nostril that could indicate a problem in the nasal cavity or guttural pouches. Assess for nostril flaring. Assess any discharge, noting amount, type and frequency. Serous nasal discharge is common early in the course of a viral respiratory infection, and a mucopurulent discharge is more likely with bacterial infection.
- **Frontal/maxillary sinuses** Look for swelling, and percuss to determine whether fluid is present/or there are signs of pain. Anatomical knowledge of the borders of the sinuses is essential (Figure 12.5.2). Fluid will result in a dull sound on percussion. This is sometimes easier to hear with a stethoscope, and opening the animal's mouth can help accentuate the sounds.
- **Larynx** Palpate for asymmetry or pain. Gently squeeze at the junction of the larynx and trachea; if a cough is elicited it can indicate that the upper airway is inflamed and irritated.
- **Auscultation** Auscultate both the upper, larynx/trachea (Figure 12.3.1) and lower respiratory tract, lungs (Figure 12.3.2). Not all conditions will produce changes in the lungs.

> A quiet environment is required so that even slight changes can be detected; this takes practice and knowledge of what 'normal' sounds like.

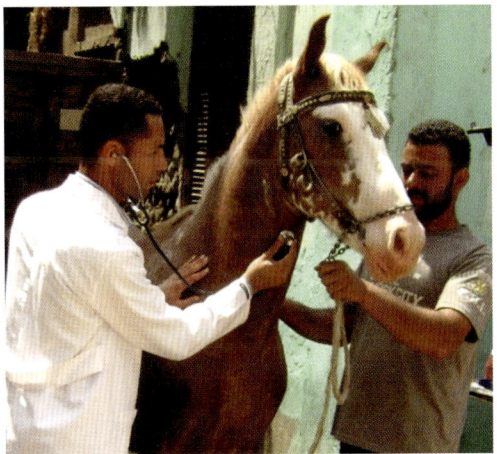

Figure 12.3.1 Auscultation of the larynx and trachea.

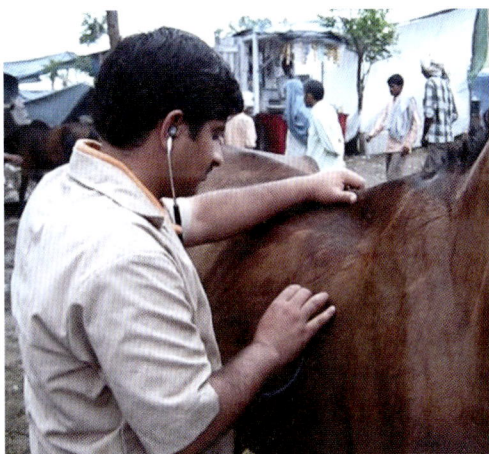

Figure 12.3.2 Auscultation of the lung field.

The normal margins of the lungs

- **Basal border** A line from the costochondral junction of the 6th rib, crossing the middle of the 11th/12th rib, to the margin of the ventral back muscles at the 16th inter-costal space
- **Dorsal border** From the caudal border of the scapula to the tuber coxae
- **Cranial border** Tricipital margin from the caudal border of the scapula to the olecranon

Auscultating many equids' lungs not only forms part of a good clinical examination but improves the perception of normal lung sounds allowing more accurate determination of abnormal lung sounds.

12 THE RESPIRATORY SYSTEM

When training other veterinarians in auscultation skills it can be useful to outline the lung field on the side of the animal (Figure 12.3.3).

Abnormal (adventitious) lung sounds

- **Wheezes** Continuous noise both on inspiration and expiration indicates inflammation usually without associated fluid, e.g. in chronic allergic conditions.
- **Crackles** Discontinuous sounds can indicate fluid is present, e.g. in pleuropneumonia or disorders causing lung oedema.
- **Friction rub** Often heard as a squeak or a grating sound. This occurs when inflamed serous surfaces rub together. This usually arises in cases of pleuritis, caused by friction between the visceral and costal pleurae. When auscultated in the region of the heart, with the rub sound occurring at the same time as the heartbeat, it is indicative of pericarditis.

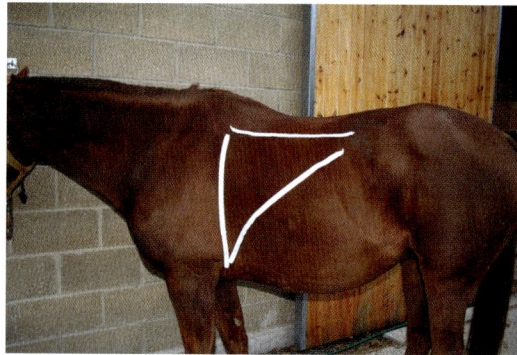

Figure 12.3.3 Delineating the lung field with tape or washable ink can assist in the training of veterinarians.

> **An understanding of the anatomy and physiology of the equine respiratory system allows effective interpretation of sounds to place them in the context of the most likely pathological condition.**

For example, increased lung sounds in the cranio-ventral region may be indicative of a bacterial pneumonia, whereas abnormal lung sounds in the caudo-dorsal region may occur as the result of allergic conditions.

Percussion of the chest

Chest percussion can detect **fluid or pleural pain**. This can be done using a thumb and middle finger to flick the chest. Work around the chest in a systematic manner so the entire lung fields are percussed. Dull areas indicate consolidation near the lung surface or the presence of fluid.

Use of a re-breathing bag

A plastic re-breathing bag can be used to **increase the rate and depth of breathing** by decreasing oxygen availability. This aids auscultation by **accentuating subtle lung changes**. Areas of pneumonia/lung consolidation may not have air passing through, and so will be silent on auscultation.

However, there are instances where a re-breathing bag should definitely not be used and, at all times, the animal's welfare is the first priority. Using a re-breathing bag can cause further respiratory distress in an already compromised animal, and taking deeper breaths, with painful conditions such as pleuritis and pleuropneumonia, will only add to the animal's suffering for the sake of a diagnosis.

> **In foals the lung sounds can be easily auscultated through the thin thoracic walls so it is unnecessary to use a re-breathing bag.**

Another complication when using a re-breathing bag is paroxysmal coughing which can occur in equids with a sensitive airway, e.g. in chronic respiratory allergies.

To use a re-breathing bag Loosely cover both nostrils with a plastic bag for approximately 30 seconds; the respiratory rate is increased. Auscultate the lungs once the bag is removed and the equid takes several deep breaths. Stop the procedure if at any time the animal becomes distressed.

Peculiarities of the donkey

Please refer to the paper (Thiemann and Bell 2001) for further information.

- Donkeys **rarely cough** when suffering respiratory disease and may display only subtle clinical signs. Cases are often presented only once the disease is advanced and severe.
- Their lung sounds are generally **more audible** than horses'.
- Donkeys have **narrower airways** and a pointed epiglottis, so take care when intubating to avoid damage or haemorrhage. Use an endotracheal tube size 21.6 mm (size 16) or 18.6 mm (size 14); use a naso-gastric tube size 9.5 or 13 mm outer diameter.

> Throughout a clinical examination and diagnostic work-up it is essential to consider the welfare of the horse, donkey or mule.

Clinical signs of respiratory disease 12.4

Clinical signs of respiratory disease are varied; consider the signs in context with respiratory tract anatomy when making a diagnosis.

Symptoms of respiratory disease can include the following:

- **Cough**
- **Nasal discharge** (Figure 12.4.1)
- Trouble breathing (*dyspnoea*)
- Increased respiratory rate (*tachypnoea*)
- **Respiratory noise** (inspiratory or expiratory)
- **Abdominal** movement when breathing, or a heaves line (Figure 12.4.2)
- Stance with **abducted limbs** and elongated neck (Figure 12.4.3)

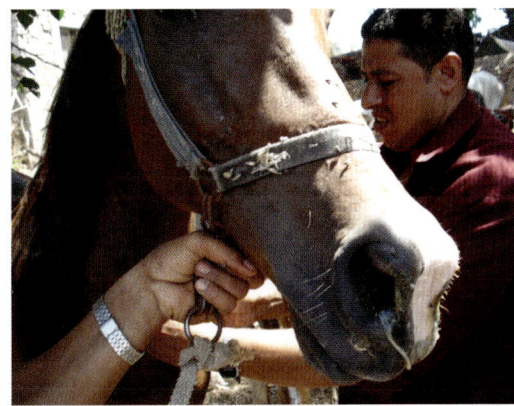

Figure 12.4.1 Nasal discharge.

12 THE RESPIRATORY SYSTEM

- Pyrexia and other systemic signs
- Associated **ocular** pathology
- Poor **mucous membrane** colour
- Poor body **condition score** in chronic cases

Examples of respiratory disease relevant to working equids
- Infectious disease – viral and bacterial
- Allergic conditions
- Sinusitis
- Guttural pouch pathology
- Aspiration pneumonia/foreign bodies
- Parasitism

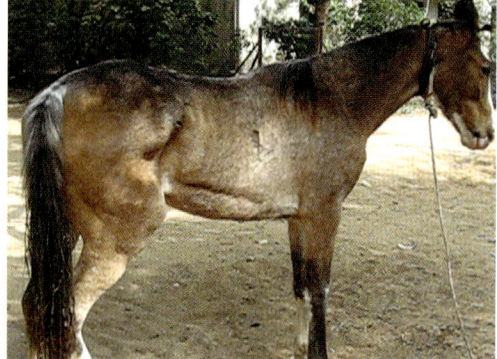

Figure 12.4.2 Heaves line visible on the lower abdomen.

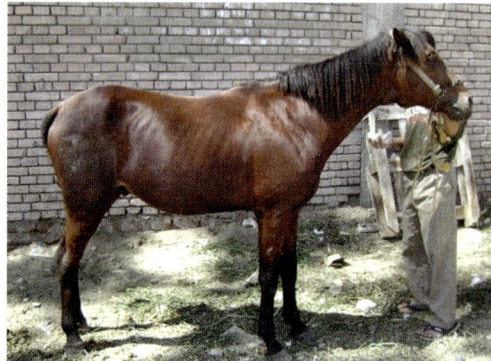

Figure 12.4.3 Extended neck in a horse with strangles.

12.5 Disorders of the upper respiratory tract

Conditions affecting the nasal passage

There are many conditions affecting the nasal cavity in working equids. Due to the difficulty of definitive diagnosis in the field, **without endoscopy,** in most cases it is important to try to manage the symptoms and remove the underlying cause if possible.

Examples of nasal passage problems
- **Trauma** – primary or iatrogenic e.g. via passage of a naso-gastric tube or inappropriate drenching
- **Infection** – sinusitis, ethmoid necrosis
- **Foreign body**

DISORDERS OF THE UPPER RESPIRATORY TRACT 12.5

- Nasal **septum** abnormalities
- **Neoplasia**
- **Polyps**
- **Congenital** malformation

Clinical signs of respiratory disease

- Nasal discharge – in a range of colours and thickness (see Figure 12.5.1)
- Epistaxis (bleeding) (see Section 12.10)
- Foul odour coming from mouth or nostrils
- Alteration/uneven air flow from nostrils
- Respiratory noises

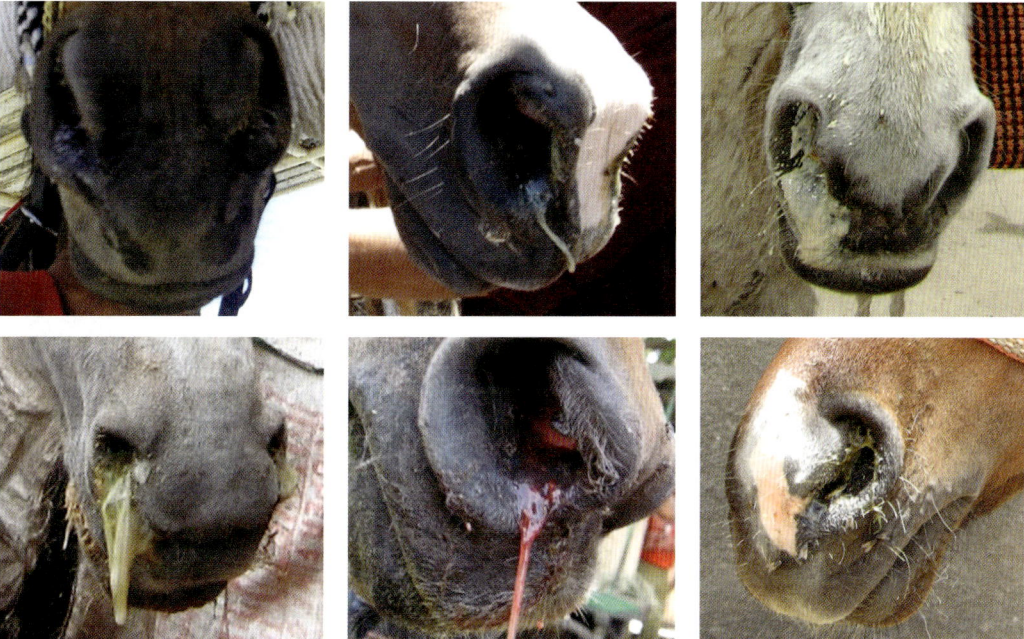

Figure 12.5.1 Nasal discharge comes in a range of colour and thickness dependent on the pathology, from serous, mucous, purulent, food-stained to blood-stained.

Treatment

- **Nasal foreign bodies** Remove with forceps if visible through the nostrils.

- **Tumours or polyps** Surgical removal of tumours or nasal polyps requires good access to the nasal cavity, involving bone flaps or trephination. Without the use of radiography and endoscopy the extent of pathology is difficult to determine which makes planning the surgery problematic. A common complication of nasal surgery is profuse bleeding, so this type of surgery is rarely done in the field.

- **Bacterial infections** A prolonged course of antibiotics is required as well as rest from work.

12 THE RESPIRATORY SYSTEM

Sinusitis

The maxillary and frontal sinuses are connected to the nasal cavity and, as a result, upper respiratory problems can extend into these areas. The last four upper cheek teeth also extend into the maxillary sinus (Figure 12.5.2), so tooth root infections can present as secondary sinusitis.

Clinical signs

- Chronic, persistent unilateral nasal discharge (mucopurulent)
- Discharge – may be bilateral but more commonly only affecting the sinuses on one side
- Difficulty breathing which worsens with exercise
- Concurrent upper respiratory tract infection
- Dull sound on percussion over the sinus area indicating fluid
- Pain on percussion or palpation
- Smell from mouth and difficulty eating (if a tooth root abscess is the primary cause)

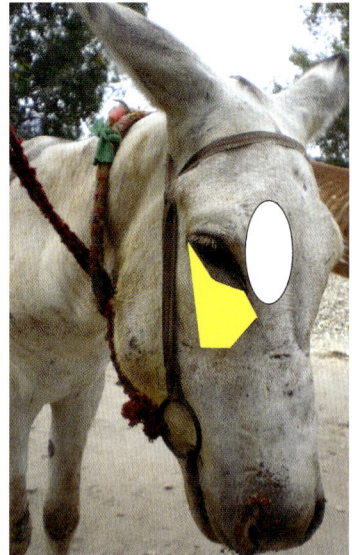

Figure 12.5.2 The white oval is overlying the frontal sinus and the yellow polygon is overlying the maxillary sinus (approximate areas).

Rare events in chronic cases

- Distortion of the facial bones
- Neurological dysfunction from infection extending beyond the frontal sinus

Treatment

> **Sinusitis can be frustrating to treat given the difficulty of access to the sinuses and low penetration by drugs. Infections often recur, so warn the owner.**

- Long-term antibiotics, often weeks of treatment, are required. Penicillin is the most effective medication.
- If a trephine is available, and the attending veterinarian has the relevant experience, fluid can be drained from the sinus. Drainage of the sinus with a catheter through a small trephine hole may be beneficial in the short term. It is essential to study the sinus anatomy in detail to ensure accurate placement of the catheter. Sedate the animal and inject 5 ml of local anaesthetic subcutaneously at the site of trephining. For placement of a lavage catheter a diameter of 7 mm is sufficient. Close the trephine portals with subcutaneous and skin sutures. The catheter can be secured in place if repeated flushing is required. Pain relief post-operatively is essential. Bone flaps are not recommended for field situations.
- A thorough oral examination is essential to determine whether dental problems exist (see Section 10.4).

Please refer to the dentistry chapter (Chapter 10) for more information on the treatment of suspected teeth problems.

Guttural pouch infections

> Guttural pouches are air-filled diverticula of the auditory tube.

The pouches are connected to the pharynx through 'slits' which open when the animal swallows. Guttural pouches are lined with a thin mucous membrane which offers little protection to the vital structures that cross the dorso-caudal aspect of the pouch. These structures are very vulnerable to damage if the guttural pouches are infected, and this can result in life-threatening pathology (refer to guttural pouch mycosis under epistaxis in Section 12.10 of this chapter).

These vital structures include:

- Cranial nerves – VII, IX, X, XI, and XII (see Section 18.2 for more information on the cranial nerves)
- Cranial sympathetic trunk
- Internal carotid artery

> Guttural pouches are prone to pathology as a result of secondary infection extending from the nasopharynx.

Externally, the location of the guttural pouches can be seen in the region of **Viborg's Triangle**. See Figure 12.5.3 in which an abscess within the guttural pouch has ruptured through the outer wall.

The landmarks are as follows:

- **Rostral border** Vertical border of the ramus of the mandible
- **Dorsal border** Tendon of insertion of the sternomandibularis muscle
- **Ventral border** Linguofacial vein

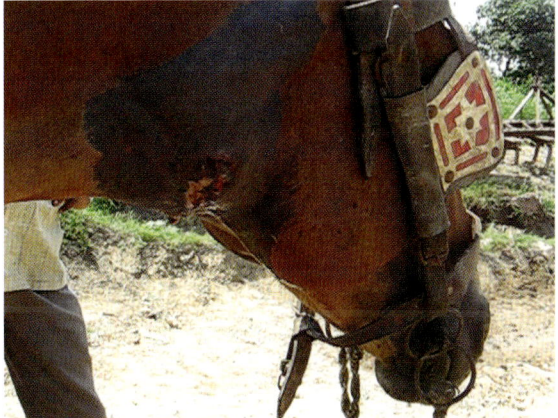

Figure 12.5.3 A ruptured abscess in the region of the guttural pouch.

A study of guttural pouch anatomy in the donkey, including a diagram of Viborg's Triangle, can be found by referring to the paper (Alsafy *et al.* 2008).

Clinical signs

- Nasal discharge (unilateral or bilateral), usually increasing when the animal swallows or lowers its head
- Distension in the region of Viborg's Triangle (not always present)
- Endoscopy can be used to diagnose guttural pouch infection; however, observation of signs can support an initial suspicion without requiring further diagnostic tools.

12 THE RESPIRATORY SYSTEM

Treatment

- *Streptococcus* spp. (including *S. equi*) are the most common bacteria to cause guttural pouch infection. If strangles is suspected, isolate the animal and carry out appropriate disinfection as a priority. Treat with penicillin only if systemically ill.
- Guttural pouch lavage can be performed with warm fluids over several days, placement of the catheter may be difficult without use of an endoscope. *See other equine anatomy texts for landmarks.*
- Severe infections require specialist surgical drainage through Viborg's triangle – care must be taken to avoid vital structures, e.g. vagus and glossopharyngeal nerves and the internal carotid artery.

12.6 Viral respiratory disease

Respiratory viruses affecting equids include equine **influenza, equine herpes viruses** (EHV) and **rhinoviruses**. The symptoms are very similar and it is not always necessary to distinguish between them for clinical purposes. Viral respiratory disease is common in younger animals, although all working equids can be susceptible, especially when kept together in groups as respiratory viruses are very contagious.

> **Respiratory viruses are transmitted by aerosol as well as by direct contact with nasal secretions.**

Remember the potential for secondary bacterial infection to occur.

Suspect a viral cause even in cases with a *small* amount of bilateral watery nasal discharge.

Clinical signs (These vary from mild to severe.)
- Nasal discharge (small amounts, watery, serous)
- Lethargy
- Fever (39–41°C)
- Poor appetite
- Ocular discharge and conjunctivitis
- Abortion and ulceration of the oral mucosa sometimes seen in EHV-1 and EHV-4

Within 24–48 hours
- Development of a harsh, dry cough in the case of influenza
- Harsh lung sounds
- Nasal discharge becomes thicker and more profuse (mucopurulent), with the colour changing to grey or yellow. In severe cases, pneumonia may develop.

Diagnosis

> **Suspect a viral pathogen based on clinical signs and the numbers of animals infected.**

- Virus isolation is not performed in most cases, as disease is self-limiting.
- In severe outbreaks a definitive diagnosis is necessary (e.g. to initiate a control programme). Check with local laboratories for available testing methods and which samples are required. Serological testing is the most common. A paired sample, at least 14 days apart, is usually necessary. ELISA (Enzyme Linked Immunosorbant Assay) field kits may be available in some countries. Nasal swabs are only useful if PCR (Polymerase Chain Reaction to detect viral DNA) or other virus-isolation technology is available and often require special transportation.

Treatment

- The best treatment is to allow resolution of the infection by the animal's own immune system. Rest, warmth and good food will usually ensure recovery in 7–10 days if there is no secondary bacterial infection.

> **Isolate affected animals.**

- As discussed in Section 12.1 ensure that there is no nose-to-nose contact or shared air space with other animals. Do not share tack or equipment with others.
- Symptomatic treatment may help but will not cure the virus.
  Administer:
  - NSAIDs for the pyrexia and airway inflammation
  - Mucolytics, e.g. eucalyptus oil, steam
  - Antibiotics if secondary infection is present, e.g. trimethoprim-sulphonamide

Prognosis

Good for a full recovery but acquired immunity is short-lived so recurrence is possible. In the case of equine influenza virus, the virus itself is constantly changing so immunity to one strain does not prevent infection from another. The severity of disease is reduced in vaccinated animals.

Prevention

Several killed/modified live virus vaccines are available. Vaccinations tend to protect against certain virus strains (equine influenza 1, 2 and EHV-1, 4 are most common) so diagnosis and knowledge of the actual virus responsible for outbreaks is required.

> **Immunity against equine respiratory viruses is short acting so any vaccinated animals will require a regular booster for vaccine efficacy.**

Regular vaccination is not always achievable in the working equid situation. However, if there is a good relationship with owners who understand, a reliable vaccine supply and an effective cold chain, regular vaccination may be applicable.

12 THE RESPIRATORY SYSTEM

It is better to manage animals so that the **immune system is strong enough** to fight viruses easily. **Immediate isolation** of affected animals helps to prevent spread of disease, as does **reduced movement** and mixing of animals. Ensure segregation of populations during markets or fairs. Ensure adequate rest allowing animals to recover and prevent a prolonged and severe clinical course of the disease.

It has been stated that working equids are more at risk of contracting influenza, increased severity of clinical signs, delayed recovery and secondary bacterial infections due to the additional stresses on their body and weakened immune system (Abd El-rahim and Hussein 2004). Figure 12.6.1 shows a horse continuing to work while infected with influenza.

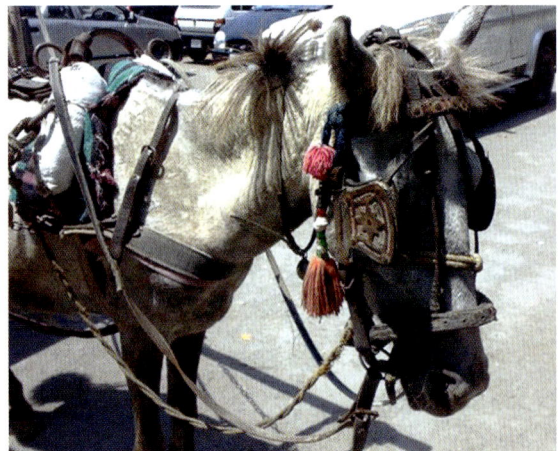

Figure 12.6.1 Equine Influenza was diagnosed in this working horse in India.

Equine influenza

- **Spread is rapid, morbidity is high.** Uncomplicated infections tend to improve in 4–7days, but a dry cough can persist for several weeks.
- Complications include secondary bacterial infection, cardiomyopathy, and persistent fatigue.

Equine herpesvirus 4

- EHV-4 is a major cause of acute respiratory infection worldwide. Most equids are affected in the first 2 years of life.
- Infections tend to be less severe and have a lower morbidity than equine influenza.
- Latent infection with EHV-4 and EHV-1 is possible, and reactivation can occur in times of stress or corticosteroid administration.

Equine herpesvirus 1

- EHV-1 can cause respiratory disease (as EHV–4). However, it can also cause abortion. Abortion occurs 2 weeks to 3 months after infection, usually between the 7th and 11th month of pregnancy. Future reproduction is unimpaired.
- In some cases a neurological condition is associated with EHV-1 caused by a viral myeloencephalitis. Ataxia with a history of a viral respiratory disease is a common presenting sign. Infrequently EHV-1 can lead to severe neurological signs such as recumbency and eventual death. Loss of bladder function is also a feature and this may persist in the long term.

Notifiable viral respiratory disease
African Horse Sickness
Cause

This disease is caused by an *orbivirus* of which there are nine serotypes.

The virus is spread by **arthropod vectors**, usually a *Culicoides* midge. It is important to realise that African Horse Sickness (AHS) is not contagious between individual equids but will spread in a population from the biting vectors, hence the importance of vector control.

Distribution

AHS is a **seasonal** disease endemic to Sub-Saharan Africa and parts of southern Africa. There have been historical reports of outbreaks in North Africa, Spain, India and Pakistan; however, there is no ongoing clinical disease in these areas. Consult the OIE WAHID interface for up-to-date information on outbreaks. **Horses have the highest susceptibility**, followed by mules, with donkeys usually showing mild or subclinical signs (Figure 12.6.2). Wild equine species (i.e. zebras) are resistant but may be involved in transmission because they attract *Culicoides* midges. AHS mainly occurs in warm, rainy climates/seasons when *Culicoides* midges are plentiful.

Clinical signs

All breeds of equids are affected (**mortality rate 70–90%**). There are a number of different manifestations of this disease depending on which form is present.

- **Acute (horses) – Lung form**
  - Has a short incubation period of usually 3–5 days
  - High fever
  - Laboured breathing/head down, coughing and profuse frothy nasal discharge
  - Mortality rate is high. Up to 95% of horses die within a week, often from 'drowning' in their own pulmonary secretions.

- **Cardiac or subacute (donkeys)**
  - Has an incubation period of 7–14 days
  - Fever followed by swelling over the head, eyelids, lips, cheeks and under the jaw
  - Conjunctival swelling which can be significant, even blocking vision
  - Mortality rate is about 60%, death results from heart failure.

- **Mixed**
  - A combination of the above two types
  - The incubation period is between 5–7 days and is indicated initially by mild respiratory signs which progress to the typical swellings of the cardiac form.

- **Mild or Horse Sickness Fever form**
  - Seen in zebras and African donkeys, this form is suspected with mucosal congestion and conjunctivitis (Figure 12.6.2). Animals usually recover.

Diagnosis

A presumptive diagnosis can be made based on clinical signs or post-mortem lesions in areas with a known vector presence. Laboratory virus isolation from infected tissues is available in some countries. Collect samples for serological tests 3 weeks apart to show a rising antibody titre associated with current infection. Serological ELISAs are available in South Africa. Animals often die before mounting an effective immune response.

Treatment

Currently no specific treatment exists; supportive therapy is the only course. Horses with the extreme acute form may have to be euthanased on welfare grounds.

Prevention

AHS is notifiable in many countries; report suspected cases to the relevant governing bodies. AHS is an OIE-listed disease. It is the responsibility of government veterinary services to report outbreaks to the OIE.

> It is the responsibility of the veterinarian to know and recognise diseases that are notifiable and to ensure all suspected cases are reported at the earliest opportunity.

Live attenuated vaccines are available commercially in South Africa; these vaccines are polyvalent but may not contain the serotype causing a local outbreak. It is essential that the vaccines are administered annually. Viable vaccines at point of use are dependent on an effective cold chain. Ethiopia has a government subsidised vaccination program following a series of recent outbreaks (Aklilu *et al.* 2012).

Ensure vector control is maintained in endemic areas by covering animals with rugs or providing fly-proof shelter (especially in the evenings when midges feed) and using repellents such as citronella or other locally available substances that are not harmful to equids.

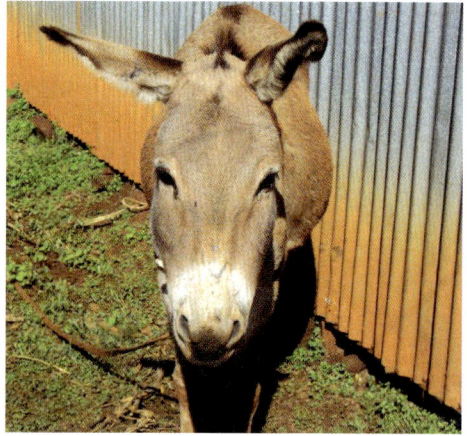

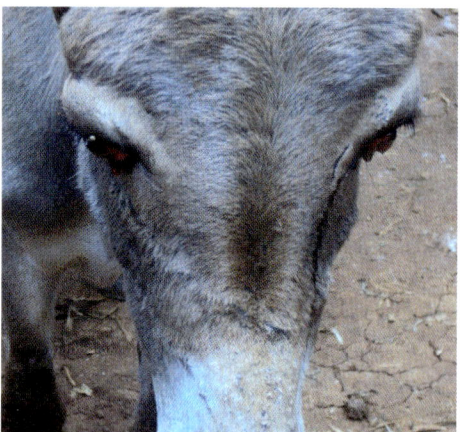

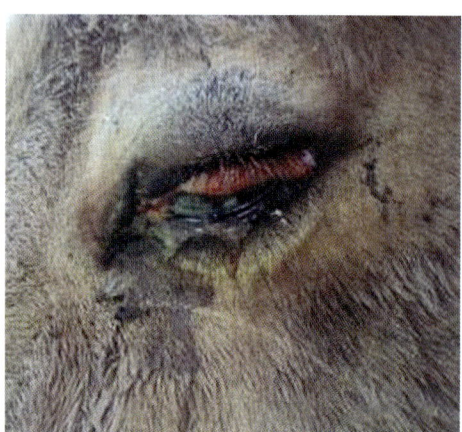

Figure 12.6.2 Clinical signs of African Horse Sickness in donkeys in Kenya.

If **vaccines** and a **virus testing** facility are available this is the preferred protocol:

- Eliminate affected animals, by isolation initially and then euthanasia on confirmation of infection.
- Vaccinate non-infected equids with a polyvalent vaccine.
- When the virus has been serotyped re-vaccinate these animals with the homologous vaccine.
- Make housing for equids insect-proof.

For a good review of AHS, including prevention and control, please refer to (Mellor and Hamblin 2004).

Myths

The following will **not** achieve adequate vector control:

- **Smoking drums around stables** This has no effect on midge activity and will have a detrimental effect on the respiratory function of equids and humans in the vicinity.
- **Repellents alone** Using repellents is not enough to reduce midge contact; covering or stabling animals during high risks periods is strongly advised.
- **Garlic supplements** There is no scientific evidence to support this.
- **Moving equids to higher altitude** Midges can tolerate altitude, providing other environmental conditions are adequate.

Bacterial respiratory disease

Bacterial involvement is common in respiratory disease. It can be a **primary** infection, for example in strangles, or **secondary** infection to any viral or systemic disease causing the immune system to be compromised, including transport or overcrowding. Many different bacteria may be involved; it is not always necessary to know the primary pathogen.

> Suspect bacterial involvement with any bilateral muco-purulent nasal discharge.

Bacterial pneumonia

This is one of the most common causes of disease affecting the lower respiratory tract of equids.

Causes

- Primary bacterial disease, e.g. strangles
- Secondary to upper respiratory tract problems (viral or otherwise)
- Secondary to generalised systemic disease

- Inhalation of foreign material (aspiration pneumonia), e.g. food as a result of dysphagia, inappropriate drenching techniques (oral administration of medication, such as paraffin), home remedies (see Section 4.1)
- Predisposing factors are those that suppress the pulmonary immunity: strenuous exercise, long-distance transport, and general anaesthesia.

Clinical signs

- Bilateral mucopurulent nasal discharge (Figure 12.7.1)
- Coughing
- Increased respiratory rate and effort
- Reduced exercise tolerance and lethargy
- Pyrexia and poor appetite
- Harsh lung sounds including pleural friction (see earlier in this chapter)
- Dullness of lower lung areas on percussion
- Pale or cyanotic mucous membranes in severe cases

Treatment

- The first line treatment of choice is Trimethoprim-sulphonamide; followed by procaine penicillin and gentamicin if unsuccessful. Use metronidazole if an anaerobic infection is suspected.

Ensure that owners are willing to comply with the necessary prolonged duration of treatment.

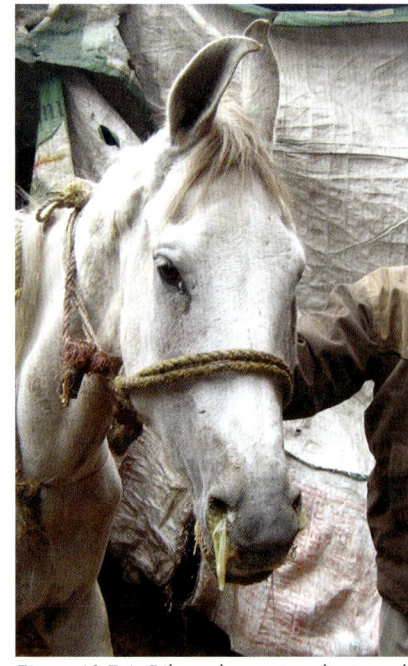

Figure 12.7.1 Bilateral mucopurulent nasal discharge.

- Duration would be for at least 7 days, cessation of treatment is dependent on resolution of clinical signs which may take weeks or even months.
- Rest in a clean, dust-free environment. Ongoing stress whilst an animal has bacterial pneumonia is one of the most frequent causes of severe complications, e.g. pleuropneumonia. Offer a high quality palatable diet.
- Reduce pyrexia with the administration of NSAIDs. It is important NSAIDs are discontinued before stopping the antibiotic therapy – these medications can give a false impression of improvement.
- Corticosteroids may be administered in severe cases including aspiration pneumonia. One or two high doses will reduce inflammation. Always use in conjunction with antibiotics as steroids depress the immune response to infection.

Prognosis

The prognosis depends on the inciting cause: guarded for bacterial pneumonia, poor for inhalation pneumonia, contingent upon the amount of permanent lung damage.

BACTERIAL RESPIRATORY DISEASE 12.7

Prevention

- Allow animals with viral respiratory disease to **rest and recover** properly before starting work again.
- Provide **early treatment** of secondary bacterial infections.
- Avoid or take extreme care when drenching equids (see Section 4.1 and the case study at the end of this chapter) or treating for oesphageal choke (Section 11.4).

Pleuropneumonia

Pleuropneumonia is defined as infection of the **lungs** and **pleural space**. This may occur as an extension of severe pneumonia, if an animal is not rested to allow recovery, or from the rupture of an abscess into the pleural space. Rarely, a penetrating injury to the thorax is the inciting cause of a pleuropneumonia. This condition is often accompanied by a **pleural effusion**; fluid builds up in the pleural space which is normally under negative pressure.

Clinical signs

- Respiratory distress – due to the pleural effusion
- Acutely painful (pleurodynia) – grunting on inhalation, abducted elbows, guarded behaviour when coughing, or flinching on percussion of the chest
- Nasal discharge – mucopurulent, bilateral. May be foul smelling if anaerobes are involved
- Inappetance
- No lungs sounds heard ventrally on auscultation
- Percussion – dull resonance ventrally

Treatment

- Long-term antibiotic therapy, as for pneumonia. Do not stop antibiotics before a complete recovery is made.
- Include metronidazole in the treatment protocol if anaerobic involvement is suspected. Anaerobic organisms are usually isolated in pleuropneumonia cases of greater than 5 days' duration, and have been associated with poor prognosis for survival (Raidal 1995).
- Rest and supportive care
- IV fluids
- NSAIDs
- Good nursing care and nutrition are important in the recovery phase (see Chapters 21 and 22).

Prognosis

Guarded; especially if there is foul odour to the breath

> **Remember:** Differential diagnoses for pleural effusion in equids include pleuropneumonia, neoplastic effusion, congestive heart failure, thoracic haemorrhage, chylothorax and pulmonary hydatidosis.

12 THE RESPIRATORY SYSTEM

Strangles

Strangles is very contagious and can **spread rapidly through a group of equids**.

Younger animals are more susceptible, and the disease is often thought to be introduced to a native population by the arrival of new animals which are incubating the disease or have become carriers. *Streptococcus equi* sub-species *equi (S. equi)*, is currently the most frequently diagnosed infectious disease of horses worldwide, responsible for high morbidity and occasional mortality of infected animals. Refer to the ACVIM Consensus statement for a detailed description of the treatment, control and prevention of strangles (Sweeney *et al.* 2005).

Transmission

- **Inhalation** of infected droplets in the air
- Direct contact with **nasal discharge** or pus from discharging abscesses
- **Fomites** on the ground, in feed, water troughs, equipment and on human hands/clothes

The incubation period is between 3 and 10 days.

Clinical signs (acute in onset)

- The first clinical sign is often pyrexia. If an animal has been exposed to a strangles case, monitoring the temperature will give an indication of whether an infection is developing.
- Swelling in the submandibular area, lymphadenopathy (Figure 12.7.2) which may progress to abscessation of lymph nodes (Figure 12.7.3). Thick pus is often produced when these rupture.
- Poor appetite and dysphagia (can result in aspiration pneumonia)
- Coughing
- Thick purulent nasal discharge (Figure 12.7.1)
- Increased respiratory rate and effort

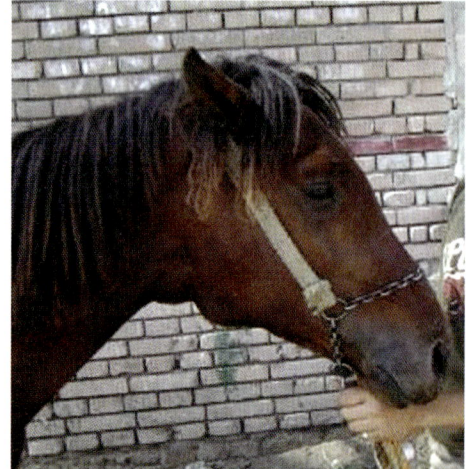

Figure 12.7.2 Swelling of the submandibular area.

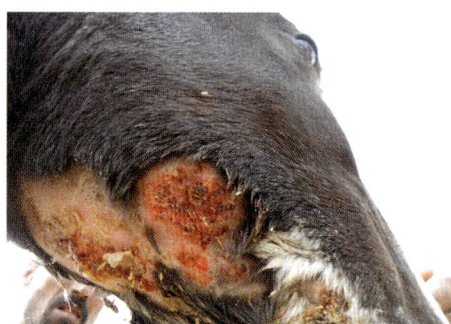

Figure 12.7.3 Resolving submandibular abscesses which ruptured following infection with strangles.

Signs that an animal may have had strangles in the past

- Chronic weight loss as a result of **'bastard strangles'**. This happens when abscesses have metastasised to other internal organs.
- Fibrosis in the area of the submandibular lymph nodes
- Chronic infections can develop in the **guttural pouches** and can be present without any clinical signs; animals which have this condition act as carriers, shedding bacteria and infecting others.

Diagnosis

- Look for clinical signs, especially if lymph node abscessation is present and there is history of exposure.
- Bacterial culture of swabs from the nasal discharge or discharging abscesses will show the presence of *S. equi*.
- A nasopharyngeal swab can be taken, although it is unlikely to yield a positive culture if collected within 24 hours of exposure. An elongated swab is gently inserted into the nasopharynx (via the nostril). This stimulates the animal to swallow which releases any bacteria that are trapped in the guttural pouches.

Treatment

> **Complete rest is very important.**

- The majority of strangles cases require no treatment with antibiotics; those that are treated are more susceptible to recurrence of infection. Limit the use of medication to those cases where severe systemic signs of infection are present (cost versus benefit): administer procaine penicillin at high doses (20,000 IU/kg) daily.

> **Antibiotic therapy is indicated in cases with dyspnea, dysphagia, prolonged high fever, and severe lethargy or anorexia.**

- Antibiotics, if used for treatment, *must* be **continued for 5–7 days after clinical signs have resolved**, as failure to do this may result in recurrence or development of bastard strangles.
- NSAIDs
- Apply warm compress on abscesses to encourage maturation and rupture.
- Abscesses may require drainage if they inhibit breathing or mastication. Determine the area where the skin is thinnest. Inject local anaesthetic sub-cutaneously. Clip and disinfect the region. Use a sterile scalpel blade to create an incision of up to 5 cm. Flush with warm saline. Continue flushing daily for 7 days. Remember the **purulent discharge is highly contagious**, so ensure all equipment and all personnel are disinfected before treating the next case. Drainage of the guttural pouches via Viborg's triangle is not recommended for field surgery.
- Give soft, palatable food.

Management of cases

Preventing dissemination of strangles is difficult as the disease is so contagious. Recovered animals **shed large numbers of bacteria for 2–3 weeks** after resolution of clinical signs, and intermittently for years if a carrier state is generated.

- Isolate affected animals for at least 4 weeks. Do not allow nose-to-nose contact with other equids.
- If bacterial culture is available then three negative nasopharyngeal swabs (at 4–7 day intervals) can be used as a determining factor for ending quarantine. (Intermittent shedding of bacteria occurs so this protocol increases the likelihood of detection.)

- Ensure that buckets, feeding sacks, grooming equipment, etc. are not shared with other equids.
- **Strangles can be transmitted on human hands and clothes;** it is important to observe strict hygiene measures, especially as a veterinarian or community animal health worker is likely to be handling many animals after treating an infected case.
- Disinfect all instruments and equipment (including ropes and head collars). Drain and disinfect water troughs thoroughly as the bacteria can persist for a long time in this environment.
- If draining abscesses, do not let pus collect on the ground where it will be a source of infection for other animals.
- Inform owners of the epidemiology of disease and how to avoid spread.
- Monitor the temperature of in-contact equids and isolate if the temperature increases and/ or if there is sub-mandibular swelling.

Prognosis

Good for most cases, but poor if 'bastard strangles' develops

Complications of strangles infection

Bastard strangles

This is the systemic spread, or metastasis, of *S. equi* to any other part of the body other than the lymph nodes of the head. A large range of organs can be infected, e.g. lungs, liver, spleen or kidneys. Suspect bastard strangles in any animal that is currently suffering or has recently had strangles and is showing obvious and unusual clinical signs. Signs tend to be non-specific and depend on which organ has been infected. General signs include depression, anorexia, intermittent pyrexia, chronic weight loss and intermittent colic in a case where an abdominal organ is affected.

Treatment

This comprises a prolonged parenteral course of penicillin. If a very long period of treatment is required, potentiated trimethoprim-sulphonamide antibiotics given orally are an alternative. NSAIDs are useful to control temperature, colic signs and encourage the horse to eat if inappetant.

Purpura haemorrhagica

This is an immune-mediated condition, which is more frequently seen in older horses. It is a vasculitis resulting in obvious subcutaneous oedema, mainly of the head and limbs and petechial haemorrhages of the mucosa. In severe cases the vasculitis can affect other/all internal organs and the peripheral oedema can be so severe it can result in fatal circulatory collapse.

Treatment

Corticosteroids are given to suppress the immune response and reduce the inflammation in the blood vessels. Treatment with penicillin, although there are concerns that this may release more of the antigen that initiates the immune-mediated vasculitis, is still currently recommended (Pusterla *et al* 2003). Supportive care – such as leg wraps, light walking exercise, and palatable food.

Rhodococcus equi infection of foals ('rattles')

See Section 18.1.

BACTERIAL RESPIRATORY DISEASE 12.7

Notifiable bacterial respiratory infections
Glanders (*Burkholderia mallei* infection)

Distribution

Asia, Africa and the Middle East

> Glanders is very contagious to other equids and it can be transmitted to humans (zoonotic).

The lungs, nasal cavity, lymphatic system and skin (a variant condition called farcy) are affected with nodular abscesses. A sticky, purulent discharge is released once these nodules ulcerate. Skin exudates and respiratory secretions contain large numbers of bacteria that are easily spread by direct contact, fomites and environmental contamination.

Clinical signs

- **Acute form** predominantly affects mules and donkeys in which death may occur within a few days.
- **Chronic form** predominantly affects horses; the infection may persist for years.

Clinical signs of acute glanders are largely respiratory and more often seen in mules and donkeys.

- High fever
- Depression, anorexia, coughing
- Swollen nostrils with septum ulceration and a thick, mucopurulent haemorrhagic discharge (Figure 12.7.4)
- Multiple nodules and ulcers developing in the respiratory tract
- Swollen/ulcerated mucous membranes; the ulcers healing to form a typical star-shaped scar in those that survive
- Swelling and abscessation followed by rupture of regional lymph nodes
- Lung consolidation and pneumonia – round, firm greyish nodules developing in the lung tissue
- Severe respiratory distress
- Death within a few days

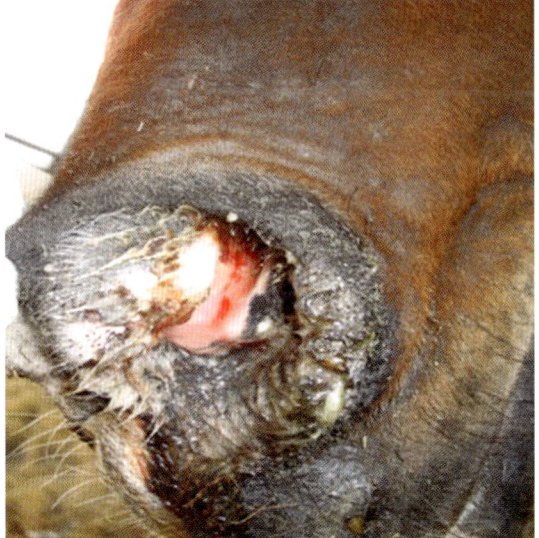

Figure 12.7.4 Nasal discharge and abscess seen in a horse with glanders.

Farcy – cutaneous form of glanders

- Develops secondary to skin injury or respiratory disease
- Superficial and/or deep subcutaneous abscesses form with or without ulceration and inflammation of the local lymph nodes.

12 THE RESPIRATORY SYSTEM

- Skin nodules can reach up to 2.5 cm diameter and may rupture releasing an infectious purulent discharge.
- Nodules develop on the head, neck, thorax, ventral abdomen and legs (Figure 12.7.5).
- Lymphatic vessels can become infected and abscessated, resulting in visible 'farcy pipes', or develop nodules – 'farcy buds' (Figure 12.7.6).
- Causes weight loss

> Horses with chronic or latent infections often maintain the disease within the population as they act as reservoirs of infection.

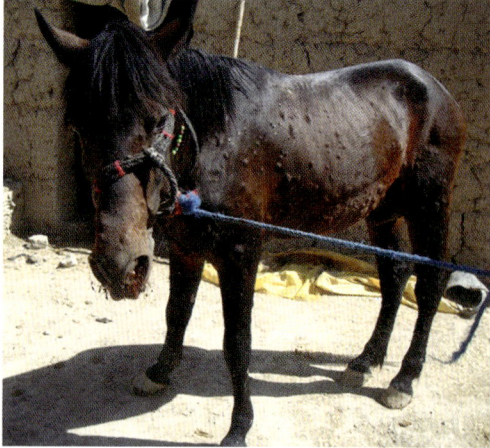

Figure 12.7.5 A case of glanders in a horse in Afghanistan, showing the respiratory and skin (farcy) forms of the disease – note the respiratory discharge and the skin nodules.

Diagnosis

- Microscopic examination of a gram-stained smear of fresh material may reveal gram negative rods. The bacteria are non-sporolating and non-encapsulated.
- Bacterial culture is not recommended unless sent to a specialist laboratory due to the zoonotic nature of the pathogen. Be aware of the capabilities of the local diagnostic laboratory.

Be aware that handling infected discharge containing the bacteria can result in infection; wear gloves at all times. It is important that laboratory technicians are made aware of the risks when handling infectious material.

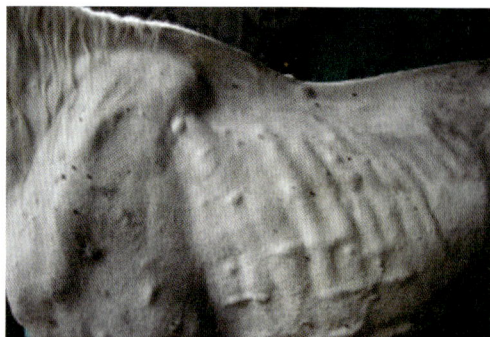

Figure 12.7.6 Farcy cords – note the linear swelling along the lymphatic vessels.

Mallein test

- The mallein test relies on a delayed hypersensitivity reaction in animals infected with glanders (Figure 12.7.7). This test is particularly useful in subclinical cases and is used as a prescriptive test for international trade. The protein is commercially available.
- Intrapalpebral injection of mallein protein derived from *Burkholderia mallei* bacteria
- Equids infected with glanders, and/or farcy, develop marked eyelid swelling, fever and occasionally a purulent ocular

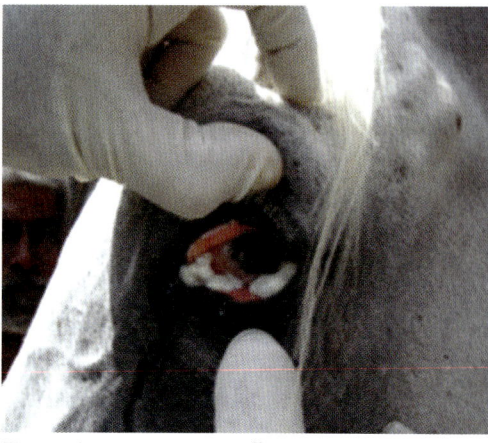

Figure 12.7.7 A positive mallein test.

discharge within 24 to 48 hours (Figure 12.7.7). Eyelid swelling is minimal in uninfected animals.

- This is a rapid field test for equids. Prompt confirmation of positive cases is crucial in infectious disease control to allow early intervention to limit spread.
- The mallein test is almost 100% specific although only 76% sensitive (see Section 4.2 for definitions of specific and sensitive) so there are likely to be more false negative results compared to false positives. It is essential to implement the isolation protocols for a suspected glanders case, pending further testing, even if negative in the mallein test.
- If the mallein protein is inadequately purified there are likely to be a greater number of false positives (de Carvalho Filho et al. 2012).

> **In countries or areas where there are no diagnostic facilities, then a diagnosis has to be made based on clinical signs alone.**

Treatment

Euthanasia is recommended as recovered animals remain a source of infection for others, including humans.

> **OIE lists glanders as a notifiable disease. Follow the prescribed protocols in countries with legislation regarding the control of glanders. It is essential that veterinarians are aware of local control policies.**

In India, for example, there is a Glanders and Farcy Act 1899 which outlines that the nearest Government Veterinary Officer (GVO) should be notified of suspected cases. A GVO will carry out the sampling (nasal swab and serum) for diagnosis and send this to the National Research Centre on Equines (NRCE). If glanders is confirmed by laboratory diagnosis the affected equid is euthanased by government authorities and compensation is paid to the owner. The animal is disposed of hygienically, the area is disinfected and animals which have been in contact are assessed.

In countries with no legislation or diagnostic facilities it is essential to implement the following protocol:

- Do not touch the animal with bare hands.
- Use face masks/disposable gloves and isolate the animal immediately.
- Dig a 2-metre-deep hole in the ground, euthanase the animal and bury it; OIE recommends burning the animal prior to burial.
- Clean and disinfect the area where the animal was living and working. Iodine is an effective disinfectant.
- Destroy harness and grooming equipment.
- Monitor any in-contact animals and humans. Early signs of glanders infection would include a high fever and the eruption of nodules.
- Isolate suspect cases.
- Attempt to notify the government and OIE of the case and inform local human health authorities.

12.8 Allergic respiratory disease

Allergic respiratory disease is extremely common in working equids due to continuous exposure to dusty and polluted environments (Figures 12.8.1, 12.1.1 and 12.2.1).

Those at most risk are:

- animals working in urban or peri-urban environments
- brick kiln animals constantly exposed to brick dust
- animals fed dry, dusty food from a sack/nosebag, or stabled next to feed stores (see Figure 12.8.1)
- animals kept on dust, hay or sawdust
- animals suffering smoke irritation from being housed close to cooking fires.

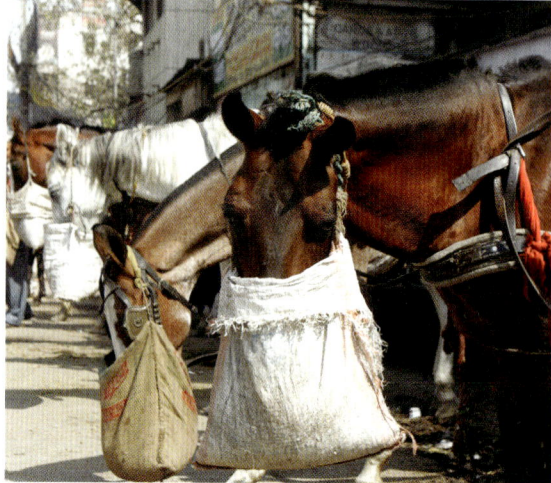

Figure 12.8.1 Feeding practice has an impact on the respiratory system.

Clinical signs

These vary in severity and may be intermittent. The clinical signs are similar to those seen for infectious disease as the immune system reacts to allergens in a similar way to pathogens.

- A **chronic cough**. May be more prevalent at certain times of the day when allergen exposure is greatest, e.g. at night, if caused by smoke irritation
- Increased respiratory **rate and effort**, even at rest
- A **'heaves'** line which is common in animals with Recurrent Airway Obstruction (RAO) also known as Chronic Obstructive Pulmonary Disease (COPD)
- Flaring of the nostrils
- Lethargy and reduced exercise tolerance
- Harsh lung sounds on auscultation – can be exacerbated with a re-breathing bag
- Possible nasal or ocular discharge
- Usually normal appetite and no fever (unless secondary bacterial infection is present)
- Can present as acute attacks; respiratory distress with an increased respiratory rate and effort occurs suddenly. These can be severe and result in the animal's obvious distress.

Management

> **Remove the equid from the irritating environment to alleviate the signs of allergic airway disease.**

As this is not always practical, long-term management of the disease may include some of the following:

- Change feeding practices to prevent inhalation of dust (e.g. feed pelleted rations rather than a mix). Soak mouldy hay to reduce inhalation of fungal spores (balance this against soaking for too long and losing considerable nutritive value of the feed).
- Improve bedding/resting environment if dust or smoke is excessive.
- Bronchodilators (e.g. clenbuterol, theophylline, aminophylline) may be useful in early stages if available; however, these medications are not as effective in severe cases and tolerance to clenbuterol develops over time and doses need to be increased (Read *et al.* 2012).
- NSAIDs or antihistamines may help.
- Corticosteroids (e.g. dexamethasone) are effective and cheap; they improve the condition, but long-term use may have side effects (see Section 5.4).
- Administer antibiotics if bacterial infection is present.

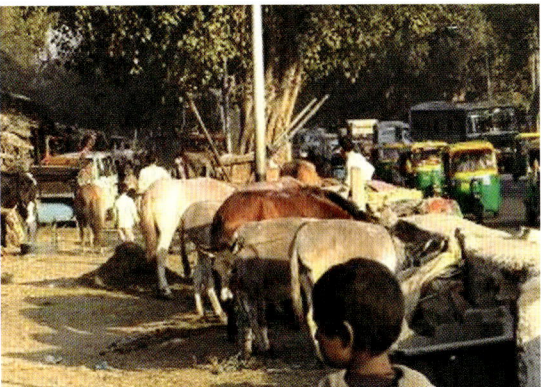

Figure 12.8.2 Animals living in polluted, dusty environments are at risk of allergic respiratory disease.

Prognosis

Without elimination of the allergen the prognosis is poor.

12.9 Parasitic respiratory disease

Lungworm – *Dictyocaulus arnfieldi*

Lungworm causes inflammation of the bronchioles in adult equids. **Donkeys rarely suffer clinical signs of lungworm**, but they act as a **reservoir** of infection for horses.

Clinical signs in horses

- Persistent chronic cough
- Slightly increased respiratory rate and lung sounds
- Non-progressive condition

Diagnosis

Patency (larvae in the faeces) is rare in horses. A bronchial lavage can be used to collect larvae for a definitive diagnosis.

Ivermectin or moxidectin are effective. Lungworm can recur if pasture contamination is present. Treat donkeys that are resident with horses, even if they do not show signs, as they can be a source of continued infection.

Parascaris equorum

Migrating larvae cause lung damage in foals.

Clinical signs

- Frequent coughing
- Greyish-white nasal discharge
- Possible fever
- Other signs of worm infestation, e.g. weight loss, poor coat, colic

Treatment

Broad-spectrum anthelmintics are effective.

Prognosis

The prognosis is good, but the disease can recur.

Epistaxis

12.10

Epistaxis is **bleeding from the nose** (Figure 12.10.1). In many cases the source of the blood can be difficult to determine, especially without specialist equipment such as endoscopy. Blood can discharge from one or both nostrils and can vary from a slow drip or intermittent to profuse and life threatening.

> It is important to note the characteristics of the discharge as this can indicate potential causes.

- **Overt blood** This is often seen with trauma of the nasal passages or lesions within the guttural pouches.
- **Sero-sanguinous fluid** This is often associated with chronic inflammatory changes and occurs alongside haemorrhage, e.g. abscess, sinusitis, neoplasia.

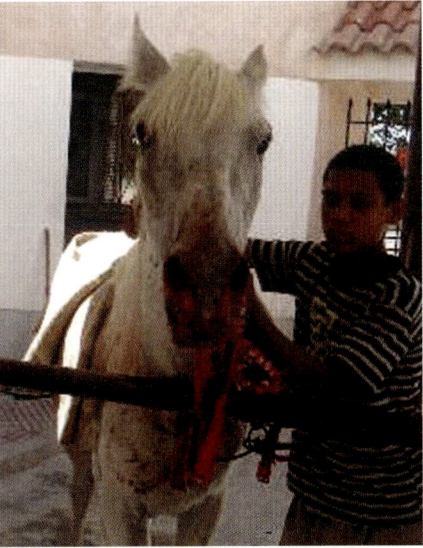

Figure 12.10.1 Blood coming from both nostrils.

It is important to note any other associated clinical signs, e.g. fever, depression, inappetance.

Bleeding from the nasal cavity

- **Trauma** Apply pressure where possible to stop haemorrhage and promote clotting. Careful repair of a damaged nostril is important to prevent deformities which may limit inspiration, particularly if the muscles responsible for dilation are injured.
- **Infection resulting in erosion (sinusitis, fungal infections, granulomas)** Fungal infections are relatively rare but are more common in tropical/subtropical climates. Clinical signs include mucopurulent malodorous discharge, dyspnoea, abnormal respiratory noise and swelling of the head and lymph nodes of the throat. Culture of nasal discharge can help with diagnosis. In advanced cases, cream-coloured plaque accumulations can progress into ulcerated granulomatous lesions.
- **Neoplasia**
- **Foreign body** In addition to epistaxis, this can present as head shyness and obvious pain. A foul-smelling discharge is common. Sedating the animal will allow gentle removal of the foreign body whilst causing the least possible damage to the delicate nasal mucosa and nasal septum.

Bleeding from guttural pouch

Guttural pouch mycosis

This is a **fungal infection** of the guttural pouches. The guttural pouches contain numerous vital structures (including the internal carotid artery and the vagus/glossopharyngeal nerves) which run across the caudal border of the guttural pouch, only protected by a thin mucous membrane. Fungal infections over these areas are often erosive and can damage these structures.

Clinical signs

- Intermittent spontaneous epistaxis of fresh arterial blood that can be extremely profuse and life threatening. A smaller episode of haemorrhage may precede the fatal bleed by 24 hours to 3 weeks. It is important to warn owners of the potential severity of even a small amount of blood at the nostrils.
- **Dysphagia** Difficulty swallowing as a result of damage to the vagus and glossopharyngeal nerves. Equids will cough and may have food/water coming out of their nostrils.
- **Horner's syndrome** Characterised by variable degrees of ptosis, prolapse of the third eyelid, enopthalmas or unilateral sweating. Horner's can be the result of damage to the cranial cervical sympathetic ganglion within the guttural pouch.
- **Facial paralysis** The facial nerve has been damaged.

Treatment

- In field conditions, treatment is impossible.

> **If a live threatening epistaxis occurs, or severe dysphagia, advise euthanasia on welfare grounds.**

If an equid shows signs of profuse epistaxis of fresh arterial blood there is potential for a fatal bleed. If fungal mycosis is present this event will usually occur within 3 weeks of the initial bleed.

Empyema

This is the term for purulent material within the guttural pouches. It is the result of an infection that either ascends up the auditory tube or through lymphatic spread. The most common cause of this is strangles (see Section 12.7).

Clinical signs

- Intermittent nasal discharge worsening when the head is lowered
- Lymph node swelling and pain in the parotid region
- A sequalae of strangles is the formation of chondroids within the guttural pouch. These solid balls of inspissated pus are difficult to remove. This can lead to a carrier state with intermittent shedding of bacteria, often without demonstrable signs of illness.

Treatment

- In the field environment treatment is limited, especially for chondroids. These can be removed endoscopically or surgically, neither of which is possible in the field context.
- Encourage lowering of head for drainage, e.g. feed from the floor.
- Treat primary infection.

CASE STUDY – ASPIRATION PNEUMONIA **12.11**

Bleeding from the lungs

Exercise-induced pulmonary haemorrhage

Epistaxis is associated with **strenuous exercise**. The pathogenesis is not fully understood.

Clinical signs

Epistaxis during or following strenuous exercise. Poor performance or exercise intolerance, seen as a reduced ability to work. Excessive swallowing and or coughing after exercise as blood is being swallowed.

Treatment

Rest if possible, ideally in a dust-free environment. Advise the owner to do less strenuous/fast work to prevent recurrence. Antibiotics can be helpful if a secondary bacterial infection develops.

Pulmonary abscess. See treatment for pneumonia (see Section 12.7).

Neoplasia in the thoracic cavity is rare in equids and is most commonly due to metastases from distant sites. Weight loss is common and older equids are more often affected. In working equids, diagnosis is usually based on clinical signs alone. The condition is untreatable and, if an animal's welfare is compromised, advise euthanasia.

Severe bacterial pneumonia or fungal pneumonia (see Section 12.7).

Case study – Aspiration pneumonia **12.11**

Area Pakistan

Attending veterinarian Dr Mohammad Iqbal Khan

Summary
This is a description of a case of pneumonia. It is assumed that this is a secondary infection as the result of aspiration when the donkey was drenched with local medication. The animal was treated with broad-spectrum antibiotics and anti-inflammatory medication.

History
A 13-year-old entire male donkey was presented to a static clinic with a 2-day history of coughing and nasal discharge (Figure 12.11.1). The donkey had been drenched (oral administration of fluids) with eggs, mustard oil and locally-available herbal masala.

12 THE RESPIRATORY SYSTEM

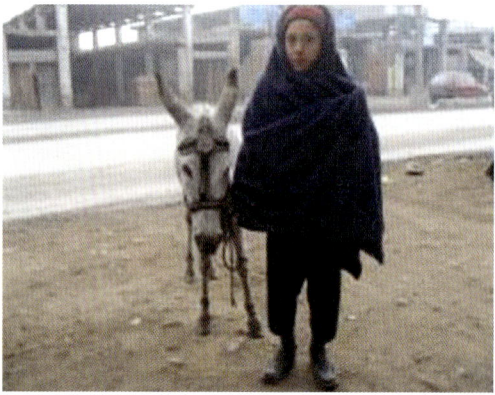
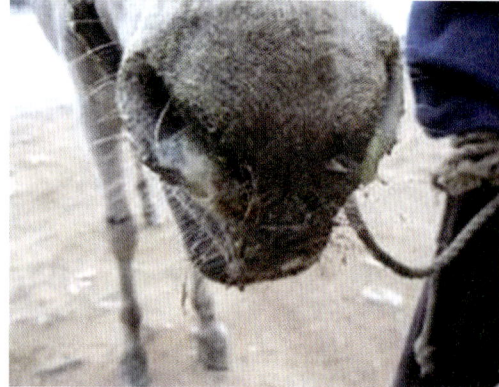

Figure 12.11.1 Presentation of the donkey at the clinic; note the bilateral purulent nasal discharge.

Clinical findings

- Bilateral, muco-purulent nasal discharge (Figure 12.11.1)
- Elevated body temperature (39°C)
- Coughing
- Poor appetite
- Pale mucous membranes
- Watery discharge from the eyes
- Increased respiratory rate and effort
- Harsh lungs sounds on auscultation (Figure 12.11.2)
- Depressed and lethargic/less tolerant of exercise

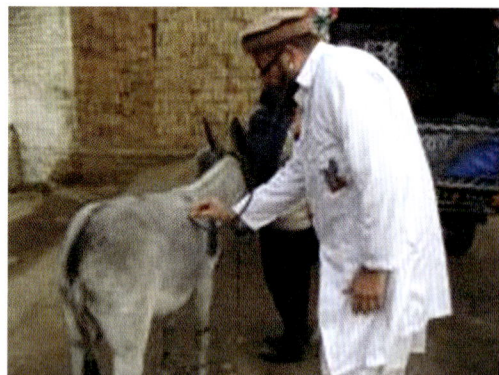

Figure 12.11.2 Dr Iqbal examining the patient.

Diagnosis
Aspiration pneumonia on the basis of history and clinical signs

Treatment (Figure 12.11.3)

- Procaine penicillin twice daily for 7 days
- Dexamethasone injection, single dose on the first day
- Ammonium chloride daily to act as an expectorant and mucolytic
- Pheniramine maleate antihistamine, administered 3 x daily as an oral tablet

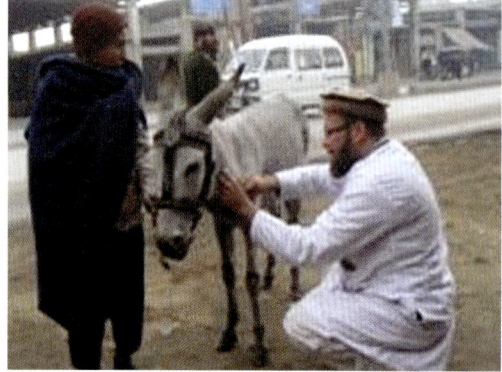

Figure 12.11.3 Dr Iqbal administers treatment to the patient.

CASE STUDY – ASPIRATION PNEUMONIA 12.11

Outcome
Although the donkey returned to work in the community he suffered from a low exercise tolerance and reduced work capacity. The owner sold the donkey at a fair.

Discussion
Owners may attempt to treat an animal using an oral drench. This may be carried out to provide the animal with energy, e.g. with milk and eggs. In this case the technique was used to administer a local treatment, herbal masala. These local medicines are also used for human patients and may be provided by a local healer.

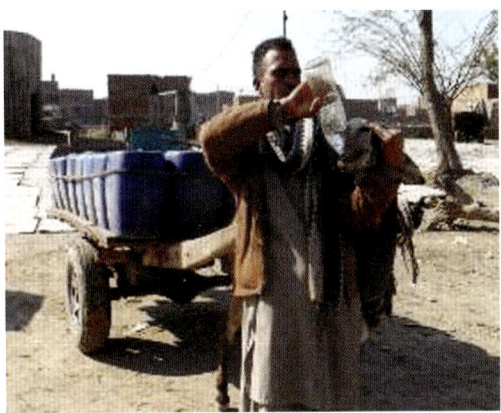

Figure 12.11.4 A donkey receiving water by drenching. It would be preferable to allow the donkey to drink from a bucket.

If drenching is carried out while the tongue is being held and the head lifted, the equid will be unable to swallow effectively and some of the liquid will pass into the trachea. Thick and oil-based fluids are not suitable for drenching.

Advise owners to feed equids a sufficiently energy-dense fodder to cope with strenuous work instead of drenching with bizarre cocktails to provide extra energy. Provide water in a bucket and allow the equid sufficient time to drink, 4–5 times a day, rather than drenching with water (Figure 12.11.4). If working equids are unwell they should be taken to a veterinarian or trained community animal health worker (CAHW) if available. If drenching is carried out, advise on an appropriate technique so that the equid does not struggle and is able to swallow the liquid (see Section 4.1).

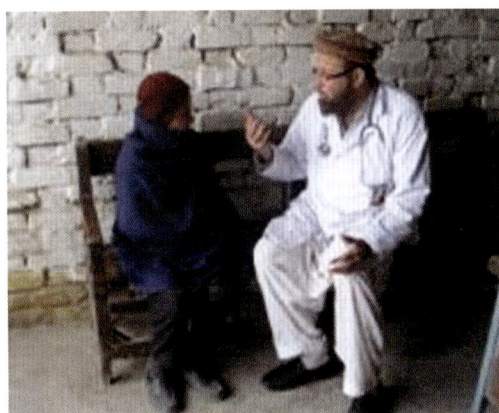

Figure 12.11.5 Dr Iqbal follows up the treatment by providing advice to the owner on the appropriate methods of drenching animals, if necessary.

Changing an owner's attitude and management is important in resolving such problems and preventing re-occurrence. Remember, establishing a good relationship with the owner is crucial (Figure 12.11.5).

12.12 References

Abd El-Rahim, I.H., Hussein, M. (2004) An epizootic of equine influenza in Upper Egypt. *Revue Scientifique et Technique Office International Epizooties*. 23 (3) 921–930.

Aklilu, N., Batten, C., Gelaye, E., Jenberie, S., Ayelet, G., Wilson, A., Belay, A., Asfaw, Y., Oura, C., Maan, S., Bachanek-Bankowska, K., Mertens, P.P. (2012) African Horse Sickness Outbreaks Caused by Multiple Virus Types in Ethiopia. *Transbound Emerg Dis*. Article first published online: 22 Oct 2012.

Alsafy, M.A., El-Kammar, M.H., El-Gendy, S.A. (2008) Topographical Anatomy, Computed Tomography, and Surgical Approach of the Guttural Pouches of the Donkey. *J. Equine Vet. Sci*. (4) 215–222.

de Carvalho Filho, M.B., Ramos, R.M., Fonseca, A.A. Jr, de Lima Orzil, L., Sales, M.L., de Assis Santana, V.L., de Souza, M.M., Dos Reis Machado, E., Filho, P.R., Leite, R.C., Dos Reis JK. (2012) Development and validation of a method for purification of mallein for the diagnosis of glanders in equines. *BMC Vet. Res.* 2; 8 (154).

Mellor, P.S., Hamblin, C. (2004) African Horse Sickness. *Vet. Res*. 35, 445–466.

Pusterla, N., Watson, J.L., Affolter, V.K., Magdesian, K.G., Wilson, W.D., Carlson GP. (2003) Purpura haemorrhagica in 53 horses. *Vet. Rec*. 153 (4) 118–121.

Raidal, S, L. (1995) Equine Pleuropneumonia. *Brit. Vet. J*. 151 (3) 233–262.

Read, J.R., Boston, R.C., Abraham, G., Bauquier, S.H., Soma, L.R., Nolen-Walston, R.D. (2012) Effect of prolonged administration of clenbuterol on airway reactivity and sweating in horses with inflammatory airway disease. *Am. J. Vet. Res*. 73 (1) 140–145.

Sweeney, C.R., Timoney, J.F., Newton, J.R., Hines, M.T. (2005) *Streptococcus equi* infections in horses: guidelines for treatment, control, and prevention of strangles. *J. Vet. Intern. Med*. 19 (1) 123-134.

Sweeney, C.R., Holcombe, S.J., Barningham, S.C., Beech, J. (1991) Aerobic and anaerobic bacterial isolates from horses with pneumonia or pleuropneumonia and antimicrobial susceptibility patterns of the aerobes. *J. Am. Vet. Med. Assoc*. 198 (5) 839–842.

Theimann, A.K., Bell, N.J. (2001) The Peculiarities of Donkey Respiratory Disease. In: *Equine Respiratory Diseases*, Lekeux P (Ed). Publisher: International Veterinary Information Services, Ithaca, New York.

World Animal Health Information Database (WAHID) Interface
http://www.oie.int/wahis_2/public/wahid.php/Wahidhome/Home

REFERENCES 12.12

Further Reading

African Horse Sickness Trust booklet, 2012/13. Available online at *www.africanhorsesickness.co.za*

Dvorak, G.D., Spickler, A.R. (2008) Glanders. *J. Am. Vet. Med. Assoc.* 233 (4) 570-577.

OIE (World Organisation for Animal Health). Animal Disease Information Summaries, 'Glanders', Available online at *http://www.oie.int/en/for-the-media/animal-diseases/animal-disease-information-summaries*.

OIE African Horse Sickness Information (Aetiology, Epidemiology, Diagnosis, Prevention and Control). Available online at *http://www.oie.int/fileadmin/Home/eng/Animal_Health_in_the_World/docs/pdf/AFRICAN_HORSE_SICKNESS_FINAL_01.pdf*

Timoney, J.F. (1993) Strangles. *Vet. Clin. N. Am. Equine.* 9 (2) 365–374.

The urinary and reproductive systems

13

Examination and diagnostic aids for the urinary tract	**13.1**
Diseases of the urinary tract	**13.2**
Examination of the reproductive system	**13.3**
Common reproductive disorders experienced In working equids	**13.4**
Case study – Urinary tract infection	**13.5**
References	**13.6**

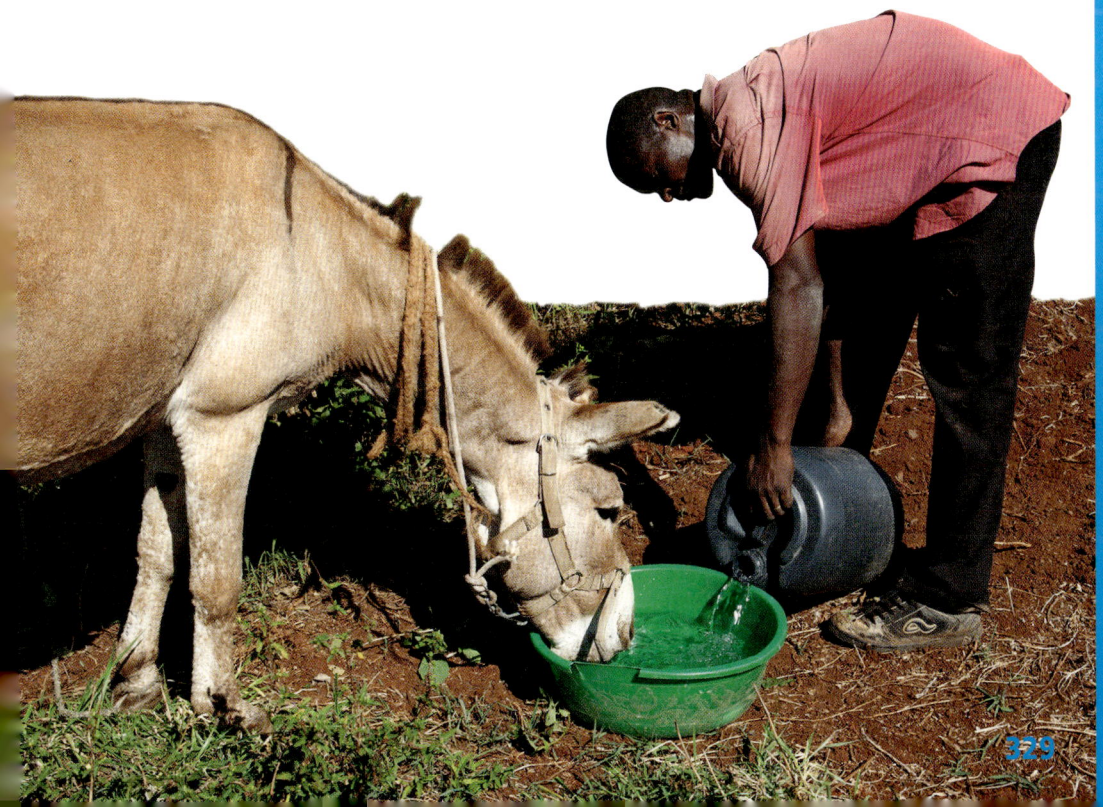

13.1 Examination and diagnostic aids for the urinary tract

History

> A complete history should be taken in order to gain a broader understanding of the problems underlying a presenting sign.

Owners will readily report changes in the colour or frequency of urination as this is an obvious clinical sign, but may not initially describe general changes such as lethargy and weight loss. Urinary tract disorders are more likely to present with non-specific signs. Signs such as haematuria, polydypsia and polyuria can be caused by non-urinary diseases, so it is important to include general history questions.

Typical urinary system related questions

- When did the equid last drink?
- How often is water offered in a day? How much/often does the equid drink in a day?
- Does the equid appear to strain or attempt to urinate frequently?
- How often does the equid urinate?
- What is the approximate volume of urine? (Urine output can be difficult to estimate but owners may have noticed recent changes.)
- What is the colour of the urine? Is the urine a light yellow colour or darker? (This gives an indication of the hydration status.) Is it red/pink/brown? (Pigmenturia is discussed later in this chapter.) Are there any blood clots?
- If there is blood in the urine does it appear at the beginning, throughout or at the end of the urine stream?
- Has the equid lost weight or had colic symptoms recently?
- Is there a history of respiratory disease or abortion?

Physical examination

A full clinical examination should be conducted.

The following conditions may be observed in an equid with a urinary tract disorder:

- Oral examination: signs such as ulcers, halitosis and plaque can be observed as the result of uraemia in chronic renal failure.
- Hair loss on the inner hind legs or ulceration of the perineum due to urine scalding may indicate incontinence.
- Observe urination if possible.
- Check for ventral oedema which may develop in cases of protein-losing nephropathy.

Following a general examination, a more detailed urinary tract examination can be conducted. Refer to this paper (Wilson 2007) for a thorough review of examination of the urinary tract; some of the techniques are advanced and not applicable to field situations.

EXAMINATION AND DIAGNOSTIC AIDS FOR THE URINARY TRACT 13.1

Urinary tract physical examination

Male equids Examine the prepuce and penis for swellings or oedema, wounds, discharge and evidence of tumours or habronemiasis (red skin ulcerations).

Sedation with ACP or xylazine will result in penile protraction and ease of examination (see Section 7.1 *Sedatives and anaesthesia* for appropriate dosages).

Remember the very small reported risk of prolonged or permanent penile prolapse with the use of ACP in stallions (Driessen *et al.* 2011).

Female equids Examine the vulva and perineum, both visually and manually, to check for urine scalding, vaginal urine pooling, wounds or abnormal discharge.

In extreme circumstances, a rectal examination can be carried out to assess the bladder for wall thickness, evidence of calculi (stones) or presence of abnormal masses. The pelvis can be palpated for evidence of trauma such as fractures. The caudal pole of the left kidney can be palpated to assess for size and pain. Remember the risks involved in rectal examination (see Chapter 11 *The gastrointestinal system*).

Catheterisation of the bladder

> This is useful for the collection of sterile urine samples for bacteriology. If the equid is having difficulty urinating (stranguria) then this technique can be used to ascertain the patency of the lower urinary tract.

Procedure

1. Ensure the safety of the animal and operator; use stocks if available.
2. Sedate geldings/stallions with an alpha-2 agonist (see Section 7.1) to encourage relaxation of the penis so the catheter can be inserted.

   a. **Male equids**
      - a.i. Holding the penis in one hand, wash the glans with *dilute* povidone-iodine.
      - a.ii. Wearing sterile gloves take the male urinary catheter out of the packaging (sterile) and lubricate.
      - a.iii. Gently insert the catheter into the urethra and push upwards. After approximately 60 cm the catheter should be in the bladder. Urine does not always flow freely; apply suction to the end of the catheter using a syringe or inject 60 ml of air from a sterile syringe.

   b. **Female equids** It may be necessary to sedate mares, mule mares and jennies prior to catheterisation.
      - b.i. Wash the perineum with dilute antiseptic.
      - b.ii. Insert a lubricated gloved hand into the vagina and locate the urethral opening on the floor of the vagina, about 10 cm inside.
      - b.iii. Using the index finger, guide the tip of a sterile, lubricated catheter into the urethra and advance gradually.

13 THE URINARY AND REPRODUCTIVE SYSTEMS

Haematology and serum biochemistry

> In field situations it is often not possible to carry out blood analysis as the machinery is expensive and difficult to maintain. Reporting results and providing further treatment may also be problematic in some contexts when individual animals cannot be traced.

Outlines of the expected changes

Haematology Increased white blood cells (WBC)/globulins indicates infection. A Packed Cell Volume (PCV) count or haematocrit is useful if presented with a patient with blood-stained urine.

Serum biochemistry Azotaemia is defined as an increase in urea nitrogen and creatinine. The kidney has a huge reserve capacity and around 75% of function is lost by the time azotaemia is diagnosed in horses (Wilson 2007).

1. *Pre-renal azotaemia* Primary cause is 'before the kidneys'; often secondary to dehydration or hypovolemia.
2. *Renal azotaemia* Primary cause is 'within the kidney' such as tubular damage.
3. *Post-renal azotaemia* Primary cause is 'after the kidney' within the urinary tract itself, including obstruction (urolithiasis) or a ruptured bladder (most commonly occurs in foals).

Acute renal failure (ARF) – hypocalcaemia and hyperphosphataemia are reported.

Chronic renal failure (CRF) – hypercalcaemia and hypophosphataemia are reported.

Hyperkalaemia – with ARF, obstruction and uroperitoneum (foals) is reported.

Hyponatraemia and hypochloraemia are also reported with renal disease (Wilson 2007).

Metabolic acidosis is common with renal failure.

Urinalysis

What to consider when collecting a urine sample

Samples can be collected as a 'free catch' (collect urine when the animal is naturally urinating) or via catheterisation (which will require sedation). Catheterisation is necessary for the collection of a sterile sample for culture and also in cases of suspected obstruction.

> Consider the cost versus benefit to the welfare of the animal when deciding whether a catheterisation procedure is necessary.

Place the urine straight into a sterile container. Note the colour of the urine; normal equine urine is often cloudy due to the presence of calcium carbonate crystals.

The urine sample can be used to assess kidney function and to identify abnormalities of the urine including cells, pigments or bacteria.

1. Normal urine pH 7.5–8.5 (adults) (Robinson and Sprayberry 2009), and 5.5–8.0 (foals). The pH decreases with starvation and can be acidic after exercise (Wood *et al.* 1990).
2. A urinary dipstick is a semi-quantitative method for the detection of several conditions such

EXAMINATION AND DIAGNOSTIC AIDS FOR THE URINARY TRACT 13.1

as proteinuria, haematuria and pigmenturia. The dipsticks should be stored correctly and used within the recommended lifespan. Normal urine should not contain protein, glucose or bilirubin; however, false positives are common with protein due to the alkaline urine of equids.

Positive pigment results can indicate overt blood (whole erythrocytes), haemoglobin (heme pigments secondary to haemolysis) or myoglobin (muscle breakdown). In order to distinguish haemoglobinuria and haematuria, centrifuge the sample or leave it to stand for at least an hour. In the case of haematuria the red blood cells will settle to leave a clear urine sample; in haemoglobinuria the protein will remain suspended in the sample which will continue to appear as a red/pink colour.

There is no test to differentiate haemoglobinuria from myoglobinuria. Assess the case to reach a diagnosis. If there is a history of trauma or myopathy it is more likely to be myoglobinuria. If the equid has pale mucous membranes and a low and/or decreasing PCV (packed cell volume/haematocrit) then the discolouration of the urine is more likely to be the result of haemoglobinuria.

3. **Cytology** This will require a centrifuge for urine sedimentation.

   Pyuria = > 5 WBC per high power field

   Haematuria = > 5 RBC per high power field

4. **Sediment examination** Normal findings are calcium carbonate (common in adults), calcium oxalate in foals, mucus strands and transitional epithelial cells (Wilson 2007).

5. **Specific gravity** (SG), measured with a refractometer, is used to estimate the solute concentration of the urine. The SG may be inaccurate in the presence of high levels of glucose or albumin.

> *Hyposthenuria* (urine less concentrated than plasma) < 1.008
> *Isothenuria* (similar concentration to plasma) 1.008–1.012
> *Hypersthenuria* (urine more concentrated than plasma) > 1.012
> Normal adult horses should have hypersthenuric urine.

If azotaemic and hypersthenuric = Pre-renal. Water is retained by the kidneys in cases of dehydration and hypovolaemia.

If azotaemic and hyposthenuric = Renal. The kidneys are unable to concentrate urine.

6. **Bacterial culture** The urine sample must be collected aseptically. (See *Catheterisation of the bladder,* page 331.)

13.2 Diseases of the urinary tract

This section describes some urinary tract disorders encountered in equids, and is not exhaustive. Refer to other equine veterinary texts for a comprehensive review.

Cystitis and pyelonephritis

Bacterial urinary tract infections (UTI), also described as cystitis with bladder involvement, are generally caused by contamination from skin or gut flora. UTIs are **un**common in equids and are usually associated with disorders that disrupt urinary flow, such as bladder paralysis or urolithiasis.

Pyelonephritis is the term used for bacterial infection which has spread from the lower urinary tract to affect the kidneys. Septicaemic foals may develop a septic nephritis. The likely organisms involved in UTI/cystitis and pyelonephritis include *E.coli*, *Enterococcus* spp., and *Streptococcus* spp. (Clark *et al.* 2008). The samples for the Clark study were collected from cases at a Canadian University clinic; the bacterial spectrum may differ in other contexts although faecal contaminants are likely to dominate. Note that contaminating bacteria may be cultured from free-catch samples collected from healthy horses (MacLeay and Kohn 1998). Therefore a definitive diagnosis should be based on the culture of > 10,000 colony forming units/ml (Reed, Bayly and Selon 2004) and ideally samples for culture should be collected by sterile catheterisation.

Certain problems will predispose an equid to a UTI

- Late gestation/post-partum infection
- Repeated urinary catheterisation (iatrogenic)
- Secondary to a bladder/urinary tract problem such as an obstruction
- Neurological (atonic bladder) – signs of dysuria/stranguria also present

Clinical signs

- Frequent attempts to urinate. (Stranguria is not frequently observed in cases of pyelonephritis.)
- Blood-stained urine (haematuria)
- Pyuria (neutrophils in the urine) observed in severe pyelonephritis
- Dribbling or urine scalding of the perineum and back legs in the mare or front legs in the stallion
- Equids with pyelonephritis will be pyrexic, depressed and anorexic.

Diagnosis

- Clinical signs are not always indicative; collect urine for analysis. A small bladder with a thickened wall may be palpated during a rectal examination, and other signs may be present such as neurological signs or anuria.

Treatment

- Treat the primary underlying disease.

DISEASES OF THE URINARY TRACT 13.2

- Consider hydration status – in dehydrated animals the 'flushing effect' that clears bacteria will be diminished.
- In mild cases resolution of the primary cause may be sufficient to treat the UTI/cystitis.

> - Antibiotic treatment should be based on urine culture and sensitivity. Trimethoprim-sulphonamide treatment is the first-line treatment, followed by penicillin if this is unsuccessful. These antibiotics are preferable as the active ingredient is excreted in the kidney and concentrated in the urine.

Haematuria, haemoglobinuria and myoglobinuria

Haematuria is the presence of whole red blood cells in the urine.

Haemoglobinuria is found when a pathological process has induced a breakdown of red blood cells and the haemoglobin is excreted in the urine.

Myoglobinuria is found when a pathological process has caused a breakdown of muscle and the myoglobin is excreted in the urine.

The latter two conditions can be classified as pigmenturia and may be difficult to distinguish.

Causes of haematuria

- **Haemorrhage** in the urinary tract: If the blood originates in the kidneys, ureters or bladder, haematuria is voided throughout the urine stream. Haematuria is observed at the start of urination if haemorrhage occurs from the bladder neck or distal urethra; and at the end of urination if there is haemorrhage from the proximal urethra. Urethral tears in stallions and geldings will present with haematuria; these defects may resolve without treatment.
- Bleeding after exercise frequently occurs with cystoliths (see later in this chapter).
- A severe case of pyelonephritis or cystitis will result in haemorrhage from the urinary tract (see the case study Section 13.5).
- Urinary tract neoplasia is a rare cause of haematuria.
- Habronema infestation of the urethral process will cause haematuria. Ivermectin and corticosteroids can be used for treatment (see Section 16.1 *Internal parasites*).
- Verminous nephritis is a very rare condition and is the result of parasitic invasion of the kidneys by *Halicephalobus gingivalis* or *Strongylus vulgaris*. This may present as haematuria due to damage induced by the parasites. Cases of *H. gingivalis* are often associated with neurological disease (Pathology in Practice 2012).

Causes of haemoglobinuria

This is often associated with a haemolytic anaemia; the haemoglobin is filtered by the kidneys, which excrete it in the urine.

- **Babesiosis** Haemolysis of infected RBCs results in haemoglobinuria. Diagnosis is by microscopic examination of a blood film. Treat with imizol (see Section 17.7 *Blood-borne parasites*).
- **Leptospirosis** In equids this infection more commonly presents as abortion or uveitis.

Both babesiosis and leptospirosis are zoonotic infections.

13 THE URINARY AND REPRODUCTIVE SYSTEMS

Causes of myoglobinuria

If there is access to blood biochemistry this condition can be distinguished from other forms of pigmenturia if the muscle enzymes are very elevated above the reference range.

Equine Rhabdomyolysis/Tying up Equid presents with stiffness and pain. (See Section 14.9 *Common conditions affecting the muscles of working equids*.)

Trauma to large muscle mass or prolonged recumbency may also cause myoglobinuria; include relevant questions when taking the history.

Bladder prolapse

Causes

Bladder prolapse is almost exclusive to mares after foaling as the result of vaginal trauma. The bladder is visible on the outside of the vulva, the surface will be shiny and smooth. There is a risk of bladder rupture and in these cases the intestines may prolapse through the bladder wall. Mares will show signs of colic and straining.

> **How to differentiate a prolapsed bladder and a prolapsed uterus?**
>
> The bladder will be smaller and with a smoother surface, usually the urethral opening can also be observed.
>
> Both of these conditions can occur after foaling (see Section 13.4 *Common reproductive disorders experienced in working equids*).

Treatment

- Sedate and administer a caudal epidural (see Section 7.2 *Local anaesthetics*).
- Clean the mucosal surface of the bladder with saline solution.
- Drain the bladder of urine by aspiration.
- Place a Foley catheter to avoid contamination of the peritoneal cavity with urine.
- Replace bladder in normal position, starting at the urethra. Apply gentle pressure.
- Administer post-operative antibiotics for 5–7 days.
- In cases of bladder rupture it will be necessary to euthanase the mare.
- Straining and re-prolapse is a common complication.

Acute renal failure

Acute renal failure is the sudden and rapid decrease in the glomerular filtration rate with a resulting azotaemia.

Causes

- Exposure to nephrotoxic substances – most commonly aminoglycoside antibiotics (gentamicin) and NSAIDs, especially if the animal has been suffering from dehydration or diarrhoea before treatment commences (see Chapter 5 *Medicines*) Other examples include exposure to heavy metals (lead poisoning) or to local toxic plants, and haemoglobinuria/myoglobinuria secondary to blood parasites or rhabdomyolysis.

- **Haemodynamic** – shock with secondary renal failure such as with acute diarrhoea, bacterial septicaemia from pneumonia or endotoxaemia from other causes
- **Obstructive** – urolithiasis, neoplasia, trauma, infection, dehydration

Clinical signs
- Signs of a primary disease which may compromise the cardio-vascular system; acute diarrhoea, colic, endotoxaemia
- Depression, anorexia
- A history of exposure to toxic substances
- Signs of a urinary tract disorder or severe dehydration (straining, etc.)
- Reluctance to move (myopathy, colic, laminitis, etc.)
- Haematuria may be present in cases of NSAID toxicity.

Diagnosis
- USG 1.008–1.012 (isothenuric = same concentration as plasma)
- Definitive diagnosis can be difficult in the field without access to blood biochemistry. A presumptive diagnosis can be made with the support of clinical signs and evidence from the history.

Treatment
- Remove or treat the primary cause (if known).
- Correct fluid deficits and maintain urine production. Administer IV or nasogastric tube fluid therapy 20–50 ml/kg/day until the animal begins to eat and drink voluntarily.
- Ensure that there is no overload to the kidneys, especially if anuria is suspected due to urine blockage/ bladder rupture.

Prognosis
- Toxicities have the best response to treatment.
- The prognosis is usually determined by assessing the response to fluid therapy. If a positive response is seen within the first 24–48 hours the prognosis is good otherwise the prognosis is guarded.

Urethral concretion

Smegma accumulates in the penis sheath. This generally does not create problems but, if it becomes hard and causes inflammation or difficulty urinating, then it requires removal. Please note that urethral concretion is a problem within the *sheath only*; however, the clinical signs can appear similar to urolithiasis (obstruction of the *urethra*).

Clinical signs
- Adult males show frequent attempts to urinate and may extend penis while urinating.
- Urine staining/scalding is present.
- Sedate with xylazine, (remember the risks of parphimosis; see Section 7.1 *Sedatives and anaesthesia*) and examine the penis. Accumulations of foul-smelling concreted smegma can be palpated around the sheath and urethral orifice.
- Differential diagnoses include habronemiasis, injury (stallions) or neoplasia.

13 THE URINARY AND REPRODUCTIVE SYSTEMS

Treatment

While the animal remains sedated, gently clean the penis, prepuce diverticulum and around the urethral orifice to remove the smegma, including any concreted 'peas' within the small spaces around the urethral orifice. A diluted antiseptic such as chlorhexadine or povidone-iodine may be used. Regular cleaning may be required to prevent recurrence.

Urolithiasis

Calculi can be found in the kidneys, bladder, ureter and urethra, usually resulting in urinary tract obstruction. Urolithiasis is more common in males, attributed to the anatomical differences between the male and female urethra. Urethral obstruction is described; calculi in other locations are problematic to diagnose and treat in the field.

Causes

- **Urinary component** High crystalluria, high mucoprotein concentrate, high mineral content $CaCO_3$
- **Diet** Feed/water high in mineral content may predispose equids to this condition.
- **Other** Urinary stasis, decreased water intake, bacterial infections

Clinical signs

- Usually occurs in male equids; the uroliths pass through the female tract more easily.
- Restlessness, colic – more severe in cases of complete obstruction
- Straining – small amounts and increased frequency of urination
- Unusual stance
- Discoloured urine or blood in urine, haemorrhage from urethral orifice
- Hindlimb lameness
- Anuria present in cases of complete obstruction
- In severe cases of obstruction the bladder or urethra can rupture. Signs of colic and discomfort will subside and the equid will become depressed and anorexic.

Diagnosis

- Clinical signs
- Obstruction to passage of urinary catheter (see below)

> **When passing a urinary catheter in cases of urethral blockage, the urethra may rupture if excessive force is applied.**

Treatment

Calculi may be expressed manually if palpated in the distal portion of the urethra. The equid must be sedated, and an epidural may be required, as this is a painful procedure. To expel the calculi use gentle manipulation and flush sterile saline through the urinary catheter. In mares it may be possible to remove stones from the bladder manually. Small calculi may be flushed out in a normal urination stream if the equid is sufficiently hydrated. Bladder lavage is indicated in cases of sabulous urolithiasis (accumulations of crystalloid material in the bladder).

Euthanasia should be considered if the obstruction cannot be removed.

Complications of urethral obstruction include urethral scar formation, a persistent cystitis or a ruptured bladder (this can be diagnosed by rectal examination or a peritoneal tap).

Examination of the reproductive system   13.3

History

Determine if the animal has been used for breeding and, if so, obtain a full breeding history. Enquire about any previous problems with the reproductive system and treatments.

External examination

Male equids Sedation will assist safe and thorough examination of the penis and scrotum/testes. (Remember the risks of paraphimosis, see Section 7.1 *Sedatives and anaesthesia*). Note any swelling, injury, tumours, cutaneous habronemiasis or vesicles/pustules (Colahan *et al.* 1999). Palpate the testes for swelling or pain.

Female equids Examine the external genitalia. The vulval mucous membranes will vary depending on the stage of oestrus: pink-red and moist during oestrus, pale and dry throughout anoestrus. Red mucous membranes indicate inflammation.

Internal examination

Male equids Rectal examination (with adequate restraint) can reveal abnormalities in the region of the inguinal rings and the accessory glands (prostate and vesicular). Describe these abnormalities.

Female equids Rectal examination can reveal abnormalities within the ovaries, uterus and cervix; stages of the oestrus cycle or pregnancy can be ascertained with this examination. Vaginal examination may reveal injury/trauma or tumours/cysts (Colahan *et al.* 1999).

Sampling

Pre-breeding tests can be used in the diagnosis of bacterial diseases such as *Streptococcus*, *E. coli*, *Pseudomonas*, *Klebsiella* and *Taylorella equigenitalis* (Contagious Equine Metritis). The Horserace Betting Levy Board produces a voluntary code of practice setting out recommendations to prevent and control specific diseases in horses (HBLB Code of Practice). *Taylorella asinigenitalis* has been isolated from male donkeys and horse mares and stallions. It has not been demonstrated that this bacterium causes disease and it is only possible to differentiate *T. asinigenitalis* from *T. equinigenitalis* by PCR (OIE Terrestrial Manual 2012).

13.4 Common reproductive disorders experienced in working equids

Although equine reproduction is unlikely to form a large part of practice with working equids, there are some communities who breed equids and also individual owners with animals who may need assistance. The following conditions have been highlighted as those most common in the field of working equine medicine:

Pregnancy diagnosis

Pregnancy diagnosis is not an emergency intervention, although in certain circumstances it will be necessary to determine whether a mare or jenny is in foal, for example prior to the use of certain teratogenic or abortive medications. The detection of pregnancy by rectal palpation is accurate at 60 days' gestation when the size of the embryonic vesicle is 10–13 cm (Davies Morel 2008).

Rectal examination should only be attempted for pregnancy diagnosis in (mares) horses.

Do not attempt rectal examination in ponies or donkeys as the potential harm far outweighs any benefit of diagnosis. See Section 11.5 for indications and care when carrying out rectal examinations for any reason.

External signs an animal is pregnant

- Enlarged abdomen (differential diagnosis includes parasitism or oedema)
- Mammary enlargement and slight ventral oedema (usually in the last 48 hours but can occur for up to 2 weeks before foaling)

Rectal examination

Knowledge of normal reproductive anatomy in the mare is essential as the signs will be difficult to differentiate in the early stages of pregnancy.

- Increased uterine and cervical tone may be palpable in the early stages of pregnancy (15–20 days' gestation). However, this is not a definitive sign of pregnancy and so it would be preferable to conduct a single rectal exam on day 60 for an accurate diagnosis.
- Unilateral distension of a uterine horn – The degree of distension will depend on the stage of the pregnancy and, as the foetus grows, the uterus will descend over the pelvic brim and may be difficult to palpate. In the later stages of pregnancy (from 200 days' gestation) the foetus and uterus will become palpable within the pelvis once again.

The workload in pregnant mares and jennies should be decreased or stopped, especially in the last 3 months. Good nutrition is important for foal development and lactation; owners should be informed of this at the time of diagnosis.

Abortion investigation

Abortion (Figure 13.4.1) can be associated with single or common occurrences in an individual mare or a group.

COMMON REPRODUCTIVE DISORDERS EXPERIENCED IN WORKING EQUIDS 13.4

Reasons for abortion

- **In a particular mare** Age, bacterial endometritis or ascending infection, chronic fibrosis in the uterus affecting the mare's ability to carry a foal to term, twinning, nutritional problems/deficits, overwork, stress

- **In a group of animals** Infectious disease such as EHV (see Section 12.6) causing abortion in the last trimester, or leptospirosis. Poisoning or toxicity is another potential cause, e.g. from plants, contaminated feed. (Single animals can also be affected, but suspect these causes if many owners from a particular area are complaining of abortion.)

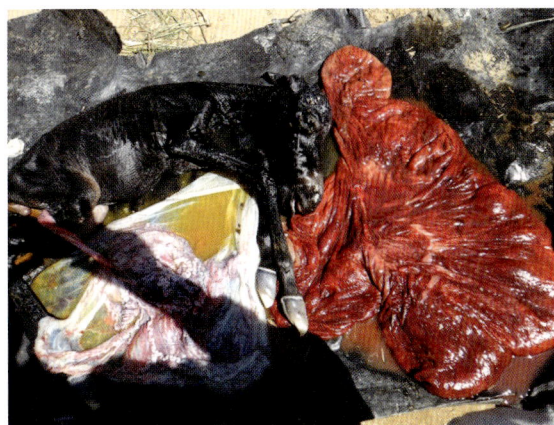

Figure 13.4.1 An aborted mule foetus at 7 months gestation. The placenta is thickened and haemorrhagic.

Abortion investigations start with an in-depth history of the animal, both in terms of reproductive history (age, how many foals, healthy foals, etc.) and general history (nutritional status, feeding of pregnant mares, workload and stress). Host factors which impair reproductive defence mechanisms will predispose to pathogens. In groups of animals, a holistic approach must be taken with examinations of the group/community management as a whole; for example, when naïve animals have been recently mixed with a new population.

Infectious causes of abortion in equids

Refer to relevant texts for diagnosis of the following conditions (Givens 2008):

Streptococcus zooepidemicus, *Taylorella equigenitalis*, brucellosis, leptospirosis, equine herpesvirus, equine viral arteritis, mycotic abortion, *Trypanosoma equiperdum* (dourine), *T.evansi* (surra), Babesiosis (See Section 17.8 *Blood borne parasites* for further description of the last three conditions.)

> **Leptospirosis and brucellosis can cause infections in humans; they are zoonotic.**

Leptospira are predominantly spread via the urine but contact with infected abortion material may also result in human infection. An equid infected with leptospirosis will often suffer from 'moon blindness', recurrent uveitis, 2–4 months following the initial infection (see Section 9.6 *Common eye diseases of working equids*).

Brucellosis is a rare cause of late term abortion in equids. Exposure to the aborted material and also consumption of infected milk may transmit the infection to humans. Equids with a brucellosis infection will more commonly present with 'fistulous withers' or 'poll evil' (see Section 14.10 *Common conditions affecting the synovial bursae of working equids*).

It is important to wear gloves and dispose of the abortion material appropriately when dealing with these cases.

13 THE URINARY AND REPRODUCTIVE SYSTEMS

Treatment

In an individual mare, abortion due to a primary problem with the reproductive tract is neither diagnosable nor within the scope of field operations. The exception is a purulent discharge from the vulva indicating a uterine infection which could be treated with lavage and antibiotics. Where a placentitis is suspected, treat as for *Retained foetal membranes* (see later in this chapter).

> For groups of affected animals, the aim is to diagnose and manage the cause of abortion. By applying knowledge, of population health and disease epidemiology to advise communities, it may be possible to reduce the number of abortions.

If many mares are aborting, consider a herd health approach to attempt a diagnosis and control plan. Examine other animals in the area (including non-pregnant, other species and males) to observe for signs of respiratory or other systemic disease or toxicities. Isolate the affected equids, particularly from other pregnant mares and jennies.

Dystocia

Unlike in cows, the second-stage labour in equids is rapid (15–20 minutes) so there is limited time to correct dystocias in equids.

It is best to examine a suspected dystocia by sedating with alpha-2 agonist and butorphanol (if available). Animals sedated with xylazine are still capable of kicking violently. General anaesthesia may be required for lengthy and involved procedures. Clean the perineum and vulva with antiseptic and lubricate well.

- **Retained forelimb** It may be possible to reach in and pull the forelimb out, or to use rope placed below the fetlock.
- **Retained head** Position a rope through mouth and back around foal's ears.
- **Oversize** is rare. If both shoulders don't fit through the vulva it is likely that the foal cannot be removed without damaging the mare or jenny.
- **Dog sitting position** This occurs when both hindlimbs are flexed and lying under the foetus, the pelvis forms a wedge preventing extraction of the foal. The head, two front legs and chest can be exteriorised but parturition does not progress past this stage. In these cases the foal is rarely delivered alive; manipulation of the foal during attempted delivery may result in uterine rupture and death of the mare. This malpresentation may be corrected by repelling the foetus and, if there is adequate space, repositioning the hindlimbs into a normal extended position. Heavy sedation or general anaesthesia is essential. Clenbuterol should be administered as a uterine muscle relaxant. Adequate pain relief must be provided to the mare. Euthanasia should be considered if attempts to deliver the foal are unsuccessful after 30 minutes.

> Dystocia correction is difficult – prolonged manipulation frequently results in metritis and laminitis and any manipulation over 30 minutes should be reassessed. Euthanasia should be considered if the foal cannot be removed, particularly if there is a lack of hospital facilities and adequate infection control.

COMMON REPRODUCTIVE DISORDERS EXPERIENCED IN WORKING EQUIDS 13.4

Fetotomy may be attempted if the foal is dead (Frazer 1997). This procedure carries a huge risk of uterine tears and infection and should only be employed if the operator is experienced in the technique and the correct equipment is available.

Uterine torsion

The presenting signs of a uterine torsion may include initiation of parturition but a failure to progress past the first stage; the mare may then stop trying to foal. Evidence of labour may not be observed at all (this is highlighted in the following case study) (Barber 1995). If the torsion occurs prior to parturition there may be signs of colic, depression and anorexia. A uterine torsion can be palpated on rectal examination; a taut broad ligament is palpable coursing transversely. During a per vagina examination the cervix appears to remain partially closed and the vaginal wall is twisted round into a corkscrew.

Non-surgical correction is feasible (Wichtel, Reinertson and Clark 1988). The method involves rolling the anaesthetised mare to correct the torsion. This technique is used frequently in cattle. If the torsion is clockwise the mare should be placed in right lateral recumbency and rolled on her back over to the left. If the torsion is counter clockwise initiate the procedure on the left. Refer to Yorke, Caldwell and Johnson (2012) for further guidance and helpful diagrams.

It is not appropriate to attempt a caesarean section if limited resources are available; the operation is unlikely to be successful and may result in particularly poor animal welfare.

The risk of mortality in both the mare and the foetus is high in cases of uterine torsion.

Uterine prolapse, rupture and haemorrhage of uterine arteries

These conditions are all sequalae to complicated foal deliveries.

A uterine prolapse is observed as severe straining and a soft, red, wrinkled mass extending from the vulval opening (can be distinguished from a bladder prolapse where the surface is smooth and pale).

Treatment

- Keep the uterus moist, and clean thoroughly using a sugar/dextrose solution to decrease oedema.
- Sedation and an epidural are mandatory.
- Administer tetanus anti-toxin and broad-spectrum systemic antibiotics.
- Replace the uterus gently, avoiding tearing the delicate inner surface.

> - Do not attempt to replace a uterus if it has been out for more than 2–3 hours, or if it has been damaged in any way, as equines are extremely susceptible to metritis (unlike bovines) and it is unlikely an infection will be controlled after this time.

Causey *et al.* 2007 describes a case study of uterine prolapse in a mare.

If the uterus is ruptured either during foaling or following a prolapse, euthanasia will be necessary.

Postpartum haemorrhage of the uterine artery is another, often fatal, consequence of foaling and will usually require euthanasia if haemorrhage cannot be alleviated. There is no treatment

13 THE URINARY AND REPRODUCTIVE SYSTEMS

for this condition but, if the mare or jenny is kept quiet and still, a clot may form and the haemorrhage cease.

Retained foetal membranes (RFM)

Retained foetal membranes (RFM) is less common in equids than in cows although it is often a sequel to abortion or to other birthing difficulties. The membranes are normally rapidly expelled in equines and, if this does not occur within 3 hours of foaling, treatment should be initiated.

> RFMs for longer than 6–8 hours is an emergency in equids as endotoxaemia and laminitis are common – systemic signs are very serious.

Treatment

In the first instance use oxytocin at 20IU IM or IV and wait 30–60 minutes to see if the placenta is expelled. Repeat the dose up to 3 times. Large boluses (more than 100 IU) cause abdominal discomfort, sweating and colic, so a good alternative is to administer oxytocin as an IV infusion. Place 100 IU of oxytocin into a one-litre bag of saline and infuse slowly (1 drop/3 seconds) over an hour, via a catheter. Decrease the flow rate if signs of discomfort are observed; usually only about 500–750 ml is required to expel the placenta.

What to do if oxytocin is unsuccessful in expelling the membranes?

- If over 1–2 hours the membranes are not expelled, manual removal will be necessary. This must be done carefully as any portion of membrane, however small, left internally may cause infection or haemorrhage. Never pull membranes forcefully, it is better to twist the external part around a long object held horizontally then gently rotated, wait for the tension to decrease, and rotate again to detach safely.

- Always give systemic NSAIDs and antibiotics such as trimethoprim, penicillin and gentamicin, especially if membranes have been retained for over 6 hours. Complications of RFMs include metritis, septicaemia and laminitis. Indications of a metritis include a foetid chocolate-coloured discharge, depression, pain, increased HR and RR.

Prognosis

Good if treated early and membranes are expelled with oxytocin. Guarded if membranes have been retained for longer than 6 hours, and extremely poor if there are signs of endotoxaemia or the membranes have been retained for longer than 12 hours. It will be necessary to discuss euthanasia with the owner in these cases.

Castration

The surgical technique for castration is out of the scope of this manual so please refer to equine surgical texts. Castration has nevertheless been included here to highlight a number of points pertaining to the welfare implications of poor technique and some considerations before undertaking this procedure.

- Castration of donkeys should never be attempted using the *standing technique* since their tendency to bleed requires the spermatic vessels to be tied off (Sprayson and Theimann 2007).

- Stallions > 3 years of age must also be castrated under GA, never standing, as they too have a tendency to bleed once mature.

- Burdizzo castrators used for cattle castration are not acceptable for equines as they will not stem the blood flow sufficiently; only attempt castration if equine emasculators are available.

Complications of castration include:

- **Excessive haemorrhage** A small amount of blood dripping from the castration wound normally stops within 30–60 minutes upon completion. If this is in a steady stream, or is prolonged, it requires further exploration. If packing of the scrotum is unsuccessful, it is essential to locate the source of the haemorrhage and ligate the vessel (Railton 1999).
- **Scrotal swelling** Inadequate post-operative care by the owner is a large contributing factor to scrotal swelling. It is more common after standing castrations; a large incision will allow drainage. It is important to provide clear post-operative instructions to include 10–15 minutes of daily exercise and NSAIDs SID for 5–7 days.

> - It is imperative that the animal does not start work again for 3 weeks. If owner compliance is unlikely it may be necessary to decline to perform the surgery.

- Local infection requires BID trimethoprim-sulphonamide or procaine penicillin; the infection can progress to scirrous cors (ascending infection from spermatic cord) swelling, purulent discharge and possible spread to the intra-peritoneal section of the spermatic cord causing lameness and colic – a condition which may ultimately result in euthanasia.
- Eventration is a rare occurrence. It is seen as small intestines appearing from the inguinal canal within a few hours to a few days of surgery. Euthanasia is necessary.

> As can be seen from the above considerations, equine castration is more complex than in other species and should never be undertaken lightly. It involves particular equipment, good owner communication and a certain amount of risk – always weigh up the harm versus benefits and only operate if there are serious, multiple welfare implications of leaving the animal entire.

Cryptorchidism There is a 2–8% prevalence of cryptorchidism in horses, and cryptorchidism also occurs in donkeys. Both testicles should be located within the scrotum when the colt foal is born (Amann *et al.* 2007), although some surgeons advise waiting at least 18 months prior to cryptorchid surgery to allow ample time for the cryptorchid testicle to descend. A single testicle should never be removed if the other cannot be located; the animal may remain fertile and this could lead to serious welfare implications if mares and jennies are impregnated.

Cutaneous habronemiasis

Larvae burrow into the urethral process and can look like a squamous cell carcinoma with swelling and discharge around the prepuce and a granulomatous reaction/ulceration if chronic. Treat with ivermectin (see Sections 9.6 and 16.1).

Hydrocoele

Causes

This condition is common in working equids as it is often seen in hot weather and can be secondary to infection and malnutrition. It is a non-painful abnormal amount of fluid in the testes resulting in a swollen appearance (Figure 13.4.2).

Diagnosis

Scrotal palpation reveals a large fluid-filled area which is *not painful*.

Treatment

Attempts to drain the fluid have only a limited success as the fluid soon accumulates again. Allow the swelling to subside. This condition may interfere with breeding ability.

Penile paralysis

Prolonged penile protrusion can result in paralysis, e.g. that seen with trauma, or after ACP or xylazine administration in stallions. The penis appears engorged, partially erect, with oedema due to congestion of blood. Observe for other neurological signs.

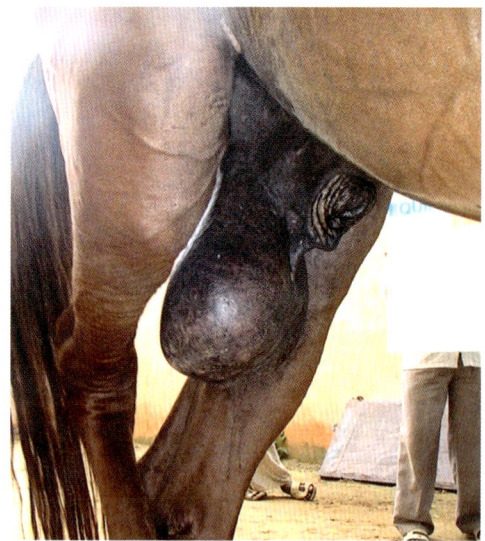

Figure 13.4.2 Swelling of the scrotum in a working horse, observed in the hot humid months in Northern India.

Treatment

Local anti-inflammatory therapies such as massage, 'sling' support and cool hosing. A sling prevents blood stasis. Slings can be created using a soft mesh/netting material so that the stallion should still be able to urinate. Systemic NSAIDs are indicated if the stallion is in pain, and antibiotics if infection or necrosis is evident. The animal may require urethral catheterisation if anuric.

Prognosis

Good if the penis can be returned into the prepuce and there are no secondary complications. Poor if it remains prolapsed for a number of days causing serious swelling and anuria. Euthanasia should be considered.

Testicular torsion

Cause

If the torsion is only 180°, diagnosis is usually only incidental during examination. Acute 360° torsion is rare and causes signs of severe colic and scrotal swelling. Differentiate this condition from tumours and injury.

Treatment

Castration is recommended for 360° torsions or if clinical signs are evident. If it is an incidental finding on clinical examination, there is no need to castrate the animal initially but inform the owner to watch for signs of discomfort.

Case study – Urinary tract infection 13.5

Area Meerut, India

Attending veterinarian Dr Amit Pandey

Summary
This report describes the diagnosis, treatment and outcome of a horse that presented with loss of condition, stranguria and subsequently discoloured urine.

History
The mare had previously been successfully treated for babesiosis. After 3 weeks the animal started showing symptoms including frequent urination of a small quantity, a reduced appetite, reduced water intake, loss of body weight and apathy.

Clinical findings
Temperature 37.8°C, heart rate 36–40 beats/minute, pale and dry mucous membranes, CRT 2 seconds, respiration rate 30 breaths/minute

Urinalysis: The colour of the urine at the beginning was straw-coloured but progressed to red.

Laboratory findings: Neutrophilia (92% in Differential Leucocyte Count), blood urea 57 mg/dL (ref range 8–27), serum glutamic oxaloacetic transaminase (SGOT or AST) 806U /L (ref range 205-555)

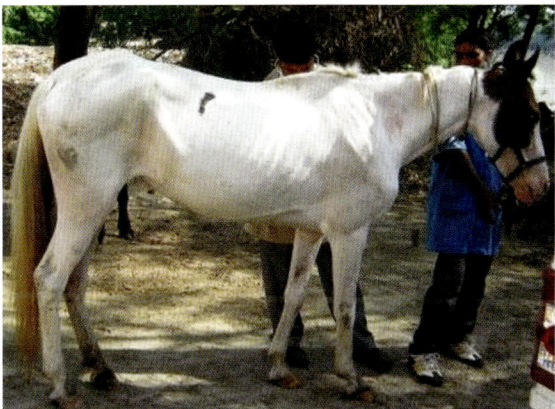

Figure 13.5.1 The mare at presentation.

Diagnosis
Acute bacterial infection of the urinary tract

Treatment
Antibiotics (trimethoprim-sulphonamide 30mg/kg), IV fluids (lactated Ringer's solution), oral and nasogastric hydration (oral rehydration salts – ORS) for 5 days

Outcome
The animal responded to treatment from the second day and recovered after one week.

Discussion
In this report a case of suspected urinary tract infection has been described. This

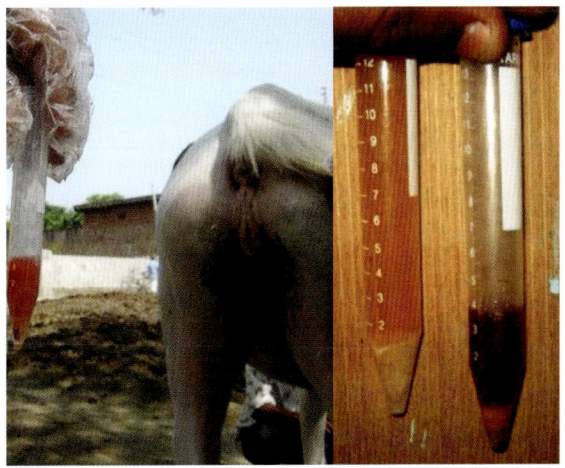

Figure 13.5.2 Discolouration of urine from the mare.

347

has not been confirmed by urinary culture but is assumed based on clinical signs and the subsequent response to antibiotic treatment. This horse had been treated for babesiosis previously. A babesiosis infection also presents with discolouration of the urine as the consequence of haemoglobinuria. In the case of a UTI the discoloured urine is due to red blood cells in the urine (haematuria) as the result of bleeding from the inflamed surface of the urinary tract. These conditions can be differentiated by centrifuging the urine sample or leaving the sample to stand for at least an hour as described in Section 13.1.

It is possible that the previous infection with babesiosis predisposed this mare to pyelonephritis as the result of kidney damage when filtering the heme protein, or that reduced urine flow allowed contaminating bacteria to establish an infection in the urinary tract. The prior babesia infection would have resulted in a general debilitation which would be likely to affect the immune system leading to opportunistic infection.

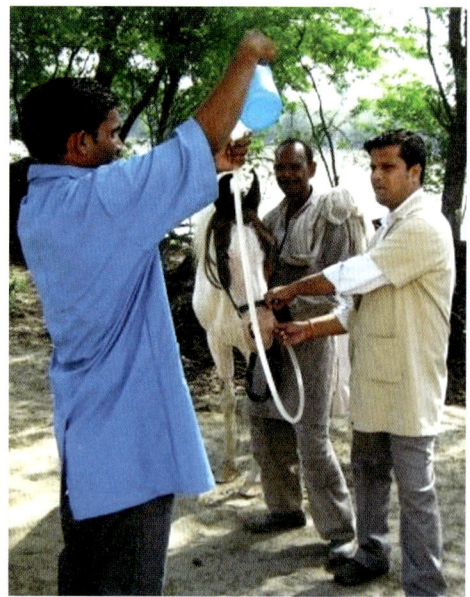

Figure 13.5.3 Administration of rehydration fluids by nasogastric tube.

13.6 References

Amann, R.P., Veeramachaneni, D.N. (2007) Cryptorchidism in common eutherian mammals. *Reproduction*. 133 (3) 541–561.

Barber, B. (1995) Complications of chronic uterine torsion in a mare. *Can. Vet. J*. 36, 102–103.

Causey, R., Ruksznis, D., Miles, R. (2007) Case Report: Field management of equine uterine prolapse in a Thoroughbred mare. *Equine Vet. Educ*. 19 (5) 254–259.

Clark, C., Greenwood, S., Boison, O.O., Chirino-Trejo, M., Dowling, PM. (2008) Bacterial isolates from equine infections in western Canada (1998–2003) *Can. Vet. J*. 49 (2) 153–160.

Colahan, P.T., Mayhew, I.G., Merritt, A.M., Moore, J.N. (1999) *Manual of Equine Medicine and Surgery*. Mosby, Inc. Missouri. 285–359.

Davies Morel, M.C.G. (2008) Equine Reproductive Physiology, Breeding and Stud Management. 156 (Chapter 14).

Driessen, B., Zarucco, L., Kalir, B., Bertolotti, L. (2011) Contemporary use of acepromazine in the anaesthetic management of male horses and ponies: a retrospective study and opinion poll. *Equine Vet. J*. 43 (1) 88–89.

Frazer, G.S. (1997) Review of the Use of Fetotomy to Resolve Dystocia in the Mare. *AAEP Proceedings. Reproduction II.* 43, 262–268.

HBLB Code of Practice. Available online *http://codes.hblb.org.uk*

MacLeay, J.M., Kohn, C.W.J. (1998) Results of quantitative cultures of urine by free catch and catheterization from healthy adult horses. *Vet. Intern. Med.* 12 (2), 76–78.

OIE Terrestrial Manual (2012) Contagious Equine Metritis. Chapter 2.5.2. Available online at *http://www.oie.int/fileadmin/Home/eng/Health_standards/tahm/2.05.02_CEM.pdf*

Pathology in Practice-*Halicephalobus gingivalis* (2012). *J. Am. Vet. Med. Assoc.* 241 (6) 703.

Reed, S.M., Bayly, W.M., Selon. D. (2004) Equine Internal Medicine. Philadelphia. 1253–1289.

Robinson, N.N., Sprayberry, K.A. (2009) Current Therapy in Equine Medicine 6. 751.

Sprayson, T., Theimann, A. (2003) Clinical approach to castration in donkeys. *In Practice.* 29 (9) 526–531.

Wilson, M.E. (2007) Examination of the urinary tract in the horse. *Vet. Clin. N. Am. Equine.* 23 (3) 563–575.

Wichtel, J.J., Reinertson, E.L., Clark, T.L. (1988) Nonsurgical treatment of uterine torsion in seven mares. *J. Am. Vet. Med. Assoc.* 193 (3) 337–338.

Wood, T., Weckman, T.J., Henry, P.A., Chang, S.L., Blake, J.W., Tobin, T. (1990) Equine urine pH: normal population distributions and methods of acidification. *Equine Vet. J.* 22 (2) 118–121.

Yorke, E.H., Caldwell, F.J., Johnson, A.K. (2012) Uterine Torsion in Mares. Compendium: Continuing Education for Veterinarians. Available online at: *https://s3.amazonaws.com/assets.prod.vetlearn.com/5f/772fb02e6411e29e50005056ad4736/file/PV1212_Yorke_CE.pdf*

Further reading

Abutarbush, S. (2005) Large Animal Clinical Rounds. 5 (2). Available online at *www.canadianveterinarians.net /larounds*.

Auer, J.A., Stick, J.A. (2012) Equine Surgery. Uterus and Ovaries, Embertson, R. 833.

Emberston R. (2012) Uterus and Ovaries 933. In: *Equine Surgery.* Ed: Auer and Stick

Givens, M.D., Marley, M.S.D. (2008) Infectious causes of embryonic and fetal mortality. *Theriogenology.* 70 (3) 270–285.

Marshall, J.F., Moorman, V.J., Moll, H.D. (2007) Comparison of the diagnosis and management of unilaterally castrated and cryptorchid horses at a referral hospital: 60 cases (2002–2006). *J. Am. Vet. Med. Assoc.* 231 (6) 931–934.

Railton, D. (1999) Complications associated with castration in the horse. *In Practice.* 21, 298–307.

The musculoskeletal system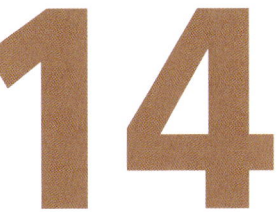

Introduction – Challenges of lameness and gait abnormalities	**14.1**
Lameness examination and diagnostic techniques	**14.2**
Hoof anatomy and conformation	**14.3**
Trimming and shoeing	**14.4**
Conditions affecting the hoof	**14.5**
Conditions affecting the bones	**14.6**
Conditions affecting the joints	**14.7**
Conditions affecting the tendons and ligaments	**14.8**
Conditions affecting the muscles	**14.9**
Conditions affecting the synovial bursae	**14.10**
Case study – Malignant oedema	**14.11**
References	**14.12**

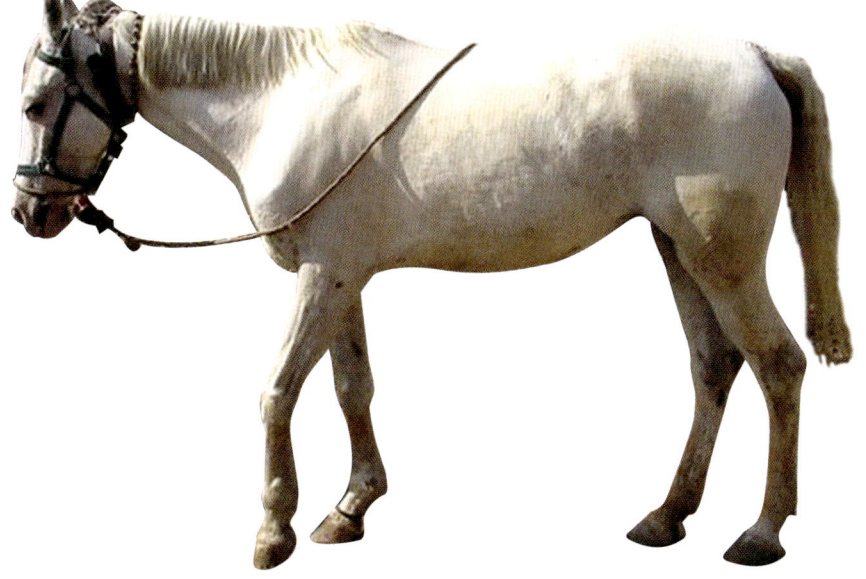

14.1 Introduction – Challenges of lameness and gait abnormalities

> The musculoskeletal system consists of structures which move the body or maintain its form: muscles, tendons, ligaments, bones and joints.

Lameness/gait abnormalities are perhaps the most common presenting sign to working equine veterinarians. Data from the welfare assessment of 4,903 working equids (Pritchard *et al.* 2005) suggest that over 99% of animals surveyed show gait abnormalities. Lameness can be very frustrating to treat, especially as many cases are chronic and may have many contributing factors (Broster *et al.* 2009). Long-term rest is often the most effective treatment but this is usually impractical for the owners of working equids.

Golden Rule 1 Basic knowledge of anatomy is essential for a confident diagnosis.

Golden Rule 2 Think holistically: 'management' rather than 'treatment'.

Golden Rule 3 The direct cause may be difficult to identify.

1. Think about which structures are under the skin in the affected area.
2. Think about what could be happening to those structures and why:
   - Acute or chronic?
   - Bone, joint, tendon, ligament or muscle?
   - Infected or sterile?
   - Single or multiple limbs?
3. Link it back to history and clinical examination to make an informed decision.

The lack of radiography, ultrasonography or other 'high-tech' diagnostic aids is no barrier to a thorough work-up. In most cases, lameness examination coupled with a good knowledge of anatomy and a detailed history will help identify the most likely problem (Figure 14.1.1), with prognosis depending on response to management in the first week. When dealing with this system, be aware of the vast amount of terminology: osteomyelitis, tendonitis, septic arthritis, osteoarthritis, synovitis, cellulitis.

> In a medical context, the suffix '-itis' almost always implies inflammation of that particular anatomical area.

Remember that infection may or may not be present with inflammation.

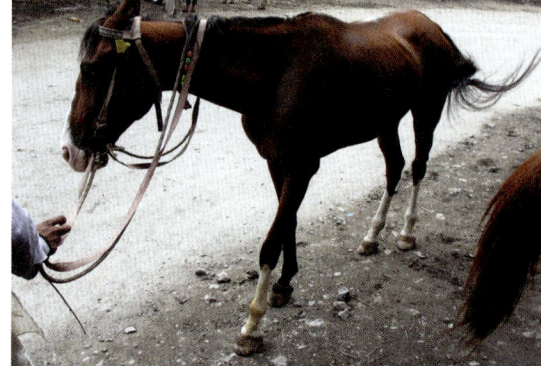

Figure 14.1.1 Lameness in working equids is a common presentation. Here the left forelimb is resting on the toe and not fully weight-bearing, indicating pain in that limb.

Lameness examination and diagnostic techniques 14.2

Lameness is any abnormality in the gait. This may be a mechanical lameness due to a healed injury, or poor conformation which has affected function, or lameness due to pain and dysfunction of the area. It is a sign that the animal is protecting the area from further damage and injury although, in very chronic or subtle lameness, the owner may not notice anything wrong.

Why should a lameness examination be conducted?

> The objective of the lameness examination is to identify whether the animal is lame, where the lameness is coming from and the most likely cause.

Classic lameness examinations are described in most textbooks; however, these are often not feasible for working equids and improvisation is frequently necessary. For example, the notion of 'trotting on a lead rope' is difficult if the animal is normally driven from behind and, unless the trotting movement is fluid and consistent, it is difficult to gain any real diagnostic information. Dragging/pulling the animal along restricts its head movement and will make evaluation more difficult. If the animal is unable to trot in hand do not force it.

History

- Exactly what is the problem that concerns the owner?
- When did it start?
- Was there any specific incident that started it?
- Is the lameness getting better, worse or staying the same? (This is often key to prognosis.)

Physical examination

> Perform the following examinations in a systematic, consistent way so that nothing is missed. If the significance of a finding is not obvious, compare both sides of the animal (but remember that the problem may be bilateral).

Look at the standing, resting animal.

- **Unequal weight bearing** It is not normal for an equid to point or rest a *foreleg* (as seen in Figure 14.2.1); however, it may normally 'rest' a hindlimb. Observe any abnormal stance (pointing forelimb, knuckling of fetlock, dropped elbow) or obvious wounds or swellings whilst the animal is still at rest.

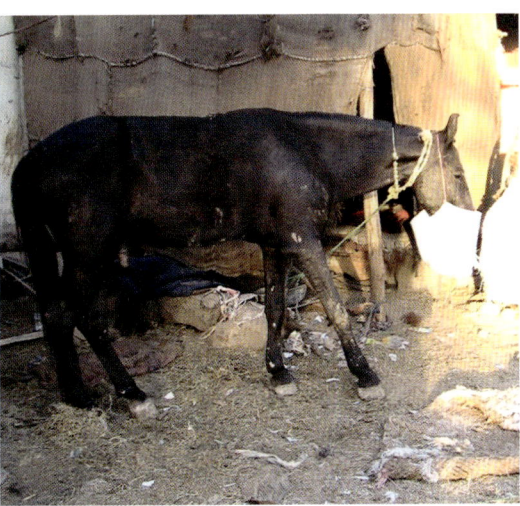

Figure 14.2.1 Unequal foreleg weight bearing. The right forelimb is placed forwards reducing weight bearing and indicating a right forelimb lameness.

14 THE MUSCULOSKELETAL SYSTEM

▌ **Conformation** Alignment of limbs with body, cow hocks, unequal foot size, etc. Look at the symmetry of the skeleton and evidence of muscle atrophy.

Note the poor hindlimb conformation of severe sickle hocks in the animal in Figure 14.2.2. Think about the implications for work such conformation could have, and the possibility for predisposition to wounds and lameness in future. Broster *et al.* (2009) showed that sickle hock conformation was significantly associated with lameness in working horses. This study also showed that conformation traits such as broken forward hoof-pastern axis was associated with pain on flexion of the carpal joint in that limb, and upright pasterns were associated with pain on palpation over the digital flexor tendon area and suspensory ligament in that limb (Broster *et al.* 2009).

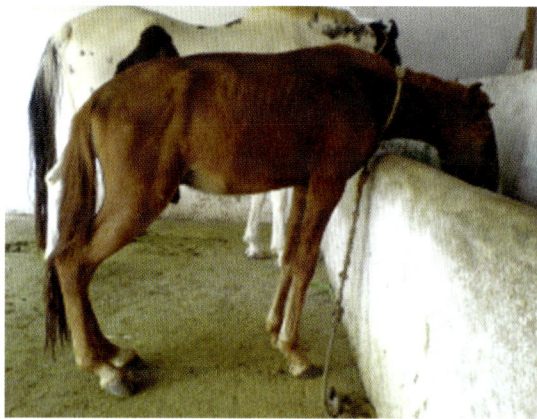

Figure 14.2.2 Poor conformation – severe 'sickle hocks' seen in this horse.

Examine the moving animal from a variety of directions.

> **Do not examine a moving animal if the lameness is severe/non-weight bearing. Do not cause unnecessary pain, fear and distress in a case where the lameness is obviously severe.**

Observe from in front (forelimb lameness) Look for a head-nod as the animal walks or trots forwards (Figure 14.2.3, first picture). If the equid is lame on a fore leg, the head will nod downwards when the *sound* fore leg hits the ground.

Observe from behind (hindlimb lameness) As the equid trots away, look for asymmetrical movement of the pelvis. The hip will raise more or 'hike up' as the lame leg *leaves* the ground.

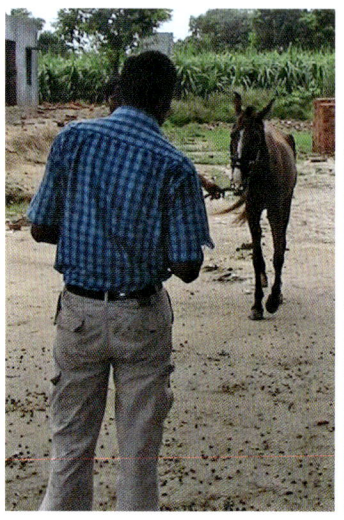
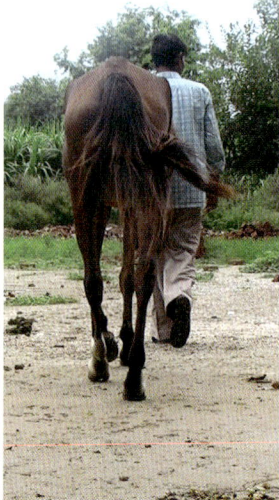
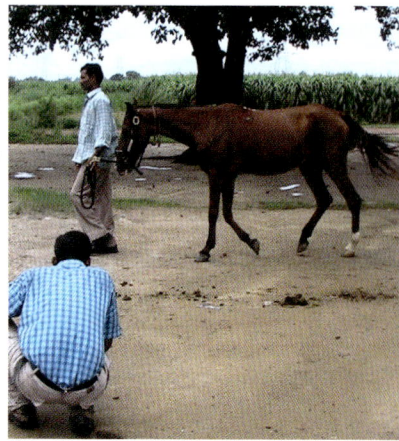

Figure 14.2.3 Examining for lameness from in front (far left), behind (left) and the side (above).

Put tape markers over the hip joint or tuber coxa on both sides – the lame side will have greater movement.

Observe from the side The lame leg will have a shorter stride length. In more severe cases, the toe may drag instead of being lifted properly, or 'dig' into the ground at the end of the stride. A shortened stride may indicate a problem with the upper part of the limb; 'high limb lameness', e.g. shoulder.

Move in a circle Lameness is more pronounced when an equid is led in a circle. The inside leg will be subjected to increased twisting and pressure forces that do not occur when walking or trotting in a straight line.

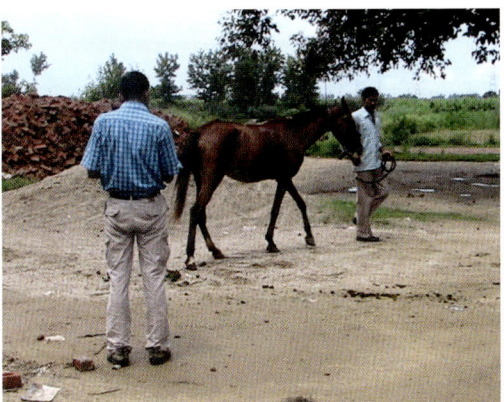
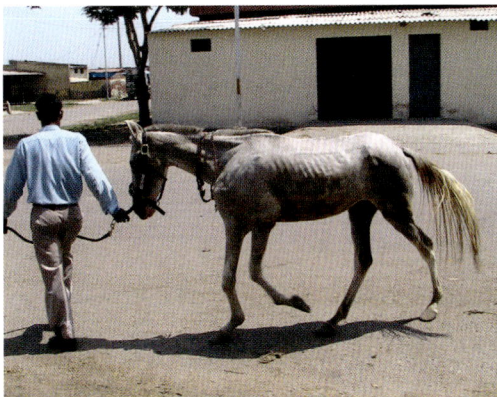

Figure 14.2.4 Observe the animal moving in a circle in both directions.

Close examination

> 'The foot is the cause of lameness unless proven otherwise.'
> (Hodgson 2000 – original quotation unknown)

Foot Always start at the foot and progress upwards, even if there is obvious muscle atrophy or joint swelling further up the leg. Assessing the hoof demonstrates the effect of lameness on the animal's movement, overgrowth and over wear show the *current* forces on that leg, despite what is often a chronic lameness, and helps to determine prognosis.

- Discharge
- Smell
- Foreign body
- **Size and shape** Compare with opposite foot, although beware of bilateral problems (Figure 14.2.5).
- **Size, fit, quality of shoes** and degree of wear (if present) (Figure 14.2.6 – see over)
- Quality of frog, sole and wall horn and any abnormalities like cracks, bruises, infection

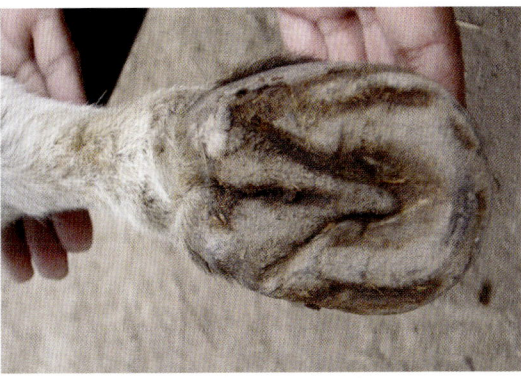

Figure 14.2.5 Examination of the solar surface of the foot.

14 THE MUSCULOSKELETAL SYSTEM

- **Check digital pulse** for rate, strength and quality (Figure 14.2.7 – see opposite).
- **To detect pain,** use the following three techniques in a methodical manner; digital pressure, hoof testers, and a small percussion hammer (Figures 14.2.8 and 14.2.9).

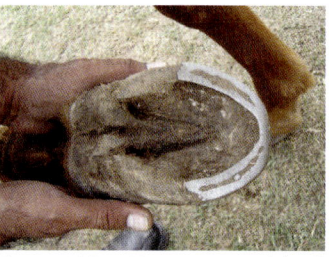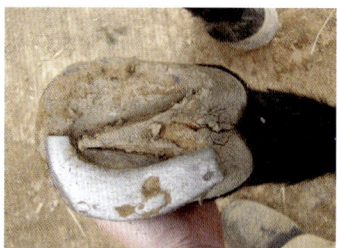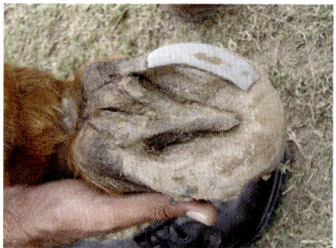

Figure 14.2.6 Examination of the shoe for uneven wear.

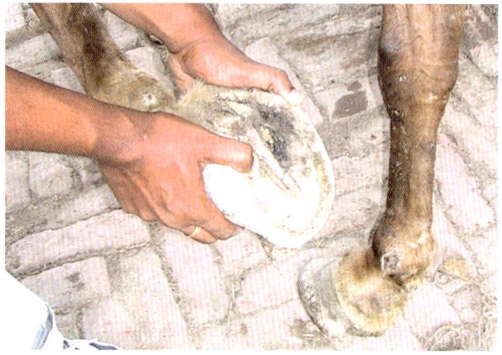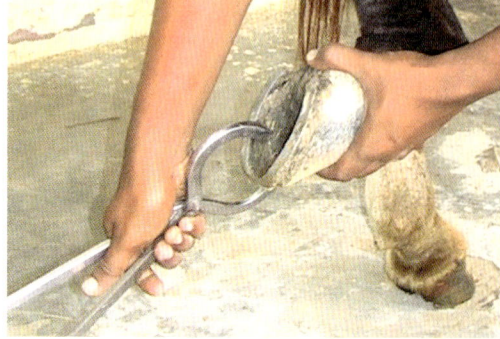

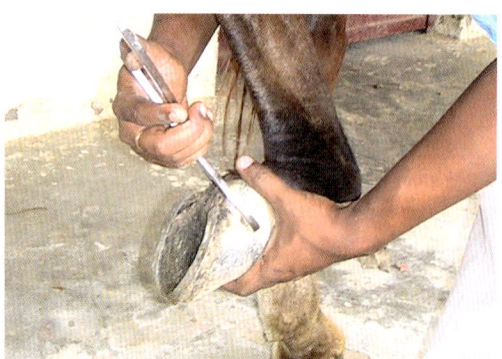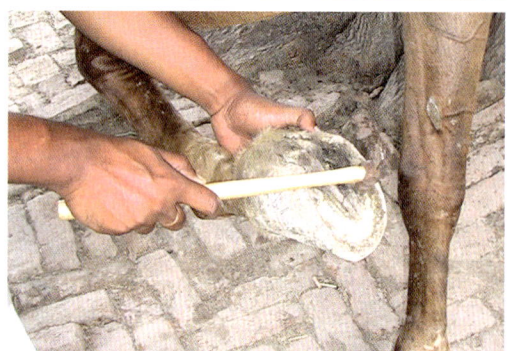

Figure 14.2.8 Testing the sole, heels and external hoof wall for pain, using digital pressure, hoof testers and a percussion hammer.

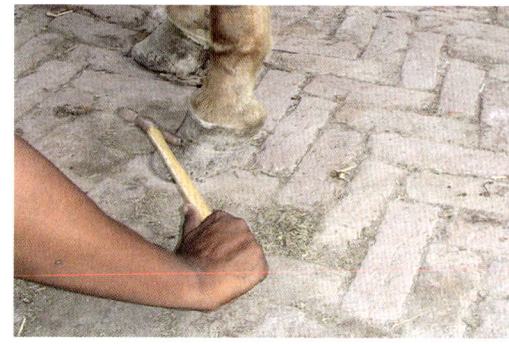

356

LAMENESS EXAMINATION AND DIAGNOSTIC TECHNIQUES 14.2

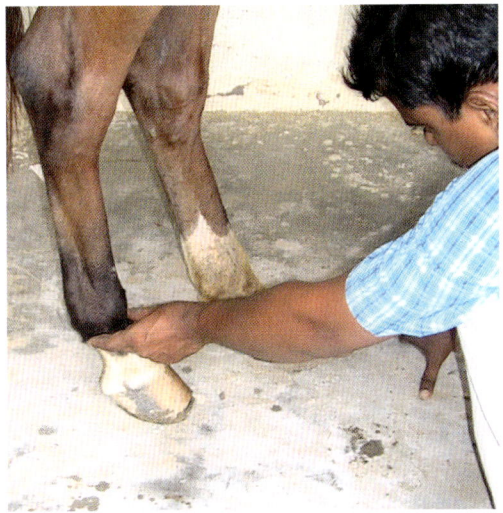

Figure 14.2.7 *Palpation of the digital pulse.*

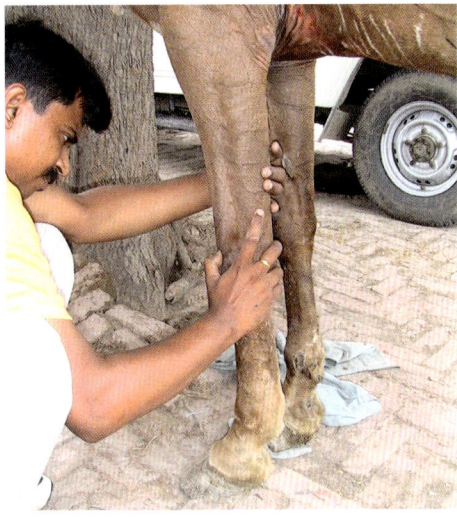

Figure 14.2.10 *Examine the limb in a methodical manner, e.g. from distal to proximal.*

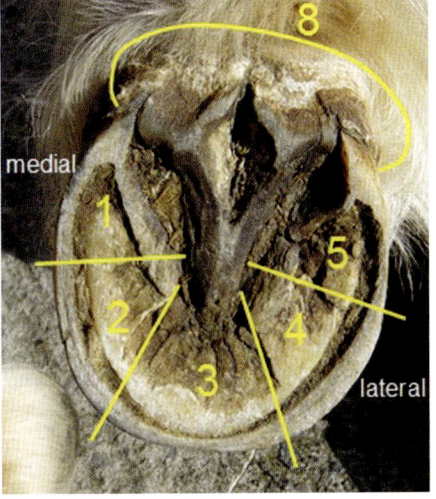
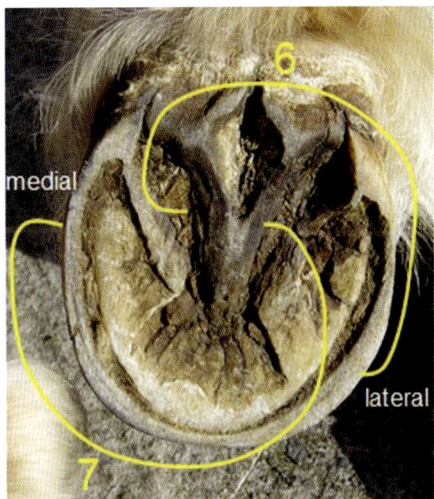

Figure 14.2.9 *Systematic examination of the hoof – yellow numbering indicates positioning of the hoof testers across different areas of the foot.*

If there are no abnormal findings on examination of the foot then palpate the joints, tendons and muscles of the lame leg for:

- swelling
- pain
- injury.

Tendons Palpate tendons both in a weight-bearing position and off the ground. The latter relaxes the tendons which can allow better examination. Feel for any swelling, heat or pain on gentle palpation. Assess tendon sheaths, particularly the large digital flexor tendon sheath, for swelling (effusion) heat or pain.

357

14 THE MUSCULOSKELETAL SYSTEM

Joints Examine all joints for swelling (effusion) or bony protuberances, both of which can reflect osteoarthritis. If the horse is not in too much pain, flex and extend joints to assess range of motion and/or pain associated with this.

Stop the lameness examination if the animal is feeling excessive pain or showing other signs of distress; analyse the cost to the animal versus the benefit of continuing the diagnosis to a deeper level.

Flexion tests

> The purpose of the flexion test is to exaggerate lameness by putting more stress on the joints, ligaments and surrounding structures before asking the animal to move.

Flex the joint for one minute then walk or trot the animal (Figure 14.2.11). Often an animal will be more lame in the affected limb after this, signalling a positive result. The test is not very specific to an individual joint or structure. This is especially true in the hindleg where, due to the reciprocal apparatus, the stifle and hock joints cannot be flexed individually.

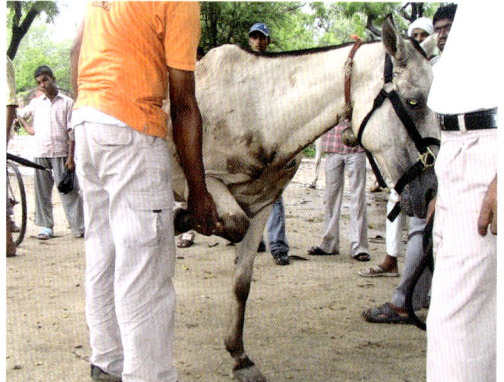
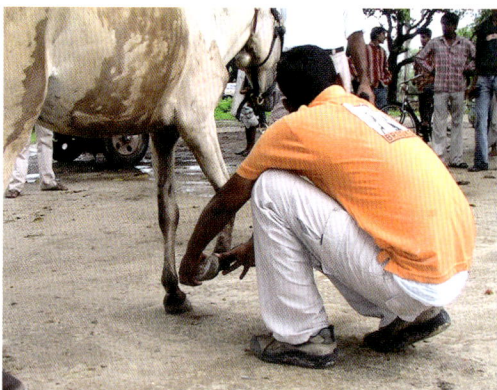
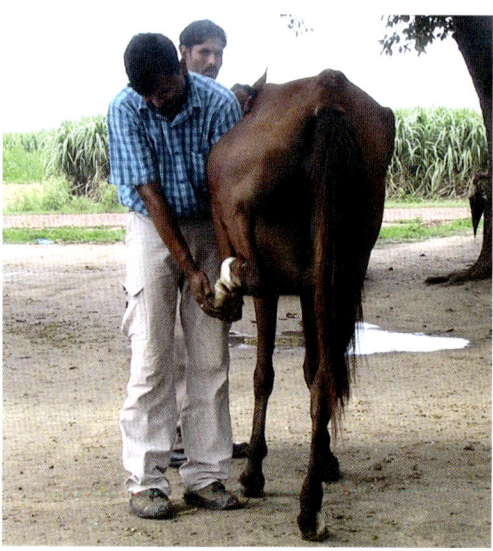
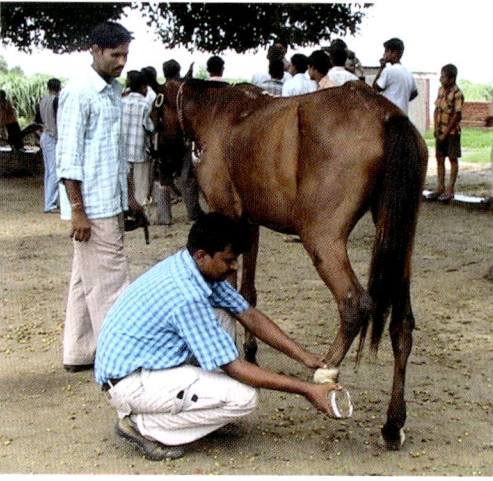

Figure 14.2.11 Flexion tests for the lower foreleg, upper foreleg, lower hindleg and full hindleg.

Some would argue flexion tests are of limited use in working equids as many animals have multiple problems and chronic arthritis. Do not attempt flexion tests if the animal shows obvious discomfort as this signals potential arthritis.

Grading of lameness

It is useful to assign a grade to the severity of lameness, using a scale. This gives a more accurate documentation of a lameness examination, thereby allowing changes between subsequent examinations to be recorded more objectively.

> **Overall Lameness Score** (based on the American Association of Equine Practitioners (AAEP) Scoring System)
>
> **Grade 0** No lameness
>
> **Grade 1** Difficult to observe; not consistently apparent regardless of circumstances (e.g. carrying weight, circling, on an incline, hard surface, etc.)
>
> **Grade 2** Difficult to observe at a walk or trotting in a straight line; consistently apparent under certain circumstances (e.g., carrying weight, circling, incline, hard surface, etc.)
>
> **Grade 3** Consistently observable at a trot under all circumstances
>
> **Grade 4** Obvious lameness, marked nodding, hitching or shortened stride
>
> **Grade 5** Minimal weight bearing in motion and/or at rest; inability to move

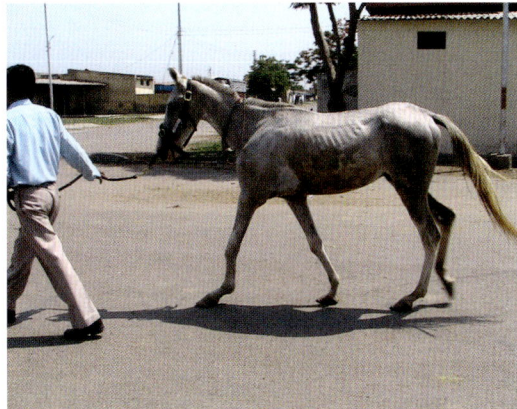

Figure 14.2.12 Grading of lameness helps with re-assessment to see if there has been an improvement.

Nerve blocks (perineural anaesthesia)

This is the use of local anaesthetic to relieve pain so that lameness will be reduced or hidden in a positive result. See Section 7.2 for further details on local analgesia. To pinpoint the site of pain, nerve blocks can be applied in a logical sequence from distal to proximal regions until the equid becomes sound. These blocks can also be used when suturing wounds, or for desensitisation of the hoof for treatment of abscesses or other painful exploratory procedures in the hoof.

> **Prepare sites for nerve blocks in a sterile fashion (clip and scrub with antiseptic) to avoid excessive swelling and possible infection post-examination.**

It is absolutely imperative that veterinarians carrying out nerve blocks know the exact location of the nerve and are aware of the location of adjacent structures to avoid iatrogenic damage/injection into adjacent synovial structures. Accidental injection of synovial structures is likely to result in synovial sepsis that will not only finish the animal's working life but would warrant euthanasia on welfare grounds. It is important to have practised injection of coloured dye into cadaver limbs before injection into a live animal (Figure 14.2.13 – see over); the skin on the

14 THE MUSCULOSKELETAL SYSTEM

cadaver can be dissected back to reveal if the injection/dye was placed in the correct position.

Palmar/plantar digital nerve block

This block desensitises the palmar aspect (frog and heel areas) of the sole and is very good for painful procedures such as paring out a hoof abscess. Always wait at least 15 minutes and test with a pen prick as it can take a long time to work. The common point of needle insertion for this block is just above the most proximal part of the lateral cartilages, close to the edge of the deep flexor tendon where the neurovascular bundle can be palpated (Figure 14.2.14). Inject 5 mls of lignocaine perivascularly.

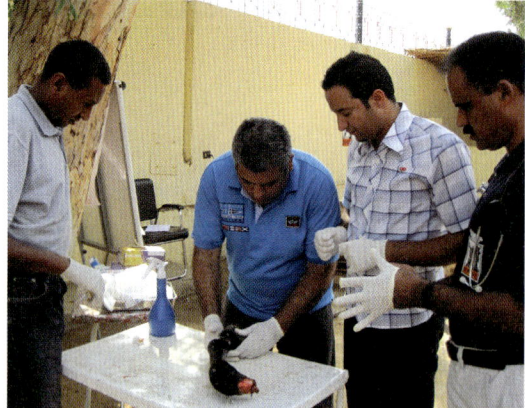

Figure 14.2.13 Take advantage of practising on cadaver limbs before injecting into a live animal for the first time.

> Take great care and attention to avoid inadvertent injection of the digital flexor tendon sheath which runs close by this injection site.

Abaxial sesamoid nerve block

This is used to desensitise all structures distal to the fetlock joint, and some of the sesamoids, and is also useful when assessing the hoof and distal phalanx joints for lameness or painful conditions over the whole sole (a palmar digital nerve block will not desensitise the toe).

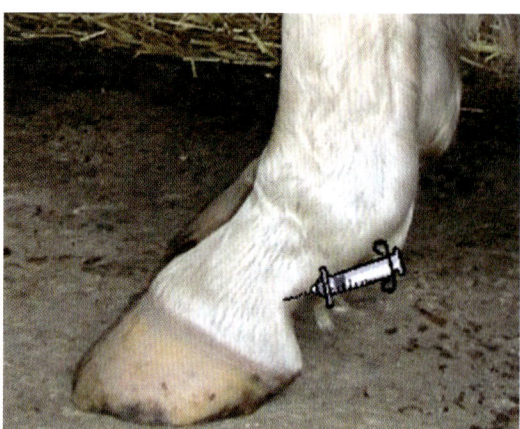

Figure 14.2.14 Site for injection of local anaesthetic for a palmar digital nerve block.

Feel for the nerve bundle over the distal extent of the abaxial sesamoids either side of the fetlock joint (Figure 14.2.15) and infiltrate SC local anaesthetic via a 25G needle into the area (2–5 mls lignocaine).

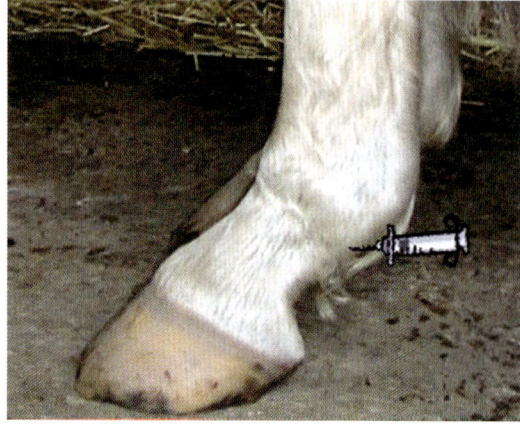

Figure 14.2.15 Site of injection of local anaesthetic for an abaxial sesamoid nerve block.

Hoof anatomy and conformation 14.3

Hoof anatomy

Figures 14.3.1 and 14.3.2 show the following parts of hoof anatomy:

Sole Seen when the foot is lifted (Figure 14.3.1). Sole horn is softer than hoof horn and more prone to injury caused by stepping on stones and other foreign objects. Ideally the sole itself should not make contact with the ground (it is concave); the frog and the wall should be the structures touching the ground in a healthy hoof.

Frog Elastic 'V'-shaped cushion at the back of the sole (Figure 14.3.1). It should be the first part of the foot to hit the ground. The elastic properties allow the foot to expand during weight bearing. It should be symmetrical and seated within deep grooves either side; known as the frog sulci. Poor conformation of the frog may be due to inadequate foot care or inappropriate farriery, such as excessive trimming of the frog.

Heel bulbs These are caudal to the heel where the frog merges with the skin.

White line Junction where the sole meets the wall on the ground surface of the foot. This represents where the sensitive laminae meet the insensitive laminae and is a natural weak spot of the hoof where bacteria can occasionally penetrate.

Bars Parts of the hoof wall that angle forward at the heel either side of the frog sulci. These should be well developed.

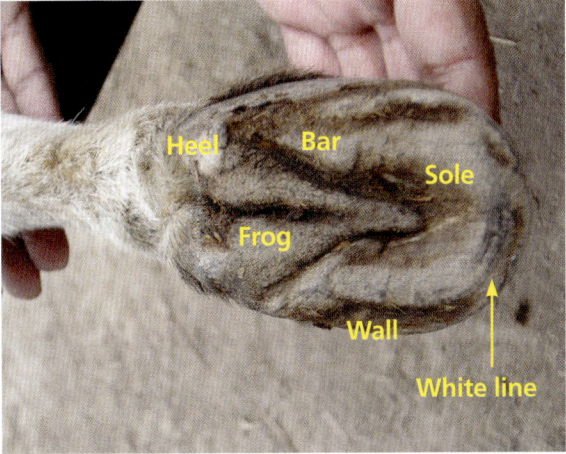

Figure 14.3.1 Solar surface of the forefoot of a working donkey.

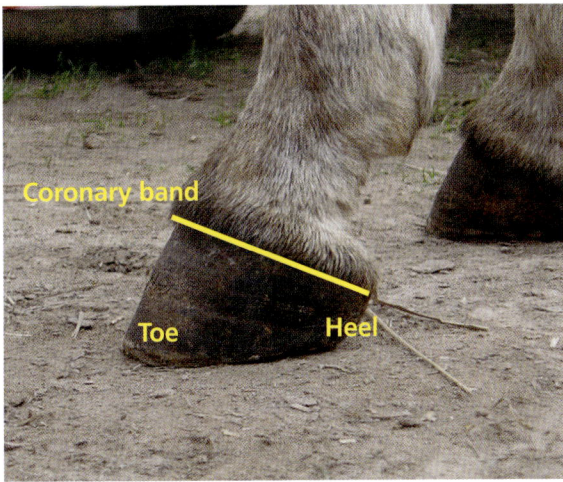

Figure 14.3.2 Lateral view of the hoof wall of a working donkey.

Coronary band Junction between hoof and skin. This area is responsible for hoof growth so, if injured, subsequent hoof growth can be affected.

Wall The hard keratinised outside capsule of the hoof (Figures 14.3.1 and 14.3.2) seen when the foot is on the ground. The wall is formed at the coronary band so injuries to this area will affect its structure and growth rate. It takes 9–12 months for the wall to grow from the coronary band to the ground. For this reason, diseases of the wall often take many months to correct; this should be explained to owners when attempting corrective trimming.

Internal structure of the foot

There are many important structures inside the hoof. A good knowledge of anatomy is important; if a nail penetrates the sole of the foot it is essential to know what might be damaged.

Bones
P1 First/proximal phalanx or long pastern bone
P2 Second/middle phalanx or short pastern bone
P3 Third/distal phalanx or pedal bone
Distal sesamoid or navicular bone

Joints
Pastern joint Proximal interphalangeal joint
Coffin joint Distal interphalangeal joint

Tendons
SDFT Superficial digital flexor tendon
DDFT Deep digital flexor tendon

Laminae
Highly vascular interlocking ridges that hold the hoof wall on to P3

Blood vessels
Digital plexus and associated veins and arteries which supply the highly vascular laminae

Foot conformation

Foot conformation is absolutely critical as any imbalance will impact the rest of the limb.

Foot axis

The angle of the dorsal hoof wall
  Forelimb = 45–50 degrees
  Hindlimb = 50–55 degrees

Hoof pastern axis

> A line drawn through the centre of a metacarpophalangeal (MCP)/metatarsophalangeal (MTP) (fetlock) joint passes straight through the centre of the proximal interphalangeal (pastern) and distal interphalangeal (coffin) joints.

- This should be a straight line with no angulations between each joint.
- It should also be parallel with the hoof axis.
- Feet should be trimmed to keep the hoof pastern axis (HPA) as straight as possible – even if the hoof axis is not at the correct angle as a result.

HOOF ANATOMY AND CONFORMATION 14.3

- An ideal HPA:
  - The HPA is parallel with the dorsal hoof wall and the heels.
  - A vertical line from the middle of the fetlock joint should align with the back of the heels.
  - A vertical line from the centre of the coffin joint should divide the hoof into two equally sized halves; this allows weight to be carried evenly.
  - Figure 14.3.3 shows the HPA in a horse, with almost straight HPA.

A broken forward HPA has been significantly associated with pain on flexion of the carpus of the same limb (Broster *et al.* 2009) in a study of 224 working horses in India and Pakistan.

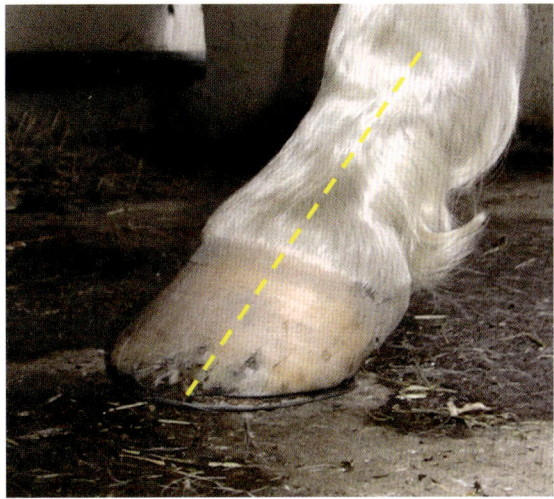

Figure 14.3.3 Hoof pastern axis shown by the yellow-dashed line.

Broken back HPA

> The angle of the dorsal hoof wall is behind the slope of the pastern (Figure 14.3.4).

This is a very common malformation which results in a number of different pathologies and lameness as a result of the incorrect strains placed on a limb. This foot conformation predisposes to navicular disease.

In a study by Broster *et al.* (2009) of 224 working horses from India and Pakistan, 81% of forelimbs and 47% of hindlimbs showed this conformation.

- The long toe delays break over.
- The low heel strains flexor tendons.
- Heel bruising
- Navicular disease
- Quarter and heel cracks
- Dorsal sole bruising
- Separation of the toe from the wall
- A broken back HPA should always be corrected even if the animal is currently sound. If left it will lead to pathology and lameness.
- This cannot be corrected in one trimming and requires multiple small trims to improve the conformation.

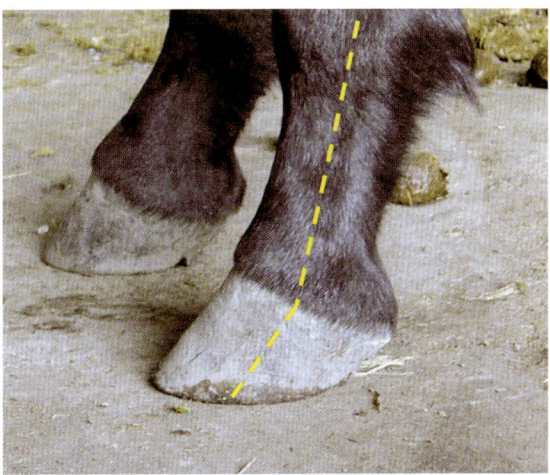

Figure 14.3.4 A broken back HPA

14 THE MUSCULOSKELETAL SYSTEM

- Trim the toe to reduce the toe length, leave the heels as much as possible to allow them to grow.
- If shoeing, ensure heels of shoe are extended to the position they are meant to be – e.g. level with the bulbs of the heel – not where the foot stops.

Broken forward HPA

> **The angle of the dorsal hoof wall is in front of the slope of the pastern (Figure 14.3.5).**

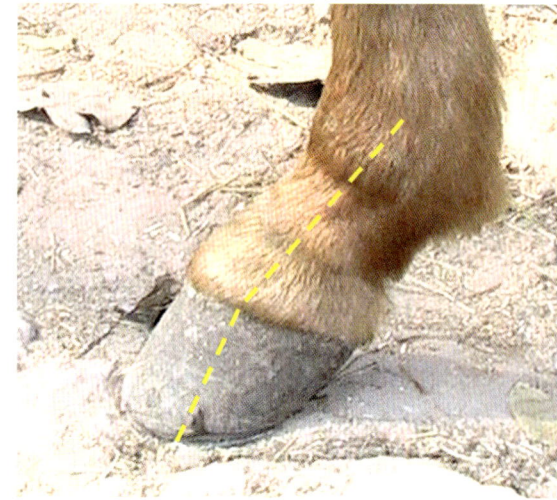

Figure 14.3.5 A broken forward HPA.

- Short toe
- High heel
- Places strain on the deep digital flexor tendon, proximal suspensory ligament, navicular bone and navicular bursa
- Injury to the extensor process of the pedal bone
- Osteoarthritis of the coffin joint
- Pedal osteitis (see Section 14.5 *The foot – Care and disease*)
- This cannot be corrected in one trimming and requires multiple small trims to improve the conformation.
- Gradually reduce heel to correct the conformation.

'Toe-in' and 'toe-out' conformation'

A line drawn through the centre of the dorsal aspect of the fetlock to the centre of the toe (in hindlimbs – plantar aspect of the fetlock to the centre of the heel) dividing the hoof into two equal parts should normally be a straight line (Figure 14.3.6). Problems arise with the toe-in and toe-out conformation.

Toe-in The axis slopes inwards, the medial side being longer and more sloping than lateral side.

Toe-out The axis slopes outwards, the lateral side being longer and more sloping than medial side (Figure 14.3.7).

Toe-out conformation has been reported by Broster *et al.* (2009) as significantly associated with pain on flexion of the MCP joint (in a study of 224 working horses in India and Pakistan).

Medial lateral foot balance

This is the balance of the medial (inside) hoof wall compared to the lateral (outside hoof wall) (Figure 14.3.8). Ensuring there is good medio-lateral balance is challenging and is an art that good farriers must master.

> **The aim of good medio-lateral balance is to ensure the animal's weight is loaded centrally over the foot.**

HOOF ANATOMY AND CONFORMATION 14.3

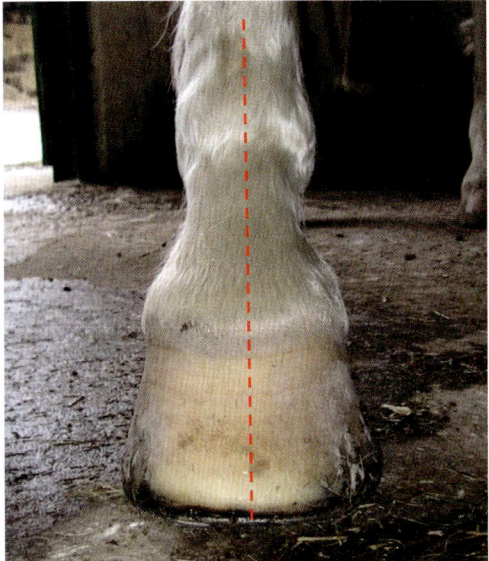

Figure 14.3.6 HPA of the forelimb from the dorsal (cranial) view.

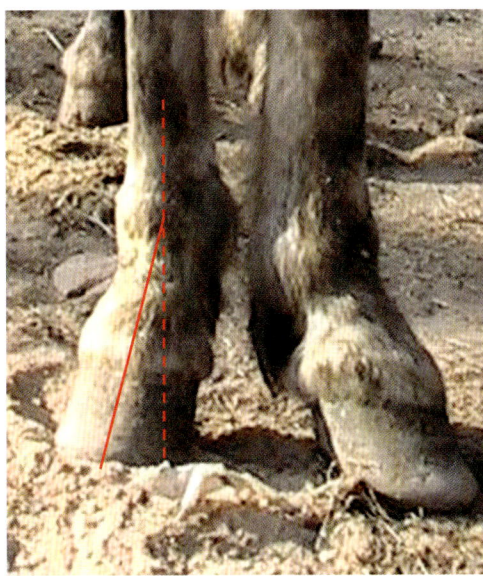

Figure 14.3.7 Bilateral toe-out in a working horse.

Altering the relative heights of the sides of the foot shifts the position of the hoof beneath the limb and changes the loading of the foot.

Lowering the inside of the foot will increase the load on the outside wall and, conversely, lowering the outside wall will increase the load on the inside wall.

Uneven loading of the foot has repercussions for the entire limb as the forces up the limb will also be uneven; this puts increased strains on joints, tendons and muscles.

> **The medial and lateral walls of the foot should strike the ground at the same time.**

To achieve this, trim the hoof so the ground surface is perpendicular to the midline of the horse.

Make the following checks:

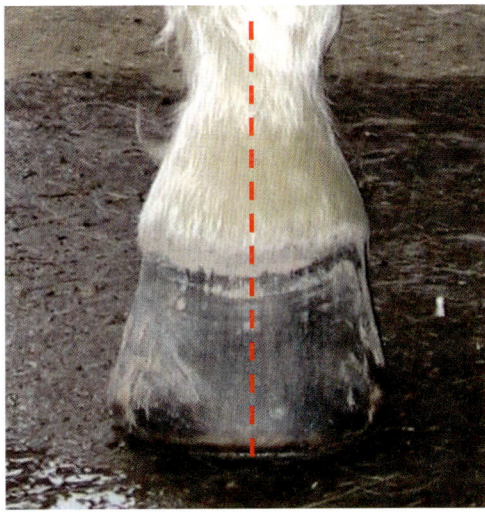

Figure 14.3.8 Foot showing medio-lateral foot balance – remember the foot should land as flat as possible to encourage even weight bearing.

- Pick up the foot and hold the leg by resting the cannon gently in one hand – so the foot is not being supported but is hanging down. This allows the trimmer to **assess the weight-bearing surface of the foot** and takes into account any natural conformational deviations the horse may have.

- The medial and lateral sides of the foot should look even – so the weight-bearing surface is flat.

- Always watch the equid walking.
- Watch the equid walk away and back to see if one side of the foot is landing before the other. If this is happening, trim the side that is landing first slightly shorter so the foot lands flat on the floor.
- Re-check the hoof landing when walking.
- Some equids' conformation means their foot will never land flat. In these cases overzealous trimming to achieve this can be very counterproductive. Therefore, correct the foot as far as possible but do not necessarily expect it to be perfect. Make any changes gradually over a number of trimmings.
- Assessing the hoof wear prior to trimming can also be helpful – if one side is much shorter than the other side make sure less is trimmed off this side.

Imbalance of the feet of working equids has been reported in one study by Upjohn *et al.* (2012). Of 312 working horses in Lesotho, 52% in the forefeet and 37% in the hindfeet had either medio-lateral or dorsopalmar/plantar imbalance. In another study of 214 working horses in India and Pakistan by Broster *et al.* (2009) hoof imbalance was reported in as high as 92% of forefeet examined. Differences in these studies were seen in a number of areas: fewer than 25% of horses in Lesotho were shod, whilst 85% of horses in India and Pakistan were shod, possibly indicating a link between shoeing and poor foot balance. Also the horses in India and Pakistan were urban and more likely to be working longer, harder hours and over tougher terrain than the rural horses in Lesotho.

Donkey and mule feet

Differences exist between the feet of horses and donkeys (Walker *et al.* 1995; Thiemann *et al.* 2013). A donkey's feet are smaller and more 'boxy' (Figure 14.4.2); the angle of the hoof wall is more upright than that of the horse. A donkey's hoof is more prone to becoming deformed as the result of a higher moisture content in the hoof wall. Radiographic anatomy differs between horses and donkeys (Collins *et al.* 2011). There is a paucity of information available on mule feet; however, texts indicate that they should be cared for in the same way as donkey feet (Svendson 2008).

Trimming and shoeing

14.4

Study the anatomy and conformation of the hoof first (see Section 14.3).

Responsibility of the owner

> A healthy foot is vital to the fitness of an equid and its ability to work. Encourage owners to carry out daily foot checking and cleaning as part of a complete preventative healthcare programme.

Owners need to be aware of what signs to look out for to identify foot problems early; emphasise that any penetrating injury to the sole requires immediate attention and a tetanus prophylaxis (consisting of tetanus antitoxin and tetanus toxoid). Repeat the tetanus toxoid 4–6 weeks later in animals with no known vaccination history.

The importance of good farriery cannot be overstated. If animals are shod, encourage owners to replace shoes that are worn, broken or too small. Regular inspection by a good farrier for trimming/shoeing should be encouraged; urge owners to seek out and strengthen existing farriery services in the local areas.

Responsibility of the veterinarian

The longer a foot problem is present the more difficult it is to correct. Advice given to owners and farriers when foot abnormalities are mild can prevent painful lameness and irreversible arthritis in the future. This is a crucial time when welfare can be improved.

Examine the feet of every equid irrespective of its presenting problem.

Early identification and correction of foot abnormalities may prevent chronic changes. Many causes of lameness affect more than one foot even if the animal only appears to be lame on one leg. When examining an animal check all four feet so that early signs of disease in the other feet are treated at the same time.

Demonstrate foot care to owners and farriers as this has more impact than verbal instructions. Clear advice to farriers can help prevent problems from recurring although, in some cases, it may be impossible to return the foot to a pain-free and functional state. Have a good knowledge of the availability and quality of farrier services in the area and, if necessary, advise the regional government or animal health NGOs of the potential for strengthening local services.

Foot problems and lameness must be tackled on a holistic basis. In order for there to be a decrease in such problems, owners and farriers need to be able to apply many of the preventative measures available. If owners do not have the option of a good farriery service, the local animal health provider has a responsibility to help rectify the situation.

Trimming the foot

Farriery is not a task routinely carried out by veterinarians; however, it is essential that poor trimming is recognised and addressed. Trimming should be done regularly every 6–12 weeks depending on the rate of hoof growth and wear. The trimming approach for each hoof differs, and it is important to attend a farriery course if this work is to be carried out regularly.

Outlined below are the basic steps to trimming a normal hoof. For further information consult other texts (e.g. Ross and Dyson 2003).

1. **Sole** Remove the flaky/chalky material of the sole so that the sole callous is observed in the toe area. The sole callous is the raised area just inside the hoof wall. The sole is naturally cupped from side to side as well as from front to back. The shape should be slightly concave and the correct thickness is when very slight movement can be felt with thumb pressure.

   Trimming the sole is critical to foot balance and it is essential that the correct amount is removed. Remove too much and the sole will be thin resulting in bruising, remove too little and the sole will be too thick. This limits foot expansion and the hoof's ability to act as a shock absorber. In normal feet very little sole needs to be removed; continuously check with digital pressure to ensure that the sole is not too thin. The sole should never bleed during routine trimming. The bars are trimmed only to remove overgrown or deformed horn.

2. **Hoof wall** Rasp or nip back the hoof wall to just above the level of the sole callous. Continue this round on each side of the toe. At this point if the toe is overly long it, too, should be trimmed back appropriately. Trim the toe last. Trim the wall using the hoof pastern axis and the angle of the wall at the coronary band as a guide. Always keep the plane of the cut parallel to the ground – a common fault is to cut the wall at 45 degrees or more so that the sole inside the white line is bearing all the weight. This is called 'dumping the toe' (the second photo Figure 14.4.6), and will cause pain and lameness. *When trimming the wall of the foot ensure that both sides are the same height* by carefully comparing one to the other; this will keep the foot level and symmetrical.

3. **Heel** Flatten the heel so that each side is equal (and at the same level as the frog buttress). The sole is then rasped back for one or two strokes only so it is flat and level ensuring medio-lateral balance.

4. **Frog** The frog is trimmed to remove loose and overgrown flaps which trap dirt and are prone to thrush. The cleft of the frog can be trimmed to reduce bacterial infection. Trim back the sulci to the frog so that mud can fall out and isn't trapped. Trimming the rest of the frog is not recommended as the frog should touch the ground when the animal is standing although the majority of the weight bearing is through the wall and the bars. *The frog should contact the ground first;* over-trimming the frog is a common and serious problem which leads to pain, thrush and contracted heels and contributes to arthritis by increasing concussion.

5. **Dorsal hoof wall** Rasping of the outer hoof wall may be necessary to form a straight line from top to bottom but it is important that the white line is not breached. The wall should be straight from the coronet to the floor surface with no indents or curves (wall flare). Bring the foot forward to dress wall flare. Use a rasp to smooth the edges but do not rasp a lot of horn from the front of the wall or it will be too thin and brittle to bear weight. If the dorsal hoof wall is so overgrown that it is turned up at the toe it will require several trimmings to correct it. Never cut it all back at once as this will cause imbalance and pain; the sole needs time to grow out to allow normal weight bearing on the dorsal wall.

6. Rasp the rim of the hoof wall to remove sharp edges.

TRIMMING AND SHOEING 14.4

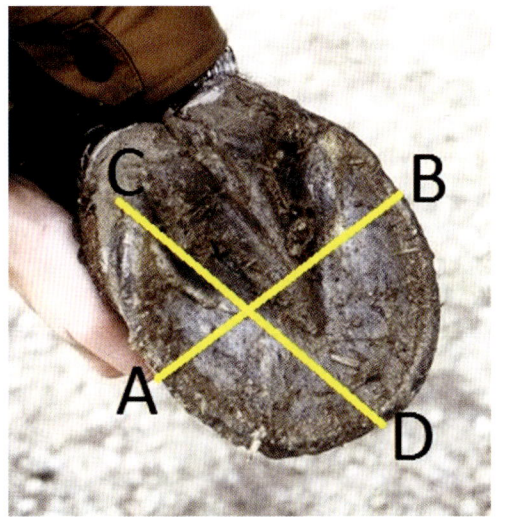

Figure 14.4.1 The line A–B indicates the width of the foot at the widest part, and line C–D indicates the length of the foot from the corner of one heel to the midpoint of the toe.

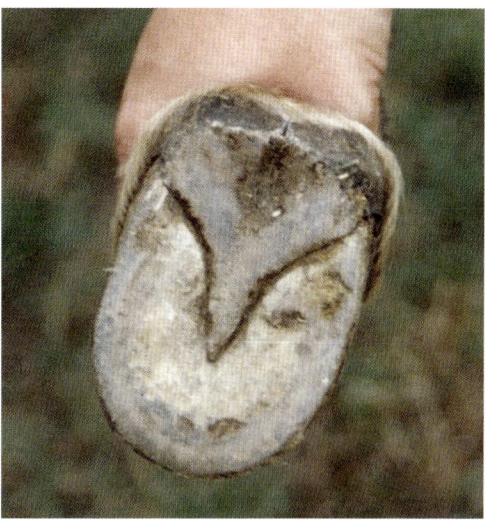

Figure 14.4.2 A normal donkey foot.

When trimming a hoof wall, shape the underside of the foot and follow the natural outline of the coronet band. As an approximate guide to the shape of the solar surface (Figure 14.4.1):

- **Front feet** The line A–B should be equal to C–D.
- **Hind feet** The line A–B should be slightly shorter than C–D (as hindfeet are slightly narrower).
- **Donkeys** The feet are always narrower (see Figure 14.4.2).

Work in the field

Trimming in the field (Figure 14.4.3) can present a number of challenges:

- **Animals may have received very little or no farriery or trimming and therefore hoof conformation can be extremely poor and overgrowths dramatic.**
  - It is not possible to correct this in one trimming – changes need to be made gradually as dramatic trimming can cause increased stress and lameness/injuries.
  - Owner education is critical – encouraging owners to have feet trimmed regularly is essential.

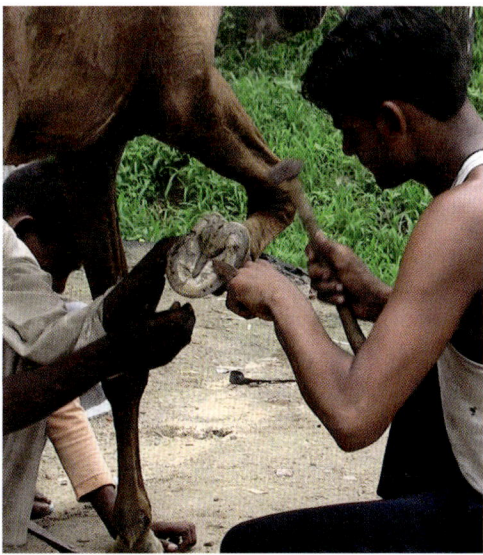

Figure 14.4.3 A hoof being trimmed in the field in India.

14 THE MUSCULOSKELETAL SYSTEM

▍ **Feet can be very hard and difficult to trim.**
  - Source sharp hoof knives, locally whenever possible, and keep them in good condition.
  - If feet are very hard, soaking them in warm water for 10 minutes prior to trimming can help soften them.

▍ **Hooves are often in very poor condition with brittle, poor quality hoof horn.**
  - Owner education about proper nutrition is essential as this will greatly improve horn quality.
  - Teaching owners how to pick out and clean hooves can make a marked difference to hoof health. Encourage them to incorporate it as part of a daily grooming routine – simple prevention and management can greatly reduce the incidence of diseases such as thrush.

Figure 14.4.4 depicts untrimmed feet with poor foot care showing overgrowths which will be putting increased stress on the joints. Notice that the horn quality is also poor and brittle with cracks in both toes. Figure 14.4.5 shows a well-trimmed, balanced foot where the horn quality looks good and healthy with no cracks.

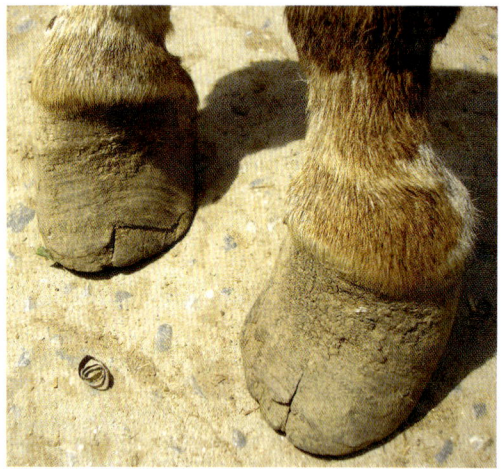

Figure 14.4.4 These hooves are overgrown and show poor conformation.

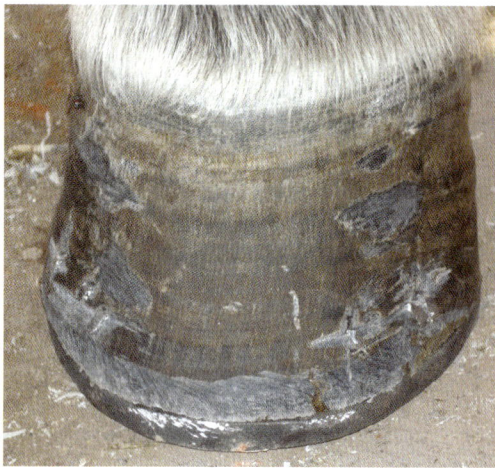

Figure 14.4.5 A hoof that is well balanced after trimming.

'To shoe or not to shoe?'

▍ While many people rely on shoeing, poor or incorrect shoeing can do a great deal of damage (Figures 14.4.6, 14.4.7 and 14.4.8).
  - **Nail placement must be very accurate** and go via the insensitive laminae only. If a nail pricks the deeper sensitive laminae underneath the horn this will be very painful and allow the introduction of infection, ultimately resulting in a foot abscess. For more information on nail bind and hoof abscess see Section 14.5.
  - **Shoes must be fitted accurately**. Shoe placement determines where on the foot weight is distributed. If the shoe is in the wrong place, or is too large or too small, weight will not be distributed evenly around the wall, and areas such as the sole might, as a consequence, be weight bearing. This will inevitably lead to lameness and will also distort future growth of the hoof resulting in deformed hooves with very poor conformation.

- **Shoes must be changed regularly.** To avoid complications, shoes should be replaced every 4–6 weeks. Shoes need to be removed as the hoof grows so that the feet can be trimmed to maintain an accurate fit. Moreover, in working animals shoes will wear out and, once wear has occurred, they should be replaced.

> Many equids cope well without shoes and, if they are coping well and are not working a lot on tarmac roads, most are best left unshod.
>
> If owners are already using shoeing it is vital that they are educated about hoof care and the requirement for regular replacement and trimming.

Figure 14.4.6 shows a shoe that is placed too far palmar (caudal/to the back) on the foot and does not follow the circumference of the hoof wall. This will be distributing the horse's weight incorrectly and will result in foot pain and lameness.

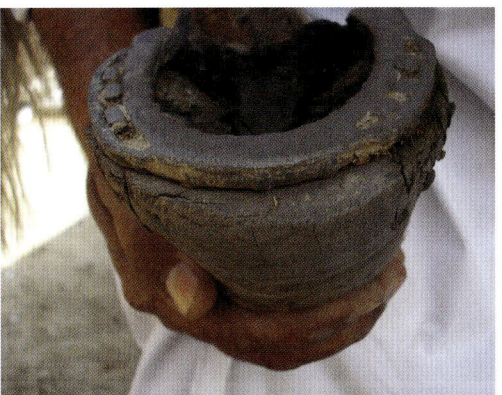
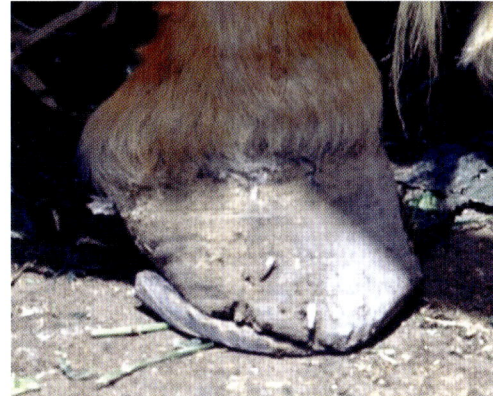

Figure 14.4.6 Poorly fitted shoes.

Figure 14.4.7 shows shoes that have been half worn away. This will be result in unbalanced loading of the hoof. Shoes should be replaced regularly to avoid reaching this stage of wear. This will greatly reduce foot pain and lameness and therefore is a great benefit for the equid and also the owner.

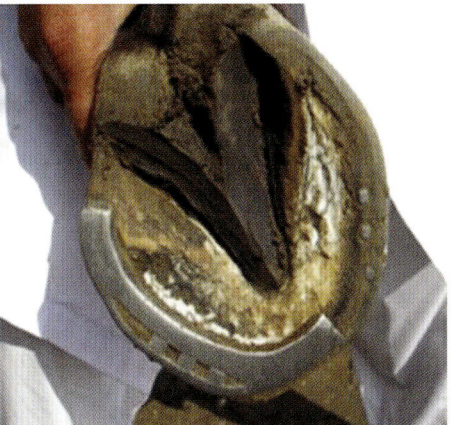
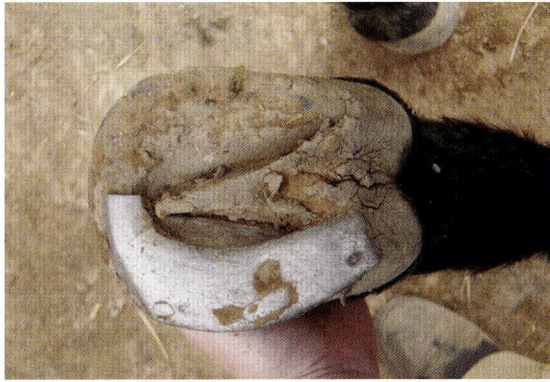

Figure 14.4.7 Shoes that have been half worn away or cracked.

Figure 14.4.8 shows a horse shod in Afghanistan with a shoe that crosses over at the heel. This will produce an imbalanced foot, placing unequal stress on the limb.

Figure 14.4.9: Note in this well-trimmed and shod foot the frog has not been trimmed back too far but the frog sulci (grooves either side of the frog) are clean and tidy. The frog expands into these sulci when the foot bears weight and this is part of the shock absorbing mechanism that reduces the impact on the joints in the limb.

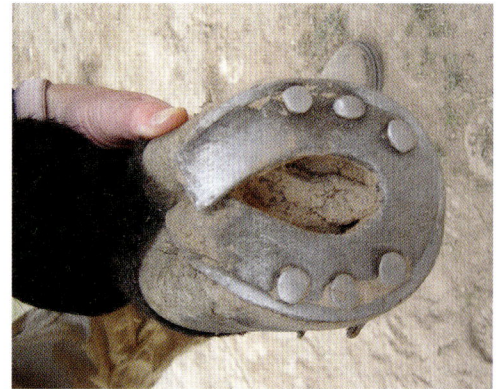

Figure 14.4.8 A horse shod in Afghanistan with a shoe that crosses over at the heel.

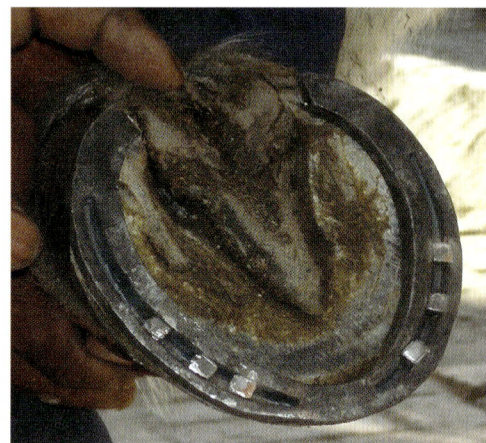

Figure 14.4.9 A well-trimmed foot and correctly placed shoe.

Conditions affecting the hoof 14.5

> 'No hoof, no horse' (or mule, or donkey!)

The equine foot is subject to continuous concussion which causes wear on both internal and external structures.

> Poor hoof care and farriery predisposes the animal to injury and infection, and can result in changes to the size, shape and function of the hoof.

The foot is a common site of both acute and chronic pain leading to lameness. Untreated diseases and abnormalities of the foot can create long-term problems in other parts of the leg due to changes in gait and weight bearing.

Conditions affecting the hoof wall

Overgrowth/overwear

If an animal has normal conformation and no shoes (unshod), there should be a balance between growth and wear of the wall.

Overgrowth occurs:

- when unshod animals are kept on soft ground
- in shod animals, when shoes are left on too long or the feet are not trimmed properly (Figure 14.5.1)
- in animals with poor conformation/injuries/lameness as the weight is not distributed evenly over the whole hoof.

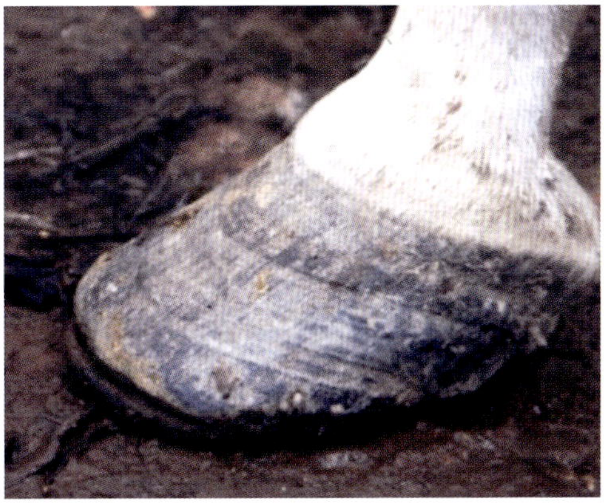

Figure 14.5.1 The shoe has been left on too long and the hoof wall is overgrown. This shoe should be removed and the hoof trimmed.

Overwear occurs:

- when unshod animals are worked excessively on hard ground (Figure 14.5.2)
- when pain, poor conformation, poor hoof balance or bad shoeing cause the animal to land unevenly on the foot
- when the shoe frequently wears or cracks in one particular area.

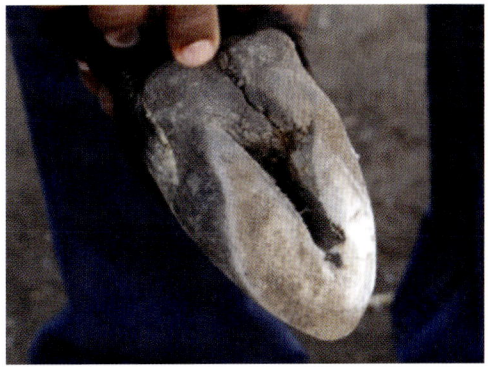

Figure 14.5.2 An example of an overworn hoof.

373

Treatment

- Identify and correct the underlying problem. Removing the cause of pain will correct mild overwear as the animal starts to bear weight evenly again.
- Correct moderate to severe uneven wear with trimming. If the problem is permanent (e.g. arthritic pain or poor conformation) trim the feet regularly (see Section 14.4 *Trimming and shoeing*)
- Returning the hoof to a perfect balance may not be possible.
- Never over-trim the wall to compensate for abnormal foot wear.

Hoof cracks: 'Grass cracks' or 'sand cracks'

Hoof cracks are classified as 'grass cracks' if they start from the ground (Figure 14.5.3) or 'sand cracks' if they start from the coronary band. Sometimes cracks can cover the whole extent of the hoof wall from the coronary band to the ground surface (Figure 14.5.4).

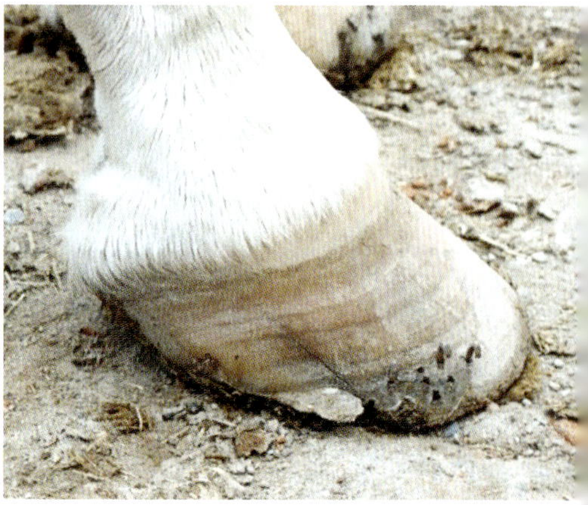

Causes

- Dehydrated and brittle hoof horn
- Damage from shoe removal
- Excessively overgrown feet
- 'Seedy toe' (see 'laminitis' later in this chapter)
- Abnormal foot shape or poor shoe placement
- Damage to the coronary band

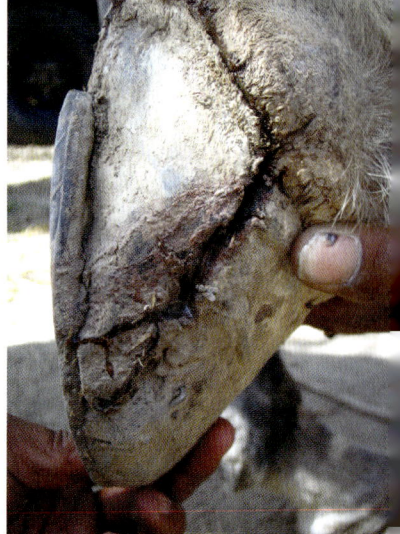

Figure 14.5.3 A grass crack in the lateral quarter of the hoof extends from the ground to approximately halfway up the hoof wall.

Diagnosis

Most cracks do not cause lameness as the full thickness of the wall is not penetrated. Lameness and a pain response are seen with deeper cracks as these can become infected or pinch the sensitive laminae. Swelling, heat and pain are present at the coronary band as infection tracks up the wall.

Treatment

The aim of treatment is to stabilise the crack and keep it clean and dry. If dirt fills the crack it will put pressure on the edges forcing it further apart. For deep hoof cracks, with infection and lameness, treat as for a hoof abscess (see later in this chapter). Stabilise the crack using quarter clips either side or with the use of adhesives to limit hoof expansion during weight bearing to **reduce movement across the crack**. When cracks occur in the area of the quarters, trim the wall near the heels so that the wall

Figure 14.5.4 A severe crack passing from ground surface through the coronary band.

either side of the crack is non-weight bearing. This allows the heel and the frog to bear the weight rather than the cracked area. Do not make a horizontal groove in the horn across the top of the crack as this weakens the hoof.

Prognosis

Good for cracks that are not infected and do not reach the coronary band. Healing of infected cracks depends on complete removal of all necrotic tissue. Permanent damage to the laminae can result in abnormal horn growth, separating the wall from the underlying tissue and causing further cracking. Cracks that originate from the coronary band have a poor prognosis as normal horn will not re-grow. Prevent hoof cracks with good farriery and good nutrition. Soak dry or brittle hooves in water, and coat in hoof grease to retain moisture.

Hoof avulsion

Avulsion of the hoof occurs when there is separation of the hoof wall from the internal structures. Exposure of the sensitive laminae and pedal bone results in severe pain and lameness, infection and osteitis.

Causes

- Trauma
- Severe febrile diseases
- Laminitis
- Administering corticosteroids to a laminitic patient (iatrogenic)

Treatment

Damage to the coronary band affects horn growth so the prognosis is poor. If the area of separation is small, attempt treatment by flushing the area, bandaging and administering antibiotics and NSAIDs.

> The most humane treatment, especially in total hoof avulsion, is euthanasia. Explain to the owner that the horn will not re-grow.

Club foot

An abnormally shaped upright foot (Figure 14.5.5)

Causes

- Congenital or acquired flexural deformity of the deep digital flexor tendon
- Prolonged disuse or chronic limb pain (a common example is from a hoof abscess) causing tendon contraction, pulling the pedal bone into a more upright position

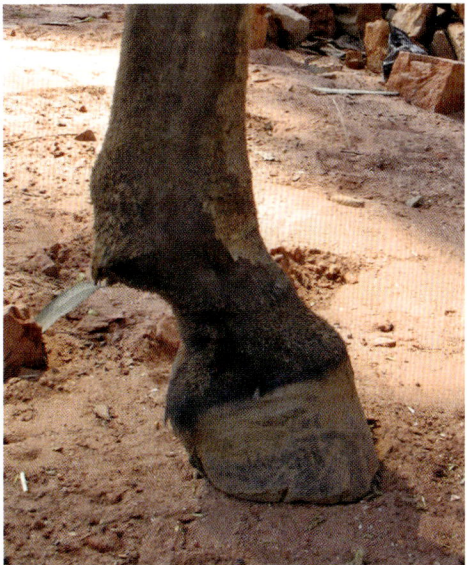

Figure 14.5.5 An upright or club foot.

Diagnosis

Club foot is diagnosed if the axis of the toe exceeds 60 degrees; the foot will also have high heels as a result. Often only one foot is affected; bilateral conditions tend to be congenital. In acute cases the heel will not touch the ground – 'walking on the toe'. If the club foot is chronic, the heels become overgrown and contracted and the dorsal hoof wall will be concave. Lameness is variable; some animals adapt their gait and are not lame.

Treatment

For acute cases, identify and remove the source of pain (e.g. hoof abscess) and use NSAIDs to encourage relaxation of the tendons. The prognosis for return to normal shape is guarded. If the club foot is chronic, trim the hoof regularly and keep the foot balanced. Do not try to return it to the 'correct' shape, as this will cause lameness; when the heel is lowered dramatically this puts a great deal of pressure and stretch on the flexor tendons. Toe abscesses are common, so protect the toe region from over wear.

Conditions affecting the sole and frog

All of these conditions are exacerbated by inadequate attention to:

- hoof hygiene; removing stones, mud or faeces (Figure 14.5.6)
- contamination of standing areas with sharp objects and stones, dirt, faeces and urine.

Demonstrate to owners how to check and clean the feet and keep the frog area clean and dry. Address any signs of frog abnormality or a foul smell immediately.

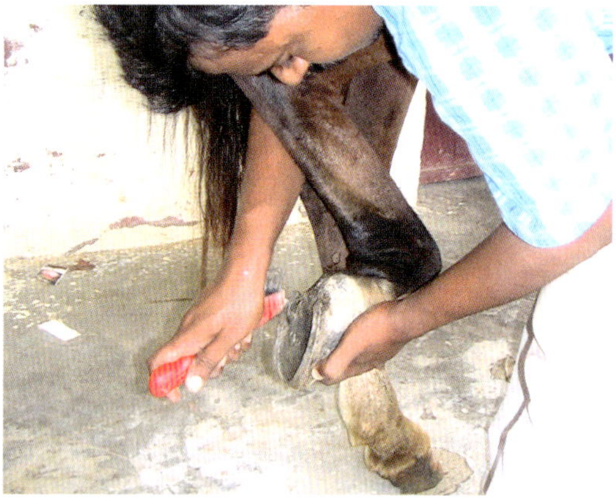

Figure 14.5.6 Basic hoof hygiene is simple but often neglected.

Puncture wounds and hoof abscesses

Causes

- Stone and foreign bodies, e.g. nails (Figure 14.5.7), can pierce the sole, leading to the introduction of anaerobic bacteria and abscess formation.
- Faulty/defective attachment of the shoe can result in 'nail prick' when the nail punctures the sensitive tissues of the hoof, or 'nail bind' when the nail applies pressure to the lamellae without directly touching the tissues.

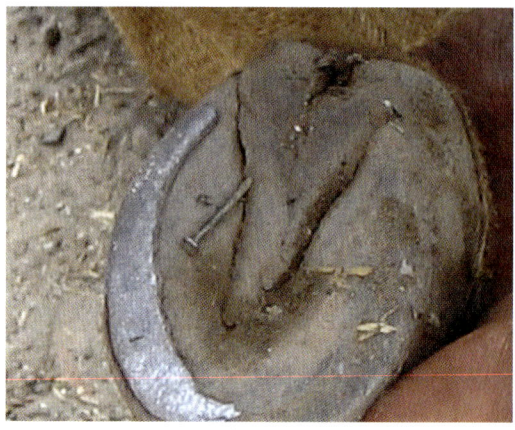

Figure 14.5.7 Nail found penetrating the frog.

Diagnosis

Severe, acute lameness; this can be mistaken by the owner as a fracture. There is often increased heat in the foot with a 'bounding' digital pulse. Following a puncture wound, infection may run up the white line or under the sole and break out at the coronary band or heel bulbs. With a penetrative injury the foreign object may still be in the sole when the equid is examined.

> **The location and depth of penetration will greatly affect prognosis.**

A penetrative injury to the middle third of the frog is the most serious as it can easily pierce the navicular bursa and/or coffin joint. This may lead to an unresponsive infection resulting in severe lameness. In such cases recommend euthanasia on welfare grounds.

Treatment

Carefully remove the foreign body if present; ensure adequate drainage through the site of penetration. Pare out the hole if the diameter is very small to prevent sealing over and abscess formation. For a suspected abscess remove the shoe and use hoof testers around the wall, sole and frog to localise the site of pain. Pay particular attention to the nail-holes, which may be the site of pain or infection ('nail-prick' or 'nail-bind').

Use a hoof knife to pare the sole and white line until they are clean, looking for a black spot at the site of penetration. Follow the black area until the origin of the abscess is opened (Figure 14.5.8). Paring the sole can be extremely painful; in this case an abaxial nerve block may be given. The foot will then be desensitised so hoof testers are no longer useful. Ensure that the location of the tract is clear before the block is performed.

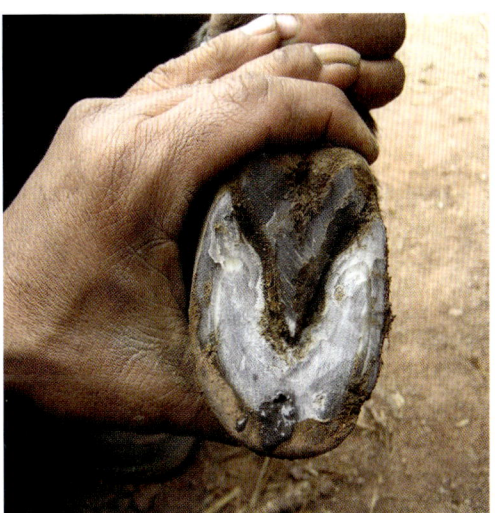

Figure 14.5.8 Foot abscess with sole pared to release purulent material.

Stop paring the foot if fresh blood appears. Paring out the wound removes contamination and allows aeration, thus reducing anaerobic bacterial infection.

> **Antibiotics are not necessary and will not work if the infection is localised, due to poor blood supply to the sole tissue. The equid must be vaccinated against tetanus as the hoof could easily become contaminated with dirt containing *Clostridium tetani*.**

If the animal is not vaccinated, or the vaccination history is unknown, then administer tetanus prophylaxis.

In all cases, drainage is most important for successful treatment.

Soak the whole foot for 10 minutes in a bucket of water containing magnesium sulphate or dilute povidone-iodine. Ask the owner to repeat this twice a day until the animal becomes sound. It may be appropriate to keep the wound covered/bandaged until fully healed to prevent re-infection. Change this dressing daily to keep the wound fresh and dry.

In rare cases, a deep puncture wound to the central zone of the foot, near the frog, can cause fracture of the navicular bone or septic navicular bursitis (see Section 14.6). If an animal develops severe lameness within a few days following a puncture of this nature, and does not respond to intensive therapy, the prognosis is very poor; discuss euthanasia with the owner.

White line disease

This is an infection of the white line – the junction of the insensitive laminae of the hoof wall and the horn of the sole. This is a natural weak region of the hoof; poor, brittle or soft horn will result in a defect at the white line and subsequent infection. Damp or very dry conditions will also predispose the animal to white line disease.

Diagnosis

The white line may appear widened and is often packed with necrotic material. If left untreated, infection can track up to the coronary band.

Treatment

Remove the necrotic horn. The foot can then be stood in magnesium sulphate solution or dilute povidone-iodine as for foot abscesses. Keep the foot clean and dry. Show the owner how to clean the white line and repeat the soaking if necessary.

Solar bruising

Solar bruising is the result of an impact to the sole that causes haemorrhage in the solar chorium. This may occur if the animal is working on stony or rocky ground or if the soles are thin as the result of poor farriery or regular work on hard surfaces.

Diagnosis

- A dark red or purple area on the white sole, seen after light paring with a hoof knife
- Pain response to hoof testers
- Mild to moderate lameness, usually worse on hard/rough ground. Lameness may be unapparent when the ground is soft.

Treatment

NSAIDs and rest to reduce pain. Treatment with formalin will toughen the solar surface; however, this chemical is dangerous to human and environmental health. Good prognosis for full recovery if the initial cause can be identified and managed.

Prevention

Discourage fast work over rough or stony ground as this exacerbates the problem. Excessive paring of the sole by the farrier makes it thin and susceptible to bruising.

Corns

Corns are bruises between the bars and the hoof wall, usually as a result of poor shoe maintenance, and are most common on the medial side of the front feet. Corns are caused when the shoe is too small or narrow at the heel – common when standards of farriery are poor. Also, when shoes are left on too long, the growth causes the shoe to be pulled forward and the shoe branch then impacts on the region most prone to corns.

Diagnosis

Lameness of varying degrees, and pain when pressing the area. Paring will reveal a soft, red/purple area between the bars and wall (Figure 14.5.9). Secondary bacterial infection may occur.

Treatment

Remove the old shoe and replace; the corn will self-heal if there is no infection. If infection is present, treat as a sole abscess (described earlier in this chapter).

Prognosis

Good, but the discoloured horn will take several weeks to grow out. Demonstrate the cause of corns to owners and farriers. Emphasise the importance of using large shoes with wide-set heels, fitting shoes correctly and replacing them regularly.

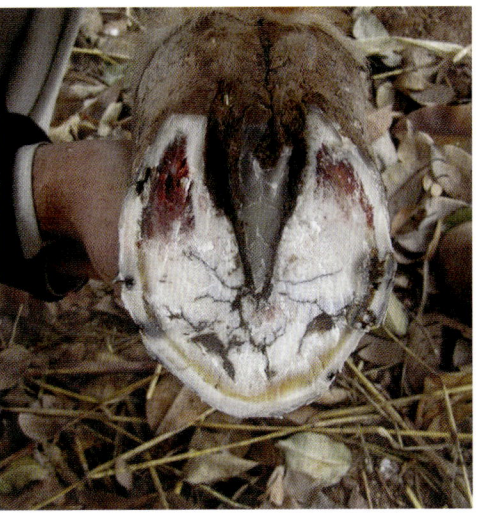

Figure 14.5.9 Corns present on medial and lateral heel angles.

Thrush

This is a bacterial infection of the grooves (central or collateral sulci) of the frog (Figure 14.5.10). The infection usually occurs when the condition of the frog degenerates as the result of a dirty environment and irregular cleaning. Excessive trimming of the frog and contracted heels result in a small deep-set frog with poor air circulation to the area. The predominant infective pathogen is *Fusobacterium necrophorum*.

Diagnosis

Lameness occurs only in severe cases; milder forms are usually unnoticed by owners. A characteristic foul smell comes from the frog due to anaerobic bacteria. The thick black discharge in the sulci may be hidden by flaps of overgrown frog.

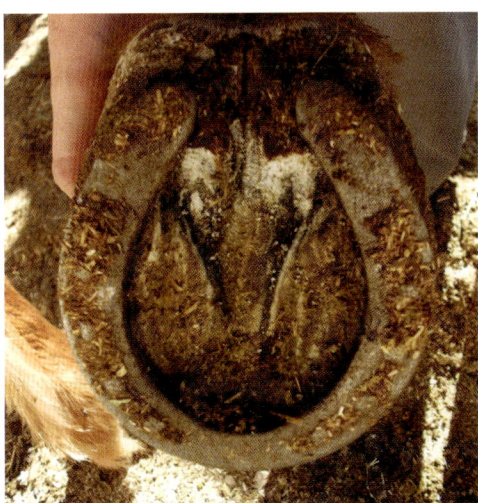

Figure 14.5.10 A thrush infection in the central and collateral sulci of the frog.

Treatment

Trim any horn flaps and improve the foot shape to allow more air to reach the sulci. Clean with dilute povidone-iodine, repeat daily until the infection is cleared. Do not bandage the foot as it is important to aerate the affected area. Antibiotics are unnecessary unless deeper structures are affected.

Prognosis

Good, but thrush will recur if the underlying problems are not corrected. Demonstrate the cause to owners and farriers. Encourage farriers to trim heels correctly and ensure that the frog comes into contact with the ground/is bearing weight.

> **Advise the owner to clean the feet daily and keep the horse on a dry standing area (remove faeces, urine and damp bedding daily).**

Canker

Cause

Canker is a proliferative dermatitis that occurs as the result of a chronic infection of the frog and surrounding tissues by *Bacteriodes* spp., spirochetes and possibly bovine papilloma virus. This condition may initially be confused with thrush but can be differentiated by a foul, necrotic odour and the presence of granulation-like tissue. It is common in animals standing for long periods in wet, dirty conditions and in warm climates.

Diagnosis

- Frog horn loosens to reveal foul-smelling, proliferative granulation tissue (Figure 14.5.11).
- Instead of the usual flat, uniform horn, filamentous fronds of horn develop.
- Thick, cream-coloured exudate
- Pain and associated lameness
- Bleeds easily and is very susceptible to screw-worm maggots

Treatment

The treatment is likely to be difficult and prolonged. Debride the granulation tissue thoroughly; this may require a nerve block and a tourniquet. Apply topical metronidazole and bandage to keep the foot dry. Change daily for 10 days.

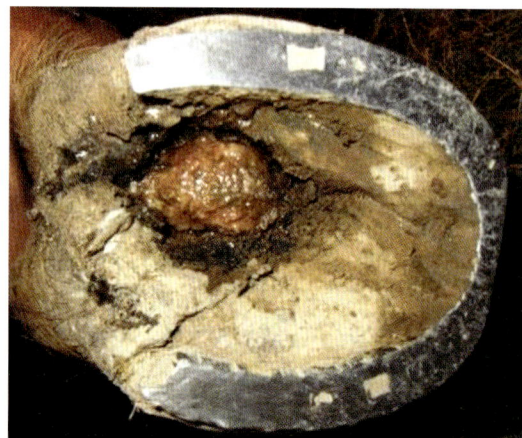

Figure 14.5.11 Canker present in a foot of a working equid.

Prognosis

Recurrence is common and treatment requires veterinary attention over a long period. Treatment may be successful if initiated early in disease course.

Conditions affecting the heels

Traumatic heel wounds

The heel is susceptible to traumatic injuries such as laceration with sharp sheet metal, or from kicking a sharp object. Often there is profuse bleeding, especially if a digital artery has been severed at the pastern.

Treatment

Ligate the artery if there is severe bleeding. Clean, debride and apply a pressure bandage; 'proud flesh' is very common following injuries in this location. Decrease motion and stabilise the hoof. Suturing is contra-indicated due to the high rate of wound breakdown in this area.

Prognosis

Usually good unless cartilage has been damaged. If the lateral cartilages are damaged there may be delayed healing or quittor (chronic infection of the cartilaginous extension of the pedal bone). If the digital flexor tendons are involved and have been cut, the prognosis for return to work is extremely poor (see Section 14.8).

Contracted heels

Cause

- Shoes that are too small and narrow at the heel prevent natural expansion as the foot hits the ground.
- Excessive paring of the frog prevents it from contacting the ground and induces frog atrophy.
- Inadequate trimming of the heels leads to an upright foot with a broken-forward hoof-pastern axis.

Over time, repeated placement of a small, tight shoe causes the foot to become smaller and more upright, with a very concave sole and small ineffective frog (Figure 14.5.12). This contributes to other foot and leg abnormalities.

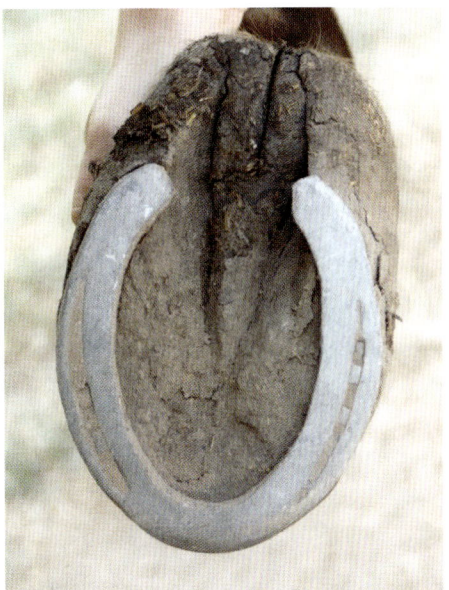

Figure 14.5.12 *The heels have narrowed creating a more oval-shaped hoof in this horse, with a diminished and ineffective frog.*

Treatment

Only good regular farriery will improve contracted heels. Shoes which are slightly larger laterally at the quarters and heels encourage hoof wall expansion (they may need to be custom-made for an individual). The frog should not be trimmed except to remove small ragged pieces.

Prognosis

Depends on severity and duration of heel contraction. It is poor in severe chronic cases where the joints and tendons have been secondarily affected by the abnormal hoof shape.

14 THE MUSCULOSKELETAL SYSTEM

Sheared heels

When one heel is longer than the other, the heel bulbs are subjected to a shearing force which can cause a breakdown of the tissue that normally holds the two heels together. This is usually the sequelae of faulty shoeing/trimming where one heel is left longer than the other.

Diagnosis

When an equid loads the foot, the heels move independently of each other as one heel bears all the weight. In severe cases the skin between the heels can be damaged by this movement and lesions or granulomas may develop. This imbalance can also lead to heel or quarter cracks.

Treatment

Allow the shorter heel to grow longer and match the other side. Good farriery can help support the heels and minimise further movement.

Heel dermatitis/'greasy heel'

Causes

- Wet, dirty standing conditions
- Hobbling with dirty rope or cloth
- Chorioptic mange (caused by Chorioptes mites)
- Photosensitisation on white lower legs

Diagnosis

Skin lesions are seen at the palmar or plantar aspect of the pastern and heel. The dermatitis is characterised by scab formation, moist/greasy exudate and erythema (Figure 14.5.13). The skin lesions are irritating and painful, although this condition rarely causes lameness. In chronic cases granulomatous round grape-like growths can develop, triggered as a result of persistent inflammation.

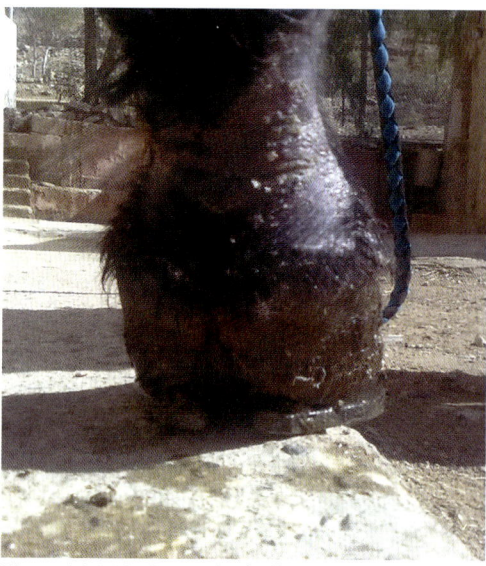

Figure 14.5.13 Greasy heel affecting a limb.

Treatment

Early diagnosis and treatment is essential to prevent the involvement of deeper structures. Clip hair from the area and clean twice a day with dilute povidone-iodine, removing all grease and scabs. Dry thoroughly and do not bandage; the aim is to dry out the skin. Antibiotics are not necessary as pharmacological penetration to this area is limited and good hygiene should resolve secondary infection. Administer antibiotics if cellulitis is present (see Section 15.3).

Prognosis

Good if the underlying cause is removed. Encourage owners to provide a clean, dry standing area and groom the legs daily to remove dirt. Dry heels with a cloth after equids have worked in wet conditions. It is important that hobbles, if used, are kept clean and well maintained.

Brushing and over-reaching

Both conditions are due to poor conformation or poor hoof balance resulting in an abnormal gait.

Brushing is an injury to the inside of the pastern/fetlock as the result of one hoof striking the other during movement (Figure 14.5.14). This may be exacerbated by poor placement of nails on shoes or poor conformation. Equids with 'cow hocks' will have brushing on the medial hocks.

Over-reaching is when the front heels are struck by the toes of the hindfeet during movement.

Treatment

Clean the area. These injuries often lie close to the fetlock joint; think about the potential for joint infection with chronic injury. Correct the underlying cause to prevent recurrence. Ensure the feet are balanced, the shoe is correctly placed, and the nails are knocked flat. In cases of over-reaching, shortening the toe of the front feet may speed break-over allowing the front feet to 'get out of the way' more quickly (Ross and Dyson 2003). Fit locally-made protection over the fetlocks and pasterns, such as a 'brushing ring' of twisted cloth or rubber around one fetlock to protect it from contact with the opposite foot. Working the animal too young (< 3 years) will contribute to poor carpal and hock conformation, as the bones are still developing.

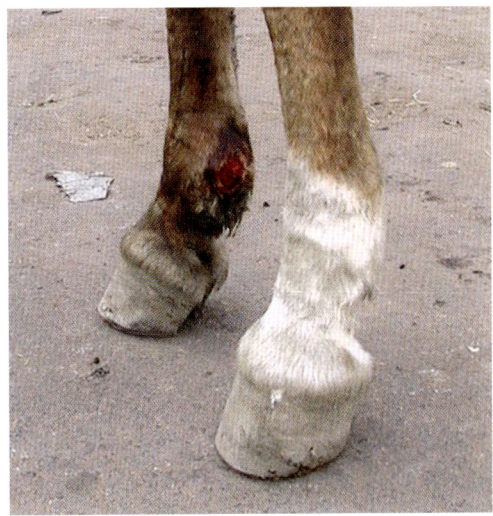

Figure 14.5.14 An example of a brushing injury.

Pedal osteitis

Pedal osteitis strictly refers to inflammation of the distal phalanx. However, it has been used to describe radiographic changes, principally demineralisation at the solar margin of this bone. Whether this is a proven disease and a cause of lameness is controversial (Ross and Dyson 2003).

Causes

Pedal osteitis is a result of persistent inflammation of the foot. It can be caused by a number of problems including: chronic solar bruising, chronic corns, laminitis, puncture wounds, deep untreated abscesses, etc. In some cases where infection is present, e.g. with a deep, chronic abscess, the pedal bone can be infected. However, the condition can occur without infection as a result of long-term persistent inflammation.

Diagnosis

Persistent lameness with a persistent reaction to hoof testers. Confirmation of diagnosis can be achieved with radiographs; however, observation of clinical signs can support an initial suspicion, without requiring further diagnostic tools.

Treatment

Prevent by the diagnosis and treatment of inflammatory conditions of the foot. Once pedal osteitis has developed treatment is limited so identify and treat the inciting cause.

14 THE MUSCULOSKELETAL SYSTEM

Laminitis

Severe inflammation and necrosis of the sensitive tissues (laminae) attaching the hoof to the pedal bone (P3)

Causes

- **Mechanical overload**
  Over-exercising on hard ground. Excessive weight bearing on one leg following lameness on the opposite limb. With any lameness examine the contra-lateral limb for signs of laminitis.

- **Bacterial endotoxin release into the blood**
  High carbohydrate intake. Iatrogenic veterinary-administered corticosteroids to treat a different condition or owner-administered corticosteroids to increase muscle and condition of animals.
  Systemic infection (toxaemia) from retained placenta (septic metritis), mastitis, enteritis, colitis, gastrointestinal torsion, pleuropneumonia, etc.

Pathogenesis

Laminitis is characterised by a failure of attachment of the epidermal laminae to the dermal laminae. The precise pathophysiology is yet to be determined. A vasoconstriction theory of laminitis aetiology, based on vascular pathology resulting in ischemia of the lamellar tissues, has been largely supplanted by the enzymatic theory in which matrix metalloproteinase enzymes (MMPs) are activated. MMPs at normal levels are responsible for enzymatic remodelling; when over-active, this enzyme causes destruction of lamellar tissues and separation. There are many experimental studies which attempt to determine the pathophysiology of laminitis. Reviews by Pollit (2004) and Eades (2010) provide a good overview.

Diagnosis

Characterised by an acute onset of severe lameness. Affected equids adopt a characteristic stance, most often the front limbs are affected and so the hindfeet are placed as far forward as possible with the forelimb pushed forwards to relieve weight bearing (Figure 14.5.15). The lameness in acute cases is severe; weight will be shifted from one side to the other, and affected equids are likely to spend long periods of time recumbent, sometimes with the legs stretched out. It can be difficult to examine the animal as there is often a refusal to walk or to lift the foot as this will increase pressure on the affected contra-lateral limb. Extreme pain is manifested as elevated respiration and heart rate.

On examination of the foot with hoof testers there is pain all over the sole,

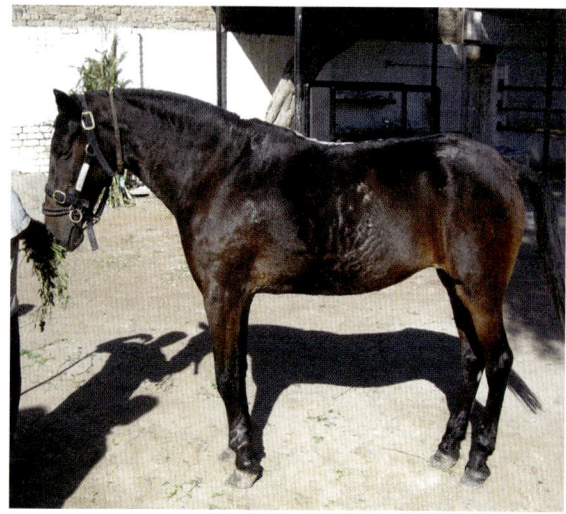

Figure 14.5.15 This horse has signs of chronic laminitis in all four feet. However, the typical leaning back stance is not seen due to joint changes in the forelimb fetlocks preventing this; note the firing over the four fetlock joint areas.

especially at the point of the frog. Bounding digital pulses (increase in amplitude) are palpable in most cases, and the feet will be hot in the early stage. Separation between the wall and underlying pedal bone causes sinking and rotation of P3 which can penetrate the sole in severe cases, seen as a creamy-white, blood-stained area in front of the frog. A depression at the coronary band may be observed as a result of the sinking and shearing forces as the pedal bone drops or rotates. In the working equid context, detection of this sign can give a useful indication of pedal bone movement when radiography is not available.

It is important to differentiate cases of acute laminitis from colic, both of which are painful conditions. Conduct a full examination. Hoof abscesses may also present with similar signs to laminitis; however, an abscess is likely to be unilateral.

Treatment

> **Acute laminitis is an emergency. If left untreated, the pedal bone may rotate through the sole in a few days, necessitating euthanasia.**

- Treat the underlying cause (retained placenta, systemic infection, grain overload, etc.).
- Do not move the animal anywhere, even to the mobile clinic, as concussion on the foot during movement will cause more sinking and rotation of the pedal bone.
- Complete rest is essential, in a confined area on a thick bed of sand, straw or any soft, conforming material to cushion the feet. It is imperative that rest is continued until soundness has completely returned once NSAID treatment has ceased.
- Working an animal too soon will re-trigger the laminitis which is likely to be more serious if it recurs. Convey this message clearly to owners.
- Mechanical foot supports for the distal phalanx; reduce concussion by applying thick padding firmly taped onto the frog/sole. Replace the foot supports as they become flattened. Frog supports are probably inappropriate for donkeys; cover the entire sole with a thick soft dressing.
- It may be necessary to nerve block the foot (abaxial sesamoid block) in order to apply frog supports.
- Do not walk the animal whilst feet are anaesthetised.
- In shod equids, ideally remove the shoes, as they concentrate the weight loading on the outside of the foot, closer to the laminae. Remove the shoes carefully to minimise concussive forces.
- Administer NSAIDs to ameliorate foot pain and suffering. Animals should be on complete rest whilst on medication.
- Corticosteroids have been linked to the development of laminitis in certain situations; avoid the use of these medications.
- Sedatives such acepromazine can be administered to encourage recumbency and reduce weight bearing and concussion within the hooves (van Eps 2010). A dose of 0.02–0.04 mg/kg intramuscularly or intravenously 4 times a day has been recommended for 3–5 days after the acute onset. It has been suggested that acepromazine is beneficial as a vasodilator. However, as the vasoconstriction theory of laminitis aetiology is unproven, this beneficial effect remains hypothetical.

- Administer **IV fluid therapy** if there are signs of shock.
- If the laminitis has been induced by a **grain overload**, pass a stomach tube to allow for reflux and to prevent gastric rupture. Then administer mineral oil/liquid paraffin. Ensure all grain is removed from the diet, feed a high fibre diet. Do not starve.
- **Cold-therapy** of the legs and feet has proven preventative experimentally. It appears to provide some analgesia and prevent progression of the laminitis. This can be achieved by standing an animal in buckets of cold or iced water or standing in a nearby stream.
- **Euthanasia** is recommended if the pedal bone has come through the sole, or if prolonged signs of pain cannot be alleviated by NSAID medication.

For further information on treatment refer to van Eps (2010).

Prognosis

> A severely rotated pedal bone is a very serious condition that is life threatening.

The outcome of treatment depends on many different aspects including:

- The animal's weight
- Degree of pain
- Degree of pedal bone rotation
- Degree of white line separation
- Sub-solar infection development
- Thickness of sole
- Environment animal is kept in
- Willingness of owner to treat and rest the animal

Permanent changes to the foot structure from a single bout of laminitis make the individual prone to repeated or chronic laminitis. Classic signs of chronic laminitis include: 'slipper-shaped' hoof, with low heels and a concave dorsal wall, and distinct rings of wall horn representing bouts of laminitis. Hoof growth is affected by laminitis – the heel is spared and grows faster than the toe. Divergent growth rings appear (Figure 14.5.16) which are normally parallel to the coronary band. A flat sole with indentation around the coronary band indicates movement of the pedal bone. A dark purulent discharge from the coronary band occurs after abscess formation between the separated lamellae. Bruising of the sole occurs due to movement of the pedal bone resulting in compression of the solar tissue. 'Seedy toe' appears as a wide area of crumbly horn at the dorsal white line which can become impacted with dirt and small stones. Animals with seedy toe are prone to white line abscesses and cracks in the dorsal wall. Pare out and trim the area regularly until the damaged horn has grown out completely.

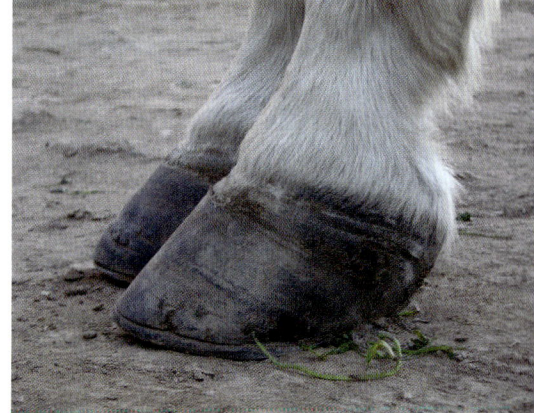

Figure 14.5.16 Typical growth patterns of chronic laminitis, where growth is faster at the heels than the toes leading to diverging lines around the hoof.

Trimming a chronic laminitic foot

> The basic principle of trimming a laminitic foot is to realign the pedal bone with the hoof wall after rotation. Trimming alone cannot force realignment but it does enable normal growth patterns to be re-established.

The main aims of therapeutic trimming are to reduce the distractive forces on the dorsal laminae in weight bearing and break over; to stabilise the pedal bone within the hoof capsule and unload the areas of pressure. Any abscesses that have formed must be drained.

Key principles

Reduce the heel area very gradually. If too much is removed in one trimming it will result in a great strain on the deep digital flexor tendon; this can lead to damage and encourage further rotation. It can be helpful to trim the toe from the ground surface to reduce the pressure on this region. The area just in front of the apex of the frog should not be trimmed. Therapeutic trimming needs to be regularly repeated every 4–6 weeks, sometimes for the rest of an animal's life.

Prevention of laminitis

Inform owners how to recognise the early symptoms of acute laminitis, as treatment in the first 24 hours will greatly decrease the likelihood of permanent damage or euthanasia. Avoid excessive or fast work on hard roads. Keep feet well-trimmed and balanced. Keep a high ratio of roughage to grain in the diet, with changes introduced slowly. Avoid heavy or long-term use of corticosteroids, a major cause of laminitis in some countries is due to owner administration of long-acting steroids (for example, this occurs with the wedding horses in India). This is a good example of the importance of working with all stakeholders on appropriate drug usage as a means of prevention.

Conditions affecting the bones 14.6

> Conditions affecting bones are usually serious. All bone conditions require complete long-term (weeks to months) rest, with a thick bed of sand or straw to lie on, to allow the bone to heal.

Even after recovery, the equid will need to be worked slowly and for shorter periods to prevent the problem recurring.

Young animals should pull a lighter load, work more slowly and for shorter periods than mature animals, to allow bones to grow and adapt to the work. Do not introduce an animal to a full load and full day's work until it is at least 3 years old.

Fractures

Causes

Most commonly, fractures are caused by trauma from accidents, kicks or falling. Fractures may occasionally be pathological due to tumours, infection or poor nutrition. However, this is rare in equids.

Diagnosis

Although radiographs will definitively diagnose fractures, observation of one or more of the following signs can support an initial suspicion, without requiring further diagnostic tools:

- Sudden onset of lameness, often **severe** or **non-weight-bearing**
- Heat, swelling and **pain** on palpation
- **Crepitus** (grating noise from the fractured ends of the bone). Auscultate with a stethoscope while gently manipulating affected limb.
- **Deviation** or alteration in the normal shape of the limb
- **Fractured ends** of the bone penetrating through the skin

How do bones heal?

An understanding of the fracture healing process will help in decisions about treatment and prognosis when dealing with a fracture:

1. **Reactive phase** Formation of blood clot and granulation tissue in the first few days post-fracture, similar to tissue healing

2. **Reparative phase**
   a. 'Bony callus' formation where the periosteum provides two important precursor cells for callus formation
      a.i. Chondroblasts – precursor to hyaline cartilage
      a.ii. Osteoblasts – precursor to woven bone
   b. The hyaline cartilage and woven bone knit together and unite, eventually covering the bone defect between the two ends of the fracture.
   c. Endochondral ossification is the 'mineralisation' of the woven bone/hyaline cartilage scaffolding.

3. **Remodelling phase** Trabecular bone formed during endochondral ossification is replaced by permanent, strong 'compact bone'. Eventually the healed bone remodels to a shape and strength closely resembling the original bone.

In order for a bone to heal the following requirements must be met:

- **Immobilisation** of the whole area (including the joint at either side)
- **Fracture ends in contact** for extended periods (6–8 weeks). Constant movement will continuously break the callus and prevent healing.
- **Good blood supply** to provide sufficient nutrients and oxygen for bone healing
- **No infection** (implication for open fractures)
- Limited contact of fracture ends with other structures such as joints
- **Age** – a younger animal is more likely to heal.

CONDITIONS AFFECTING THE BONES 14.6

It is usually unrealistic to fulfil these requirements, particularly in the context of a less developed country and in equids required to work.

Long bone fractures (femur, tibia, humerus, and radius)

Adult (mature) equids

> These will never heal effectively because of the weight of the animal and difficulty immobilising the fracture site for long periods.

Surgical treatment requires specialist hospital facilities and there is a high likelihood of contralateral limb laminitis if treatment is attempted. Limb amputation is not acceptable for a working equid. Euthanase to prevent prolonged suffering (Figure 14.6.1).

Foals (immature) equids

Closed, non-displaced long bone fractures can be contained within a Robert-Jones bandage or cast, extending from the ground as high up the leg as possible. Ensure thick padding under the heel and keep lower joints flexed. This prevents normal weight-bearing forces from displacing the fracture. Plenty of thick padding must be used over the whole limb, especially tendons and joints, to prevent damage and pressure sores from the cast or splint. The splint will need to be in place for at least 6 weeks with deep bedding for the foal to lie on. If the animal is older, e.g. a yearling, it could possibly be cross-tied standing, but young animals are unlikely to tolerate this and it may cause other developmental orthopaedic problems. The animal must not work for 4–6 months. The prognosis is guarded, as the fracture may fail to heal or, when healed, the limb may be weak or deviated preventing a good working life in future.

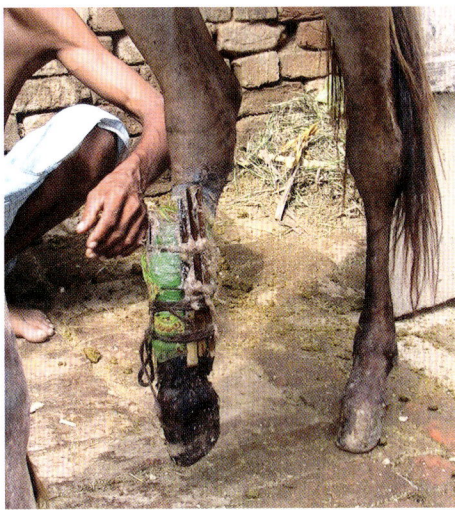

Figure 14.6.1 Fractured right hindleg with owner-applied splint (this horse was euthanased on humane grounds).

> When considering whether to treat a long bone fracture in a young animal, always remember welfare cost versus benefit.

- What are the physical/mental welfare implications of long-term confinement?
- Will regular veterinary visits be possible to ensure the bandage/cast is not causing pressure sores, infection, swelling or even necrosis of the encased limb?
- Is the owner willing to allow the animal to rest for the long period required for healing?

> Never attempt to treat an open fracture. Euthanase these cases straight away.

14 THE MUSCULOSKELETAL SYSTEM

Non-displaced fractures

If the fracture is not displaced (for example in a metacarpal bone), diagnosis can be difficult without radiography. Consider the following when reaching an informed decision about how to proceed:

- **Severity** of lameness
- **Duration** of lameness
- **History** of how it developed
- Physical and mental **welfare status** of the animal – Alert? Eating?
- The **owner's attitude**
- **Response** to treatment

In most cases if there is a positive response to complete rest and pain relief it is unlikely that a fracture has occurred. Table 14.6.1 demonstrates the non-displaced fractures that can be confused with other conditions.

Type of fracture	Can look like…	Suspect fracture if…
Pedal bone	Laminitis, hoof abscess	Trauma to the foot
Navicular bone	Laminitis, hoof abscess	Penetrating injury in frog area, trauma, severe pain on foot manipulation (due to movement of the deep flexor tendon)
Splint bones	Discharging sinus, generalised fetlock/cannon swelling	Trauma, brushing injuries
Carpal bones	Carpal osteoarthritis, joint infection	Carpal hyperextension/fatigue, e.g. from fast work, hard ground Evidence of falling, e.g. knee lesions
Olecranon (elbow)	Capped elbow	Direct trauma (kick, accident) 'Dropped elbow' stance Fatigue – slipping when forelimb out in front (avulsion fracture)
Scapula	'Sweeney' (muscle atrophy of the shoulder area due to damage to the suprascapular nerve, if chronic)	Direct trauma to the area
Patella	Stifle osteoarthritis, joint infection	Direct trauma, stiff hindlimb gait
Pelvis	Early tetanus, neurological problems	Direct trauma/falling/knocking pelvis on cart or gate
Spine	Neurological disease, collapse	Very severe trauma

Table 14.6.1 Differential diagnoses for fractures accompanied by aspects of history and clinical signs.

CONDITIONS AFFECTING THE BONES 14.6

If treatment is not an option, which will be very common with the working equid, then advise euthanasia as early as possible to alleviate pain and suffering. If an injured equid needs to be moved, ensure that adequate support and protection is given to the limb to avoid further pain, and that analgesia is administered.

Emergency splinting and bandaging

> If a fracture is suspected, splint the leg immediately following examination (Walmsley 1999); the position of the splint depends on the site of the fracture.

Light **sedation** may be required. The joints above and below the fractured bone need to be immobilised. A 'Robert-Jones' is a multi-layered bandage that will provide a degree of support. This bandage comprises many **layers of cotton** wool applied sequentially and held in place with an **elastic bandage**. Each layer should be at least 2.5 cm thick and should be applied more tightly than the last. The bandaged limb should be **three times the thickness** of the contra-lateral limb. Once a Robert-Jones is completed a splint can be applied, the position of which depends on the site of the facture. A splint should be light but strong and not bend; a broom handle cut to an appropriate length is ideal. Firmly tape to the leg with non-elastic tape.

Sequestra

> A sequestrum is a small piece of bone that has become detached from its blood supply usually as the result of trauma, e.g. avulsion or a comminuted fracture.

Diagnosis

- History of **trauma**
- Evidence of a **sinus tract** discharging pus through the skin, often recurring

Treatment

- Identify bone piece(s) by palpation.
- Remove the bone, if easy to access, under local, regional or general anaesthesia.
- Extreme care must be taken to avoid synovial structures when removing sequestra.
- Debride and flush the wound thoroughly. Administer a 7–10 day course of penicillin, and NSAID medication as required.
- Tetanus prophylaxis is essential.

Prognosis

Depends on the site of the sequestra and how effectively all **necrotic tissue** has been removed. In some cases (e.g. fractures of the pelvis) it will not be possible to remove the sequestra. There is likely to be a continuous discharging tract, and infection may spread to neighbouring tissues.

14 THE MUSCULOSKELETAL SYSTEM

Periosteal regrowth – 'splints' and 'bucked shins'

> 'Splints' refer to periostitis or fractures of the 2nd or 4th metacarpal/tarsal bones ('splint bones' Mc/t II and IV).

> 'Shin splints/bucked shins' refer to dorsal periostitis (stress microfractures) on the dorsal aspect of the 3rd metacarpal (cannon bone, McIII).

Periosteal new bone growth in both of these areas occurs as the result of inflammation (periostitis); this can be due to abnormal **stress**, direct **trauma** (e.g. brushing) or excessive **work**. Stress microfractures in McIII occur commonly in young horses running at speed. This work exceeds the ability of the bone to re-model and adapt to this stress. Large amounts of new bone growth on McII and IV may interfere with the **suspensory ligament** (interosseous) and can even lead to fractures of the splint bones if severe.

Clinical signs of forelimb periosteal growth

- **Acute phase** Variable amount of swelling, heat and pain on palpation; the animal may show lameness which increases with further work.
- **Chronic phase** Mild to severe, cold swelling; the animal shows no lameness.
- If severe signs are present, a splint bone may be fractured. Microfractures predispose McIII to complete fractures.

Treatment

In the acute phase, rest the animal for as long as possible, ideally **one month**, to minimise the periosteal reaction. Use systemic (and topical, if available) NSAID medication to reduce the lameness and soft-tissue swelling. Chronic splints are a cosmetic problem only and do not require treatment. Correct the underlying cause if possible.

Sesamoiditis

Cause

Inflammation of the proximal sesamoid bones as the result of tearing of the suspensory ligament fibres at the insertion. The suspensory ligament undergoes severe strain during fast work. The other structures of the fetlock (ligaments, tendon sheath, cartilage and soft tissue) may also be affected.

Clinical signs

- Sudden onset of moderate to severe **lameness**
- Diffuse **swelling** around the sesamoids, with pain on palpation and fetlock flexion
- **Distension** of the fetlock joint capsule

The ideal treatment is to apply a strong support bandage for 2 months and rest the animal for up to a year. This, however, is impractical in working equids which cannot be rested for such a long period; in this case rest as long as possible and use support bandaging and NSAIDs to reduce inflammation and pain.

CONDITIONS AFFECTING THE BONES 14.6

Pathology involving the navicular bone and bursa

> Navicular syndrome is chronic idiopathic osteitis of the navicular bone.

> Acute navicular bursitis/fracture is infection and inflammation of the navicular bursa due to a penetrating injury in the frog area.

Cause

Different theories have been discussed about the underlying cause and pathogenesis of navicular syndrome; however, acute navicular bursitis or fracture is often the more likely presentation in working equids. The end result is degeneration and pain in the navicular bone with accompanying lameness.

Clinical signs of navicular pathology

- Mild, slow-onset forelimb lameness
- Unequal foot size
- Positive response to palmar digital nerve block
- Pointing of the toe in the front feet

Expert radiography and interpretation is needed to confirm diagnosis. Without access to further diagnostic aids an informed decision is based on history, clinical signs and knowledge of anatomy.

Treatment

There is no cure for navicular disease; treatment is management-based with the use of long-term daily pain relief and hoof trimming to achieve a correct hoof-pastern-axis. Treatment of navicular bursitis is rarely successful, and euthanasia is recommended if the lameness and pain is severe.

Osteomyelitis/osteitis

> Osteomyelitis is inflammation and infection of bone and marrow.

> Osteitis is inflammation of bone only.

Pedal osteitis Inflammation of the pedal bone P3. The significance of this condition is controversial.

Causes

Haematogenous spread (via the bloodstream). This occurs in young foals at the physis (growth plate) of subchondral bone, as the blood flow in these vessels is slow. A localised osteitis can develop after **trauma**, from the spread of infection from local structures.

Diagnosis

- Lameness is seen in the initial phases. However, if the condition becomes chronic, lameness may no longer be apparent.

- In osteitis secondary to trauma, there is often a purulent discharging sinus with a non-healing wound. There may be a history of an intermittent discharge without resolution.
- In haematogenous osteomyelitis, the affected limb will be swollen and lame; several sites may be infected including both bones and joints.

Treatment

- If a localised bone infection is present secondary to an open wound, antibiotic therapy is of little or no value. The lesion may improve following treatment but, once this is ceased, the signs will recur.
- Debride necrotic bone, if present, with appropriate analgesia, e.g. regional anaesthesia and systemic analgesia. Only perform this operation if the sequestra are in a safely accessible area, without a large risk of iatrogenic damage. A good knowledge of local anatomy is essential.
- In haematogenous osteomyelitis, prolonged antibiotic therapy is warranted and, if the treatment is started early enough in the course of the disease, there may be a resolution. This is likely to take 3–4 weeks. In severe cases it may not be successful so warn owners before considering treatment. If an animal is not going to be treated, recommend euthanasia on welfare grounds.

14.7 Conditions affecting the joints

> Joints are complex structures that are extremely susceptible to injury in working equids (Broster *et al.* 2009).

All joints have the following characteristics:

- **Cartilage** Elastic 'shock absorber'
- **Synovial fluid** Highly viscous 'lubrication'
- **Joint capsule/tendons/ligaments** Vary according to which joint is involved but generally act as 'stabilisers'

Injury and damage to the joint results in pain, inflammation and decreased flexibility (Figure 14.7.1), all of which contribute to lameness. When treating joint disorders with parenteral medication, the limited blood supply makes it difficult to achieve articular therapeutic concentrations.

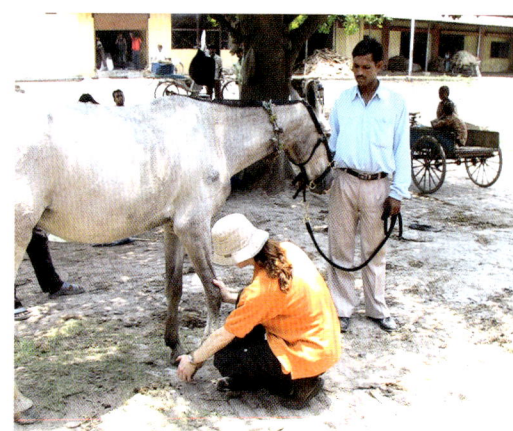

Figure 14.7.1 Ensure a full examination of all limbs and flexion of joints.

Osteoarthritis (OA) and degenerative joint disease (DJD)

The most common cause of lameness reported in horses is joint disease (Rossdale *et al.* 1985) and osteoarthritis is the most common condition. One report found that the highest cause of death or euthanasia was joint disease (Egenvall *et al.* 2006).

> OA/DJD = chronic inflammatory changes in the joint over time leading to a progressive deterioration of articular cartilage.

Causes

- 'Wear and tear' as part of the ageing process
- Secondary to **joint injury** – joint strain, articular chip fractures, joint infection
- Long-term, **excessive work** on hard roads
- Poor limb **conformation** – resulting in asymmetric stresses to joints
- Uneven **weight loads** or inappropriate weight loads
- Poor **foot care**
- **Iatrogenic** – poor, incorrectly administered joint injections

Changes that occur in the joint during development of osteoarthritis

- **Cartilage** Cracks (fissures) and decreased elasticity over time reduces the 'shock-absorber' effect.
- **Synovial membrane** Twisting, stretching or direct trauma over time results in a continuing cycle of joint damage:
  - Increased production of synovial fluid which is less viscous, resulting in less effective joint lubrication and protection
  - Increased production of enzymes and inflammatory cells, causing further tissue destruction and inflammation

Clinical signs of early osteoarthritis/DJD

- Varying degrees of lameness, usually in multiple limbs
- Pain on joint manipulation
- Decreased range of motion
- Positive response to flexion tests
- Variable joint capsule distension with synovial fluid

With *advanced* osteoarthritis/DJD, clinical signs may also include rough bony swellings (osteophytes) around the joint margins which are easily palpated and externally visible in more advanced cases (Figure 14.7.2). The metacarpophalangeal (MCP) or fetlock joint has been reported as the most commonly affected joint with OA in the horse (Cantley *et al.* 1999). There is reduced

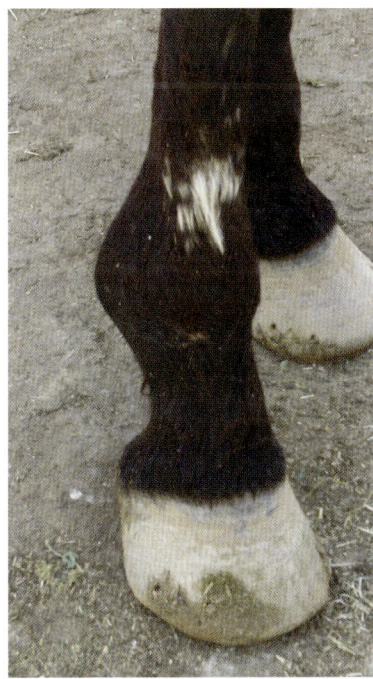

Figure 14.7.2 Ossseous growth around the metacarpophalangeal joint of the right forelimb.

14 THE MUSCULOSKELETAL SYSTEM

New bone formation (common name)	Location	Example
Low ringbone	Distal interphalangeal joint	
High ringbone	Proximal interphalangeal joint	
Bone spavin	Distal hock joint (distal intertarsal and tarsometatarsal joints)	
Fluid Distension (common name)		
Wind gall/wind puffs	Digital flexor tendon sheath (encases the flexor tendons) Incidental, unassociated with lameness	
Bog spavin	Tarso crural joint (hock)	

Table 14.7.1 Examples of other common terms that refer to osteoarthritis.

CONDITIONS AFFECTING THE JOINTS 14.7

flexion of the joint. In some cases the joint cannot be moved at all because it has become fixed (arthrodesed) by new bone formation around the joint.

'One condition, many names' – Different terms are used for osteoarthritis depending on the site (Table 14.7.1). The pathology, however, remains the same.

Treatment

> Osteoarthritis cannot be cured. Changes in the joint structure and function are irreversible, so emphasise pain management and prevention to owners: A strategic, multimodal approach is often required. It is essential that everyone (owner, vet, user, carer, animal) works as a team. Always keep the animal's best interest in mind.

Owner communication is essential for management and prevention, emphasising that osteoarthritis cannot be cured, and any visible changes to the joints (bony swellings, fluid pockets) are permanent. Instead, encourage the following:

- Reduce the speed and duration of work on hard roads.
- Attempt to rest animals for long periods if they are lame.
- Take good care of hooves – especially the frog.
- Start young working equids slowly and gently – and do not start work before 3 years of age.

Rest reduces the aggravation of the inflammation process allowing time for natural healing. When lameness and pain reduce, slow and steady exercise can begin.

Medical treatment options

NSAIDs such as phenylbutazone (PBZ) and flunixin are commonly used to alleviate the pain associated with OA. Daily NSAIDs can be administered but, in advanced cases, this is often ineffective. Remember the side-effects of long-term use on internal organs. There has also been concern regarding the negative effects of NSAIDs on cartilage (Beluche et al. 2001). NSAIDs will not treat the condition, may mask the clinical signs and make the animal more comfortable. The owner should be warned of this and it should be remembered that working an animal on NSAIDs is likely to speed the progression of the disease by increasing the wear and tear of the joint. An animal's natural instinct to protect an injured limb will decrease with pain relief, often resulting in further damage if the owner is not careful. This should not prevent the use of these medications as they have both analgesic and anti-inflammatory effects. In the early stages of disease NSAIDs should be used to full effect to stop progression.

Corticosteroids are very effective drugs for reducing inflammation. **Intra-articular corticosteroid injections** are only recommended if used very carefully in the early stages. This is usually not feasible in working equids due to the presentation of mostly chronic cases to clinics. Joint injections should be followed by 3–4 weeks of complete rest. This medication is ineffective where a lot of bony changes are already present; do not use if the joint capsule is already distended. Avoid steroids if there is a suspicion of septic arthritis. Injections must be given under strict aseptic conditions (see Section 4.1 *Drug administration techniques*).

> Weigh up the cost versus benefit – an iatrogenic joint infection as the result of poor hygiene will outweigh any benefits from the treatment.

- **Correct farriery** Correct trimming or shoeing of the feet is essential in the management of locomotion system pathology.
- **Firing and burning** *do not benefit* arthritic joints (Table 14.7.1 *Bog spavin photograph*). Offer owners alternatives such as massage or simple physiotherapy techniques.

Problems with treatment

There can be inter-animal variation of response to treatment as the result of heterogeneity of the disease. The stage of the disease affects the outcome of the treatment. Different preparations of the same drug are available; check concentration and dose rate. Expectations of the owner may be higher than is possible.

There is a poor correlation between imaging and the disease process. The use of radiography does not tend to enhance the ability to diagnose and treat. Once changes are seen on a radiograph the disease is at a very advanced stage and easily diagnosed by clinical examination. Radiography will not affect the treatment regime and management in most cases.

Synovitis

> **Synovitis is the inflammation of the synovial membrane resulting in excessive synovial fluid production; cartilage is usually unaffected.**

Causes

- Excessive concussion of the joints of young animals
- Trauma
- Poor conformation, especially hoof conformation and trimming
- Working on uneven surfaces

Diagnosis

Large fluid swellings in the joints, most commonly seen as 'bog spavin' (dorsomedial and plantar pouches of the hock joints, Table 14.7.1).

Treatment

Reduce the work load. Treat with NSAIDs in the early stages; it is important to stop inflammation early to avoid cartilage damage leading to osteoarthritis.

Septic arthritis

> **Bacterial infection of the joint(s) results in a septic arthritis.**

Causes

- Penetrating joint injury
- Iatrogenic when infection is introduced by a veterinary procedure, e.g. joint injection (especially when corticosteroids are used). It is absolutely essential that joint injections are only done aseptically in a suitable environment.

- Tracking of infection from superficial wounds or abscess in the area (e.g. brushing wounds)
- Haematogenous (joint-ill in foals)

Bacteria in the joint stimulate a severe inflammatory reaction of the synovial membrane. This produces increased amounts of synovial fluid, inflammatory cells and enzymes which further inflame the synovial membrane and rapidly destroy the cartilage. When large areas of articular cartilage are lost, the underlying bone is susceptible to bacterial exposure, leading to secondary osteomyelitis.

Clinical signs

- Severe pain and lameness which may not appear for several days after a suspected injury/corticosteroid injection (may be mistaken for a fracture)
- Marked fluid swelling of the joint, which can progress to soft tissue swelling and heat in the surrounding area
- Dullness, poor appetite, fever

Diagnosis

If trained in this procedure, collect a joint fluid sample (see Section 4.1 *Drug administration techniques*) under strict aseptic conditions. Prior to collection ensure that facilities for analysis are available, either within the clinic or at a local laboratory. The joint fluid may appear discoloured, blood-stained or cloudy. Septic joint fluid, when shaken in a tube, froths more than normal joint fluid as there is a higher protein content. If a microscope is available, examine a stained smear. A WBC exceeding 30,000/µl with a total protein exceeding 45 g/L is suggestive of an infected joint (Caron 2011). Differential cell counts are valuable; normally the neutrophils make up less than 10% of the WBC count. If this proportion increases, particularly to around 80%, the diagnosis of a septic arthritis is strongly supported.

To determine whether a laceration close to the joint has penetrated the synovial capsule, the joint should be aseptically prepared at a distant site to the injury. Following retrieval of a sample for analysis, a small volume of sterile saline can be injected into the joint capsule. If fluid flows from the site of trauma the joint capsule has been breached and should be treated as septic. Once completed, the synovial structure is typically injected with an antibiotic (e.g. 125–500 mg amikacin sulphate).

Collecting a synovial fluid sample

1. With the site identified and prepared (see Section 4.1 *Drug administration techniques*), appropriately restrain the animal and identify the location for needle insertion. Some joints may be easier to sample with the limb flexed (e.g. carpus).
2. Use a 20/21G, 25- or 40-mm needle, depending on the size of the joint and amount of soft tissue swelling. Introduce it quickly through the skin, then advance slowly until synovial fluid appears in the hub. In inflamed/infected joints, the synovial fluid is under pressure and will usually drip out, otherwise attach a 5-ml syringe and apply gentle suction to aspirate sample. This needs to be performed under strict asepsis. Do not attempt to collect synovial fluid through infected skin.
3. Immediately transfer the sample to two sterile vacutainers, one plain and one EDTA. For a bacterial culture blood culture tubes are required; these may be obtained from the laboratory.

Send the sample to the laboratory with clear instructions, or examine a stained smear under a microscope (Table 14.2.1).

Property	Normal joint fluid	Abnormal joint fluid
Appearance	Clear, non-turbid, pale yellow	Turbid; may contain lumps/particles; darker yellow; may be blood-stained
Viscosity	Viscous (stringy appearance when stretched between thumb and finger)	Less viscous (negative stringing test)
Total leukocyte count	$< 0.5 \times 10^9$ per L	$> 0.5 \times 10^9$ per L (usually much higher in septic arthritis)
Total protein (use a refractometer)	< 18 g/L	> 18 g/L

Table 14.2.1 *Microscopic properties of normal and abnormal joint fluid.*

Treatment

> **Veterinarians and owners should be aware that attempted treatment of a septic joint is a long, slow process requiring many weeks of commitment from both parties.**

- Septic arthritis is an emergency; treatment should be early and aggressive.
- Ideally for a successful outcome, septic joints should be irrigated with copious fluids, in a sterile theatre, within the first 24 hours. In the working equid context this is not possible and hence often treatment is not possible. If the joint has been septic for over 3 days, success of treatment is poor as irreversible damage occurs during this time.
- Treatment in the field may consist of a standing joint flush under sedation and long-term parenteral antibiotics.
- Antibiotics need to be administered for at least 2 weeks after the resolution of lameness.

Flushing an infected joint

Flushing (lavage) of an infected joint aims to remove dirt, bacteria, fibrin and other inflammatory products which destroy the joint cartilage and permanently damage the joint, such as in septic arthritis. Flushing should begin as soon as joint penetration is suspected; the longer the delay between infection and flushing, the less successful the treatment is likely to be. This through-a-needle technique will not remove solid fibrin or purulent material. Do not attempt this procedure if untrained in the technique.

Required materials

- Sedatives or general anaesthetic
- Local anaesthetic
- 18G to 14G needles or catheters; syringes 2 ml, 5 ml, 20 ml
- Sterile saline bags (at least 1 litre) and intravenous giving set
- Bandages/dressing materials
- Antibiotics (gentamicin or penicillin), NSAIDs, tetanus antitoxin

Flushing the joint

1. Administer prophylactic antibiotics, NSAIDs and tetanus antitoxin.
2. Shave and prepare the area aseptically as for intra-articular injection. Several needles may be placed, so prepare the whole joint area plus 3–5 cm in all directions.
3. Sedate or anaesthetise the animal as necessary. If not anaesthetised, place a subcutaneous bleb of local anaesthetic at each injection site. If anaesthetised, the joint will need to be scrubbed once the animal is positioned for the procedure.
4. Introduce needles (as for intra-articular injection) into the joint at **two** distant points, e.g. caudal and cranial pouches of the joint capsule. Synovial fluid should appear if in the correct position; collect this for laboratory evaluation.
5. Using the giving set, attach the fluid bag to one needle ('ingress') and gently distend the joint with saline until it flows out of the other needle ('egress'). Gently manipulate the joint to encourage flushing. Avoid damaging the cartilage with excessive needle movement.
6. If fluid does not flow, one or both needles may be touching the cartilage or blocked by fibrin or inflamed synovial membrane. Redirect needles or withdraw and replace with a new needle. Flush the joint thoroughly, ideally with 10 litres of saline.
7. Withdraw the 'egress' needle. Aspirate a few ml of fluid from the 'ingress' needle and inject 250–500 mg gentamicin or 125 mg amikacin before withdrawal.
8. Cover with a sterile dressing and bandage the joint. Advise the owner on hygiene of the area, and ensure a 5–7 day course of antibiotics.

Prognosis

Guarded, but early treatment can lead to good results. If the condition has been present for more than 14 days, the prognosis is very poor and euthanasia should be advised on welfare grounds.

Prevention and owner communication

Treat skin wounds over joints as a potential risk of a joint infection.

Many brushing or knee lesions are encountered on a daily basis in working equine examinations; any one of these could become a septic joint.

Encourage owners to keep wounds clean and identify/address the underlying causes.

Osteochondrosis

This is a developmental disturbance to the cellular differentiation of cartilage in growing horses (osteochondrosis has not been reported in donkeys). There is a failure of ossification that starts at the growth plates and results in cartilage defects such as a separation from underlying bone, cracking (fissures) and weak spots. Flaps of cartilage develop and can break off to form loose fragments which are referred to as osteochondrosis dessicans (OCD). Subchondral bone cysts can also form.

Causes (Ross and Dyson 2003)

Despite extensive investigations, the cause remains unclear but it is thought to be the result of excessive force on weak bone or cartilage. It is most commonly seen in large-breed fast-growing horses and is mainly seen in yearlings up to 2-year-olds. Diets that are high in energy and have a calcium phosphate imbalance have been commonly associated with the condition. Some manifestations have a hereditary component. An inappropriately high workload at a young age may also contribute to OCD development.

Diagnosis

- Joint effusion is the most common clinical sign. Several joints may be involved including phalangeal, fetlock, carpal, shoulder, tarsal and stifle joints.
- Joint lameness and pain can be present but not always.
- Subtle early changes may be visible on radiographs, although these changes are usually not definitive until the disease has reached a severe stage.
- If the cervical spine is affected this can lead to instability resulting in a neurological condition known as Wobbler Syndrome (Cervical Stenotic Myelopathy).

Treatment

- Ideally this should be treated as early as possible, so early diagnosis will improve the disease progression and prognosis.
- Horses should be rested and dietary changes made; reduce the dietary energy but ensure ample roughage remains in the diet.
- If not detected early, extensive areas of damaged cartilage can develop which will trigger the development of arthritis, and the prognosis for soundness in adult life is poor.

Sprains – sub-luxations and luxations

A sprain is the stretching or tearing of the support ligaments of a joint. In a mild sprain only a few fibres are torn and the integrity of the support is not lost.

Sub-luxation/luxation is a severe sprain where the integrity of one or more support ligaments for a joint is lost.

> A sub-luxation is the partial dislocation of a joint, and a luxation is a complete dislocation of a joint. These can be complicated by fractures such as avulsion fractures, when the stress of the ligament breaking pulls off the piece of bone it attaches to.

Clinical signs

Sprain
- Mild peri-articular swelling, and possibly some laxity of the joint when manipulated
- Lameness and weakness of joint

Subluxation/luxation
- Extensive swelling around joint and adjacent structures
- Severe lameness and weakness
- Sub-luxation (abnormal extension or flexion on manipulation)
- Luxation (abnormal posture)

Treatment

Sprain

- Cold therapy – Apply cold water and ice as soon as possible after trauma.
- Stable the equid and immobilise the limb using a support bandage and confined space. Rest until the lameness has resolved, the length of time depends on severity of sprain. Ensure the bandage is applied correctly and changed regularly to avoid pressure sores and rubs.
- Administer NSAIDs for analgesic and anti-inflammatory effects.
- The prognosis is good.

Sub-luxation/luxation

- These injuries require full immobilisation and, in the working equid context, this is rarely possible.
- Radiography is useful to assess for concomitant fractures and determine prognosis. Although, at best, these images serve as further evidence to euthanase an injured equid rather than to determine a treatment protocol.
- Treatment is by splinting or casting for a minimum of 6 weeks followed by a convalescence of up to 1 year.
- Even with full treatment and no concomitant fractures the prognosis for return to work is extremely guarded.
- Given the limitations of treatment in the working equid context, and the risk to animal welfare if treatment fails, euthanasia should be strongly advised for this condition.

Upward fixation of the patella (locking stifle)

This occurs when the medial patella ligament hooks over the medial trochlea of the femur, locking the hind limb in permanent extension.

Causes

- **Poor conformation** – straight hindlimb
- **Sudden weight loss** can predispose to locking. The infra-patella fat pad reduces in size so the patella sits deeper in the trochlear groove.
- **Loss of fitness** and muscle tone

Clinical signs

The hindlimb is locked in extension, the stifle and hock are in extension, with a flexed fetlock. The foot is dragged behind and the limb cannot bear weight. Locking can be intermittent or can remain locked for long periods. Severe/prolonged upward fixation of the patella is more frequently seen in small equids, particularly donkeys. If there is a history of upward fixation this can be induced by walking in a tight circle or walking up and down a slope. There is stifle effusion as the result of inflammation in the joint.

Treatment

- Unlock patella manually – push the horse backwards and manually push the patella medially and distally; this can be difficult to do.

14 THE MUSCULOSKELETAL SYSTEM

- NSAIDs – Adminster phenylbutazone for a few days.
- Improve the condition of the animal by increasing the muscling to hindlimbs, increase the level of nutrition, administer anthelmintics (if there is evidence of GI parasites) and corrective dentistry as required. This is particularly effective in young animals and the condition can resolve once the hindquarter muscling has increased.
- If repeated locking persists there is a risk of arthritis and joint pain as the joint surface becomes damaged.
- A medial patellar ligament desmotomy should only be considered if attempts at conservative and medical therapy have failed, the patellar continues to lock and the owner will not consider euthanasia. Consult Tnibar 2003 for further details on this procedure.

14.8 Conditions affecting the tendons and ligaments

Tendons connect muscle to bone in the equine musculoskeletal system. They are fibrous with a limited blood supply and are protected by sheaths containing synovial fluid where they pass over high motion joints such as the carpus.

> **Think of tendons as rubber bands that can stretch. If the stretching becomes too great the tendon becomes 'strained' and can eventually snap, much like an over-stretched rubber band.**

Working equids which are ridden have a greater chance of damaging the forelimb tendons due to fetlock hyperextension at high speeds. Those equids which pull carts or carriages are more likely to damage the hindlimb tendons due to excessive strain exerted when pulling a heavy load (Maranhão et al. 2006), see Figure 14.8.1. Knowledge of work type is therefore important.

Tendon healing is a very slow process due to the low blood supply common to fibrous tissues. Once damaged, tendon fibres are replaced by weaker fibrous tissue which is less flexible. The healed tendon is more prone to further damage in the future, so prevention is always better than cure.

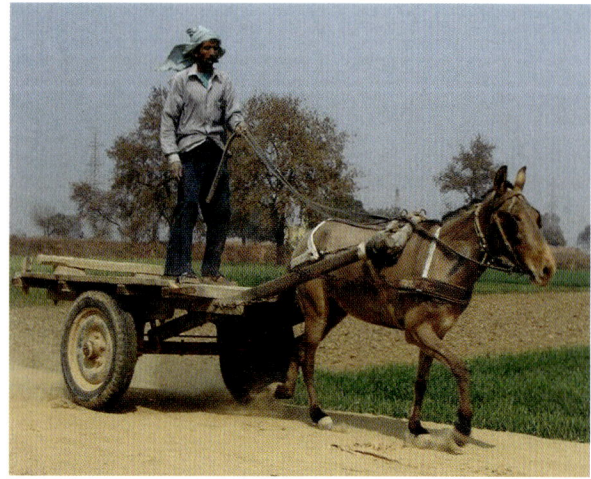

Figure 14.8.1 A mule pulling a cart in a brick kiln in Delhi. Note the hyperextension of the right hind fetlock.

CONDITIONS AFFECTING THE TENDONS AND LIGAMENTS 14.8

Strains: tendonitis and tenosynovitis

> Tendonitis/tenosynovitis = inflammation of the tendon/tendon sheath either through trauma or infection

Tendon injuries in horses are extremely common, with some tendons more prone to injury than others. The superficial digital flexor tendon (SDFT) of the forelimbs is the most commonly affected; damage to this tendon makes up 80–90% of reported tendon injuries (Williams 2001, Pinchbeck *et al.* 2004). In working horses digital flexor tendonitis was found in at least one limb in 83% of animals examined (Broster *et al.* 2009). Recent research findings show that the microstructure of the SDFT changes with age, increasing the risk of injury in older horses (Thorpe *et al.* 2012).

Causes

- **Hyperextension** (Figure 14.8.2) or other excessive force can cause straining or tearing of tendon fibres.
- **Tendon sheaths** can become distended with increased synovial fluid (tenosynovitis).
- **Infection** can also be present, for example with a penetrating injury over a tendon or a tendon sheath.

Clinical signs

Acute tendon strain

- Five signs of acute inflammation (heat, swelling, loss of function, redness, pain) occur over affected tendon. The limb should be palpated both when weight bearing and when raised to permit a thorough examination (Figure 14.8.3).
- Lameness
- Increased synovial fluid in the tendon sheath can make the tendon difficult to palpate so always compare with the opposite leg.

Chronic tendon injury

- Firm thickening of the affected tendon ('bowed tendons'), with or without synovial sheath distension (Figure 14.8.4)
- No heat or pain on palpation

Treatment of acute tendon strain

Treatment is aimed at **controlling the inflammatory response** rather than being curative.

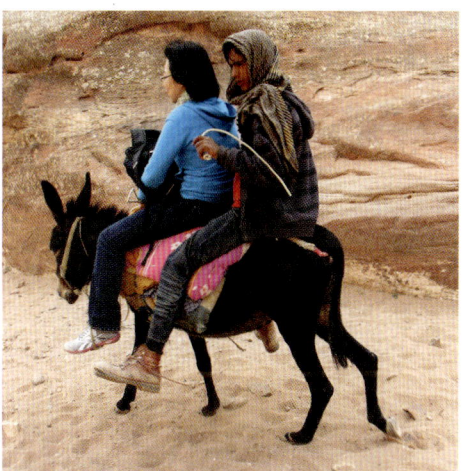

14.8.2 An overloaded donkey in Jordan. Note that the hind fetlock is hyperextended.

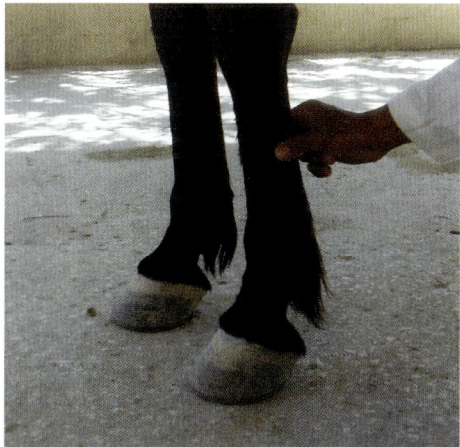

Figure 14.8.3 Palpation of tendons for the five signs of acute inflammation.

405

Cold water hosing twice daily can reduce inflammation but has a limited effect on tendon swelling. Apply a firm **pressure bandage** along length of tendon, ensuring that the top and bottom of the bandage are not too tight. Administer **NSAIDs** in decreasing dosage. Continue to rest the animal while under treatment as it may appear sound with analgesia. **Rest** over a period of **4–6 weeks** is the most effective circumstance for tendons to heal. Return to work should be slow with lighter loads to prevent recurrence.

> Firing is proven to have no effect on tendon healing. (Firing is the application of heat to burn the skin using a red hot iron; this causes scar tissue to form). Silver and Rossdale (1983) presented the first research study for evidence that firing is not an effective treatment for tendon injuries and reduces the strength of the skin in the burnt areas (Figure 14.8.4).

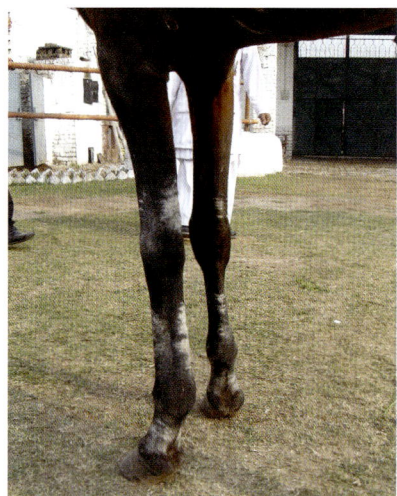

Figure 14.8.4 Chronic tendonitis left forelimb, with lesser affected right fore; scarring as a result of firing is present on both forelimbs.

Prognosis

Return to normal is unlikely due to the impracticalities of long-term rest in working equids. Permanent bowed tendons do not normally affect the animal's ability to work; however, damage to tendons will predispose to further episodes of tendonitis or rupture.

Tendon rupture

Severe damage to tendons may occur following degeneration on sudden **over-extension** or as the result of a **traumatic laceration** (Table 14.8.1).

Diagnosis

- Severe non-weight bearing lameness
- Transection of the extensor tendon will result in knuckling of the fetlock with attempts to bear weight.
- Transection of both the superficial and deep digital flexor tendon will result in the fetlock dropping significantly and the toe will rock proximally.
- In some cases the transection will be obvious, for example if there is an open wound (Figure 14.8.5). In other cases it may be less clear and diagnosis can be made on fetlock instability.

Treatment

Treat as for **open wound management**; **lavage** and debride. Long-term **supportive bandages** are essential to keep the limb immobilised. This should be a Robert-

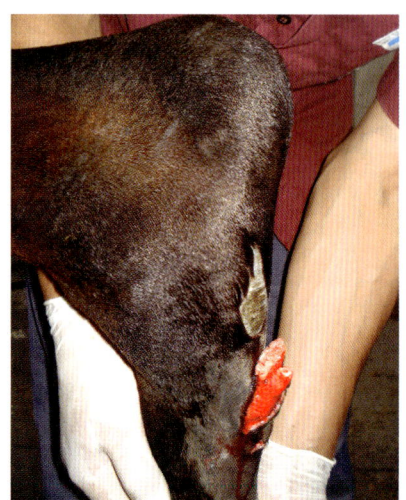

Figure 14.8.5 Lacerated flexor tendons in a hindlimb.

CONDITIONS AFFECTING THE TENDONS AND LIGAMENTS   14.8

Jones as a minimum and will require regular changes and check-ups. The owner should be aware of the long-term management and nursing required before embarking on treatment. In the working equid context this may not be possible or appropriate. **Long-term rest** and pain management is vital due to the slow healing process and must be discussed with the owner accordingly. Prognosis for return to work is poor and euthanasia should be considered on welfare grounds.

Surgical repair requires a specialist suture technique, general anaesthetic and long-term post-surgical management, all of which are difficult under field conditions.

Tendon	Cause of Rupture	Clinical Signs	Treatment	Prognosis
Extensor tendon	Trauma to dorsal cannon	Knuckling of fetlock Normal weight bearing	Open wound management NSAIDs Surgical repair often unsuccessful	Good if rested and animal learns to flip foot into correct position
Superficial digital flexor tendon (SDFT)	Kicks, wire or sheet metal trauma to back of cannon area	Slightly dropped fetlock	As for open wounds Tetanus prophylaxis Surgical repair only if clean and fresh	Guarded
Deep digital flexor tendon (DDFT)	As for SDFT rupture (usually occurs at the same time)	Severely dropped fetlock Toe raised off ground	Requires surgical intervention Raised heel extensions on shoe	Guarded/poor (Discuss euthanasia in severe cases)
Peroneus Tertius	Wounds Hock hyperextension (trapped or falling animal)	Hock does not flex on forward movement (characteristic) Hock extension whilst stifle flexed Dimpling of gastrocnemius	Rest (9–12 months) NSAIDs Do not suture (extreme load in this tendon)	Fair, although gait will always be abnormal

Table 14.8.1 Features of tendon rupture, including cause, treatment and prognosis.

Desmitis

> Desmitis = inflammation of a ligament

Ligaments connect **bone to bone**. The most common ligaments to be affected by overstrain injuries are the suspensory ligament (interosseous) and the **inferior carpal check ligament**.

Clinical signs

- Pain and swelling of:
  - proximal lateral metacarpus (inferior carpal check ligament)
  - distal metacarpus/tarsus (suspensory ligament).

  (Compare reaction with that in the opposite leg.)
- Lameness is variable, often mild.
- A loss of the sharp outline of the fetlock occurs with suspensory ligament damage, 'rounding of the fetlock'. This is often associated with sesamoiditis.

> Many animals will have signs of suspensory ligament desmitis, with or without lameness.

Treatment

As for tendonitis, with cold hosing, pressure-bandaging, NSAIDs and rest in acute cases

Prognosis

Good for mild ligament strains, but poor for severe injury to the suspensory ligament

Hygroma

See Section 14.10.

14.9 Conditions affecting the muscles

When examining the musculature of an equid, note any tremors or fasciculations before palpating the muscles to detect heat, pain or swelling. Ancillary diagnostic tests, such as measuring the muscle enzymes, serum creatinine kinase and aspartate aminotransferase, may be helpful when diagnosing muscle damage or necrosis. However, the clinical signs alone are likely to be supportive of a diagnosis.

CONDITIONS AFFECTING THE MUSCLES 14.9

Exertional rhabdomyolysis ('tying up', 'Monday morning disease')

Exertional rhabdomyolysis (ER) is defined as acute muscle cell damage following exercise. In severe cases, equids can die from this condition as the result of necrosis of the muscle and **kidney failure** following filtration of high levels of myoglobin. ER is a complex syndrome with multiple causes.

This condition frequently occurs following exercise preceded by a **long period of rest**, hence the term 'Monday morning disease'. An increase in work can have the same effect. An increased risk has been associated with **carbohydrate overload** and selenium deficiency. The mechanism of this is not completely understood. It is thought that high carbohydrate diets result in increased glycogen storage. During exercise there is a sudden breakdown of glycogen in muscles causing a local acidosis and muscular vasoconstriction which leads to muscle cramping and damage. Electrolyte imbalances may also predispose to this condition.

Clinical signs

- Generalised **stiffness** and reluctance to move shortly after a period of exercise
- Muscle tremors or spasms, particularly over the back and hindquarters
- Muscles, particularly of the hindquarter, feel **tense and solid**. Affected muscles are painful on palpation.
- Elevated heart rate and respiratory rate
- **Sweating**
- Anxiety and a tucked-up appearance
- Red-brown urine (**myoglobinuria**)

Treatment

- Administer **NSAIDs** to reduce inflammation and alleviate pain.
- Acepromazine (see Section 7.1) is used for muscle relaxation but ensure that the animal is not dehydrated prior to treatment with this medication as acepromazine has profound hypotensive properties.
- Administer **IV fluids** (at least 10–15 litres) to address dehydration but also to improve glomerular filtration rates in the face of myoglobin filtration by the kidneys.
- In severe cases corticosteroids may be administered.
- Vitamin B, Vitamin E and selenium may help muscle recovery.
- Avoid moving the animal if possible. Do not force the animal to walk if it is reluctant.
- Reduce grain intake and replace with abundant **high fibre diet**, such as hay.
- When restarting work do so **gradually and slowly**. Reintroduce grains once the animal is working again.

Prognosis

This is good in most cases, although recovery may take days to weeks. Advise the owner to return the animal to work slowly, especially after rest periods. Some cases may show a number of consecutive episodes, particularly if the animal has not been adequately rested before restarting work.

14 THE MUSCULOSKELETAL SYSTEM

Exhaustion and muscular cramping

> In some circumstances, working equids are given little opportunity to rest. This is detrimental to the health and welfare of the animal and will shorten its working life.

High workloads combined with energy, water and electrolyte deficiencies can easily overcome the coping strategies of a stoic working equid (Figure 14.9.1).

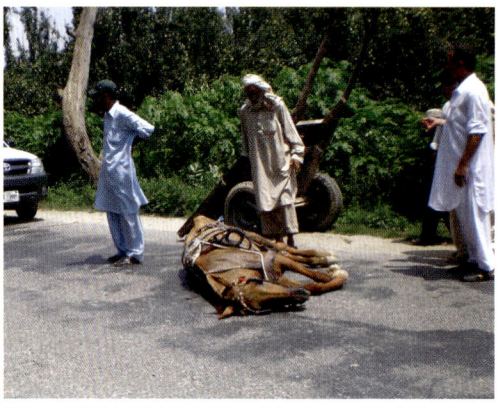
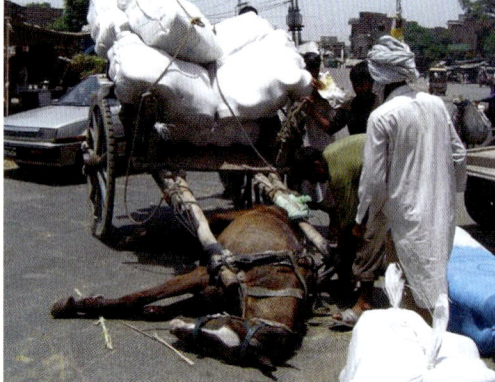

Figure 14.9.1 Collapsed working horses in Pakistan.

Clinical signs

- Depression, lethargy, collapse
- Little interest in food/water
- **Muscular cramping**
- Mild colic signs
- Synchronous diaphragmatic flutter – Diaphragm contractions occur due to electrolyte deficiencies. It may appear as though the animal is hiccuping.
- Reduced sweating; sweat sticky rather than watery
- Increased heart rate and respiratory rate

Treatment

- Offer water. If the equid will not drink, administer fluids through a stomach tube or give at least 10–15 litres of sterile fluids intravenously (see Chapter 6 *Dehydration and fluid therapy*).
- Rest
- To prevent reoccurrence add half a tablespoon of salt and half a tablespoon of potassium chloride (KCl) to feed when equids are undergoing long or strenuous exercise.

Malignant oedema (Clostridial myonecrosis)

> Malignant oedema is an acute, frequently fatal toxaemia affecting all species and ages of animals and is usually caused by the contamination of wounds with soil.

Infection with **Clostridium** *septicum, perfringens* or *chauvoei* via wounds, surgery or contaminated needles

Clinical signs

- Characterised by a **rapid clinical course** with signs appearing from just a few hours up to 48 hours following an injury or injection
- Extensive **pitting oedema** with gas formation under the skin (**subcutaneous emphysema**)
- Pain over affected area
- Rapid progression to massive **swelling** and **muscle necrosis** with jelly-like exudate
- Fever, anorexia and depression
- Myoglobinuria
- Generalised toxaemia; increased pulse and respiratory rates, injected mucous membranes (dark pink to red colour)
- A stained smear of the exudate, or aspirated fluid, may show large Gram +ve rod-shaped bacteria.

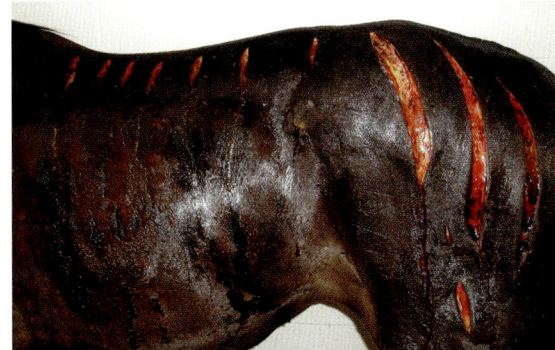

Figure 14.9.2 A case of clostridial myositis that was treated with a myotomy procedure as well as supportive antibiotic therapy. The horse recovered although the iatrogenic wounds took months to heal. (Image provided by Klara Saville)

Treatment

- Very high doses of penicillin for at least 10 days
- At least 10–15 litres intravenous fluids; continue fluid administration over several days if possible. This is particularly important if the animal has myoglobinuria to reduce the risk of renal failure.
- Surgical drainage of the site if localised
- The early use of a myotomy/fasciotomy procedure has been described to expose the anaerobic bacteria to oxygen (Figure 14.9.2). This procedure is associated with an improved prognosis. However, the iatrogenic deep muscle wounds take a long time to heal and require intensive management (Peek, Semrad and Perkins 2003).
- NSAIDs

Prognosis

Clostridial myonecrosis is usually fatal in a few days. Sequelae of this condition include laminitis and colic as the result of the toxaemia.

It is essential to ensure hygiene when injecting animals; encourage colleagues and para-professionals to change needles and follow good clean practice.

Hypocalcaemia

Cause

Calcium depletion, for example in **lactating mares** (milk fever, eclampsia), or following hard work or transport (transit tetany). This is a very satisfying and easy condition to treat. However, the signs are often not recognised in time by owners and veterinarians alike which can result in the death of the animal.

Clinical signs

- **Stiff gait**
- **Muscle fasciculation** (twitching, particularly around the jaw and the back of the upper forelimb)
- Dysphagia (difficulty eating) as the muscles of the jaw are affected
- Ataxia (unsteadiness)
- Profuse sweating
- Pyrexia
- Thumping noise in time with breathing, caused by abnormal function of phrenic nerve (synchronous diaphragmatic flutter). The equid can appear to be hiccuping.
- Seizures, coma and death if untreated

Treatment

Calcium borogluconate: 250–500 mls per 500 kg body weight. Dilute the calcium solution in 4 x the volume of saline; administer this mixture by slow IV infusion. Calcium borogluconate should be readily available in most countries as it is the same formula as that used to treat cattle with 'milk fever' (hypocalcaemia).

Prognosis

Good with early treatment. If hypocalcaemia recurs it may be helpful to supplement the diet with calcium.

Muscle atrophy

Muscle atrophy is defined as the decrease in mass of a muscle; this may be the result of poor nutrition, reduced use of a muscle (disuse atrophy) or a denervation of that muscle.

Generalised muscle atrophy is usually symmetrical and is the result of poor nutrition, cachexia, malnutrition, old age.

Localised muscle atrophy can be caused by:

- damage to the nerve innervating the muscle. Severe asymmetrical atrophy results from the loss of nerve stimulus.
- immobilisation of a limb, or chronic lameness
- injury to the muscle attachment.

Treatment

Identify and address the primary cause if possible. If a nerve is compressed it may regain function. However, if a nerve is transected and the neural sheath is not intact then the neurons will not regrow and the atrophy will be permanent.

Conditions affecting the synovial bursae 14.10

Hygroma

A hygroma is an acquired subcutaneous synovial bursa.

As hygromas are generally caused by a repetitive chronic trauma, there are certain predilection sites: the elbow, the hock, the withers and the carpus. The bursa is a small cavity filled with synovial fluid that acts as a cushion between two tendons or between tendon and bone. Hygromas are considered a cosmetic problem and are not usually associated with lameness.

Causes

- Repeated chronic **trauma**
- The majority of carpal hygromas communicate with the carpal joint. The carpal hygroma can form from a **synovial fistula** from the extensor tendon sheath or the carpal joint.
- **Infectious causes** Brucellosis is a rare cause of **fistulous withers** and **poll evil**. In working equids the most likely cause of fistulous withers is a poorly fitted harness and onchocerciasis has also been proposed as a possible cause (Doumbia 2011). However, if an equid has been in contact with infected cattle (*B. abortus*) or pigs (*B.suis*), the lesions should be considered infectious in origin. Brucellosis is a zoonotic disease; wear gloves when treating the animal and enforce strict isolation from animals and humans. Brucellosis is generally a notifiable disease; check local regulations. It is reasonable to keep equids separate from Brucella-infected cattle, and cattle separate from equids with discharging fistulous withers.

Clinical Signs

- Diffuse swelling. (Differentiate from carpal distension in which the joint will be involved.)
- No lameness
- Infected hygromas will present as an obvious wound, often discharging purulent material. There may be an associated lameness, particularly if the hygroma is connected to a joint casing a septic arthritis.

Treatment

- Hygromas are generally only a cosmetic problem.
- In the acute stages, **firm bandaging** and **NSAIDs** may reduce the swelling.
- **Drainage is ineffective** and carries the risk of infection of nearby joints and tendon sheaths.
- Infected hygromas will require more aggressive treatment involving sterile flushing and antibiotic therapy.

> - It is important to prevent these lesions occurring by reducing repetitive trauma to a particular site. (For example, improve the harness design to prevent fistulous withers, or provide soft bedding to prevent capped hock.)

Type of Bursitis	Clinical signs	Cause	Treatment and prevention
Bicipital	Painful swelling at point of shoulder	Penetrating injury at point of shoulder Chronic strain injury (conformational or compensatory)	Puncture wounds: treat aggressively with debridement, antibiotics/joint flushing, NSAIDs and rest.
Calcaneal 'capped hock'	Fluid swelling at point of the hock (between gastrocnemius and SDF tendons)	Kicking the cart Trauma from lying down on hard floors without sufficient bedding/padding	Unnecessary if sterile, otherwise treat aggressively. Pad front of cart/protect hock to prevent further injury. Beating will contribute to problem as animals kick in response. Ensure a soft area is provided for the animal to lie down.
Olecranon 'capped elbow'	Fluid swelling at the elbow	Repeat trauma to point of elbow (e.g. pressure from shoe when animal lying down)	Medical treatment unnecessary if sterile, otherwise treat aggressively. Ensure good hoof care/shoeing technique. Ensure a soft area is provided for the animal to lie down in when resting.
Carpal hygroma	Fluctuant swelling over the carpal joint	Repeated trauma to the knees e.g. falling/stumbling on uneven ground Kicking a stable door	Medical treatment unnecessary if sterile, otherwise treat aggressively. Ensure a soft area is provided for the animal to lie down in when resting. Ensure feet are kept well-trimmed to minimise stumbling and do not work at fast speeds.
Atlantal 'poll evil'	Deep discharging sinus midline behind the ears	Ill-fitting headgear Infected wound Brucellosis	Difficult due to position (requires daily flushing). Sedate and clean. Prolonged systemic antibiotics (continue 5 days after signs disappear). Often recurring – warn owner.

CONDITIONS AFFECTING THE SYNOVIAL BURSAE 14.10

Type of Bursitis	Clinical signs	Cause	Treatment and prevention
Supraspinous fistulous withers	Swelling and pain in wither region, can rupture to discharge pus in severe cases. Secondary osteomyelitis	Ill-fitting harness or saddle **Onchocerca** **Brucellosis**	Clean and debride. Administer systemic antibiotics if deep. Advise owner on prevention. Keep harness off wound, use a 'doughnut bandage' until healed. Prognosis is poor if osteomyelitis present.
Navicular	Severe lameness following sole/frog injury. Pain response to hoof testers across heels	Deep puncture wound to frog or middle third of sole	Poor response to antibiotics/flushing. Complications can include navicular fracture. Prognosis is usually hopeless.

Table 14.10.1 *Common bursal injuries in working equids, including cause, treatment and prevention.*

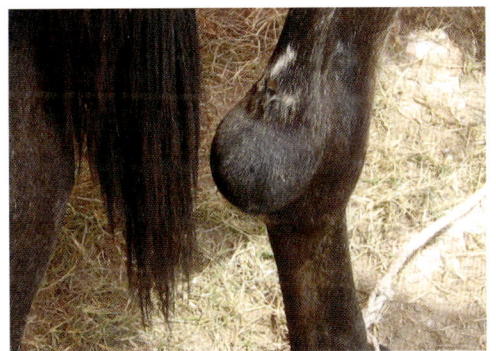
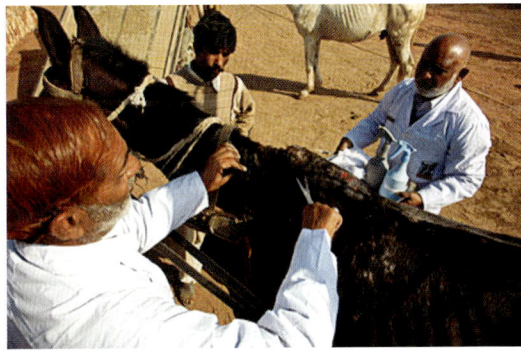
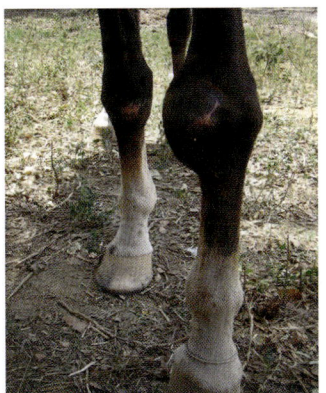
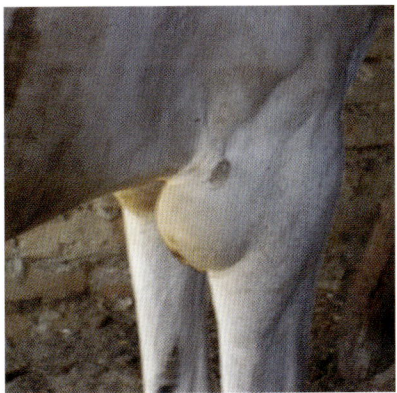

Figure 14.10.1 *Illustrations of common bursal injuries in working equids: calcaneal 'capped hock', supraspinous 'fistulous withers', carpal hygroma and olecranon 'capped elbow'.*

14.11 Case study – Malignant oedema

Area India

Attending veterinarians Dr Dharmendra and Dr Alok Shukla

Summary Successful management of a Clostridial infection (malignant oedema) in a stallion

History
A 6-year-old skewbald stallion presented with a history of a ventral swelling that had developed over 3 days. The stallion had been treated by a local unqualified healer, with injections in the neck, using an old needle.

Clinical findings
Ventral oedema was prominent on lower abdomen, neck, scrotum and penis (Figures 14.11.1 and 14.11.2). The horse would not eat or drink. On palpation sub-cutaneous emphysema was present. Oral mucous membranes were congested, with a CRT of 3 seconds. The respiration rate was 28 breaths per minute, and the heart rate 64 beats per minute. Rectal temperature 39.1°C.

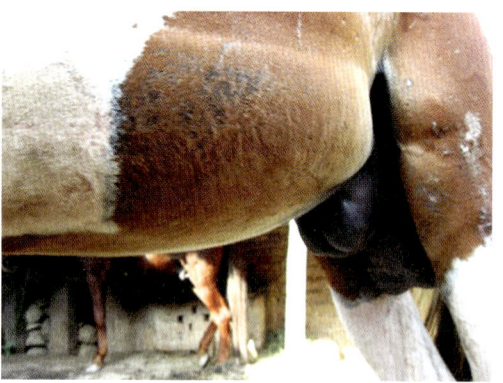

Figure 14.11.1 Ventral oedema affecting abdomen, prepuce and scrotum.

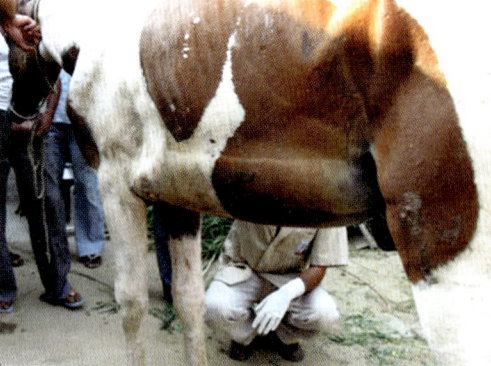

Figure 14.11.2 Severe ventral oedema.

Diagnosis
Based on history and clinical examination the disease was diagnosed as malignant oedema (Clostridial myonecrosis) which is caused by *Clostridium* spp., a gram positive anaerobic bacteria.

Treatment
1. Procaine penicillin 20,000 IU/kg BID IM in combination with metronidazole 10 mg/kg BID IV for 7 days
2. A fasciotomy/myotomy procedure was used to minimise the anaerobic environment. This involved making incisions in several sites across the oedematous area.
3. Flunixin 1.1 mg/kg SID IV for 7 days
4. Intravenous fluid therapy
5. Palliative care was provided by the owner; feed and water were raised off the ground to reduce the oedema (14.11.3). Soft bedding and good green feed were provided.

CASE STUDY – MALIGNANT OEDEMA 14.11

Preventive messages discussed with owner:

- Always ask local healers to use a new (sterile) disposable syringe and needle.
- When an animal is unwell it is preferable to seek advice from a veterinarian or a trained local healer.

Outcome
The recovery was uneventful and animal well again after 10 days (Figure 14.11.4).

Discussion
Malignant oedema, also known as Clostridial myonecrosis, is an acute, generally fatal toxaemia of cattle, equids, sheep, goats and pigs usually caused by *Clostridium septicum*. Other Clostridia implicated in wound infections include *C chauvoei, C. perfringens, C. novyi*, and *C. sordellii*.

In a retrospective case series, malignant oedema (Clostridial myonecrosis) was diagnosed in nine horses with signs of illness that included fever, depression, painful muscular swellings, and toxaemia. The infection followed intramuscular injections in eight horses and developed in a puncture wound in one horse. Treatment consisted of surgical fenestration of the involved muscle, high doses of penicillin, NSAIDs and analgesics, and supportive fluid therapy.

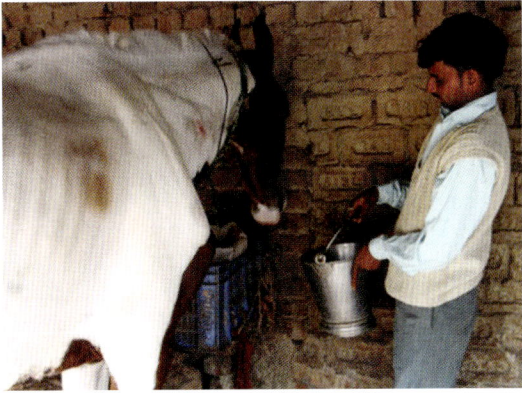

Figure 14.11.3 The owner taking good care of his recovering horse.

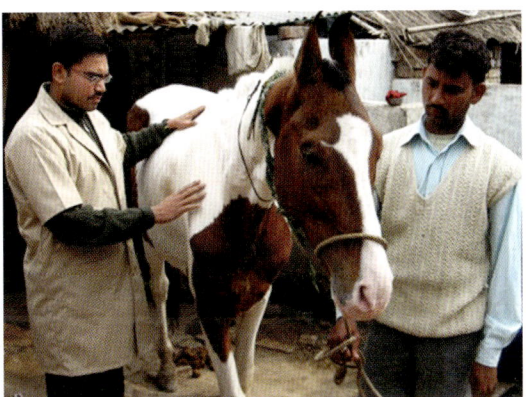

Figure 14.11.4 Dr Dharmendra examining the recovered case.

Five of the horses recovered and four died. Those that died had advanced signs of the disease at admission (Rebhun *et al.* 1985). A more recent study (Peek, Semrad and Perkins 2003) demonstrates a higher survival rate in horses treated for Clostridial myonecrosis at two equine referral centres in the United States.

The early use of a myotomy/fasciotomy procedure can improve the prognosis in cases of Clostridial myonecrosis. However, deep iatrogenic wounds are created when using this technique and it is vital that these wounds can be managed appropriately throughout the lengthy healing process. It is remarkable that the outcome of this case in India was positive considering the fatality rate of this condition and the prolonged clinical course prior to veterinary examination.

14.12 References

Beluche, L.A., Bertone, A.L., Anderson, D.E., Rhode, C. (2001) Effects of oral administration of phenylbutazone to horses on invitro articular cartilage metabolism. *Am. J. Vet. Res.* 62, 1916–1921.

Broster, C.E., Burn, C.C., Barr, A.R.S., Whay, H.R. (2009) The range and prevalance of pathological abnormalities associated with lameness in working horses from developing countries. *Equine Vet. J.* 41 (5) 474–481.

Cantley, C.E.L., Firth, E.C., Delahunt, J.W., Pfieffer, D.U., Thompson, K.G. (1999) Naturally occuring osteoarthritis in the metacorpophalangeal joints of wild horses. *Equine Vet. J.* 31, 73–80.

Caron, J.P. (2011) Septic arthritis and tenosynovitis: Diagnosis and treatment. ACVS Symposium Proceedings. Available online at: *http://www.acvs.org/Symposium/Proceedings2011/data/papers/019.pdf*

Collins, S.N., Dyson, S.J., Murray, R.C., Burden, F., Trawford, A. (2011) Radiological anatomy of the donkey's foot: Objective characterisation of the normal and laminitic donkey foot. *Equine Vet. J.* 43 (4) 478–486.

Crane, M. (2008) The Donkey's Foot. Chapter 10. In: The Professional Handbook of the Donkey. Ed: Svendsen, E.D. Whittet Books.

Doumbia, A. (2011) Onchocerciasis in working donkeys in Mali, Africa. 12th Congress of the World Equine Veterinary Association, Hyderabad, India.

Eades, S.C. (2010) Overview of Current Laminitis Research. *Vet. Clin. N. Am. Equine.* 26, 51–63.

Egenvall, A., Pennell, J.J., Bonnett, B.N., Olsen, P., Pringle, J. (2006) Mortality of Swedish horses with complete life insurance between 1997 and 2000: variations with sex, age, breed and diagnosis. *Vet. Rec.* 158 (12) 397–406.

Peek, S.F., Semrad, S.D., Perkins, G.A. (2003) Clostridial myonecrosis in horses (37 cases 1985–2000) *Equine Vet. J.* 35 (1) 86–92.

Pinchbeck, G.L., Clegg, P.D., Proudman, C.J., Stirk, A., Morgan, K.L., French, N.P. (2004) Horse injuries and racing practices in national hunt racehorses in the UK: the results of a prospective cohort study. *The Vet. J.* 167 (1) 45–52.

Pollit, C. (2004) Equine Laminitis. *Clin. Tech. Equine P.* 3 (1) 34–44.

Pritchard, J.C., Lindberg, A.C., Main, D.C.J., Whay, H.R. (2005) Assessment of the welfare of working horses, donkeys and mules, using health and behaviour parameters. *Prev. Vet. Med.* 69 (3–4) 265–283.

Rebhun, W.C. (1985) Malignant edema in horses. *J. Am. Vet. Med. Assoc.* 187 (7) 732–736.

Ross, M.W., Dyson, S.J. (2003) Diagnosis and Management of Lameness in the Horse. Saunders.

- Chapter 18 Lameness in the Sport Horse (Brushing and over reaching) 887.
- Chapter 27 The Foot and Shoeing (Natural balance trimming for a barefooted horse) 272.

- Chapter 34 The Distal Phalanx and Distal Interphalangeal Joint (Pedal osteitis: does it exist?) 321.
- Chapter 56 Developmental Orthopaedic Disease and Lameness (Pathogenesis of Osteochondrosis) 536–541.

Rossdale, P.D., Hopes, R., Digby, N.J., Offord, K. (1985) Epidemiology study of wastage among racehorses 1982 and 1983. *Vet. Rec.* 116 (3) 66–69.

Silver, I.A,. Rossdale, P.D. (1983) A clinical and experimental study of tendon injury, healing and treatment in the horse. *Equine Vet. J.* S1, 1–43.

Thiemann, A., Rickards, K. (2013) Donkey hoof disorders and their treatment. *In Practice.* 35: 134-140.

Thorpe, C.T., Birch, H.L., Clegg, P.D., Screen, H.R.C. (2012) The microstructural response of SDFT tendon fascicles to applied strain is altered with ageing. *Proceedings of the BEVA congress.* 229.

Tnibar, A. (2003) Treatment of upward fixation of the patella in the horse: an update. *Equine Vet. Educ.* 15 (5) 236–242.

Upjohn, M.M., Shipton, K., Pfeiffer, D.U., Lerotholi, T., Attwood, G., Verheyen, K.L.P. (2012) Cross-sectional survey of owner knowledge and husbandry practices, tack and health issues affecting working horses in Lesotho. *Equine Vet. J.* 44 (3).

van Eps, AW. (2010) Acute Laminitis: Medical and Supportive Therapy. *Vet. Clin. N. Am. Equine.* 26, 103–114.

Walmsley, J. (1999) Equine Practice: Emergency management of fractures in horses. *In Practice.* 21 (3) 122–127.

Walker, M., Taylor, T., Slater, M., Hood, D., Weir, V., Elslander, J. (1995) Radiographic appearance of the feet of mammoth donkeys and the findings of subclinical laminitis. *J. Vet. Radiology Ultrasound.* 36 (1) 32–37.

Further reading

Gough, M. (1998) Diagnosis of palmar foot pain in the equine forelimb. *In Practice.* 358–366.

Pollitt, C. (2008) Equine Laminitis Current Concepts. Available online at *http://hovslagarforeningen.nu/media/f_ng-compendie.pdf*

For a good overview of external and internal hoof anatomy refer to this website *http://www.thenaturalhoof.co.uk/4.html*

Tremaine, H. (2000) Infection of equine joints and tendon sheaths. *In Practice.* 22, 262–274.

Rendle, D. (2006) Equine Laminitis: Management in the acute stage. *In Practice.* 28, 434–443.

The integumentary system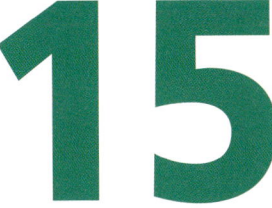

Principles of inflammation and wound management	**15.1**
Diagnosis of skin abnormalities	**15.2**
Common skin diseases of working equids	**15.3**
The long-term prevention of wounds	**15.4**
Bandaging	**15.5**
Case study – Wound management	**15.6**
References	**15.7**

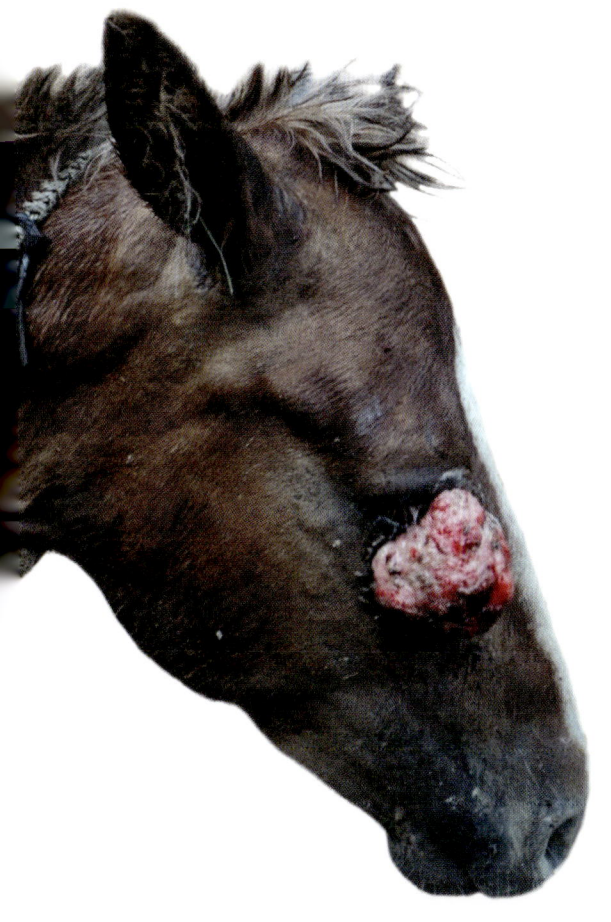

15.1 Principles of inflammation and wound management

> Wounds are an extremely common, and in many cases preventable, presentation to working equine veterinarians. Knowledge of inflammation and the healing process is required for the management of these wounds. In order to minimise the occurrence of wounds in the future, it is important to understand the underlying causes.

Phases of healing

There is overlap between each of the classic phases of healing described. The timing of each process will depend on the size and depth of the wound.

1. Inflammatory phase

This phase begins *immediately* after injury has occurred.

Haemostasis and formation of a wound matrix: haemorrhaging blood from traumatised vessels flushes the wound; removing debris and micro-organisms. This is followed by vasoconstriction and clot formation (haemostasis). Fibrin within the blood clot forms the provisional wound matrix. Cells involved in tissue regeneration begin to migrate to the site.

The inflammatory process is initiated by activation of the complement pathway within the wound. The early phase of the inflammatory response is characterised by the arrival of neutrophils. A late phase follows (day 3 onwards) with the appearance of monocytes. Phagocytosis of bacteria and degradation of necrotic tissue by neutrophils occurs for 2–5 days. Inflammation can lead to tissue damage if prolonged; this can occur in infected wounds.

> There are five clinical signs of acute inflammation: heat, redness (vasodilation), swelling (oedema), loss of function and pain (inflammatory mediators sensitise nerve fibres).

2. Proliferative phase

This phase begins *2–3 days* after injury and the duration depends on the size of the original wound.

During the proliferative phase the wound surface is covered with granulation tissue which also helps to fill the cavity. New blood vessels form (angiogenesis) to supply the granulation tissue; the healing wound is highly vascularised and easily traumatised at this stage. Excessive granulation tissue is known as proud flesh (where the tissue protrudes above the surrounding skin), which inhibits skin re-epithelialisation. Re-epithelialisation is initiated from the wound edges; this is preceded by the migration of fibroblasts to the injury site. Fibroblasts synthesise collagen forming the basis of a new matrix of connective tissue. Keratinocytes migrate across the matrix to form the new epithelial layer.

3. Maturation phase

Formation of granulation tissue gradually slows (from 2 to 3 weeks post injury), and the wound becomes stronger with the re-modelling of collagen fibres within the tissue. Angiogenic processes diminish and the blood supply to the wound reduces. Myofibroblasts induce wound contraction.

PRINCIPLES OF INFLAMMATION AND WOUND MANAGEMENT 15.1

As there is no potential for the regeneration of hair follicles the scar will remain hairless.

By understanding the process of wound healing the optimal conditions can be created to promote rapid repair of injury. This process is not only complex but fragile, and susceptible to interruption or failure leading to the formation of non-healing **chronic wounds**. Infection of a wound delays healing; it is essential to spend sufficient time cleaning and preparing wounds for effective healing.

Figures 15.1.1 demonstrate the healing process from the initial trauma with associated haemorrhage and inflammation through to granulation and epithelialisation stages.

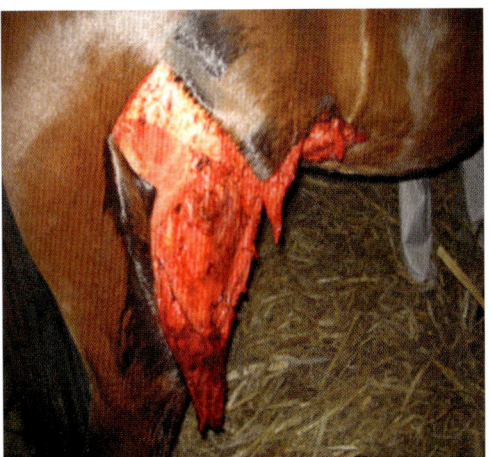 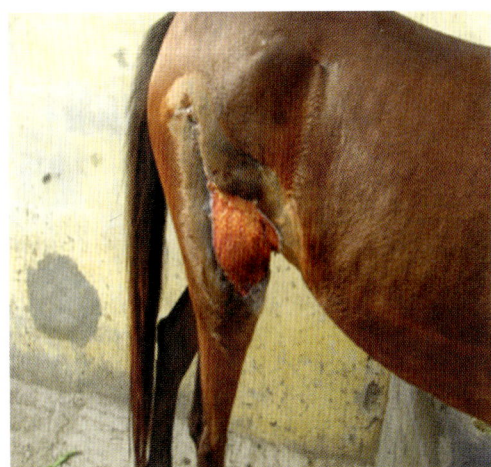

Figure 15.1.1 The wound on day 1 (left) and 2 weeks later demonstrating healthy granulation tissue with re-epithelialisation and contraction.

Factors affecting wound healing

What factors affect the prognosis of a healing wound?

When treating a wound or advising the owner on appropriate management it is important to consider whether the following factors are present, and how to alleviate or prevent them.

Infection resulting in a chronic inflammatory state. The tissue fails to progress through the normal stages giving rise to a non-healing wound.

Ischaemia and necrosis Often the result of poor perfusion or substantial tissue trauma as outlined below

Oedema Extracellular water which increases the diffusion distances of oxygen from capillaries

Tissue trauma Trauma to the wound site when the injury occurred, or subsequent trauma, e.g. caused by the vet's over-zealous surgical debridement or the owner's application of toxic substances

Foreign body The presence of foreign material within the wound induces a chronic inflammatory state if the foreign body is too large to be resolved by macrophage phagocytosis.

Corticosteroids These delay wound closure by suppressing the growth factors necessary in the proliferative phase.

15 THE INTEGUMENTARY SYSTEM

Protein deficiency Low albumin results in slower collagen formation.

Poor perfusion Reduced delivery of nutrients, leukocytes, inflammatory cytokines and oxygen to the injury site. This may be the result of damaged local blood vessels, hypovolaemia, severe anaemia, etc.

Stress Induces a physiological (as opposed to iatrogenic) increase in glucocorticoids which has negative effects on pro-inflammatory cytokines and growth factors. This factor is of particular importance for working equids (Christian et al. 2006).

Movement Pressure and movement from harnesses, tack, etc. or movement of the wound as the skin shifts over a joint will slow healing as the wound matrix breaks. New epithelial cells are delicate and a repaired wound has reduced strength even once a scar has formed.

Concurrent disease A chronic debilitating disease can cause immunosuppression and reduced nutrient supply to a healing wound.

Wound management

When an injury occurs directly over a joint (Figure 15.1.2) it is essential to establish whether a synovial membrane has been breached as, if this has occurred, the result is a septic arthritis (see Section 14.7 *Conditions affecting the joints*). Once a joint infection is established, a day or so after the inciting cause, the affected animal is likely to be severely lame. At this stage it is difficult to resolve the infection. By determining at the outset whether a joint is involved it may be possible to flush the joint and reduce the likelihood of infection.

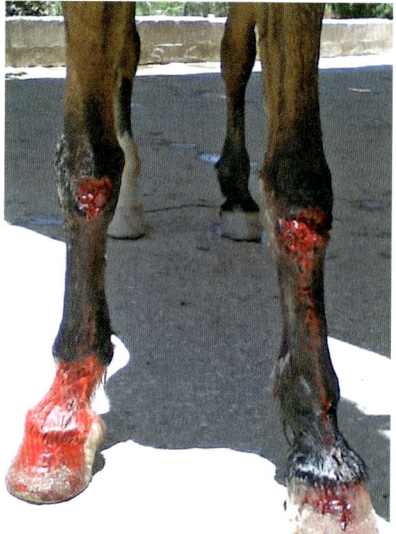

Figure 15.1.2 Open wounds over the carpus joint. The fresh blood indicates that this wound has occurred within the last few hours. There is a risk of joint sepsis in wounds directly over joints.

Clip and aseptically prepare a large area around the wound to include the skin overlying any local joints. Place a needle into the joint (synoviocentesis) at a site distant to the wound, as described for intra-articular medication in Section 4.1 *Drug administration techniques*. After collecting joint fluid for cytology, inject 5–10 ml of sterile saline through the needle to pressurise the joint capsule. If this fluid passes out though the wound this confirms damage to the synovial membrane and the joint is likely to be contaminated. Continue to flush the joint with copious (at least 1 litre) sterile fluids, place an egress needle at another site in the joint to improve flow. Following flushing remove the egress needle and inject 2–5 ml of an antibiotic suitable for intra-articular use such as amikacin sulfate (250–500 mg) or gentamicin (1 g).

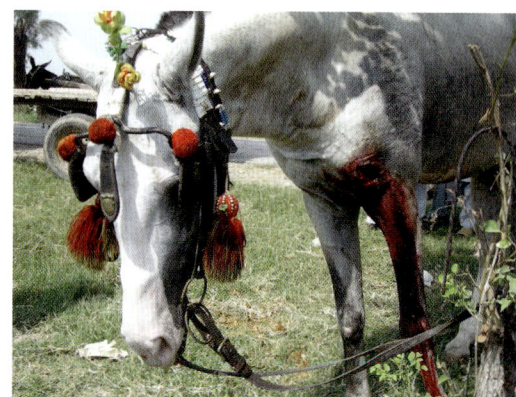

Figure 15.1.3 Fresh wound on a horse's forelimb.

PRINCIPLES OF INFLAMMATION AND WOUND MANAGEMENT 15.1

The Golden Period is a theoretical time frame of 8 hours after which a contaminated wound is described as infected (Figure 15.1.3). Within approximately 8 hours any bacteria present within the wound will adhere to the tissue surface and are unlikely to be removed by wound flushing and debridement. This has implications when determining a wound management protocol (e.g. open wound or closed wound). If more than 8 hours have passed it is preferable to allow a wound to heal by second intention. Suturing an infected wound is likely to lead to slow healing, chronic wound formation and suture breakdown.

Initial medical treatment of acute wounds

Treat with NSAIDs to provide pain relief and minimise swelling. Ensure **tetanus cover** is provided and, if the equid has not been vaccinated, administer tetanus anti-toxin. Administer a full course of **antibiotics** to equids with an infected wound. A single dose will have little effect and risks the development of bacterial resistance. If the wound is uncontaminated and sutured within 8 hours of the injury antibiotics may not be required; these cases are rare.

> Most wounds in working equids are unlikely to be suitable for suturing.

Open wound management

Wound types appropriate for open wound management are listed below:
- Dirty or infected wounds (> 8 hours old)
- All puncture wounds
- Maggot-infested wounds
- Chronic wounds
- Saddle and harness wounds
- Wounds with large skin or tissue deficits
- Wounds over joints
- Wounds below the carpus
- Sutured wounds that have broken down

Steps in managing open wounds

1. **Reduce contamination or infection:**

    - Protect the wound with moist swabs or sterile lubricant.
    - Clip or shave hair from wound edges (Figure 15.1.4).

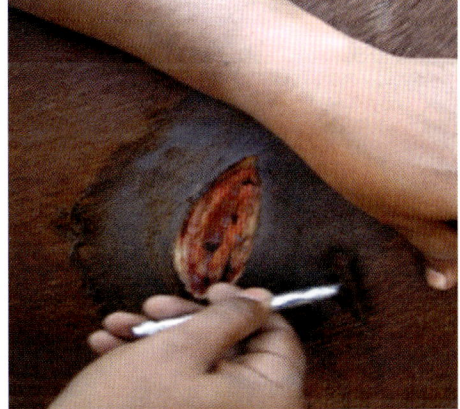

Figure 15.1.4 Shaving around a wound.

- Clean the surrounding area with antiseptic. Iodine, if used, should be the colour of weak tea. Strong antiseptics, including spirit or purple spray, result in damage to the delicate epithelial tissue.
- Remove any maggots or foreign bodies from the wound.
- Clean the wound from the centre.
- Flush with large volumes of sterile saline in a 60-ml syringe with an 18G needle.
- With sterile gloves explore the wound to establish which anatomical structures are involved.

15 THE INTEGUMENTARY SYSTEM

> 'Dilution is the solution to pollution.' A large volume of water, applied under moderate pressure, is an important factor in helping a wound to heal. Owners can continue with this treatment daily. Caution that clean boiled and cooled water must be used for flushing.

2. Debride the wound:

   1. Infiltrate a local anaesthetic to the wound edges. It is preferable to use mepivacaine or lidocaine without adrenaline. An alternative is perineural anaesthesia (see Section 14.2 *Working equine lameness examination*).
   2. Use a scalpel blade to debride the edges of the skin by sharp dissection; remove a thin margin of skin rather than just scraping the edge of the wound.
   3. Resect devitalised and necrotic tissue (black, dried, crusting).

For grossly contaminated wounds 'wet-to-dry' dressings can be used to lift the necrotic tissue and debris from the wound surface that cannot be removed by cleaning and debridement. Apply wet gauzes to the surface of the wound and bandage. Remove after 24 hours.

3. Protect the wound:

   1. Application of a sterile wound lubricant is beneficial to keep the wound surface moist. Antiseptics, antibiotic preparations or medicinal plants are unlikely to create an environment optimal for wound healing. However, honey has been used to treat human wounds and there is evidence that this has positive effects for wound healing (Noori *et al.* 2011).
   2. Corticosteroid creams should not be used in the majority of cases as it slows wound healing. The exception is with proud flesh (see later in this chapter).
   3. Keep flies and dirt away with a bandage if possible and ensure harness or padding is not over the top of the wound. A cotton sheet can be used on areas that are hard to bandage such as the withers or neck. Bandaging can also reduce swelling and oedema, in the early stages, and immobilise the affected region. 'Strikethrough', where wound exudate has seeped through the bandage, creates a channel for the migration of micro-organisms. The bandage should be changed at this stage.

Closed wound management (suturing)

Sutured wounds in equids have a high rate of breakdown, even in the absence of the aforementioned factors which delay healing.

> A wound may *only* be sutured if the following conditions can be fulfilled:
> 1. A fresh wound of less than 8 hours old ('golden period')
> 2. A clean wound with no gross contamination
> 3. There will be little tension when the skin edges are brought together.

Principles of suturing wounds

Needle choice Use a cutting needle when suturing the skin and a round-bodied needle when suturing subcutaneous tissues.

PRINCIPLES OF INFLAMMATION AND WOUND MANAGEMENT 15.1

Suture material

Absorbable sutures are used when suturing structures below the skin surface.

Subcutaneous tissue Size 2 to 3 metric, absorbable monofilament such as monocryl (poliglecaprone 25) or multifilament such as vicryl (polyglactin 910). Catgut can be used. However, natural suture materials tend to induce an inflammatory reaction and rapidly reduce in tensile strength.

Muscle Size 3 to 5 metric, absorbable monofilament such as maxon (polyglyconate)/PDS (polydioxanone) or multifilament such as vicryl (polyglactin 910). Again, catgut can be used but synthetic suture materials are preferable.

Non-absorbable sutures for the skin itself (will need removing after 10–14 days).

Monofilament is preferable as multifilament sutures may create a channel for microorganisms into the wound.

Size is important – ensure it is not going to pull through (too thin) or affect healing (too thick).

Appositional skin sutures Size 3 to 3.5 metric, non-absorbable monofilament prolene (polypropylene) or ethilon (nylon)

(Suture recommendations from Stashak and Theoret, 2009)

Suture pattern Simple interrupted, cruciate or mattress suture patterns are preferable. It is essential to use the least number of sutures necessary to appose the wound under minimal tension. Sutures are a foreign body and will induce an inflammatory response.

Tension Excessive tension can cause tissue necrosis. Wound edges should just touch; swelling continues for 24 hours following an injury. Tying the throws down over a pair of haemostat forceps will ensure that the sutures are not too tight. Tension sutures may be required to stabilise a wound over a joint. If the wound is under severe tension, mobilisation of skin, using undermining, skin incisions or flaps, has been recommended. These procedures can be technically challenging and can risk wound breakdown, refer to Stashak and Theoret (2009) for detailed instruction.

Intra-wound antibiotics are controversial but have been shown to reduce infection rates. Limit antibiotic delivery into the wound to examples with a poor blood supply. It is important to use water soluble and non-irritant antibiotics.

> **If it is unclear whether a wound should be sutured or left open, always ensure cleanliness and leave to heal as an open wound.**

Surgical drains

Dead space is the potential space underlying an incompletely closed wound. This space is created as the result of a deficit in the muscle or subcutaneous tissue that has not been closed or where it has not been possible to directly appose tissues. Accumulation of blood or serum within this space will delay healing. A surgical drain placed within the wound allows drainage of the accumulating fluid, and eventually closure of the space. A Penrose drain (soft rubber tube) is most commonly used; the fluid drains along the sides of this tube rather than through the centre. Gauze or bandage in the wound is not recommended as drainage is poor, and this material can act as a 'wick' for infection.

The drain should be placed in the wound and attached by a suture through the skin. Exit the drain through a separate stab incision at the most ventral part of the cavity, below the suture line, attaching with a second skin suture. Do not exit the drain through the wound or suture line as this will prevent healing. Remove the drain after fluid has stopped leaking from the wound (usually 2–3 days). The drain should not be left in for longer than 3–4 days.

Proud flesh (excessive granulation tissue)

Wounds heal via **granulation** from the depth and **epithelialisation** from the edges. Usually these two act in synchrony resulting in a fast healing process.

> Proud flesh occurs when granulation > epithelialisation

This is seen as excessive pink tissue forming a large protruding growth which prevents epithelialisation (Figure 15.1.5). It is common on the distal limb but can occur anywhere.

How to manage excessive granulation tissue?

1. Using a scalpel blade, trim the excess granulation tissue back to just below the skin surface. Remember granulation tissue has an excellent blood supply, so will bleed profusely. Be careful not to disturb the newly laid epithelium around the edges of the wound.
2. The aim is to encourage epithelialisation so the wound heals. Apply corticosteroid cream to the **centre** of the wound only, to inhibit further granulation, keeping it away from the delicate edges.
3. Firmly bandage the wound – the pressure will prevent further bleeding (granulation tissue is highly vascular).
4. Apply the corticosteroid cream to the granulation tissue every third day for 3–5 applications after debridement. If exuberant granulation tissue reforms, repeat the process. Do not use other chemicals such as potassium permanganate or copper sulphate.

Prevention of excessive granulation is preferable. The early treatment of wounds is essential; clean wounds thoroughly to prevent infection (Figure 15.1.6). Bandaging and immobilisation will also limit the development of proud flesh.

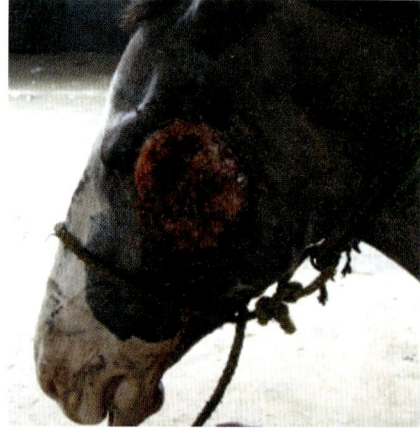
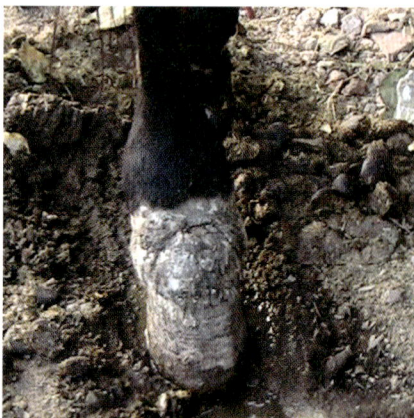

Figure 15.1.5 *Proud flesh on the face of a horse (top) and dorsal coronary band.*

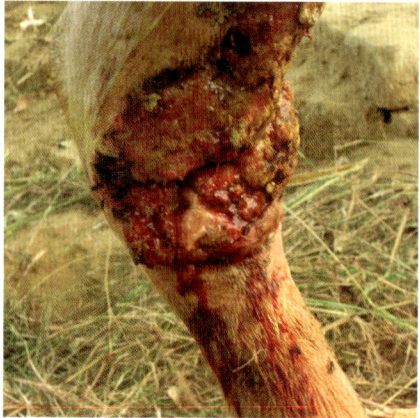

Figure 15.1.6 *This horse became entangled in barbed wire. The wound is infected and excessive granulation tissue is forming.*

Diagnosis of skin abnormalities

15.2

> A logical and systematic approach is necessary when attempting to diagnose skin disease. Many conditions may present with the same signs even though the inciting cause is different: the signs are not pathognomonic.

History

Outlined below is a **skin specific history** that can be incorporated into the initial discussions with an owner:

- When and where on the body did the problem start?
- What did the initial lesion looks like?
- Is there any pruritus (itching)?
- Have there been any skin problems before and, if so, has there been a seasonal link?
- Are any in-contact horses, donkeys, mules showing similar signs?
- Has any treatment already been given?
- Have there been any recent changes to management, diet, tack, etc.?

Primary lesions These include the following:

- **Papules** Small (< 1 cm) circumscribed solid elevations of the skin with no visible fluid. These often develop into pustules.
- **Pustules** Small and raised containing purulent material
- **Macules** Changes to the colour of the skin, neither raised nor depressed
- **Wheals** (urticaria) Raised skin lesions that are either rounded or flat-topped and often disappear in 24–48 hours
- **Nodules** Lesions that extend into the dermis or subcutaneous tissue. The term tumour is used for larger nodules.
- **Alopecia** Loss of hair. This may form part of the pathological process or could be the result of rubbing induced by pruritus.
- **Changes in skin colour**

Secondary lesions These lesions may develop from primary lesions resulting from external forces such as self-trauma, infections and treatment:

- **Excoriations** Caused by self-trauma such as the equid biting or rubbing pruritic lesions
- **Erosion** A break in the skin not penetrating the full thickness of the epidermis
- **Ulcer** A break in the skin, full thickness and revealing the underlying sub-cutaneous tissue
- **Lichenification** Thickening of the skin, usually as the result of persistent excoriation
- **Scale** Flakes or plates of peeling sheets of skin
- **Crusts** Dried plasma or exudate on the surface of the skin
- **Scars** Areas of fibrosis that replace normal skin after injury

15 THE INTEGUMENTARY SYSTEM

Further diagnostics

> It is frequently necessary to collect an appropriate sample for laboratory examination in order to make a definitive diagnosis of a skin condition.

If a microscope is available, skin brushings and scrapings are easily collected for direct examination. This is often the first stage in a skin disease work-up.

Skin scraping

Skin scrapes are usually carried out if a **parasitic skin infection**, such as mange, is suspected.

It is important to do a number of scrapes from different areas where the lesions occur. Apply a small amount of paraffin on the scalpel blade. Parting the hair of the animal, scrape the skin carefully, but firmly, to induce redness and slight bleeding. (Mites can burrow deeply under the skin. In the case of *Sarcoptes scabei* var *equi* a skin biopsy may be more appropriate.) Examine using a microscope.

Skin brushing

Several skin parasites, such as the *Chorioptes* mite, live on the skin surface. By brushing over the coat surface onto a large sheet of paper, debris can be collected for examination microscopically.

Fine needle aspirate

A fine needle aspirate (FNA) is a technique used to collect cells from skin lumps or fluid from cavities. In nodules or tumours of an unknown aetiology a diagnosis may be determined by collecting cells from within the mass by FNA and examining microscopically. This procedure can be used to differentiate an **abscess**, which may need to be drained, from a **haematoma**, the draining of which would result in further haemorrhage.

Procedure

1. Shave a small area of hair at the most dependent point of the mass.
2. Clean and disinfect the skin.
3. Choosing a small needle, quickly but gently insert it down to the hub.
4. Re-direct the needle or aspirate using a syringe to release fluid or collect cells for microscopic examination.

Cytology

This is a simple, fast diagnostic test that is underused in evaluating skin disease. It is possible to identify the presence of yeasts, fungal hyphae, bacteria, different types of inflammatory cells and even neoplastic cells.

Obtaining the smear

Direct impression smears Useful for moist areas such as the underside of crusts, areas of exudate/discharge or open pustules, vesicles or papules.

Firmly press the glass slide directly onto the skin surface. Stain with Diff-Quik (or alternative histological stain) and examine when dry (see Section 4.4 *Blood smears and staining*).

Swab smears Useful for dry, superficial areas such as crusts, hairless patches of skin or ear canals. Moisten a cotton-tipped applicator with saline and rub briskly over area to be examined. Roll the cotton tip over the surface of glass slide and examine after staining with Diff-Quik.

Sticky tape preparations Useful for dry areas. Interpretation can be slightly more difficult unless cell types/organisms are present in large numbers. Firmly press sticky tape onto the skin in a number of different areas. Place a few drops Diff-Quik onto glass slide and press tape onto slide, distributing the stain evenly underneath the tape with your fingers.

Biopsy

> Nodules and tumours will often require a histological diagnosis to discern the aetiology. Do not conduct a diagnostic test unless it will be used to inform treatment. It is essential that a laboratory facility is available and capable of processing samples before biopsies are collected.

Biopsy Surgical removal of a small sample of the lump for laboratory assessment. This is used as an investigative tool, for example to determine the margins required for a surgical removal or to establish a prognosis for the animal.

Lumpectomy Complete removal of a lump, with the objective of being curative. A specific diagnosis should be obtained prior to complete excision. Only histopatholoical examination can provide a definitive diagnosis. When this is not available lesions should be managed as malignant; remove wide margins around the tumour in order to reduce the likelihood of recurrence. When removing a tumour it is essential that it is removed completely; this also necessitates knowledge of the types of tumours which occur, and whether complete excision is possible given the size and position of the tumour, and its relation to underlying tissues.

What should be considered before attempting to remove a lump?

Is the lump suitable for biopsy/removal? Consider the following:

- What is the most likely **cause** of the lump?
- Is there evidence of **infection/inflammation** which could delay the healing process?
- Is the lump in a suitable **site** which allows for healing? Ensure it is not in a dependent or highly mobile area which would result in wound breakdown.
- Are you able to ensure **total excision**, if this is the objective?
- Do you have a suitable area in which to carry out the procedure?
- Is there access to a laboratory where analysis of the biopsy can be carried out?

> The primary responsibility of a veterinarian is to the animal, regardless of what the owner feels is possible. Consider the goal of the surgery and whether this is achievable.

15.3 Common skin diseases of working equids

> For practical diagnostic purposes, it is easier to categorise skin conditions according to the presenting signs rather than aetiological agents. Skin disease is characterised by pruritus, nodules, lumps and bumps or crusting and ulcerative lesions.

Skin diseases characterised by pruritus (itching)

Refer to Section 17.5 for parasitic skin conditions.

Pyoderma

A **secondary bacterial infection** is common in all skin afflictions, regardless of the primary cause. Many bacteria, for example *Staphylococcus* species, are **commensal** organisms. If there is a break in the integrity of the skin surface, such as a wound, these bacteria can easily colonise in the damaged tissue.

Causal organisms

- *Staphylococcus* spp. (predominant bacteria in pyoderma)
- *Corynebacterium* spp.
- *Dermatophilus congolensis* ('rain scald' – see opposite)

Causal factors

Damp skin (warm, wet weather), poor grooming, skin wounds, abrasion and pruritic conditions resulting in excoriation. Pyoderma is very commonly associated with skin contact with tack, rugs or cart equipment, particularly if sweating occurs and the equipment is dirty.

Appearance

- *Staphylococcus* infection – forms crusts in a circular pattern (similar to ringworm).
- The skin appears wet due to exudate.
- Encrusted papules and pustules are evident.
- In severe cases a deep pyoderma with ulceration develops.
- There are signs of pruritus and discomfort.
- Inflammation – causes redness, swelling and pain. (Staphylococcus lesions are usually *very* painful.)

Treatment

Clip the affected area and clean with dilute antiseptic. An application of topical anti-bacterial solution may be necessary; in severe or chronic cases systemic antibiotics may be indicated (trimethoprim sulfamethoxazole). If pyoderma is associated with tack or rugs make sure these are **removed** frequently and **kept clean**. Un-tacking and allowing air to reach the skin can greatly facilitate healing and reduce the chances of pyoderma recurring.

COMMON SKIN DISEASES OF WORKING EQUIDS 15.3

> Consider the human health risks of *Staphylococcus* infection particularly antibiotic-resistant strains known as MRSA (Methicillin Resistant *Staphylococcus Aureus*) (Yusada *et al.* 2000).

Dermatophilosis ('rain scald')

Dermatophilus congolensis (actinomycete bacteria) is spread by carrier animals; pre-disposing factors for infection include moisture and abrasion.

Appearance

- Small crusty lumps with hair standing up (paintbrush)
- Underlying skin moist and inflamed
- Impression smear of the underside of crusts – 'railroad track' cocci (bacteria joined together in a line)

Distribution

Dorsal surfaces which can become soaked with rain. Also common on the caudal pastern due to hobbles or a muddy environment. Rain scald can also affect other areas: under harness, flanks or face (Figure 15.3.1).

Treatment

Minimise exposure to wet, muddy environments. Rugs and saddle padding should be removed to avoid contact with sweaty skin. Shave or clip the affected area. Apply dilute antiseptic and leave open to the air to dry. Remove loose scabs and crusting which harbour the bacteria. Burn the removed scabs, as bacteria within this material can infect other horses. Disinfect the grooming kit and minimise grooming until the infection has resolved. Treat with penicillin or trimethoprim sulfamethoxazole for 7 days. Protect lesions on the lower limb by applying a waterproof barrier cream (petroleum jelly or hydrous wool fat). Apply a small amount before the animal begins work and remove afterwards.

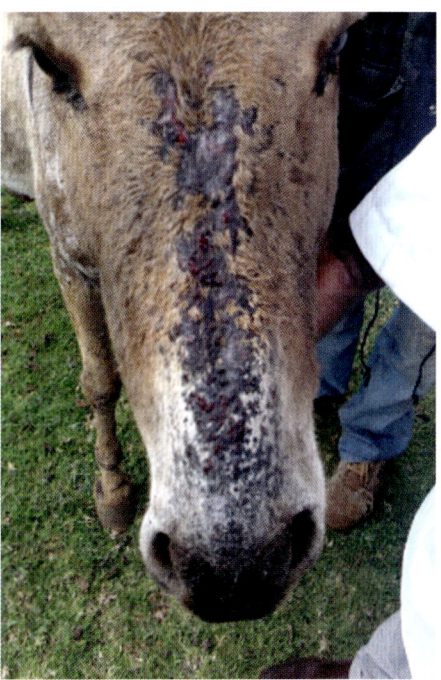

Figure 15.3.1 Dermatophilosis on the face of a donkey.

Pastern and heel dermatitis ('mud fever')

Pastern dermatitis is not a single disease but a generic skin reaction to a variety of causes. This condition is invariably associated with chronic saturation of the distal limb resulting in a bacterial folliculitis (*Staphylococcus* infection). Other causes include contact irritation, photosensitisation, mites, fungal infection and immune-mediated inflammation.

15 THE INTEGUMENTARY SYSTEM

Clinical signs

- **Inflammation** – red skin, hair loss (alopecia), initially around the skin folds of the pastern/heel bulbs
- **Exudate** – from a mild serous discharge to significant exudation with marked crusting and thick scab formation
- **Pain** on palpation – cellulitis can develop if a severe infection is present.
- Prolonged cases show chronic skin thickening, persistent hair loss and scarring.

Treatment

Debride the area to remove all scabs and necrotic skin. Soak scabs with warm, dilute disinfectant prior to removal. This is a painful procedure and may require sedation and analgesics. Rest the animal and reduce exposure to wet and muddy conditions. Apply antibiotic cream in severe cases; mild cases will heal with management alone. Severe cases may benefit from a topical steroid application on one or two occasions; repeated steroid application will delay healing. For long-term management the use of barrier creams can be helpful (petroleum jelly). Advise owners to clean and dry the legs of the equid after work.

Dermatophytosis ('ringworm')

This is most common in young or immune-compromised animals and those kept in dirty conditions. Lesions are caused by fungal species that utilise keratin, *Trichophyton* and *Microsporum*. Fungal spores can contaminate buildings and tack. The incubation period is 1–4 weeks and the infection spreads slowly amongst a group of equids.

> **Ringworm is a zoonotic skin condition; wear gloves when treating affected animals.**

Appearance

- Crusting and scaling
- Multifocal, sharply demarcated areas of hair loss, classically a coin-shaped appearance (Figure 15.3.2)
- Initial lesions appearing as raised, swollen lumps (urticaria)
- Variable pruritus

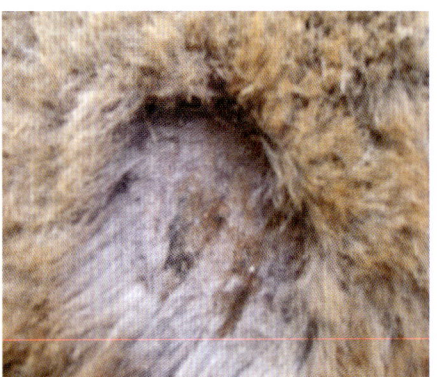
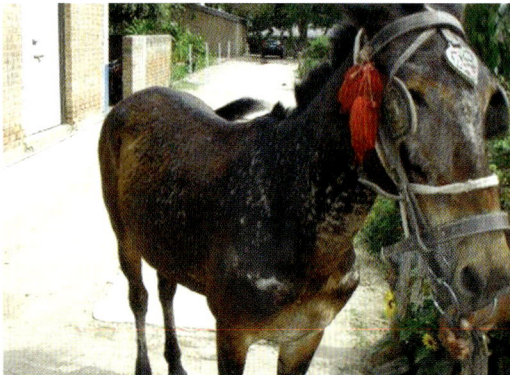

Figure 15.3.2 Clinical appearance of dermatophytosis.

Treatment

Generally equids recover over the course of several months. Affected equids are a source of infection to other animals and humans throughout recovery. If severe, topical antifungals are indicated. Follow the instructions as these medications can be toxic. Wash daily with dilute iodine (10% solution) including the harness and grooming equipment. Systemic antifungals (griseofulvin) require a prolonged treatment period for efficacy, and compliance can be problematic. Griseofulvin should not be used in pregnant mares as the medication is teratogenic. Isolate the affected animal and monitor animals in contact for signs of similar skin lesions.

Insect hypersensitivity ('sweet itch')

Any biting insect can cause this type of hypersensitivity reaction although it is predominantly induced by *Culicoides* spp. (midges). Most reactions are an immediate hypersensitivity (Type I) but also include a delayed hypersensitivity reaction (Type IV).

Appearance

- **Multiple swellings** occur over the body; urticarial (Figure 15.3.3).
- **Hair loss**/rubbed hair especially over the mane/neck and tail base; look for broken hairs.
- **Associated pruritus** and evidence of excoriation. In chronic cases the skin will be thickened (lichenified).
- **Plaques or wheals** form in some cases.

Treatment

In some cases urticaria resolves within 24–48 hours. Steroid treatment will temporarily alleviate the pruritus and skin inflammation. Anti-histamines may help prevent a hypersensitivity reaction, although there is very little evidence for its efficacy in equids. Protect from flies by stabling the affected equid and covering the affected areas. Make owners aware that insect hypersensitivity is likely to be a chronic condition which should be controlled with management appropriate to the feeding habits of the insects involved.

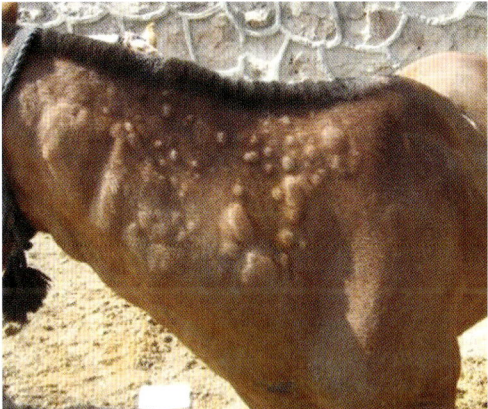

Figure 15.3.3 Urticaria on the neck of a horse.

Skin diseases characterised by nodules, lumps and bumps

Infectious nodular skin conditions

Habronemiasis (Section 9.6 *Common eye diseases of working equids* and Section 17.5 *External parasite species*)

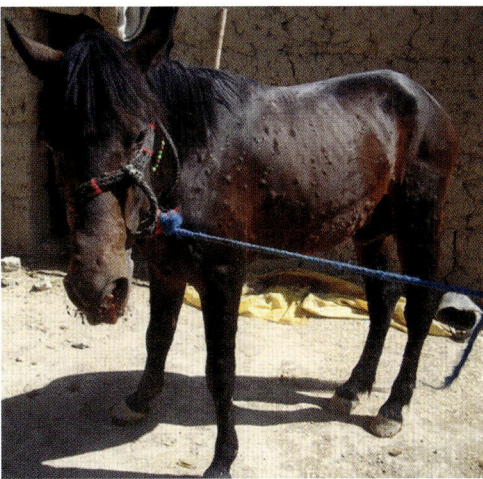

Figure 15.3.4 'Farcy' presentation of glanders.

15 THE INTEGUMENTARY SYSTEM

Corynebacterium pseudotuberculosis Multiple ventral abscesses

Glanders 'Farcy' presentation (Section 12.7 *Bacterial respiratory disease*) (Figure 15.3.4)

Sporotrichosis A (rare) zoonotic yeast infection presenting as a nodular or ulcerative skin condition (Crothers *et al.* 2009)

Epizootic lymphangitis

This is a form of lymphangitis caused by the fungus *Histoplasma capsulatum var. farciminosum*. This devastating disease is endemic in parts of Africa (with a high prevalence in Ethiopia), Asia and the Middle East and spreads rapidly among equines, particularly younger animals. It is more common in horses than donkeys. Transmission is thought to be through contamination of open wounds and by ticks and biting flies which act as mechanical vectors. Epizootic lymphangitis has been known to affect camels, cattle and even humans.

Clinical signs

The skin form Skin nodules and infected tracts along lymphatic vessels form which are similar to the lesions present in the Farcy form of Glanders (Figures 15.3.5 and 15.3.6).

Lacrimal histoplasmosis is an ocular form of the disease and is the most common form in donkeys. It presents as a granulomatous proliferation of the conjunctival sac that protrudes out of the medial lacrimal puncta. There is swelling, blepharospasm, conjunctivitis and a purulent ocular discharge (Figure 15.3.7).

Obstruction of the nasolacrimal duct causes increased discharge from the eye (Figure 15.3.8).

A pulmonary form of the disease is very rare and occurs after inhalation of the organism.

Diagnosis

Definitive diagnosis is by identification of the characteristic yeast-like cells on stained smears of purulent material. The pus from lanced abscesses has the appearance of honey. The skin form of the disease can look similar to Glanders (Farcy). The mallein test will distinguish the two diseases.

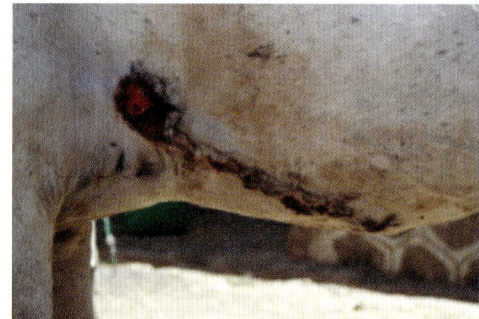

Figure 15.3.5 Cutaneous form of the disease shows an infective nodule/granulomatous lesion with an invasive tract showing spread along the lymphatic vessel.

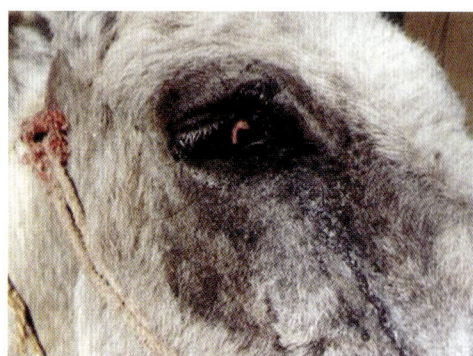

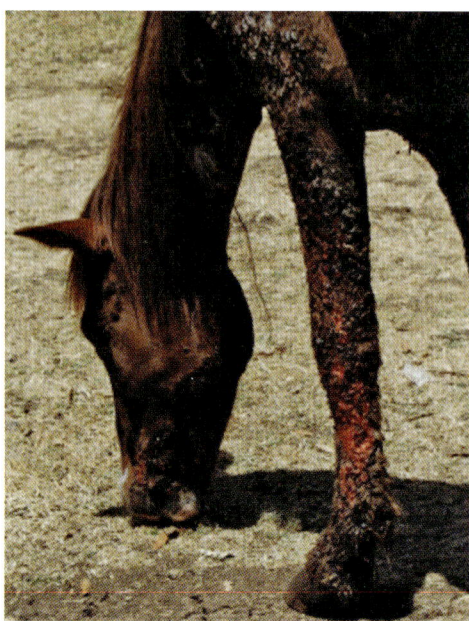

Figure 15.3.6 Lesions seen on the face and the left forelimb.

COMMON SKIN DISEASES OF WORKING EQUIDS 15.3

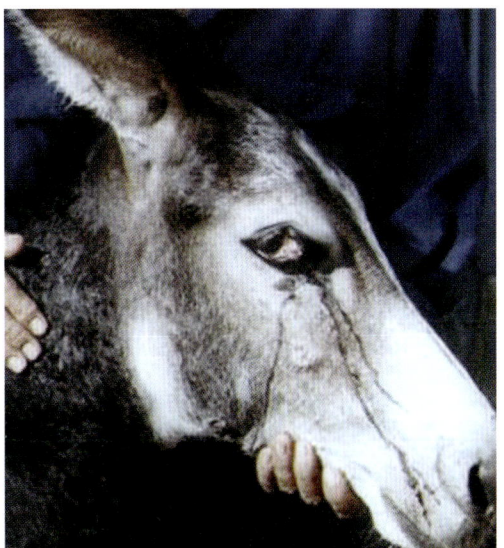

Figure 15.3.7 Conjunctival infection and inflammation associated with the lacrimal histoplasmosis.

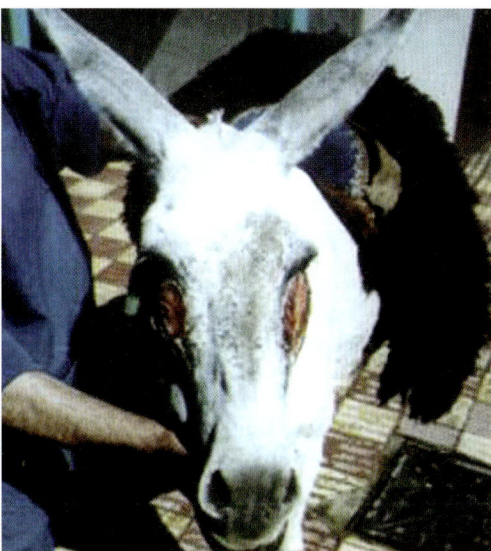

Figure 15.3.8 Lacrimal histoplasmosis has a similar presentation to Habronema infection.

The ocular form may look clinically similar to lacrimal Habronemiasis; differentiate by histopathology, identification of Habronema larvae or a treatment trial. The 'histofarcin test' was studied for diagnosis of enzootic lymphangitis (Ameni *et al.* 2006) although this is not commercially available.

Treatment

Various protocols have been trialled, including treatment with sodium iodide or oral potassium iodide. Nodules and abscesses, if in small numbers and distribution, can be treated by lancing and cleaning with iodine based antiseptics. However, the chronic weight loss and debility remains.

Sodium iodide (NaI) has been used succesfully in Ethiopia where this condition is common (Hadush *et al.* 2008). Administer 125 ml of 20% NaI solution IV once daily for 3 days. Followed by oral administration of 30 g NaI dissolved in 1 litre of clean tap water for 30 days. Although the study in Ethiopia showed this to be the most successful treatment, owner compliance was low as the cost of NaI exceeded the cost of the horse/donkey. Potassium iodide cannot be administered safely IV. Administer orally; 15 g KI in 1 litre of water, or mixed with feed such as bran, for 30 days. Heragy (2002) reported that topical ocular anti-fungal preparations were effective for the treatment of lacrimal histoplasmosis.

Prevention

- Isolate affected animals and attempt to keep flies from landing on wounds, especially where many animals are housed or there is a known case/outbreak in the area.
- Avoid and minimise wounds whenever possible as these are an entry point for the fungus. Ensure all wounds are protected against flies.
- Vaccine development has been attempted (Zhang *et al.* 1986) but the vaccines are not commercially available.
- In severe cases, discuss euthanasia with the owner as soon as possible to reduce transmission of the disease to other animals.

Papillomatosis (Warts)

Warts follow infection with papillomavirus and usually affect young equids (under 3 years old).

Appearance

Multiple raised nodules with a 'cauliflower-like' appearance (Figure 15.3.9). These are not usually associated with ulceration or exudation unless secondary infection occurs due to pressure from a harness/saddle.

Treatment

Papillomatosis is self-limiting; the animal mounts an immune response against the virus and the warts disappear over time.

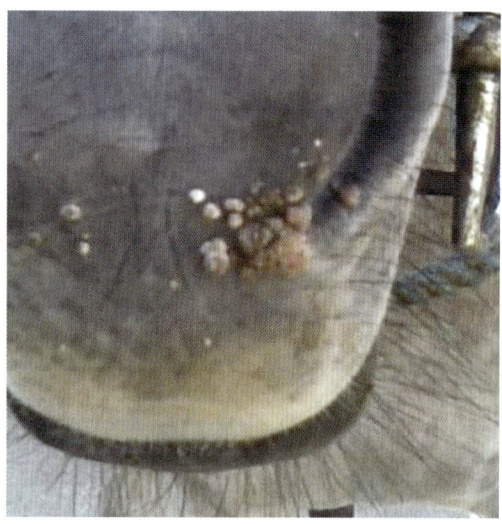

Figure 15.3.9 Papilloma on the nose of a horse.

Neoplasms

> Without adequate access to veterinary attention neoplastic lesions may grow to an unmanageable size (Figure 15.3.10) where euthanasia, rather than attempts at surgical or medical treatment, is the most appropriate option.

Definitive diagnosis of skin tumours requires sampling and cytology which is not always possible in the field situation. However, a working diagnosis can be determined through clinical signs, appearance, history and distribution.

Squamous cell carcinoma

The exact aetiology of squamous cell carcinoma (SCC) is unknown. It is thought that exposure to UV radiation is a predisposing factor. SCC is common around the eye (eyelids, third eyelid and medial canthus) and muco-cutaneous junctions such as nostrils, prepuce and vulva.

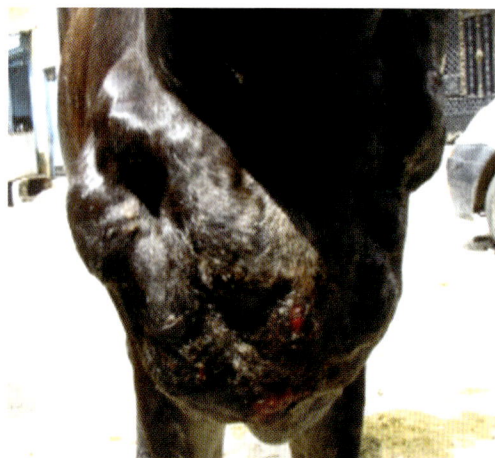

Figure 15.3.10 Neoplasms in working equids may be presented to a clinician at a late stage in the disease's progression.

Appearance

- Mild inflammation and swelling in the early stages
- As the condition progresses the masses become irregular and ulcerated with secondary bacterial infection (Figure 15.3.11).

Treatment

Surgical excision of squamous cell carcinomas is frequently unsuccessful as this tumour is aggressive. At muco-cutaneous junctions of the eye or penis it is difficult to remove sufficient marginal tissue around the tumour. If the SCC is on the third eyelid, removal is often curative and does not cause any defect to the tear film. The use of BCG vaccine infiltration has been successful (McCalla *et al.* 1992). Despite being locally aggressive, these tumours do not usually metastasise to other areas.

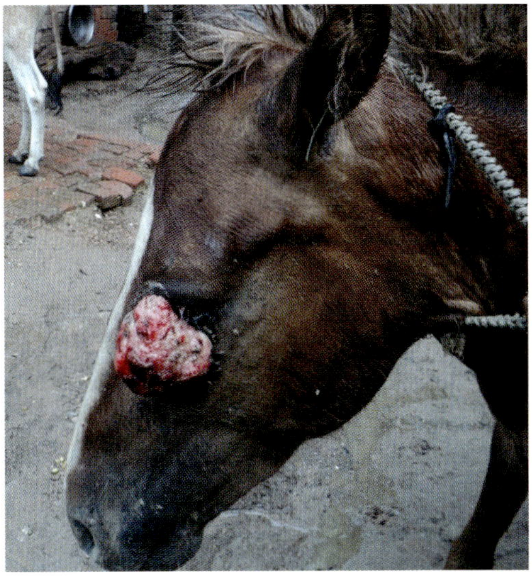

Melanoma

Melanomas are benign or malignant tumours of melanocytes, common in older (> 15 years) grey or white equids. Giemsa staining of a fine needle aspirate will show melanin granules within tumour cells. Melanomas are common in the perineal region and under the tail (Figure 15.3.12).

Appearance

- Firm, nodular pigmented swellings
- Single or multiple
- Slow growing. Some melanomas are more aggressive and metastasise quickly, including to internal organs such as the lungs and the gastro-intestinal tract.

Treatment

Surgical excision may be curative, and is necessary if the mass is interfering with harness or tack. However, there are likely to be metastatic lesions if the tumour is chronic (Valentine 1995), and the prognosis is poor.

Sarcoids

Sarcoids are common skin tumours and can be problematic to treat; they have a tendency to recur following surgical excision. There is a proposed viral aetiology for the development of sarcoids. Papilloma viruses induce hyper-proliferation of epithelial cells, usually developing into warts. It has been proposed that a bovine papilloma virus, transmitted by

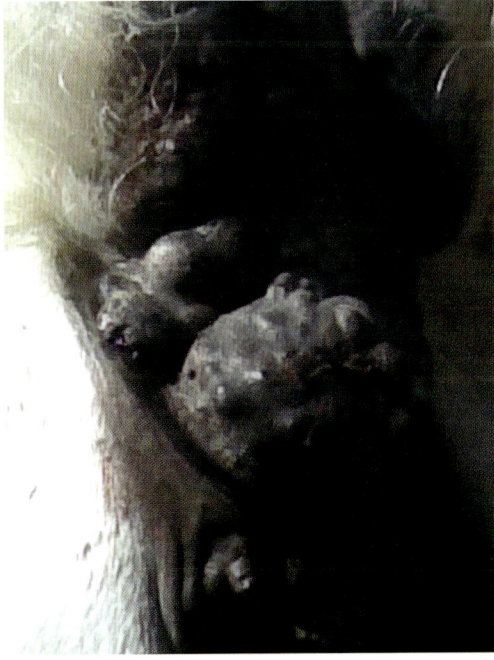

Figure 15.3.11 A suspected squamous cell carcinoma. Following surgical removal the tumour recurred; obtaining adequate margins in this region is impossible. The tumour resolved when treated with multiple BCG injections (vaccination for TB).

Figure 15.3.12 Melanomas under a horse's tail on the underside of the dock – the tail has been raised.

biting flies, infects epithelial cells to induce uncontrolled growth resulting in sarcoids. Despite being benign (they do not metastasise), sarcoids are locally aggressive and can become secondarily infected.

Clinical types include:

Verrucose Crusty and wart-like with alopecia and thickened skin around the lesion. A differential diagnosis is ringworm.

Fibroblastic Ulcerated and very vascular, lesions can have a small or large base (Figure 15.3.13). A differential diagnosis is squamous cell carcinoma.

Occult The initial lesion is a small area of alopecia that develops a crusted surface.

Nodular Encapsulated discrete masses are contained within the dermis/epidermis (Figure 15.3.14 and 15).

Mixed These are very common and are a mixture of the above descriptions.

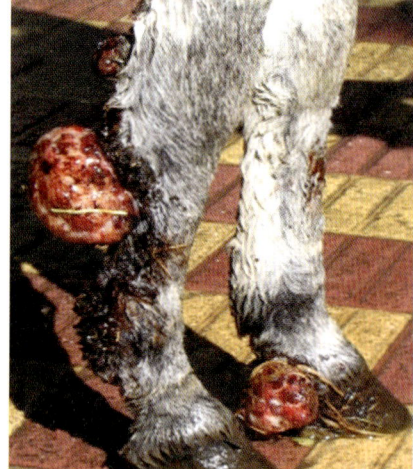

Figure 15.3.13 A fibroblastic sarcoid.

Distribution

Sarcoids can be found on any part of the body; however, they are common around the head (particularly the verrucose type), eyes, groin, ventral midline and axilla.

> Visual diagnosis is simple and safe. A biopsy can trigger further growth and should be avoided when a sarcoid is suspected.

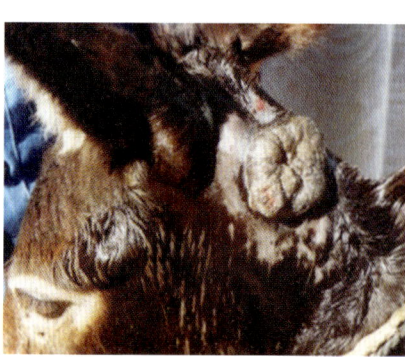

Figure 15.3.14 A nodular sarcoid.

Treatment

Leave a sarcoid alone if possible. If the lesion is small and interfering with a harness, surgical excision is possible. Lesions frequently recur following surgery, as sarcoids are locally invasive. Some studies indicate a protocol of injections with BCG. There has been a varied success rate, and there is a small risk of anaphylactic shock (Knottenbelt *et al.* 2000). Sarcoids of the limbs and axilla are more difficult to treat and have a high recurrence rate.

Lumps and swellings of the skin

Abscesses

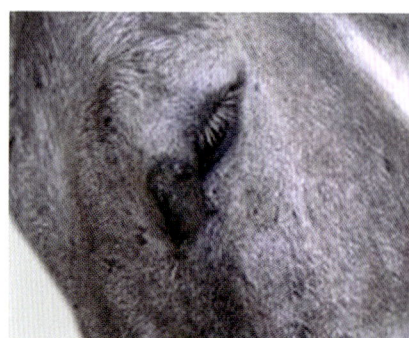

Figure 15.3.15 A nodular, periocular sarcoid.

> An abscess is an accumulation of white blood cells (predominantly neutrophils) in response either to an infectious process or to a foreign body.

COMMON SKIN DISEASES OF WORKING EQUIDS 15.3

Typically an abscess presents as a hot, swollen, painful area of the skin, and there is sometimes evidence of an injury such as a penetrating wound.

Causes

- Systemic infection (strangles, glanders)
- Penetrating injuries (wire, animal bites)
- Iatrogenic (inappropriate treatment technique) such as an injection site abscess (Figure 15.3.16)
- Continuous abrasion by poorly maintained equipment
- Foreign body (sinus tract)

Treatment

- **Mature** an abscess using hot packs.
- **Clip** or shave the area and clean with antiseptic.
- **Lance** with a scalpel blade in a **vertical** line from the centre to the most ventral part.
- **Flush** out purulent material with large volumes of warm salt water/iodine.
- **Treat as open wound**; do not suture.
- Administer **tetanus** antitoxin (TAT).
- Antibiotics are **not** a substitute for drainage and irrigation, and are not usually indicated unless there is evidence of systemic infection. Antibiotics **will not penetrate** a walled-off abscess.
- Flushing to be continued, daily for 5 days, by the owner to ensure drainage continues.

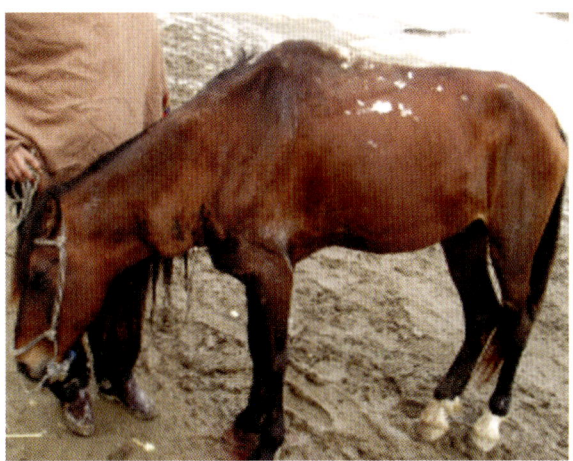
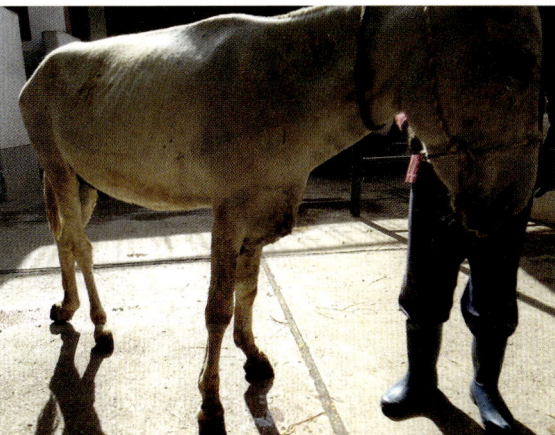

Figure 15.3.16 Iatrogenic injection site abscesses in the neck (top) and the chest.

> Before lancing it is important to ensure that the swelling is an abscess. Conduct a fine needle aspirate prior to surgery.

Hernias and ruptures

> A hernia is a swelling due to mesenteric fat and intestines protruding through a congenital opening in the body wall muscle (umbilical, inguinal).
>
> A rupture is a swelling due to mesenteric fat and intestines protruding through an acquired opening in the body wall muscle (accidents, trauma).

Appearance

- Both hernias and ruptures present as a soft swelling of varying size depending on how much abdominal content has protruded through the opening (Figure 15.3.17).
- Usually there is no heat or pain on palpation.
- Contents can be pushed back (reduced) internally; a 'hernial ring' defect can be palpated in the muscle.
- If intestine is entrapped and strangulated the animal will have signs of colic.

Treatment

Hernias may be sub-clinical if small. If a rupture is suspected, bandaging may help to retain intestines within the abdomen while the defect heals. Surgical repair of ruptures and large hernias cannot be recommended in field conditions as there is high risk of wound breakdown and peritonitis. Small umbilical hernias may be repaired in foals. An imbricating suture pattern is used to draw one muscle layer over the top of the other. It is essential that hernias and ruptures are differentiated from an abscess prior to attempts to drain the latter.

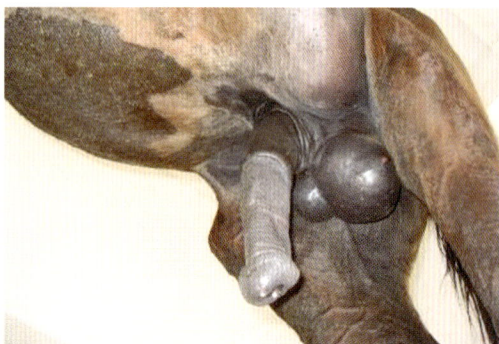

Figure 15.3.17. Examples of abdominal and inguinal hernias/ruptures.

Haematoma

A blunt trauma (fall/kick) ruptures small blood vessels under the skin, causing subcutaneous bleeding. This blood clots forming a lump over the next few days which eventually fibroses and shrinks to a small hard mass.

Appearance

- Sudden-onset swelling following a history of trauma (Figure 15.3.18)
- Heat and pain on palpation
- Blood/blood-tinged serum on aspiration
- In chronic stages the lump becomes small and hard with no fluid.

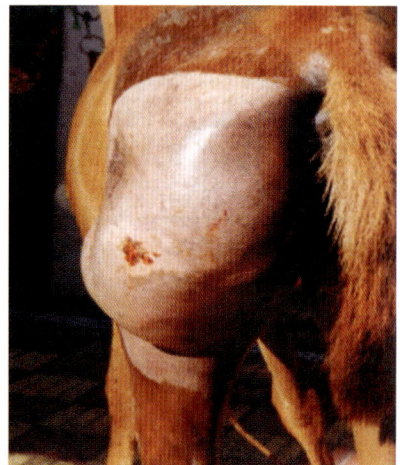

Figure 15.3.18 Haematoma on the hindquarter of a horse.

Treatment

NSAIDs reduce pain and swelling in the initial stages following trauma. Cold therapy with hosing, buckets of water or rags soaked in water can help to reduce the inflammation in the acute stages. Haematomas tend to resolve gradually. Surgical drainage is not recommended as haemorrhage is likely to continue. Antibiotics are not usually necessary.

Seroma

A seroma (pocket of serous fluid) often develops after suturing a wound or surgery, particularly if dead space has been left under the suture line. Seromas present as a fluid-filled mass in the vicinity of a surgical incision or site of trauma. Aspiration of fluid produces a clear, serous exudate (Figure 15.3.19).

Treatment

Remove one or two ventral sutures and allow to drain, or take out all sutures and allow to heal as an open wound. Drainage of a closed seroma is not worthwhile as the fluid will continue to accumulate. When suturing a wound ensure that the dead space is closed down by using a multi-layered closure.

Oedema

Oedema is a subcutaneous, interstitial accumulation of fluid. Distribution depends on the underlying cause although it is seen most often in dependent areas such as the ventral abdomen/chest, sheath and lower limbs (Figure 15.3.20). Generally, the swelling is diffuse and an **indentation is left when the oedema is pressed (pitting)**. A fine needle aspirate is unlikely to yield fluid.

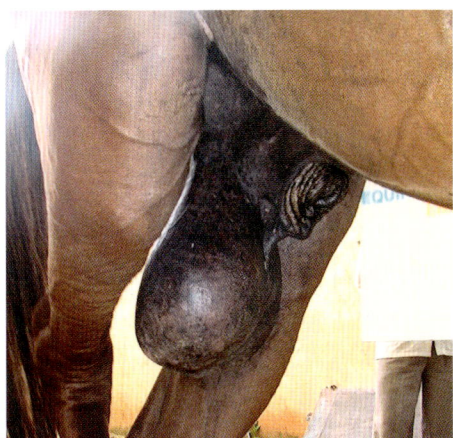

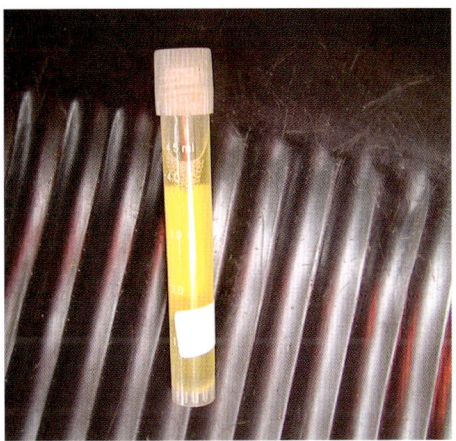

Figure 15.3.19 Severe swelling of the scrotum (top); aspiration of blood-tinged serous fluid.

Causes

- Localised circulatory disturbances
- Lower-limb swelling due to standing for long periods
- Poor venous circulation and lymphatic drainage
- Unsuitable bandaging methods
- Major circulatory disturbances such as heart failure
- Hypo-proteinaemia as the result of liver disease, parasitism or malnutrition
- Inflammation of vessels which increases permeability to fluid

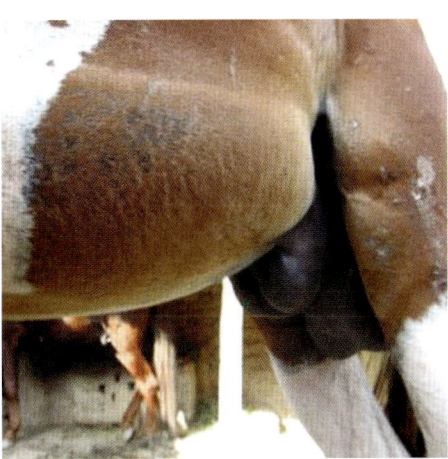

Figure 15.3.20 Ventral oedema in the horse.

Treatment

Walking the animal will help to resolve localised distal limb oedema. Cold therapy can reduce any inflammation. Generalised oedema will require a thorough clinical examination for signs of underlying systemic disease or other causes of low blood protein. Drainage is not recommended.

Cellulitis

> Cellulitis is an inflammation of the subcutaneous tissue, often associated with infection.

Recommended protocol for treatment of cellulitis

- If microbial culture is available, a swab or aspirate of the fluid should be collected.
- The recommended first-line treatment is procaine penicillin 22,000 IU/kg IM BID and gentamicin 6.6 mg/kg IV SID. At least 3 consecutive days of treatment is required. Penicillin alone may be ineffective in 60% of cellulitis cases (Haggett and Wilson 2008, Fjordbakk et al. 2008).
- Initiate pain relief therapy to prevent laminitis in the contra-lateral limb.
- The animal should not work throughout the duration of treatment. Hand walking may be beneficial.
- Prognosis is guarded and recurrences are common.

Skin diseases characterised by crusting and ulcerative lesions

Sunburn and photosensitisation

Sunburn is primary direct damage to the epidermis by intense ultraviolet light. Damage tends to be to non-pigmented skin which is more sensitive to the harmful rays.

Photosensitisation is the over-reaction to normal levels of sunlight as the result of photodynamic agents accumulating in the skin for two main reasons:

- Ingestion of plants containing photodynamic agents which are directly absorbed and circulate in the blood
- Failure of the liver to detoxify phylloerythin a by-product of chlorophyll

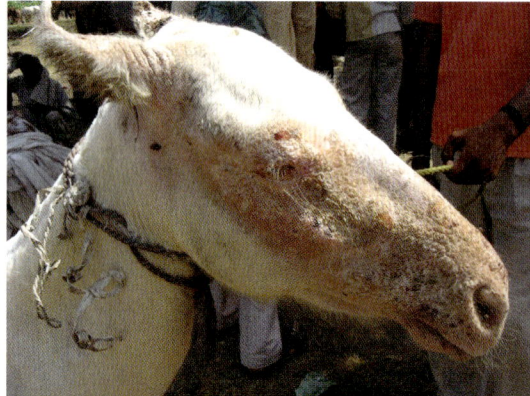

Figure 15.3.21 Sunburn on a horse's face following over-exposure to sunlight.

Appearance

Cases of sunburn present as vesicle formation and blistering, followed by rapid crusting, commonly on the muzzle and around the eyes (Figure 15.3.21). The appearance of photosensitisation is often more severe and includes erythema (redness), oedema (swelling), pain, vesicle (blister) formation leading to serum exudation, ulceration and, in severe cases, skin sloughing.

Management

- Avoid sun exposure (bring into the shade) and cover sensitive areas with mask/rug.
- Apply high-factor sunscreen, or a similar barrier cream, and provide analgesia.
- Treat secondary bacterial infections. Topical creams can be soothing and antibacterial (cold sulphadiazine cream). Emollient creams containing aloe vera will soothe the skin.

In cases of photosensitisation, in addition to the above, remove inciting cause if due to plant toxicity. In cases of severe liver disease there is a poor prognosis and any treatment is only supportive. Discuss euthanasia with the owner.

The long-term prevention of wounds 15.4

> Knowledge and recognition of the underlying causes and good owner communication is essential for the prevention of wounds.

Consider the root causes of wounds. In working equids chronic wounds are frequently the result of a poorly fitting harness (Burn *et al.* 2008), inappropriate materials used for tack (Figure 15.4.1) and a poor state of repair of equipment. Equids working in developing countries will be harnessed or saddled for several hours each day and equipment-related injuries are commonly reported (Pritchard *et al.* 2005).

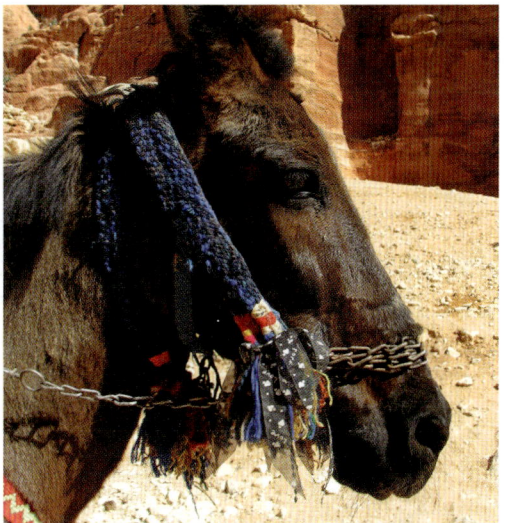 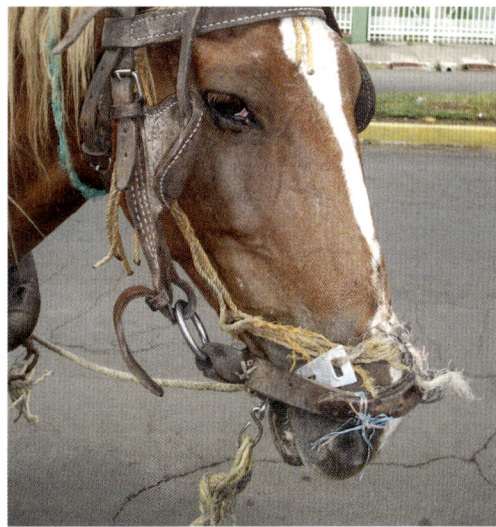

Figure 15.4.1 Nose band lesions caused by inappropriate materials such as chains or wire.

Lip lesions

In a study (Shah *et al.* 2010) in Pakistan, 70% of 512 working equids surveyed had lip lesions (Figure 15.4.2). These lesions are painful, reduce feed and water consumption and result in weight loss. To reduce such lesions it has been shown that **involvement of the whole community**, not just the equine owners, is needed (Shah *et al.* 2010). Advice may be provided to bit-makers on proper bit selection, fit and maintenance. Owners can be advised on cleaning and removing the bit when the animal is eating, drinking and not working, as well as maintaining the other parts of the harness. A study by Nawaz *et al.* (2006) showed that lip lesions in working equids in Pakistan were affected by the bit, bridle, cart and by owner behaviour and attitude, as well as by animal physiology. The highest risk factor for lip lesions was a jointed bit, **with a straight-bar bit least likely to cause damage**.

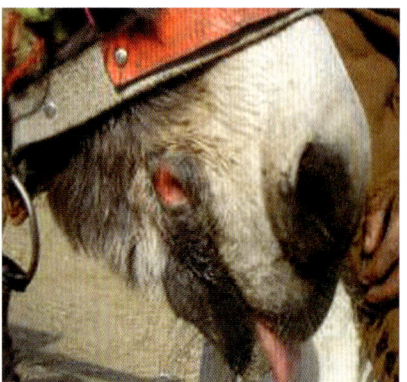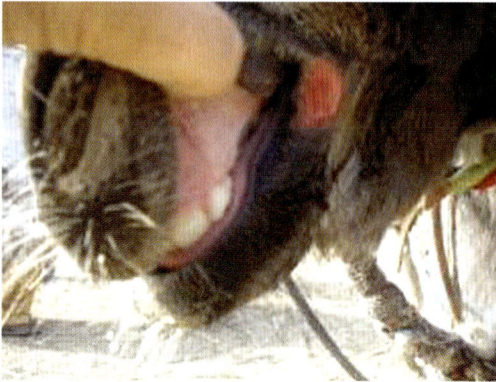

Figure 15.4.2 Harness-related lip lesions in working equids.

Tail-base lesions

Tail-base lesions are generally located underneath the tail, between the tail base and the rectum (Figure 15.4.3), and are thought to be caused by rump/crupper straps used to stop the saddle from slipping forward. A study by Burn *et al.* (2008) in Jordan found 73% of the 86 donkeys surveyed had tail-base lesions. The most **severe lesions were associated with more padded straps** used under the tail, and by those that were not clean; cotton straps were associated with more severe lesions than synthetic straps.

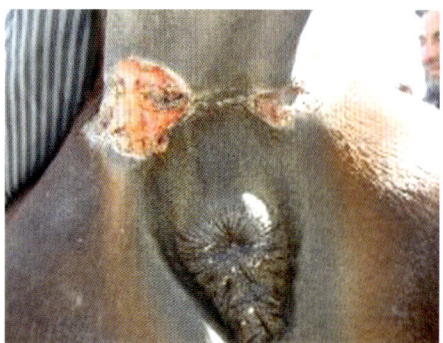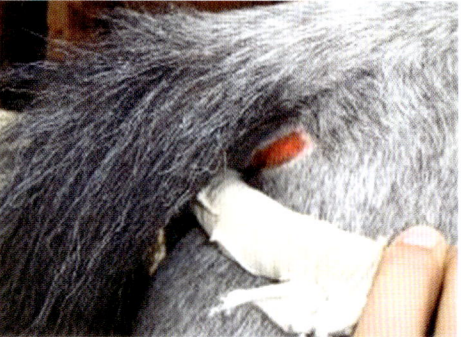

Figure 15.4.3 Harness-related tail-base lesions in working equids.

Body lesions

Withers wounds (Figure 15.4.4) have been reported as present in 52% of working equids carrying pack saddles in the brick kilns of Delhi, India (Aravindan *et al.* 2006). **Early signs of pain and hair loss** prior to lesion development were identified and can be used as indicators for owners to adopt preventive measures.

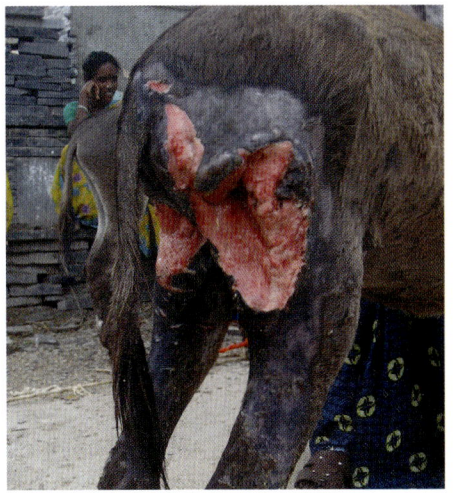
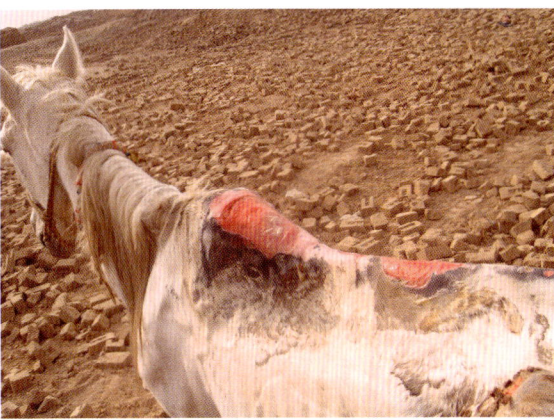

Figure 15.4.4 Harness-related body lesions in working equids. Withers lesions caused by pack saddles and hindleg lesions caused by poorly fitted breaching straps.

Prevention

Many of these lesions can be prevented by increasing owner awareness of the impact, and devising local solutions to such problems. For example, soft 'doughnuts' can be made from cloth, to raise the harness above the withers, or chain nose bands can be replaced by a softer material. This involves working with owners and harness makers.

> **Owners:** Encourage owners to be aware that a better-fitting and well-maintained harness results in fewer injuries and debilities for working equids.
> **Harness makers:** Increase the skill of using local materials and techniques to make well-fitting harnesses, and the ability to repair them affordably for owners.

Deliberate mutilations are frequently conducted in some regions and are often the result of misguided beliefs (described in brackets for each mutilation). In these situations treat the wounds and provide guidance to owners on evidence-based strategies to deal with the problems that are of concern (see Section 2.4 *Firing and nostril slitting*). Examples of mutilations and the regions where these procedures are commonly carried out are outlined:

Gum cutting or firing West Africa, India and Latin America (to 'treat' lampas, swelling of the hard palate, Figure 15.4.5) (see Section 11.4 *Conditions of the mouth and oesophagus*)

Nostril slitting East Africa, India and Pakistan (to 'improve' breathing) (Figure 15.4.6)

Ear removal/cutting India and East Africa (to 'prevent' tetanus and for identification) (Figure 15.4.6)

Setonism Threading wire or thread through the skin (often creating a chronic infected wound) (Figure 15.4.7)

15 THE INTEGUMENTARY SYSTEM

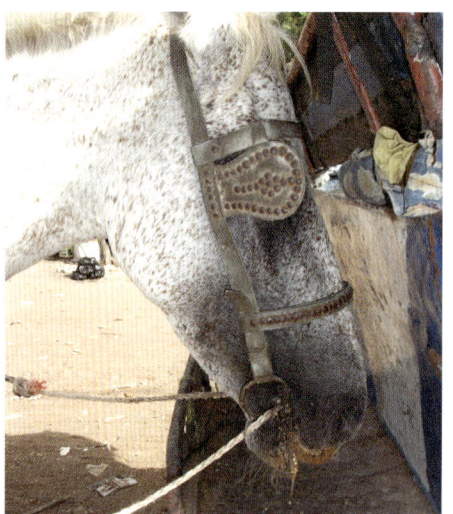

Figure 15.4.5 *This horse in Senegal had lampas (inflammation of the roof of the mouth) which the owner has attempted to treat by inserting a hot rod into the mouth. The horse is struggling to eat and drink as the result of severe inflammation.*

Firing Widely practised ('treatment' of many disorders) (Figure 15.4.8)

Tail mutilations Widespread (improved cleanliness)

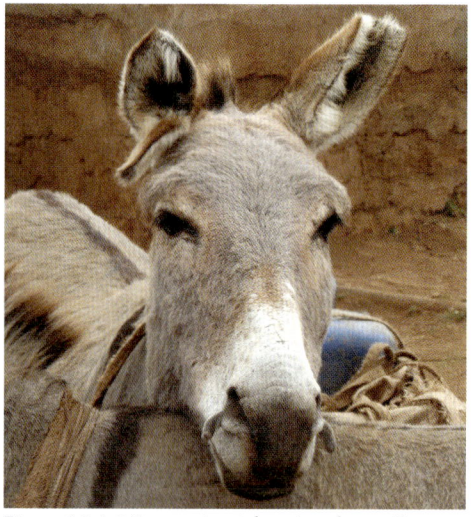

Figure 15.4.6 *Ear cutting (above) and nostril slitting (below).*

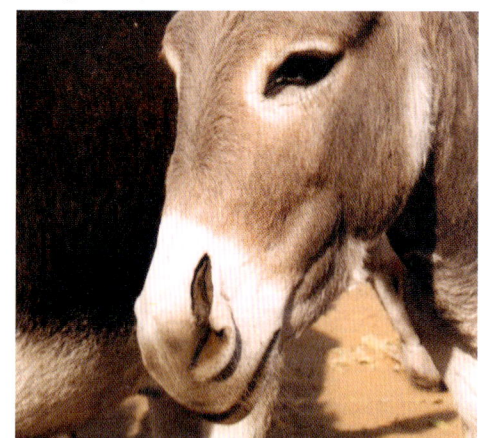

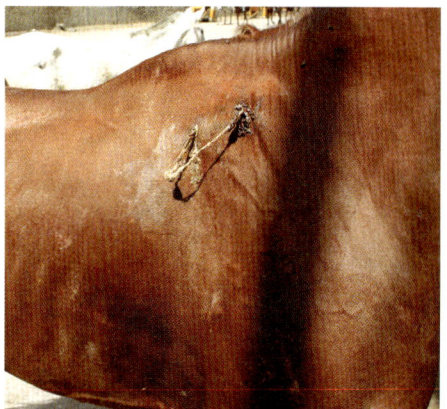

Figure 15.4.7 *An example of setonism in which thread or wire is stitched into the skin.*

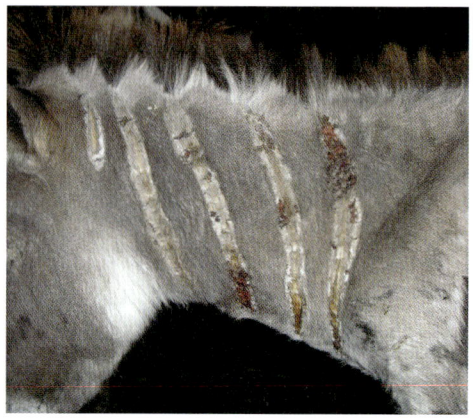

Figure 15.4.8 *An example of firing; the skin is burnt using a red-hot iron.*

448

Bandaging 15.5

> Developing an appropriate bandaging technique is vital to the management of wounds and injuries in equids.

Bandages are important for:

- controlling and reducing swelling and oedema (reducing dead space to prevent seroma formation)
- controlling haemorrhage
- protecting open wounds from contamination, flies and further trauma
- providing a favourable environment for wound healing, i.e. holding wound edges together and immobilising the area
- providing stability to injuries (e.g. tendon injuries/fractures)
- immobilising and supporting the limb to make the patient more comfortable – a useful adjunct to analgesia for pain control
- protecting a wound against harm by the patient.

However, if done incorrectly, bandaging can cause a huge amount of damage. Complications include:

Infection If a bandage is left on too long and/or becomes very dirty, bacteria can spread through the bandage and contaminate the wound.

Pressure sores A bandage applied with uneven pressure, or a bandage that slips, will cause constriction. This may result in localised areas of tissue damage.

Pressure necrosis If the bandage is put on too tightly it impedes blood supply to the area which can result in sloughing of large patches of skin and tissue.

It is essential that bandages are applied correctly and that the bandaging is well maintained. It is often necessary for an owner to replace the bandage. Provide clear, precise instructions including a demonstration of bandage application.

Materials

There are normally three layers to a bandage (Table 15.5.1); the first directly covers the wound, the second offers padding/support (the thickness of this varies, depending on the amount of support required) and the final layer holds the bandage in place and offers some protection from the environment.

15 THE INTEGUMENTARY SYSTEM

Layer	What this layer provides	Materials that can be used
Primary layer – wound dressing	This directly covers the wound. Apply aseptically after the wound has been thoroughly cleaned and debrided. This dressing should be non-stick (unless additional debridement is required) so that delicate granulation tissue is not disturbed. **Absorbent** – so any wound exudation is drawn away from the wound surface (to avoid wound maceration/inflammation) **Semi-occlusive** – to allow oxygen to reach the wound **Non-stick**	**Purpose made dressings** These have a shiny, non-stick surface, that goes against the wound, and a matt, cotton surface that faces away from the wound. **Cotton gauze/cotton wool** Avoid using cotton wool as it sticks to wounds. Adding a layer of petroleum jelly will reduce this; however it will also reduce the amount of oxygen that can reach the wound. **Absorbent dressing** Some thicker dressings are specially designed to absorb more wound exudate.
Padding layer	This provides **padding and support**. The amount of support provided depends on the number of padding layers applied. A Robert Jones bandage can have 10 layers or more and should be at least three times the diameter of the leg. The padding layer should be clean, absorbent and soft. Apply padding evenly and reasonably tightly. If more than one layer is applied use a weave bandage or crepe bandage between each layer.	**Cotton wool** This is available in most countries and is inexpensive. **Disposable nappies** Although expensive these are very absorbent and can be useful in fresh large wounds which are discharging excessively. **Towels and cloths** Although absorbent these tend to stick but can be useful if there is no alternative. These materials can be washed so are reusable.
Outer layer	The final **protective layer secures the other bandages**. This needs to be durable and strong as well as non-absorbent and waterproof. Care must be taken that this layer is applied with the **correct tension**. Too little tension and the bandage will slip, resulting in pressure rubs. Too much and this will injure the skin and deeper structures, resulting in pressure sores and pressure necrosis.	**Elasticated cohesive dressing** This is very useful and easy to apply although it can be expensive. **Adhesive dressings** Elasticated adhesive dressings can also be useful especially around the top and bottom of bandages. **A cotton bandage or strips of cotton** (e.g. cut from cloth) Cloth can be useful as it is readily available and affordable.

Table 15.5.1 The purpose and potential materials for different layers of a bandage.

Location

Different parts of the body will require different types of bandaging materials and techniques. Table 15.5.2 describes the more common areas which may require bandaging and important aspects of application and care.

BANDAGING 15.5

Types of bandage	Notes
Foot bandage	This includes the foot only and finishes around the pastern/coronet (Figure 15.5.1). This technique is commonly used for applying **poultices** to treat foot abscesses: Clean the foot thoroughly, and dry before bandaging, to prevent the development of thrush. It can be useful to put a stable bandage on the distal part of the limb above the foot bandage to keep it in place. Apply a padding layer over the foot and coronet/pastern, to alleviate pressure and rubbing on the coronet. Cover the entire foot with duct tape or other impermeable material to avoid wicking of faeces/urine/dirt. Change the bandage regularly, ideally daily.
Lower limb bandage	This extends from the coronary band to just proximal to the hock/carpus (Figure 15.5.2). The amount of padding depends on the amount of support needed. For superficial wounds very little support is required, one layer is sufficient. For more severe injuries to bone/tendon a half limb **Robert Jones** may be required. (See Section 14.6 *Common conditions affecting the bones of working equids*.)
Full limb bandage	Full limb bandages are difficult to apply and maintain, and require regular veterinary attention and re-checking. The amount of bandaging material becomes expensive. **Protect pressure point**s, such as the caudal aspect of the carpus (accessory carpal bone) and the point of the hock, either by reducing the padding over these points or applying the bandage in a figure-of-eight configuration.
Splints	A splint can be applied over the top of a bandage to offer additional support to the leg (see Section 14.6). Splints are most commonly used to stabilise fractures. There are very few fractures that are amenable to treatment in the working equid context. Consider the prognosis and welfare implications before fracture treatment is offered. Fit a splint snugly to the bandage with elastic tape.
Pressure bandage	A pressure bandage is a useful way of applying pressure consistently for a long enough period to control haemorrhage. A bandage can be applied quite tightly. Leave the bandage in place for at least a couple of hours, after which gently remove the bandage without dislodging the clot. A second bandage can then be applied to protect the wound and allow for healing. Monitor for signs of continued haemorrhage such as 'strike through' (blood seeping through the bandage). A pressure bandage should not be left on for a long period of time (maximum 6–8 hours). A bandage soaked in blood is detrimental to wound healing, and a tight bandage may cause skin necrosis.
Head bandage	The head and face can be covered with a roll of 6-inch orthopaedic stockinet. Holes are trimmed in the stockinet over the eyes and to accommodate the ears. If a tubular bandage is not available, ensure that any dressing applied is light and does not impose any restriction on head, neck and jaw movements.
Trunk bandages	These bandages are not frequently applied but may be required to protect a trunk laceration. A light bandage covered with an elasticated cohesive layer is ideal (Figure 15.5.3).

Table 15.5.2 Different types of bandages for equids.

15 THE INTEGUMENTARY SYSTEM

Bandage maintenance

> A wound cannot be easily assessed without first removing any applied bandaging. Good monitoring of the animal and the bandage is essential to avoid complications and it is crucial the owner knows and understands what to look out for.

Lameness Check the comfort of the animal at least once daily. If the lameness worsens, this could indicate wound/injury deterioration.

Strike through This is when wound exudate/haemorrhage soaks through the bandage. It indicates that all the bandage layers are saturated. Change the bandage without delay and re-check the wound.

Bandage slips If the bandage slips, replace it without delay as pressure sores and skin necrosis can develop rapidly.

Dirt Keep the bandage as clean and dry as possible.

Regular changes Change bandages regularly; the frequency depends on the location and injury. Ideally, foot bandages and wounds that are discharging copious exudate are changed daily. A bandage should not be left on for more than 5 days.

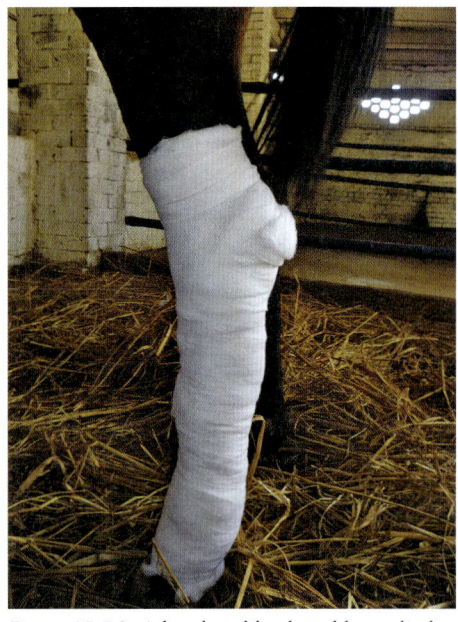

Figure 15.5.2 A bandaged hock and lower limb.

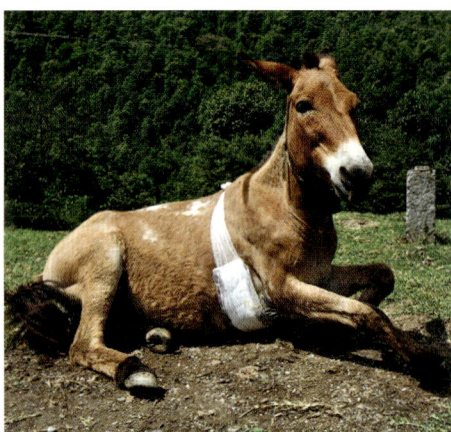

Figure 15.5.3 A light thoracic bandage.

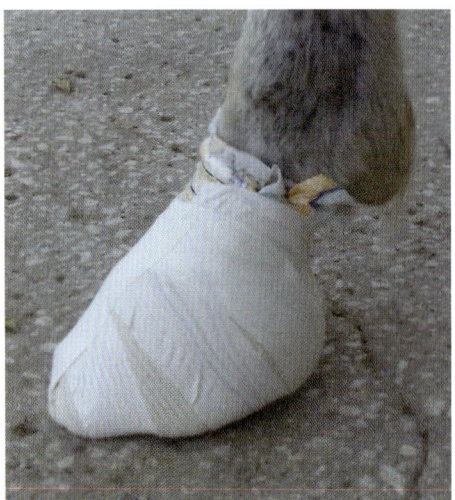

Figure 15.5.1 A foot bandage.

Case study – Wound management   15.6

Location Senegal

Attending veterinarian Francois-Xavier Laleye

History
A 3-year-old cart horse presented with a chronic history of a withers wound from a poorly fitted harness. It also had a 5-day history of wounds on the stifle and scrotum as the result of whipping with a riding crop. The horse was reluctant to move while it was being trained to pull the cart. The owner had treated the wounds with motor oil, local plant remedies and blue methyl alcohol.

Clinical findings
The withers wound was purulent, infected and 10 cm deep. The area surrounding the wound was painful and the horse was 4/5 lame. The wound was contaminated with motor oil, plant fragments and sand (Figure 15.6.1). Other wounds were observed between the front limbs, inside the thighs, scrotum, sheath and cranial aspect of the hind leg.

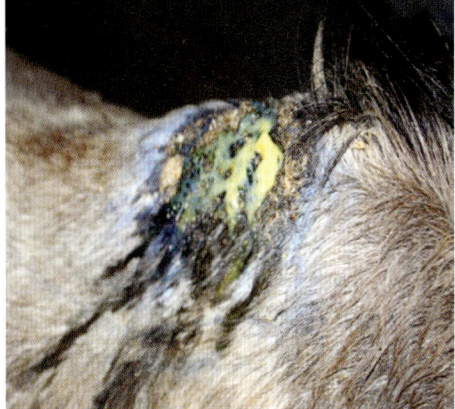

Figure 15.6.1 The wither wound at presentation with heavy contamination.

Treatment
All wounds were clipped and cleaned with dilute povidone-iodine. Shea butter was applied to the wounds twice a day until the lesions had healed. IM procaine penicillin 20,000IU was prescribed daily for 5 days. Anti-tetanus serum was given. Strict rest for one month was advised. A discussion took place with the owner regarding proper treatment of the horse in future (no beating and appropriate harnessing).

Outcome
One month later the lesions had healed (Figure 15.6.2).

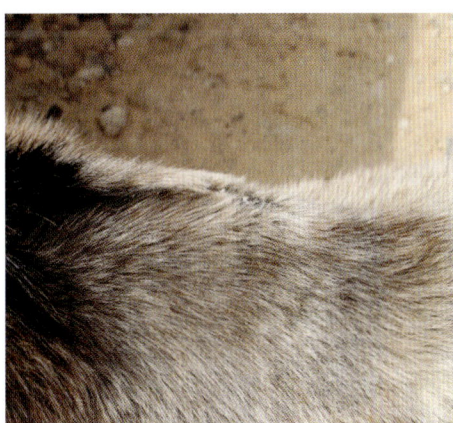

Figure 15.6.2 One month later the wither lesion had healed.

Discussion
Young animals should be trained to pull a cart by someone with expertise in this area. Advice on simple first aid techniques can easily be imparted to owners to avoid the use of unsuitable treatments such as motor oil. The use of shea butter in this case is interesting as this is a locally available resource. Application of a **sterile** wound lubricant is beneficial to keep the wound surface moist; however, ensure that topical wound treatments do not delay wound healing.

15.7 References

Ameni, G., Terefe, W., Hailu, A. (2006) Histofarcin test for the diagnosis of epizootic lymphangitis in Ethiopia: development, optimisation, and validation in the field. *Vet. J.* 171 (2) 358–362.

Al-Ani, F.K., Ali, A.H., Banna, H.B. (1998) Histoplasma farciminosum infection of horses in *Iraq Veterinarski Arhiv*. 68, 101–107.

Aravindan, M., Zaman, S.F., Roy, C., Shaw, A. (2006) Development of wither wounds in working equines of brick kilns in India. *Proceedings of the 5th International Colloquium on Working Equines*. Addis Ababa, Ethiopia, 30 October–2 November. 37–40.

Burn, C.C., Pritchard, J.C., Farajat, M., Twaissi, A.A,. Whay, H.R. (2008) Risk factors for strap related lesions in working donkeys at the World Heritage Site of Petra in Jordan. *Vet. J.* 178 (2) 263–267.

Christian, L.M., Graham, J.E., Padgett, D.A., Glaser, R., Kiecolt-Glaser, J.K. (2006) Stress and Wound Healing. *Neuroimmunomodulat*. 13 (5–6) 337–346.

Crothers, S.L., White, S.D., Ihrke, P.J., Affolter, V.K. (2009) Sporotrichosis: a retrospective evaluation of 23 cases seen in northern California (1987–2007). *Vet. Derm.* 20 (4) 249–259.

Fjordbakk, C.T., Arroyo, L.G., Hewson, J. (2008) Retrospective study of the clinical features of limb cellulitis in 63 horses. *Vet. Rec.* 162 (8) 233–236.

Haggett, E.F., Wilson, W.D. (2008) Overview of the use of antimicrobials for the treatment of bacterial infections in horses. *Equine Vet. Educ.* 20 (8) 433–448.

Hadush, E., Ameni.G., Medhin, G. (2008) Equine histoplasmosis: Treatment trial in cart horses in central Ethiopia. *Trop. Anim. Health Prod.* 40, 407–411.

Heragy, A.M. (2002) Lacrimal Histoplasmosis in the working donkeys of Luxor villages. *Fourth International Colloquium on Working Equines*. Al Baath University, Hama, Syria 20–26 April 2002.

Knottenbelt, D.C., Kelly, D.F. (2000) The diagnosis and treatment of periorbital sarcoid in the Horse: 445 cases from 1974 to 1999. *Vet. Ophthal.* 3, 169–191.

McCalla, T.L., Moore, C.P., Collier, L.L. (1992) Immunotherapy of periocular squamous cell carcinoma with metastasis in a pony. *J. Am. Vet. Med. Assoc.* 200 (11) 1678–1681.

Nawaz, S., Shah, Z., Gondal, J.I., Habib, M., Shaw, A. (2006) The influence of cart and bit characteristics on presence, size and severity of lip lesions in draught equines in Mardan/Gujranwala – Pakistan. Proceedings of the *5th International Colloquium on Working Equids*, Addis Ababa, Ethiopia, 30 October–2 November 2006. 28–36.

Noori, S., Al-Waili, Salom, K., Al-Ghamdi, A.A. (2011) *The Scientific World Journal*. 11, 766–787.

Pritchard, J.C., Lindberg, A.C., Main, D.C.J., Whay, H.R. (2005) Assessment of the welfare of working horses, donkeys and mules, using health and behaviour parameters. *Prev. Vet. Med.* 69 (3–4) 265–283.

Shah, S.Z.A., Eager, R., Nawaz, S., Khan, M., Khan, G. (2010) Minimizing prevalence and severity of lip lesions in working donkeys of Rustam community through awareness raising: a pilot project based on lip lesion risk assessment, 2006 findings. *Proceedings of the 6th International Colloquium on Working Equids*, New Delhi, India, 29 November–2 December 2010. 147–151.

Stashak, T.S., Theoret, C.L. (2008) Equine Wound Management. Chapter 4 – Approaches to wound closure. Second edition. Blackwell.

Valentine, B. (1995) Equine melanocytic tumors: A Retrospective study of 53 horses (1988–1991). *J. Vet. Intern. Med.* 9 (5) 291–297.

Yasuda, R., Kawano, J., Humiaka, O., Takagi, M., Shimizu, A., Anzai, T. (2000) Methicillin resistant coagulase negative staphylococci isolated from healthy horses in Japan. *Am. J. Vet. Res.* 61, 1451–1455.

Zhang, W.T., Wang, Z.R., Liu, Y.P., Zhang, D.L., Liang, P.Q., Fang, Y,Z., Huang, Y.J., Gao, S.D. (1986) Attenuated vaccine against epizootic lymphangitis of horses. *Chin. J. Vet. Sci. Technol.* 7, 3–5.

Further reading

Ameni, G. (2006) Epidemiology of equine histoplasmosis (epizootic lymphangitis) in carthorses. *Ethiopian Vet. J.* 172, 160–165.

Berk, W.A., Osbourne, D.D., Taylor, D.D. (1988) Evaluation of the 'golden period' for wound repair: 204 cases from a Third World emergency department. *Ann. Emerg. Med.* 17(5) 496–500.

Kearney, C., Hunt, L., Jenner, F. (2009) Management of wounds in horses. *Irish Vet. J.* 62 (7) 477–482.

Knottenbelt, D., Pilsworth, R.C. (2007) Skin Diseases Refresher – Diagnostic Methods. *Equine Vet. Educ.* 19 (9) 492–494.

Knottenbelt, D., Edwards, S., Daniel, E. (1995) Diagnosis and treatment of the equine sarcoid. *In Practice*. 17, 123–129.

Orsini, J.A., Elce, Y., Kraus, B. (2004) Management of Severely Infected Wounds in the Equine Patient. *Clin. Tech. Equine P.* 3, 225–236.

Pascoe, R.R., Knottenbelt, D.C. (1999) Manual of Equine Dermatology. Chapter 7 Bacterial Diseases. Saunders, W.B.

Pilsworth, R.C., Knottenbelt, D.C. (2007) Photosensitisation and sunburn. *Equine Vet. Educ.* 19 (1) 32–33.

Powell, R.K., Bell, N.J., Abreha T, Asmamaw K, Bekelle H, Dawit T, Itsay K, Feseha GA. (2006) Cutaneous histoplamosis in 13 Ethiopian donkeys. *Vet. Rec.* 158 (24) 836–837.

Quinn, G. (2010) Management of large wounds in horses. *In Practice*. 32, 370–381.

Taylor, S., Haldorson, G. (2013) A review of equine mucocutaneous squamous cell carcinoma. *Equine Vet. Educ.* 25 (7) 374–378.

The neurological system

16

Disorders of the neurological system	**16.1**
Case study – Tetanus in a working horse	**16.2**
References	**16.3**

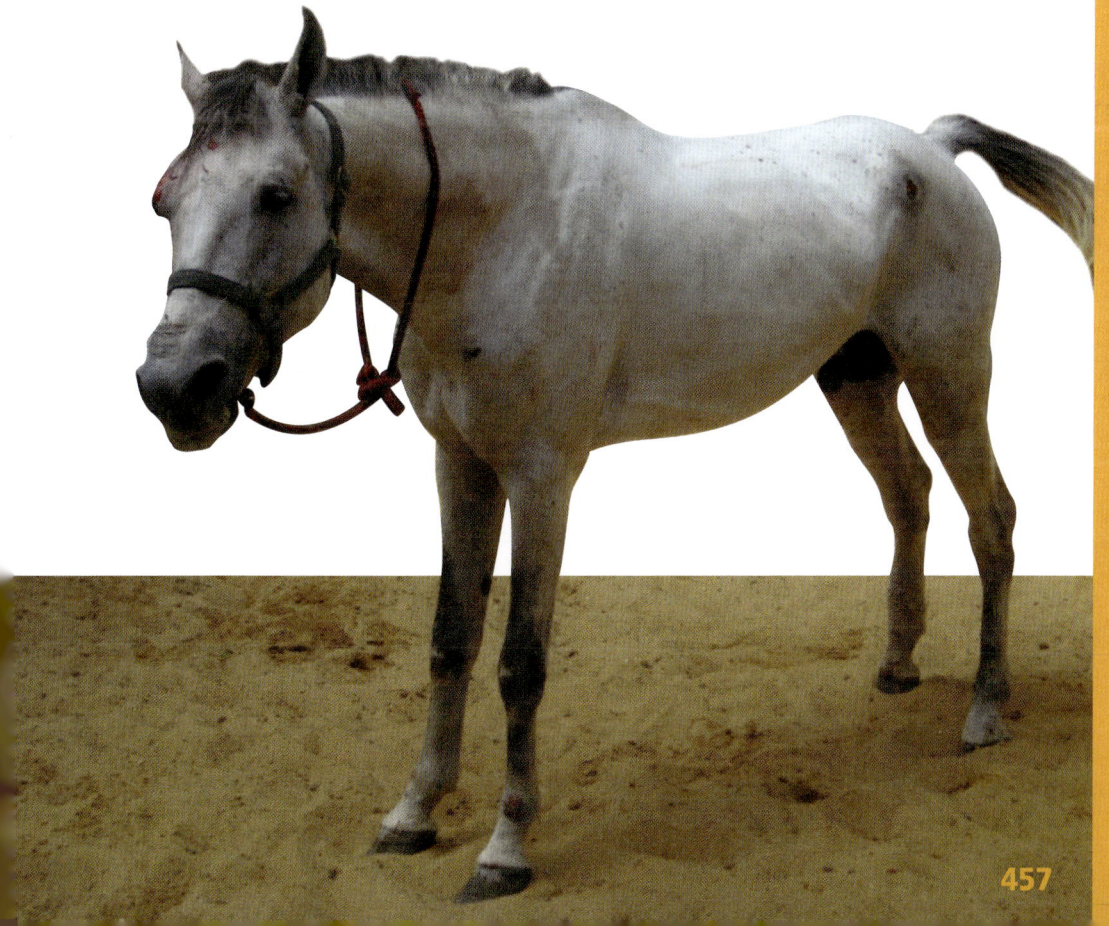

16.1 Disorders of the neurological system

Traumatic conditions

Spinal cord trauma

It is important that neurological trauma is identified and managed appropriately as equids with neurological damage can be a danger to themselves and other equids or people.

Clinical signs

- Ataxia – lack of coordinated muscle movements
- Postural deficits – wide-based stance, narrow-based stance, unstable
- Paralysis and muscle atrophy
- Weakness
- Increased or decreased muscle tone
- Hyperreflexia or hyporeflexia
- Loss of pain – superficial and deep pain. Loss of deep pain is a very poor prognostic indicator (this indicates extensive spinal cord injury).
- Loss of autonomic process – urination and defecation

The exact clinical signs depend on the location of the injury/lesion.

Treatment

Treatment is rarely recommended as the prognosis is poor for spinal cord damage. If the animal is **recumbent,** euthanasia is a necessity on welfare grounds. Recumbency will rapidly result in muscle damage from lying in one position. In cases of acute recumbency wait a minimum of 2 hours (with appropriate analgesia) before attempting to get the equid to stand. If severe neurological damage has occurred then the clinical signs will not improve in this time.

If, following an injury to the spinal cord, the animal is standing and showing gait abnormalities, euthanasia should again be considered on the grounds of welfare and safety.

If treatment is attempted, the equid should be able to stand, walk around without undue discomfort, and be able to pass urine and faeces. Rest the animal and administer steroids to reduce neurone swelling. Initiate a course of NSAIDs once the effects of the steroid have worn off to provide analgesia and long-term anti-inflammatory effects. If there is no improvement after 1–2 weeks consider euthanasia or retirement as the chances of a full recovery are much reduced. Recovery following nerve damage is often disappointing and slow.

Head trauma

Trauma to the head can result in neurological deficits if there is sufficient brain injury. Injuries to the poll commonly occur when a horse rears up and falls over backwards.

DISORDERS OF THE NEUROLOGICAL SYSTEM 16.1

Clinical signs

- Injury to the head may be visible.
- Neurological signs due to brain injury
  - Altered consciousness, e.g. coma, dullness, depression
  - Convulsions, seizures
  - Ataxia
  - Head tilt, nystagmus, circling
  - Head pressing
  - Blindness

The clinical signs depend on the location and extent of brain injury.

Treatment

If there has been head trauma but the equid is neurologically normal, treat wounds symptomatically (clean, suture, analgesia and antibiotics as required). If there are marked neurological signs the safety of those handling the animal are the first priority. Sedate the affected equid if it is a danger to itself or others and, if the neurological effects are severe, consider euthanasia. Steroids can be used to reduce brain inflammation and swelling. Administer dexamethasone at 0.5 mg/kg IV or IM as soon after the original injury as possible.

Peripheral nerve trauma

Damage to peripheral nerves (lower motor neurons) results in very specific clinical signs in only the muscle(s) that the nerve innervates. If the nerve injury has resulted in bruising or swelling, rather than complete transection, a full recovery may be possible with anti-inflammatory therapy and rest. If the nerve has been fully transected full recovery is unlikely. Treat all cases of peripheral nerve damage with anti-inflammatory medication, steroids initially, followed by a course of NSAIDs.

Facial nerve paralysis

This is commonly seen when an equid lies with its head on the buckle of the head collar. Facial nerve paralysis can be a complication of general anaesthesia and it is always recommended to remove the head collar while the animal is recumbent.

Clinical signs

- Facial asymmetry – deviation of the nose to one side, dropping of the ear, lip, and eyelid on affected side
- Muscle atrophy (wasting), if nerve damage has been present for some time

Sweeny

This is seen in equids that pull carts or farm machinery with a yoke (a ring around the base of the neck). The yoke can cause pressure and injury to the suprascapular nerve as it crosses in front of the scapula. Ensure yokes are well fitted and padded.

Clinical signs

- Prominent scapular spine due to muscle atrophy
- Lameness and weakness in the affected limb

Obturator nerve paralysis

The obturator nerve, which passes along the internal aspect of the pelvis, may be damaged during a difficult foaling. If the equid is unable to stand, euthanasia should be considered on welfare grounds.

Clinical signs

- Hindlimbs do the 'splits' (splay out either side).

Infectious conditions

Tetanus

Tetanus is a global disease caused by *Clostridium tetani*, from the soil or faeces, entering the body via wounds. Once contracted it leads to a distressing and often fatal outcome (Kay and Knottenbelt 2007). Tetanus has been shown to be more prevalent in developing countries (Reichmann *et al.* 2008). Within the anaerobic environment of a deep wound the bacteria sporolate and produce the tetanus neurotoxin. The incubation period of the disease ranges from 3 days to 3 weeks. The neurotoxin potentiates normal sensory stimuli leading to muscular spasticity, hyperaesthesia, seizures and respiratory arrest.

Clinical signs

- Recent history of a wound – If no wound has been identified do not rule tetanus out if there is a strong indication from the clinical signs.
- Vague stiffness, mild signs of colic initially
- Muscle spasms – commonly the masseter muscles (known as 'lock jaw') and also muscles of the neck and hind limbs
- Spasms and stiffness which can be elicited by external stimuli such as loud noises and tactile stimulation
- Third eyelid protrusion, flared nostrils, erect ears and tail
- Fixed pupil dilation
- Extensor rigor 'saw-horse stance' with stiff rigid legs and hindlimbs stretched out behind (Figure 16.1.1)

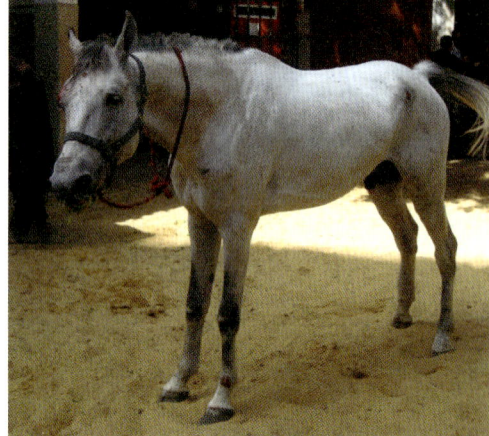

Figure 16.1.1 A horse showing classic signs of Tetanus: elevated tail, stiff-legged rigid stance.

- Collapse and death from respiratory arrest (usually within 3 to 10 days of the onset of clinical signs)

Diagnosis is based on wound history and clinical signs. The most commonly reported risk factor, in a series of affected horses, was the absence of vaccination (van Galen *et al.* 2006).

It has been suggested that donkeys have better survival rates than horses. Young animals are affected more often and more severely by tetanus than older animals. The combination of dysphagia, dyspnoea, and recumbency can be considered as an indicator of a poor prognosis in equids suffering from tetanus (van Galen *et al.* 2008).

Treatment

Treatment is sometimes successful in equids although, even with intensive therapy, mortality rates are reported at 68% and 75% in retrospective studies (van Galen *et al.* 2008, Green *et al.* 1994).

If treatment is attempted, keep the affected equid in a quiet, deep-bedded stable. Administer analgesia as muscle spasms are painful. Debride and lavage any wounds to allow oxygen into the space and reduce contamination. Administer high doses of systemic penicillin (2–3 times the normal dose rate for 7 days; however, be aware of the risks of antibiotic-induced colitis). The use of metronidazole is advocated in human treatment of tetanus (Gibson *et al.* 2009). Sedate the animal to induce muscle relaxation. Administer acetylpromazine, at a dose of up to 0.1 mg/kg body weight every 4–6 hours according to effect. Supportive therapy such as IV fluids and hand feeding will be necessary if the equid is unable to eat or drink.

If available, administer anti-tetanus toxin serum (immunoglobulin) as soon as possible after an injury, whether signs of tetanus are developing or not. These antibodies will bind the tetanus toxin before it can exert an effect on the neuromuscular junction. In human cases of tetanus, following the onset of clinical signs, intrathecal administration (spinal injection) of anti tetanus immunoglobulin is associated with higher survival rates (Kabura *et al.* 2006), although this has not been demonstrated in equids (Steinman *et al.* 2000).

If anti-toxin serum is not available, the vaccine may be administered after an injury. This will stimulate the immune system to generate anti-toxin antibodies; however, the response is unlikely to be fully protective until the booster 28 days after the initial vaccination. As the disease course for tetanus is usually less than 21 days this is unlikely to be an effective treatment in all cases.

Prevention

Tetanus toxoid is commonly administered to equids as a form of prophylaxis (Wilson *et al.* 2001). An initial course of two doses of vaccine at an interval of 4–6 weeks is required to achieve protection against tetanus for a 12-month period (Tasman and Huygen 1954). As the result of variation between individuals, a single dose may be effective in some cases but this cannot be relied upon to provide sufficient antibody levels for protection against the disease (Liefman *et al.* 1981). There is little evidence to demonstrate the duration of immunity; however, a booster every 1–2 years is recommended.

Botulism

Botulism is caused by the bacteria *Clostridium botulinum* which, in a similar way to tetanus, produces a neurotoxin. Unlike tetanus, the botulinum toxin causes flaccid paralysis. It is commonly associated with feeding silage/haylage which undergoes secondary fermentation when oxygen gains access to the forage. Rotting carcases, which may be eaten by equids browsing rubbish dumps, are another source of the bacterial toxin.

Clinical signs

- Progressive muscle weakness – which can be gradual or rapid in onset
- Difficult breathing – dyspnoea
- Tongue paralysis
- Eyelid drooping (ptosis) and pupil dilation
- Reduced anal tone, ileus, constipation, and urine retention
- Death due to respiratory paralysis or pneumonia after 24–72 hours

16 THE NEUROLOGICAL SYSTEM

Treatment

Provide supportive therapy and administer the anti-toxin, if available. Identify and remove the source of the bacterial toxin to prevent botulism in other animals. Ensure only well-kept silage is fed to equids; discard silage that has been exposed to oxygen.

Rabies

Rabies is a fatal viral infection transmitted in saliva and predominantly spread by bites from infected wild or domestic animals including dogs and hyenas, and vampire bats in Central and South America. The rabies virus can also spread if infected saliva contacts mucous membranes or open wounds, and there is evidence of transmission through droplet inhalation.

The incubation period relates to dose and pathogenicity of the viral strain, immune status of host and proximity of bite to the central nervous system. The incubation period can be up to 1 year but signs of rabies usually develop within 3 weeks to 3 months of exposure. The virus can be present in saliva for up to 5 days before clinical signs appear.

> Rabies is zoonotic and fatal to humans so extreme care must be taken when handling any suspected case (Figure 16.1.2)

All members of the veterinary team should have a course of pre-exposure rabies vaccinations. If you or any colleague suspects that they have been in contact with the saliva of a rabid animal, wash the affected area thoroughly with large amounts of soap and water and seek immediate advice from a medical doctor. Post-exposure vaccinations are recommended even if the individual had received a full course of rabies vaccinations prior to exposure.

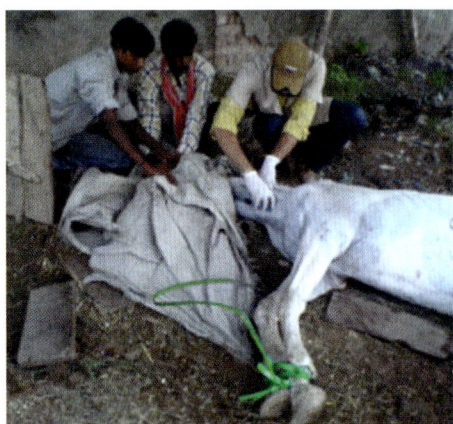

Figure 16.1.2 *Extreme care should be taken when handling any rabies case. Note the gloves, covering of the head to protect handlers from being bitten/contact with saliva, and the leg restraint.*

Clinical signs

Cerebral or furious form (Figure 16.1.3)

Aggression, photophobia, straining, inappetance, chewing seizures

Brainstem or dumb form

Depression, ataxia, pyrexia, circling, head tilt, facial paralysis, dysphagia or anorexia with increased salivation, progressive ascending paralysis, flaccid tail/anus, urinary incontinence, self mutilation. Progressing to recumbency and a comatose state with death following within 5 days.

The dumb form is reported to be more common in equids than the cerebral/rabid form.

> Always consider rabies in any rapidly progressing, multifocal neurological disorder.

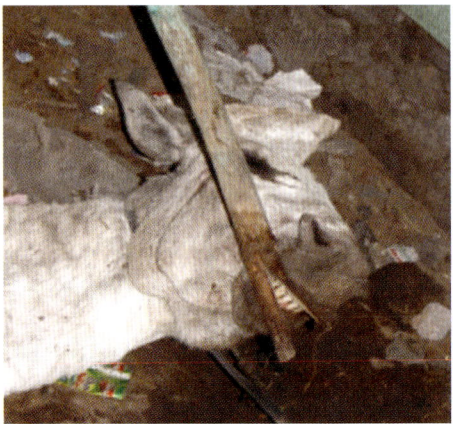

Figure 16.1.3 *The cerebral form of rabies.*

Diagnosis

There is no ante-mortem test for rabies so diagnosis is based on history and clinical signs. A diagnosis can be confirmed through histopathological examination of central nervous tissue (brain tissue). Ensure compliance with local regulations for reporting rabies cases.

Treatment

There is no treatment for rabies. If the disease is strongly suspected, euthanasia should be carried out immediately with minimal handling of the animal (Figure 16.1.4). Handlers should wear protective clothing and gloves and use sufficient restraint to ensure that they are not bitten.

If the diagnosis is uncertain, the animal should be held in a secure place, with minimal handling, for observation. Any symptomatic treatment given to the animal must not compromise the safety of handlers. Visit the affected animal at its home to avoid risk to large numbers of people and animals at a clinic. It is absolutely imperative that owners are warned of the risks to themselves and their animals so that isolation procedures are strictly adhered to.

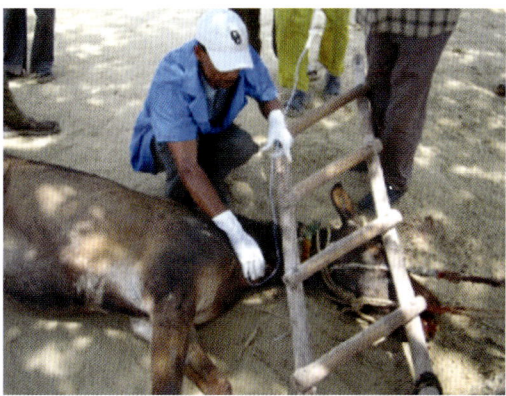

Figure 16.1.4 Carrying out euthanasia in a rabies case.

What do you do if an equid is bitten by a rabid animal?

If there is a history of previous vaccination, clean the wounds with antiseptic, revaccinate, isolate and watch for 45 days. Unvaccinated animals should be observed for 6 months in isolation, administer a course of rabies vaccinations (day 0, day 21 and day 56 following exposure).

Euthanase immediately if the bitten animal starts showing signs of rabies.

Rabies prophylaxis

Commercially available vaccines are available in many countries, and there may be government vaccination programmes in operation for the canine or wild populations. Equids should be vaccinated at 3 months old, 1 year old, then annually. Vaccinate mares before breeding rather than during pregnancy. There are a number of killed vaccines available for use in equines. Modified live vaccines should not be used.

> Any equine rabies vaccination programme will have little effect if the surrounding canine population is not effectively controlled or vaccinated.

Togaviral encephalitis

Eastern Equine Encephalitis (EEE)
Western Equine Encephalitis (WEE)
Venezuelan Equine Encephalitis (VEE)

The togaviruses are infectious, mosquito-borne diseases of equids affecting the central nervous system. Togaviral encephalitis in equids is largely confined to the Americas. All three diseases are found in Central and South America, and EEE and WEE are mostly confined to the eastern and western United States respectively. VEE can cause large outbreaks of disease over extensive geographical areas in both humans and horses. Spread of this virus into Central America has had disastrous consequences. The virus is transmitted by mosquitoes, from reservoir hosts to equids. Infection is most common during the season when vector populations are greatest. WEE and VEE may also be transmitted horse to horse through nasal secretions.

The viruses are zoonotic, although not directly contagious, and notifiable to OIE.

Clinical signs in humans include fever, headache, stupor and seizures, and can lead to death. Inform owners to minimise contact with mosquitoes, and ensure your approach to the case is consistent with existing government protocols. Human vaccination is recommended for vets in endemic areas.

Clinical signs

The severity of neurological disease varies according to the type of togavirus but will include a generalised illness and fever progressing to behavioural change, circling, blindness, seizures, coma and death. Mortality rates are very high for EEE and VEE infections (40–100%).

Diagnosis

Diagnose by virus isolation or antigen detection in clinical cases. In the case of VEE, ELISA can be used for diagnosis.

Treatment

Administer supportive treatment including NSAIDs, fluid therapy and seizure control (diazepam 0.05-0.5 mg/kg IV as required); death is common if neurological signs progress.

Prevention

Vaccination with a killed trivalent vaccine is recommended in endemic areas in late spring (protection lasts for 6 months), and in the face of an outbreak. Mares should be vaccinated 1 month before foaling. Horses with VEE can be persistently viraemic and are therefore a source of infection.

West Nile Virus

West Nile Virus (WNV) is a mosquito-borne flavivirus; equids and humans are infected as dead-end hosts as the virus generally circulates in birds. WNV is normally distributed through Central and North Africa, the Middle East, west and central Asia and Australia. However, since 1999, the virus has spread rapidly across North America.

Signs of infection in equids vary from a mild fever to severe neurological signs progressing from mild ataxia to muscle fasciculation and cranial nerve deficits. Signs of cortical brain damage are rare.

Equine Protozoal Myeloencephalitis

This neurological condition is caused by the protozoa *Sarcocystis neurona*. Equine Protozoal Myeloencephalitis (EPM) results in a wide range of neurological signs depending on the migration pattern through the central nervous system.

CASE STUDY **16.2**

Clinical signs

- Ataxia – can be severe
- Paresis, weakness and or spasticity
- Muscle atrophy
- Localised sweating
- Asymmetric pattern – The parasite migrates to a number of different locations in the nervous system.
- If untreated, it can progress to recumbency in 14 days to 6 months.

Treatment

The use of anti-coccidial agents, such as ponazuril, has been recommended (Mackay *et al.* 2008). NSAIDs can be given but corticosteroids are likely to worsen clinical signs. Consider euthanasia if signs deteriorate.

Case study – Tetanus in a working horse **16.2**

Location Uttar Pradesh, India

Attending veterinarians Dr Hridesh Yadav and Dr Nidhish Bhardwaj

History

A 10-year-old mare, used for working in brick kilns, was having difficulty moving and feeding for 24 hours. The mare had been attended by a Local Health Provider on the previous day. The mare had no history of Tetanus Toxoid vaccination.

Clinical findings

Pulse Rate 48/min; respiration rate 24/min; CRT 2 Seconds; rectal temperature 38.4°C; mucous membrane: pink; stiffness in the body and frightened attitude; erect ears and raised tail (figures 16.2.1 and 16.2.2); third eyelid 'prolapse' (figure 16.2.3)

Differential diagnosis

- Tetanus
- Equine exhertional rhabdomyolysis
- Laminitis
- Hypocalcaemia
- Rabies
- Meningitis

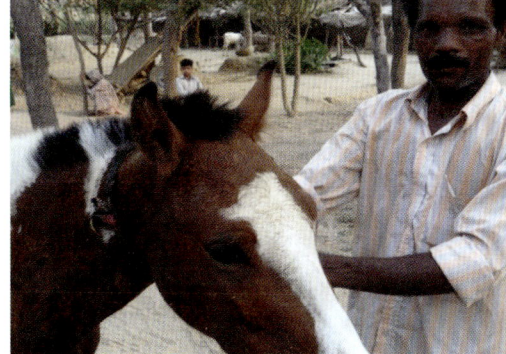

Figure 16.2.1 Erect ears.

On the basis of history and symptoms, the case was diagnosed as Tetanus.

16 THE NEUROLOGICAL SYSTEM

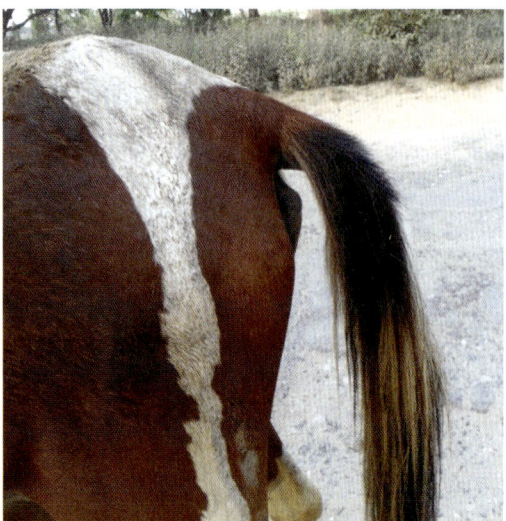

Figure 16.2.2 *Raised tail.*

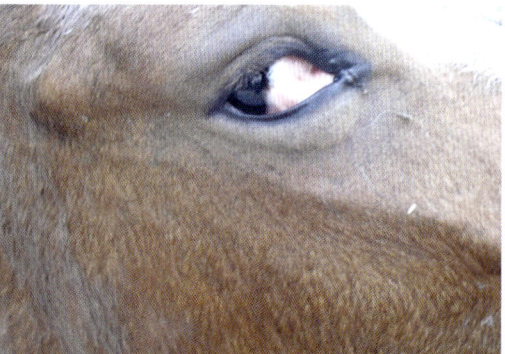

Figure 16.2.3 *'Prolapsed' third eyelid.*

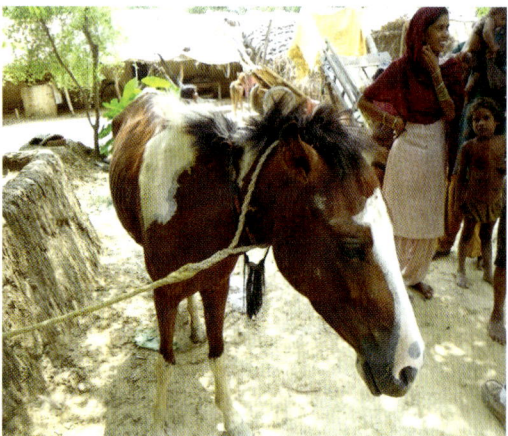

Figure 16.2.4 *The recovered horse at day 15.*

Treatment

Treatment focused on three major aspects in tetanus: killing of organisms, neutralization of toxins and relaxation of muscles to prevent asphyxiation. Procaine penicillin (20,000 IU/kg, IM BID) was administered for 7 days. Penicillin is a drug of choice for Clostridial infections. Metronidazole (15 mg/kg B IV SID) was also administered for 7 days to kill anaerobic bacteria. Ketoprofen (2.2 mg/kg IV SID) was administered for 2 days and Acepromazine (0.10 mg/kg IV) on the first day, (0.08 mg/kg IM BID) for 5 days. Fluid therapy (Normal Saline and 5% Dextrose Normal Saline) was administered IV.

The owner was advised to take specific measures while nursing the animal at home including placing cotton plugs in the animal's ears to reduce sound-induced spasms, offering hand feeding with fresh green grass and bran, keeping the animal in a dark, quiet place with plenty of space, undertaking minimal handling of the animal to avoid muscle spasms and providing soft bedding to avoid self-inflicted injury.

The owner was also advised on prevention measures including: a full course of Tetanus Toxoid (TT) vaccine, as equines are very prone to Tetanus; vaccination of broodmares 4–6 weeks prior to foaling to ensure passive immunity for the foal; protection of working equines against wounds by proper saddle management and care; regular cleaning of stable.

Outcome

Fifteen days following initial examination, on re-examination the animal was fully recovered, moving and eating normally, see Figure 16.2.4.

Discussion

This case was successfully treated without the use of ATS (Anti Tetanus Serum) as the case was diagnosed in the initial stage and treatment started immediately. The case was treated with antibiotics and supportive therapy. The toxins produced at the site are absorbed in the blood stream and attach to motor end plates. The toxins then pass to the CNS by crossing the blood brain barrier. Once the toxins are attached to the motor end plate they can never be released.

ATS intravenously, intramuscularly or subcutaneously does not cross the blood-brain barrier and has effect only on circulating toxin that has not attached to nervous system receptors. The amount of ATS applied intravenously does not have an influence on survival rates. These results are in accordance with other authors and corroborate their concern with the financial impact for poor animal owners by the use of high amounts of ATS without proven higher effectiveness (Reichmann *et al.* 2008).

ATS may be neither beneficial nor economically justifiable in the treatment of tetanus in working animals in the developing world. Early diagnosis, nursing care, high doses of parenteral penicillin and establishing aerobic conditions at the infected site are probably the most important aspects of treatment (Kay and Knottenbelt 2007).

References

Gibson, K., Bonaventure Uwineza, J., Kiviri, W., Parlow, J. (2009) Tetanus in developing countries: a case series and review. *Can. J. Anaes.* 56 (4) 307–315.

Green, S.L., Little, C.B., Baird, J.D., Tremblay, R.R., Smith-Maxie, L.L. (1994) Tetanus in the horse: a review of 20 cases (1970 to 1990). *J. Vet. Intern. Med.* 8 (2) 128–132.

Kabura, L., Ilibagiza, D., Menten, J., Van den Ende, J. (2006) Intrathecal vs. intramuscular administration of human antitetanus immunoglobulin or equine tetanus antitoxin in the treatment of tetanus: a meta-analysis. *Trop. Med. Int. Health.* 11 (7) 1075–1081.

Kay, G., Knottenbelt, D.C. (2007) Tetanus in equids: A report of 56 cases. *Equine Vet Educ.* 19 (2) 107–112.

Liefman, C.E. (1981) Active immunisation of horses against tetanus including the booster dose and its application. *Aust. Vet. J.* 57 (2) 57–60.

Mackay, R.J., Tanhauser, S.T., Gillis, K.D., Mayhew, I.G., Kennedy, T.J. (2008) Effect of intermittent oral administration of ponazuril on experimental Sarcocystis neurona infection of horses. *Am. J. Vet. Res.* 69 (3) 396–402.

Reichmann, P., Lisboa, J.N., Araujo, R.G. (2008). Tetanus in Equids: A Review of 76 Cases. *J. Equine Vet. Sci.* 28 (9) 518–523.

Steinman, A., Haik, R., Elad, D., Sutton, G.A.(2000) Intrathecal administration of tetanus antitoxin to three cases of tetanus in horses. *Equine Vet. Educ.* 12 (5) 237–240.

Tasman, A., Huygen, F.J.A. (1954) Immunization against tetanus of patients given injections of anti-tetanus serum. *Bull. World Health Organ.* 26, 397.

van Galen, G., Delguste, C., Sandersen, C., Verwilghen, D., Grulke, S., Amory, H. (2008) Tetanus in the equine species: a retrospective study of 31 cases. *Tijdschr Diergenee sk*. 133 (12) 512–517.

van Galen, G., Delguste, C., Sandersen, C. (2006) Tetanus in horses: a review of 31 cases. In: Handbook of presentations and free communications, *BEVA Congress*, Birmingham UK, 13–16 September. 203–204.

Wilson, W.D., Mihalyi, J.E., Hussey, S., Lunn, D.P. (2001) Passive transfer of maternal immunoglobulin isotype antibodies against tetanus and influenza and their effect on the response of foals to vaccination. *Equine Vet. J.* 33 (7) 644–650.

Further Reading

Barquero, N., Gilkerson, J.R., Newton, J.R. (2007) Evidence based immunization in horses. *Vet. Clin. N. Am Equine*. 23 (2) 481–508.

Holmes, M.A., Townsend, H.G.G., Kohler, A.K., Hussey, S., Breathnach, C., Barnett, C., Holland, R., Lunn, D.P. (2006) Immune responses to commercial equine vaccines against equine herpesvirus–1, equine influenza virus, eastern equine encephalomyelitis, and tetanus. *Vet. Immunol. and Immunop*. 111 (1–2) 67–80.

Piercy, R.J. (2008) Is it weak, lame or neurological? In: *Proceedings of the 47th British Equine Veterinary Congress*, Liverpool, UK. 56–57.

Parasitology

17

Internal parasites	**17.1**
Anthelmintic medication	**17.2**
Principles of a strategic de-worming programme	**17.3**
Faecal egg count	**17.4**
External parasites	**17.5**
Ectoparasite medication	**17.6**
Protozoal infections	**17.7**
Case study – Surra	**17.8**
References	**17.9**

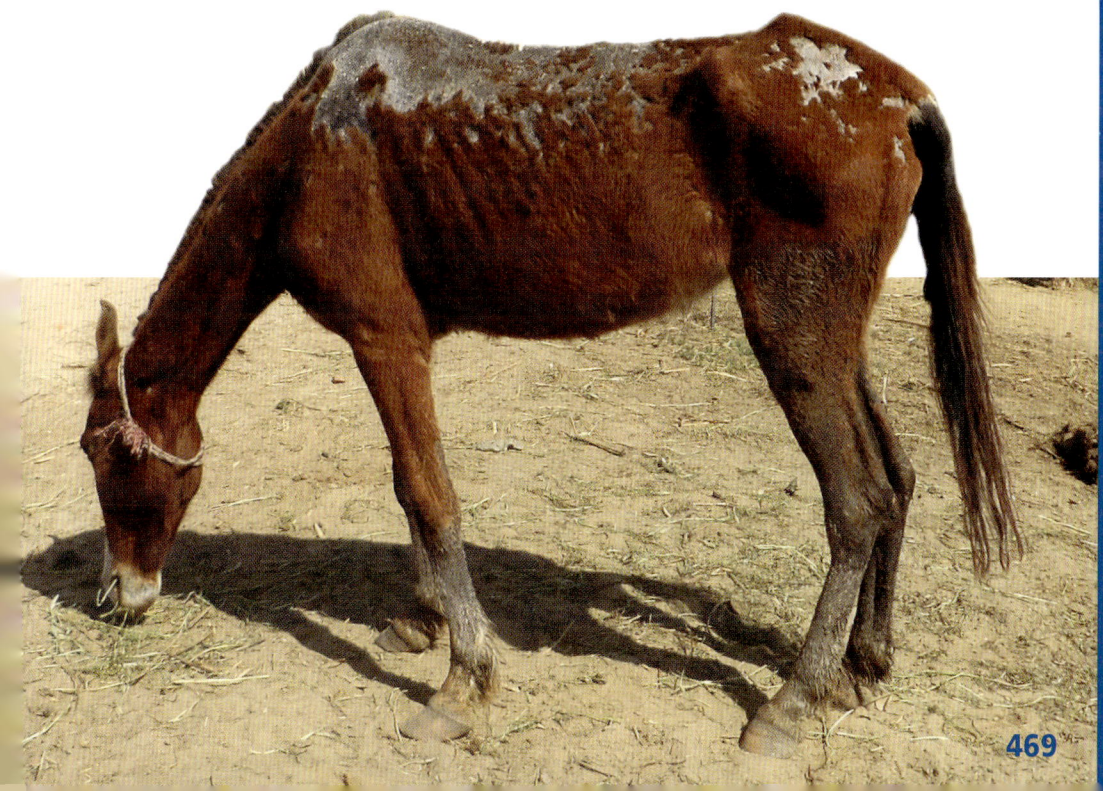

17.1 Internal parasites

Gastro-intestinal parasites of working equids

Studies have shown that gastro-intestinal (GI) parasites have been detected in a high proportion of working equids: 76% of horses and 71% of mules in one study of 532 samples in India (Singh *et al.* 2012), and 91% of animals had a positive faecal egg count (FEC) in a study of 112 donkeys, horses and mules in Mexico (Valdez-Cruz *et al.* 2006).

Type of parasite	Predilection sites
Large strongyles (*Strongylus* spp. particularly *vulgaris*)	**Adults** Large intestine **Larvae** Liver and arteries
Small strongyles (*Cyathostomes*)	**Adults** Large intestine **Larvae** Intestinal wall
Roundworms (*Parascaris equorum*)	**Adults** Small intestine **Larvae** Liver and lungs
Pinworms (*Oxyuris equi*)	**Adults** Large intestine **Larvae** Intestinal wall
Tapeworms (*Anoplocephala* spp.)	**Adults** Large and small intestine **Larvae** Forage mites
Thread worms (*Strongyloides westeri*)	**Adults** Small intestines **Larvae** Lungs and other tissues
Liver fluke (rarely causes disease in equids) (*Fasciola hepatica* - temperate *Fasciola gigantica* - tropical)	**Adults** Liver **Larvae** Snail

Table 16.1.1 Commonly found GI parasites of equids and predilection sites.

Clinical signs

Reported clinical signs for equids affected by GI parasites are varied, including poor coat health, anorexia, weight loss, diarrhoea, colic, rectal prolapse, lack of vigour, poor work performance, and productive loss (Singh *et al.* 2012).

The pre-patent period is the period between infection with a parasite and the demonstration of the parasite in the body, determined by the recovery of an infective form (for example by detecting eggs during a faecal egg count; FEC).

Large strongyles

Strongylus vulgaris

Adult nematodes vary between 1.5 and 5 cm and live in the large intestine.

Life cycle

Eggs are passed in the faeces and develop into infective larvae in the soil. Larvae are ingested, then penetrate intestinal mucosa, enter small arteries and migrate in the endothelium to the predilection site at the cranial mesenteric artery and its branches. After development, the nematodes return to the intestinal wall, via the artery lumen, to form nodules in the wall of the caecum and colon. The adults remain within the walls of the large intestine, and eggs are excreted in the faeces.

Clinical signs

> **The most significant pathology is caused by migration of the larval stage through the cranial mesenteric arteries and adjacent branches.**

Migration induces thrombus formation and thickening of arterial walls. Blockage of the blood supply to the intestine results in infarction and severe colic. If the cranial mesenteric artery is completely occluded the intestines become necrotic; this condition is fatal. A high count of large strongyles causes weight loss and anaemia.

Diagnosis

- Clinical signs
- Confirm diagnosis using an FEC.

> **The faecal egg count cannot distinguish between species of strongyle (large and small).**

- Speciation is possible by providing favourable conditions for the eggs to hatch; the larvae of each species can then be differentiated. Larval culture takes several days and this technique increases the cost of laboratory diagnosis.
- The FEC only reflects the number of egg-laying adult parasites present. Currently there is no test available that can accurately detect migrating larvae, which is the most pathogenic stage. Investigations are on-going to develop a pre-patent test (Anderson *et al*. 2013).

Treatment

All stages of the life cycle are susceptible to benzimidazoles, ivermectin and moxidectin. In equids that are regularly de-wormed, *S. vulgaris* has been largely controlled. However, working equids may not receive this treatment so large strongyles should still be considered a priority.

Strongylus edentatus

Life cycle

The life cycle of *S. edentatus* is similar to that of *S. vulgaris* except the larvae migrate through the liver. From here the larvae return to the large intestine sub-peritoneally.

Clinical signs

Migration of the larvae causes liver damage, and large numbers of adults in the intestine result in unthriftiness, weight loss and anaemia. However, the severe colic associated with intestinal infarction is not a feature.

Diagnosis and treatment   As for *S. vulgaris*

17 PARASITOLOGY

Small strongyles

Small strongyles, also referred to as Cyathostomes, have a non-migratory life cycle. There are more than 50 species in this genus infecting all equids (Eysker *et al.* 1989). Cyathostomes are generally less than 1.5 cm in length and range in colour from white to dark red.

Life cycle

Eggs are excreted in the faeces and develop into infective larvae in the soil. Larvae are ingested and invade the wall of the large intestine. Larvae develop into adults and emerge into the gut lumen.

> **Verminous enteritis:** If environmental conditions are not favourable for development (e.g. cold winter, dry season) larvae hypobiose (arrest development) and encyst in the large intestinal wall. The numbers of larvae in the large intestinal wall gradually increase over several months. When environmental conditions improve larval development is triggered. Mass emergence of encysted larvae from the gut wall causes significant damage to the large intestine.

Clinical signs

- The signs of cyathostome infection are more moderate than that of large strongyles but include loss of condition, peripheral oedema, vague malaise, weight loss, poor appetite, lethargy and disrupted intestinal motility.
- Mass emergence results in a marked pathology, 'verminous enteritis', with profuse diarrhoea, colic, weight loss, dehydration, inappetance, dullness depression and protein-losing enteropathy.
- Mortality rates can be as high as 40–70%.

Diagnosis

- Clinical signs. Examine all animals sharing grazing.
- An FEC can confirm the presence of strongyles, although large and small strongyle eggs cannot be distinguished.
- The FEC reflects only the number of egg-laying adult parasites present. Eggs are not produced by the encysted hypobiosed larvae. The FEC may be low in equids presenting with signs of verminous enteritis.
- In heavy burdens, adult worms may be visible in the faeces.

Treatment

There are three drug classes effective against the cyathostomes: benzimadazoles, pyrantel and macrocyclic lactones. Cyathostomin larvae have a low susceptibility to anthelmintics when in the hypobiosed state. Treatment and control is also complicated by the fact that there is widespread resistance to benzimadazoles (Eysker *et al.* 1989), so this medication is frequently ineffective. Ivermectin resistance is also present. Multi-drug resistance is a major problem for treatment efficacy. Paradoxically, treatment with anthelmintics is thought to trigger mass emergence and severe verminous enteritis.

Treatment for verminous enteritis

Give supportive treatment, including fluid therapy to address dehydration, and a balanced, palatable diet. Treat with moxidectin, in preference to fenbendazole, as the latter can cause severe inflammation of the colon as the larvae die off (Steinbach *et al.* 2006). Administer steroid treatment, dexamethasone or prednisolone is advised, particularly before anthelmintic treatment, to reduce the gut inflammation caused by the killed larvae. Prognosis is poor and mortality is high even with intensive treatment. If one equid has shown clinical signs of verminous enteritis then the others in the same grazing system are likely to have high burdens.

Roundworms

Parascaris equorum is one of the largest endoparasites and can grow up to 40 cm.

Life cycle

Roundworms have a direct life cycle with no intermediate host. Eggs are excreted in faeces and the larvae develop into the infective stage whilst in the egg. Following ingestion, the larvae penetrate the small intestinal wall and migrate through the liver and lungs. Larvae are coughed up from the lungs and swallowed. Development is completed in the small intestine. Adult roundworms produce high numbers of eggs, so transmission rates are high.

Clinical signs

- Mild coughing and nasal discharge in the migratory phase. Affected equids remain bright and alert.
- Light intestinal infections are tolerated well with no clinical signs.
- Heavy infections result in unthriftiness, a dull coat, poor growth in young stock, and lethargy. Younger animals can show signs of colic if a heavy roundworm burden causes a blockage of those parts of the digestive tract with a particularly narrow lumen.
- Significant clinical signs are reported predominantly in foals as adults generally develop resistance. However, *Parascaris equorum* does cause clinical disease in adult working equids, possibly due to reduced immunity as the result of physiological stress. In a recent large-scale study of working adult donkeys in Ethiopia, *Parascaris* eggs were found in 51% of the animals surveyed (Getachew *et al.* 2010b).

Diagnosis

- Clinical signs
- An FEC can confirm infection with roundworm. Parascaris eggs have a characteristic thick shell.
- Worm egg counts only detect adult egg-laying roundworm.

Treatment

Generally ascarids are readily controlled by routine de-worming with broad spectrum anthelmintics. However, macrocyclic lactone resistance has been reported. Adjust the treatment strategy to use only those anthelmintics known to be effective in indigenous populations (Reinemyer 2009). In areas where Parascaris infection is common, treat foals at 2 months, then every 2 months until 1 year of age.

17 PARASITOLOGY

Pinworm

Pinworms *(Oxyuris equi)* are a common parasite in equids but are often non-pathogenic. Female adult worms can reach up to 10 cm.

Life cycle

Adult worms live in the lumen of the colon. After fertilisation the female migrates to the anus and deposits eggs in yellowish white streaks on the perineal skin. Eggs are deposited on the pasture in the faeces, and then ingested. Larvae encyst in the large colon, develop, and the adults are released into the lumen of the colon.

Clinical signs

- Pinworms rarely cause signs of GI pathology.
- Intense pruritus around the anus can lead to self-trauma.

Diagnosis

Use sticky tape around the perineum to recover eggs for microscopic examination.

Treatment

Oxyuris equi is well controlled by all anthelmintics. Resistance to macrocyclic lactones has been reported in some populations. A small clinical trial did not find resistance when horses were treated with ivermectin and pyrantel (Reinemyer *et al*. 2010). If marked pruritus is evident, clean the underside of the tail and perineal area regularly with a disposable cloth.

Tapeworms

Tapeworms (*Anoplocephala* spp.) have an indirect lifecycle with an insect vector.

Life cycle

Eggs are passed in the faeces in a gravid segment. Following disintegration of the segment, eggs are ingested by forage mites in the soil where larval development occurs for 2–4 months. The forage mite is eaten and the adult tapeworm is released into the intestine. *Anoplocephala perfoliata* is found around the ileo-caecal junction and causes ulceration at the site of attachment.

Clinical signs

Mild infestations are considered non-pathogenic; however, moderate to severe tapeworm burdens have been associated with spasmodic colic, intussusception and intestinal rupture.

Diagnosis

Although an FEC can be used to demonstrate infection with tapeworm, this test has been shown to be unreliable (Meana *et al*. 1998). A test for circulating antibodies is available, although this has a low sensitivity (Skotarek *et al*. 2010).

Treatment

Praziquantel is an effective treatment for tapeworms (Slocombe *et al*. 2007). Control of tapeworms can difficult as there is a reservoir of infection within the forage mite population.

Liver fluke

Detection of liver fluke (*Fasciola* spp.) in working equids is generally low, particularly in arid climates (Haridy *et al.* 2002, Tavassoli *et al.* 2010). High burdens have been reported in some populations and should be considered as a differential diagnosis in cases of suspected hepatic pathology (Getachew *et al.* 2010a).

Stomach bot

The stomach bot (*Gasterophilus* spp.) is the larvae of the bot fly and is generally considered to be of little clinical significance.

Life cycle

Adult flies lay eggs on the coat of equids. Eggs are easily visible, 1–2 mm long and creamy white in colour (Figure 17.1.1). Larvae either crawl into the mouth or are ingested with grooming. Larvae penetrate the tongue/buccal (cheek) mucosa, and from here migrate to the stomach. Bot larvae tend to attach in the cardiac region of the stomach and remain for up to a year. Some species of bots will re-attach to the rectal mucosa on the passage through the digestive tract. The larvae pupate in the soil and emerge as adult flies.

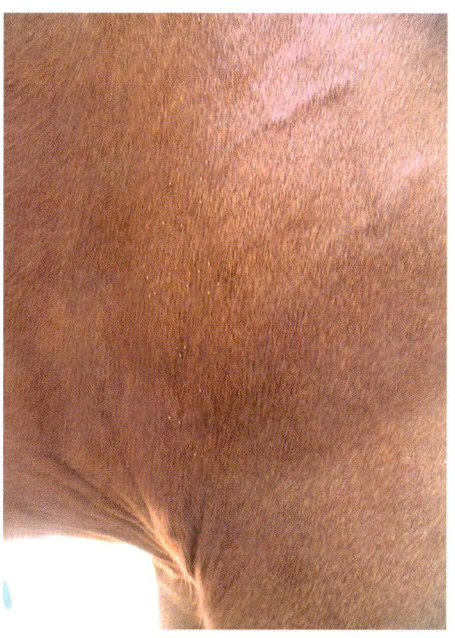

Figure 17.1.1 Bot fly eggs on the shoulder of a horse.

Clinical signs

- Presence of larvae in the buccal cavity may cause inflammation, although this is rare.
- Mild localised inflammation/ulceration can occur at the attachment site in the stomach, although the true pathogenic significance of this is unclear.
- Attachment to the rectal mucosa has been associated with rectal prolapse (Getachew *et al.* 2008).

Treatment

The only medication available for the treatment of *Gasterophilus* spp. is ivermectin and moxidectin, both of which are important for the control of nematodes. As there is little evidence for the pathogenic significance of bot fly larvae, the use of these medications for mass treatment of this condition is questionable.

> Egg removal from the coat, and fly control will minimise infection with bot fly larvae.

Lungworm (*Dictyocaulus* spp.)

See Section 12.9 *Parasitic respiratory disease*.

17.2 Anthelmintic medication

Anthelmintics are chemicals used to expel helminths (parasitic worms) from the body. Anthelmintic resistance has become increasingly important in the equine veterinary field. Resistance to individual drug classes is described in this section, and the issue of anthelmintic resistance and strategies to reduce development are addressed in Section 17.4 *Principles of a strategic de-worming programme*.

Macrocyclic lactones

The macrocyclic lactones (avermectins and milbemycins) selectively paralyse parasites which are then pushed out of the gut lumen by peristalsis. The macrocyclic lactones also treat external parasites. Commercially available avermectins include ivermectin, doramectin and eprinomectin. Milbemycins include **moxidectin** and milbemycin oxime.

Ivermectin

Indications

Used in treatment of all major helminth parasites as well as lungworm, lice, mange, cutaneous and gastric habronemiasis, thelaziasis, *Gasterophilus* spp. (bots). Effective against microfilaria of *Onchocerca* but not the adult parasites. Ivermectin does not treat tapeworm. There is questionable efficacy against encysted cyathostome larvae both at therapeutic doses (Eysker *et al.* 1992) and at higher doses (Klei *et al.* 1993). This is not as the result of drug resistance as ivermectin still shows excellent control of lumen-dwelling adults (Monahan *et al.* 1996).

Dose 0.2 mg/kg PO

Parenteral administration (introduction of medication into the body via a route other than the mouth) of ivermectin can cause severe life threatening reactions. The licence for the injectable form for horses was withdrawn in 1984 following severe reactions, including fatalities, after parenteral administration (French *et al.* 1983; Leaning 1983; Reed 1983). Studies conducted subsequently, including use in donkeys (Binev *et al.* 2005), have not reported adverse effects. IV use has been reported to be safe but is not licensed and cannot be recommended.

Pour-on (topical) formulations of ivermectin are available for the treatment of cattle. When applied to horses the plasma concentration and systemic availability of ivermectin was lower than the oral route (Gokbulut *et al.* 2010). Therefore, the use of pour-on/topical formulations is not recommended as it is likely to increase the development of resistance.

Use the ivermectin paste formulation *per os* if available. If parenteral administration is the only option, make the owner aware of possible adverse reactions and ensure correct dosing.

Moxidectin

Broad spectrum coverage of parasites with a wide safety margin in healthy adult equids. Moxidectin has a prolonged action compared with other anthelmintics.

Indications

Moxidectin has a similar spectrum of activity to ivermectin except for a reduced efficacy for treatment of *Gasterophilus intestinalis*, and an increased efficacy for encysted small strongyles (Moahan *et al.* 1996). Moxidectin does not treat tapeworm.

Dose 0.4 mg/kg PO

Moxidectin has a very long half-life in body fat, which results in a long period of suppression on equine faecal worm egg counts compared to other anthelmintics (long egg reappearance period). Young and emaciated animals have insufficient adipose tissue and are at risk of moxidectin toxicity. Symptoms of toxicity include adverse neurological reactions including prolonged coma and, in some cases, death (Johnson *et al.* 1999). Moxidectin should not be used in foals under 4 months old.

Resistance to macrocyclic lactones

Ascarids (roundworm) Decreased efficacy and resistance of ivermectin in ascarids has been reported since 2002 in North America and Europe. *Parascaris equorum* isolates have been reported to be resistant to both ivermectin (Hearn *et al.* 2003) and moxidectin.

Cyathostomins (small strongyles) Reduced efficacy of ivermectin and moxidectin against small strongyles has been reported (Lyons *et al.* 2011 and Molento *et al.* 2012).

Benzimidazoles

This class of anthelmintic acts by interfering with the energy metabolism of the parasite; decreasing the absorption and digestion of glucose. Pharmacologically, the onset of benzimidazole action is slow compared to other anthelmintics.

Fenbendazole

Indications

Large strongyles, small strongyles, oxyuris, ascarids *(Parascaris equorum)*, *Dictyocaulus arnfieldi*, strongyloides. Fenbendazole is not effective against tapeworm or bots.

Doses The licensed dose rate is 7.5 mg/kg PO

When dosed daily for 5 consecutive days, fenbendazole is effective against all stages of mucosal cyathostome larvae including early third-stage hypobiotic larvae (Duncan *et al.* 1998). However, a more recent study did not support this treatment protocol for encysted cyathostome larvae (Rossano *et al.* 2010). The efficacy of fenbendazole against cyathostomins will depend on the resistance in the population present.

Mebendazole

Indications

Treatment of strongyles, cyathostomins, mature larval *Parascaris equorum*, adult *Oxyuris equi* and *Dictyocaulus arnfieldi*. Mebendazole is not effective against tapeworm or bots.

Dose 8.8 mg/kg PO

15–20 mg/kg for 5 days for *Dictyocaulus arnfieldi* in donkeys (Clayton *et al.* 1979)

Mebendazole is safe for pregnant mares and foals, but may cause mild diarrhoea if overdosed. Pregnant donkeys should not receive the higher dose regime.

Oxfenbendazole and Oxibendazole

Indications Treatment of ascarids, strongyles, and *Oxyuris equi*

Dose 10 mg/kg PO

Triclabendazole

Triclabendazole is not licensed for the treatment of liver fluke in equids. In a case of clinical necessity, this medication can be administered at a dose rate of 12 mg/kg. Small studies have shown no adverse effects of treatment (Trawford *et al.*1996; Rubilar *et al.* 1988).

Resistance to benzimidazole

The resistance to this group of anthelmintics can be considered together, as cross resistance between medications in this class is common.

Small strongyles Resistance is documented globally and has been reported for several decades (Slocombe *et al.* 1977; Kuzmina *et al.* 2008; Slocombe *et al.* 2008). Fenbendazole resistance has been very well documented throughout America, Europe and Australia.

Pyrimidines (pyrantel salts)

Three pyrimidines are registered for use in equids: pamoate, emboate and tartrate. These medications work by causing spastic paralysis of parasites.

Pyrantel emboate

Indications

Treatment of large and small strongyles, *Oxyuris*, *Parascaris equi* and *Anoplocephala* spp. (Owen and Slocombe 2004; Marchiondo *et al.* 2006)

Dose 19 mg/kg PO

Resistance to pyrantel

Cyathostomin resistance to pyrantel was found in one-third of 102 horse farms in the UK, Germany and Italy (Traversa *et al.* 2009). Resistance of cyathostomins is even more widespread in the US where pyrantel has been available for daily feeding.

Piperazine

Indications

Treatment of *Parascaris equorum* and adult strongyles. Piperazine does not treat bots, tapeworm or any larval forms. Used alone this medication has a narrow spectrum of activity; however, piperazine is frequently used in combination with benzimidazoles for broad-spectrum activity against benzimidazole-resistant cyathostomins. The narrow spectrum of activity of Piperazine, only effective against adult stages of cyathostomins/ascarids, and low therapeutic margin have limited its clinical value.

Dose 110 mg/kg PO (EMEA 1999)

There is a risk of photosensitisation. Rapid death and detachment of Parascaris can cause rupture or obstruction of the small intestine.

Praziquantel

Praziquantel causes spastic paralysis of the parasite. It is available in some countries in combination with ivermectin and benzimidazoles for the treatment of tapeworm.

Indications Tapeworm only

Dose 1.5 mg/kg PO

Resistance of roundworms to praziquantel is low although, as FEC examination is unreliable in tapeworm, resistance is difficult to measure. A small study in Ethiopia demonstrated efficacy of praziquantel against tapeworm (Getachew *et al.* 2013).

Principles of a strategic de-worming programme 17.3

Traditional helminth control programmes rely on regular administration of anthelmintics. There are three major drug classes currently being used: benzimidazoles, pyrantel and macrocyclic lactones. Parasitic resistance to these treatments, resulting in reduced efficacy, has been documented. Several factors can influence the rate at which anthelmintic resistance develops; high frequency of treatment is the most important. To reduce anthelmintic treatment frequency significantly, it is essential to examine the efficacy of the medication routinely for each drug class and to design a **targeted** control strategy, with management changes if necessary.

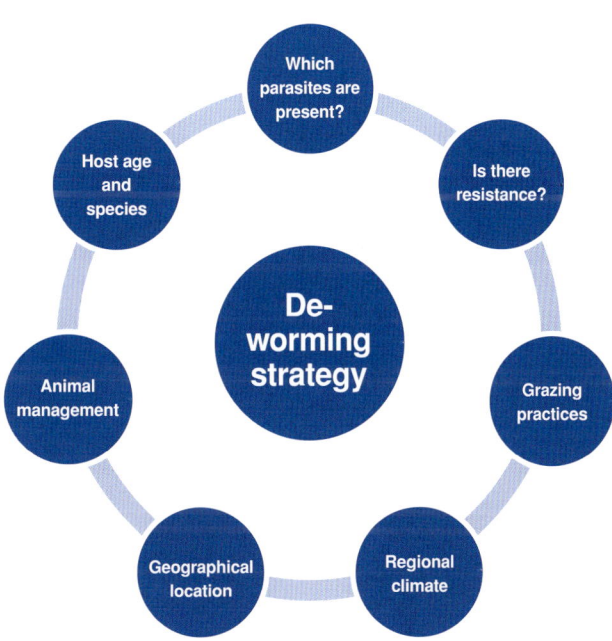

Figure 17.3.1 The epidemiological factors to consider when designing a de-worming programme.

Local epidemiology

- Which parasites are present in working equines and how common are they?
- Of these, which parasites are causing **overt disease**? (These must be the main targets of the de-worming strategy.)
- Which anthelmintic medication will be effective against these parasites?

Important helminths to consider in all de-worming strategies:

> - Strongyles – large *(S. vulgaris)*, small *(Cyathostomes)*
> - Ascarids
> - Tapeworms

European and American de-worming strategies and research focus heavily on cyathostomes as, in these countries, the large strongyle species are well controlled. In working equids this is often not the case and studies have shown that the predominant disease risk is from *Strongylus vulgaris*. Consider this difference when reading literature based on non-working equids.

Host demographics

Young equids are more susceptible to worm infestations than adults; frequently they have higher helminth burdens and increased rates of shedding. In Europe and America certain helminths, such as *Parascaris equorum and Strongyles westeri*, are thought to cause clinical disease only in young animals, as adults develop resistance. In working equids adults do not seem to develop such a strong immunity. Hard work and physiological stress may result in immune-compromise. Consequently, species such as *Parascaris equorum* may cause disease even in adulthood.

Regional climate

Larvae on pasture become desiccated in hot, dry conditions so, in this climate, pasture contamination is rapidly reduced. In warm, humid conditions the rate of larval development increases, raising the infection level of grazing equids. Consider administering de-worming treatment at the end of the dry season/beginning of the wet season to reduce worm burdens prior to a period of increased propagation.

Cyathostomes arrest development by encysting within the gut wall when environmental conditions are unfavourable, such as cold, or dry and hot weather. Schedule de-worming, if deemed necessary by an FEC, prior to the change in season to minimise the number of cyathostomes that enter arrested development.

Animal husbandry

Keep new equids in isolation for 3 weeks before introducing them to the herd. Treat with an anthelmintic and assess efficacy with an FEC.

> Remove faeces, from stable/paddocks/grazing areas, at least once a week to reduce transmission of helminths and thereby reduce the dependence on anthelmintic medication.

Grazing management

Management practices can be combined with drug intervention to minimise the spread of helminths between animals. Rest heavily grazed ground, and limit density of numbers to reduce pasture contamination.

Anthelmintic resistance

Monitor and evaluate de-worming strategies regularly using FEC, FEC Reduction and by recording clinical disease caused by helminths. If resistant parasites are detected, withdraw the use of this anthelmintic.

PRINCIPLES OF A STRATEGIC DE-WORMING PROGRAMME 17.3

> The proportion of a parasite population not exposed to anthelmintic treatment is described as 'refugia'.

Although many factors affect the rate at which resistance develops, levels of refugia are considered the most important as these parasites provide a pool of sensitive genes in the population.

It is the aim of any **responsible** worming programme to maximise the number of worms in refugia. This is done by **limiting** treatment to only those animals that require it, for example using FEC and treating young animals and those with counts above a pre-determined threshold.

In most host-parasite situations, the majority of animals in a group have relatively few parasites; environmental egg contamination comes from a minority of individuals with a heavy worm burden. In order to benefit the whole group and reduce the use of anthelmintics, identify and treat only these animals. Untreated animals will provide a pool of susceptible eggs (refugia). It is preferable to use an FEC to accurately identify equids with a high worm burden. However, clinical signs of 'intestinal parasitism', such as a poor coat, colic signs or adult worms seen in faeces, can also give an indication of the severely affected individuals.

Working equids in less developed countries do not generally receive regular anthelmintic treatments. This is likely to be due to the prohibitive costs, or a lack of access to veterinary medicines. There are very few studies investigating anthelmintic resistance in working equids (Kyvsgaarda *et al.* 2001). Resistance overall is likely to be low, and it is essential that the pool of sensitive helminths is preserved by using targeted treatments combined with improved management practices. **Minimising the dependence on anthelmintic drugs will help prevent the development of resistance.**

De-worming strategies

Programme	Dosing strategy	Comments
Targeted dosing	Regular FEC for entire herd De-worm all animals with an FEC above a set level (e.g. 1000 epg). FEC will not detect tapeworm. Perform a tapeworm faecal analysis or serology twice yearly. Alternatively, include a tapeworm treatment in the regime twice a year (interval dosing). Dose all tapeworm positive animals with pyrantel/praziquantel.	Appropriate if grazing is well managed, with predominantly adult horses and minimal new intake of animals (treated/isolated prior to introduction) Compliant owner to undertake frequent sampling Will detect high burden equids, those with a low burden will not require de-worming.
Strategic dosing	Dose only at times of year when de-worming will be most effective, e.g. with seasonal changes. Dose all grazing animals at the same time.	Regional variation in climate affects the time taken for the life cycle of parasites. Appropriate in countries/regions which have marked seasons
Interval dosing	Year-round synchronised dosing in all grazing animals. Dosing with principle anthelmintic at pre-determined intervals, based on ERP for each drug class.	Not recommended. Intensive use of anthelmintic predisposes development of resistance. It does not leave any refugia.

Table 17.3.1 Different de-worming dosing strategies.

17.4 Faecal egg count

The McMaster technique is a widely accepted protocol for the detection of nematode eggs in equine faeces. It is described below. An alternative technique is the FECPAK system (Presland et al. 2005). Here a larger faecal sample is taken giving greater sensitivity with low egg densities. Tapeworm egg counts are likely to be unreliable in both cases.

Materials

- McMaster slide (or alternative counting chamber of known volume)
- Microscope
- Clean containers with lids (such as jars)
- Wooden spatula to weigh 3 g samples
- Small sieve (such as a tea strainer or a gauze pad)
- Plastic pipettes
- Super-saturated salt (NaCl) solution:
  - Fill container with water.
  - Add table salt and shake/stir until the solution is saturated (salt settles at the bottom and will not dissolve).
  - Epsom salts, magnesium sulphate, can also be used.
- Weighing machine/scales in grams

  – or make a measuring device:
  - Draw up 42 ml water into a syringe.
  - Add the water to a jar and draw a line at the water level.
  - Add 3 ml water and draw a second line to mark 45 ml.

FEC procedure

1. Collect faecal samples from the target population/animal and label appropriately. Avoid collecting samples directly from the rectum.
2. Use fresh samples if possible and ensure air is taken out of the sample bag to stop development of eggs. Keep samples refrigerated and examine within 24 hours.
3. Weigh 3 g faeces from each sample and place in separate containers OR add faeces to 42 ml salt solution until the water level reaches the second line.
4. Mix the sample, by shaking the jar and breaking the faeces up with the spatula until they are evenly distributed throughout the water.
5. Using the sieve, strain the mixed faecal sample into another clean container.
6. Using the pipette, fill the McMaster counting chambers immediately.
7. Allow to sit for 1 minute, so that eggs float to the top, before reading.
8. Count the number of eggs (Figure 17.4.1) in each chamber and add together.

FAECAL EGG COUNT 17.4

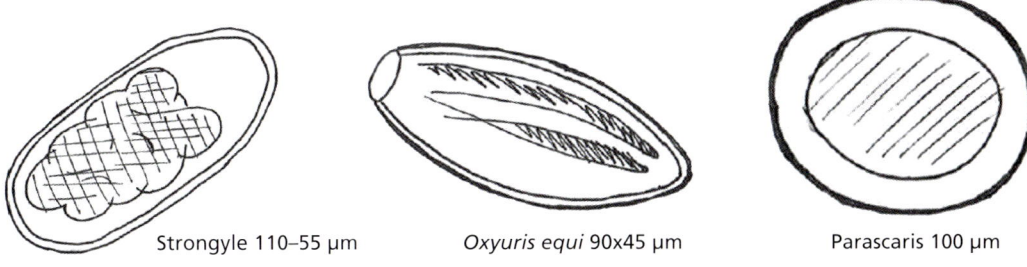

Figure 17.4.1 Commonly encountered helminth eggs. Note the distinctive operculum in the Oxyuris egg.

Larval culture to speciate strongyle eggs

It is possible to differentiate large and small strongyles by larval hatching from the faeces. In practice, if there are a large number of strongyle eggs, treatment without a precise diagnosis is acceptable.

To calculate the eggs per gram (epg), when using 3 g of faeces in 42 ml of salt solution read in a standard McMaster chamber (0.3 ml when both chambers counted), multiply the egg count by 50 (e.g. if there were four eggs the total count is 200 epg). Calculate the FEC for strongyles and ascarids separately. The strongyle count will include that for large and small strongyles as these eggs cannot be distinguished.

> There are four categories into which **strongyle epg** can be classified according to Soulsby 1982: none, low (up to 500 epg), medium (501–1,000 epg) or high (> 1,000 epg).

There is little official information on the egg counts of working equids and the level of parasite burden that causes problems for them. A study in working equids in Mexico revealed that there was no correlation between epg and body condition score (Valdez-cruz *et al.* 2013). The use of an epg 'cut off point' for anthelmintic treatment is likely to depend on local epidemiology and individual animal circumstances. Treat equids with an epg of > 1000 as they are likely to be high shedders and responsible for pasture contamination. If the epg is medium, clinical discretion is required.

Design field trials within an operational area to gain a broader understanding of the worm burdens in local equids, build a local databank of baseline information prior to de-worming.

Measuring anthelmintic resistance

In those animals that have been de-wormed (based on an medium to high epg) repeat the FEC 10–14 days after worming to test the efficacy of the anthelmintic. This is known as a Faecal Egg Count Reduction (FECR) test and is a technique for testing resistance. The FECR should be used in conjunction with the Egg Reappearance Period (ERP) to determine resistance levels effectively. ERP may be a more sensitive early indicator of resistance.

$$\text{FECR (\%)} = \frac{(\text{Day 0 FEC} - \text{Day 14 FEC}) \times 100}{\text{Day 0 FEC}}$$

FECR of > 95% for macrocyclic lactones and > 90% for benzimidazoles/pyrantel is expected for appropriate efficacy (Kaplan and Nielsen 2010).

Egg reappearance period

> ERP is the time taken for worm eggs to reappear in the faeces after de-worming. This time period reduces as resistance starts to develop.

1. Determine egg counts in faecal samples collected from six or more equids prior de-worming.
2. Treat equids with label dosage of anthelmintic. Use a weigh tape and treat at 110% estimated weight.
3. Collect faecal samples from the same horses at 2-week intervals after de-worming, until 2 weeks after the recorded ERP for that anthelmintic (6 weeks for fenbendazole and pyrantel, 8 weeks for ivermectin and 13 weeks for moxidectin).

The ERP is usually defined as the **time interval** from treatment until the mean FEC exceeds a value of 20% of the pre-treatment FEC (Kyvsgaard *et al.* 2011).

17.5 External parasite species

Arthropod parasites

Lice

Two types of lice affect equids: the biting louse *Damalinia equi* and the sucking louse *Haematopinus asini*. Both are common where equids are kept in dirty or crowded conditions without regular grooming. Lice can be transmitted by direct contact or via saddlery or grooming kits.

Clinical signs

- Itching and hair loss varies from mild to severe.
- Adult lice are small and greyish-yellow. They can be hard to find but may be seen moving in the dust and scale on the skin surface, especially over the neck and rump/flanks.
- The eggs are pale yellow and stick to the ends of the hair, especially on the neck, upper limbs, and the base of the mane and tail.

Treatment

Wash the equid with a treatment containing a pyrethroid. Repeat treatment 3 times, once every 7–10 days. Treat all in-contact animals at the same time. Wash saddlery and grooming kits to prevent re-infestation.

Mites

Several species of mange mite affect equids: *Chorioptes* spp., *Psoroptes* spp., *Demodex* spp. and *Sarcoptes scabei*. Infestation is by direct contact with an infected equid or through saddlery and grooming kits. Mites burrow into the skin so, unlike lice, they cannot be seen with the naked eye. Skin scrapings (described in Section 15.2) or a skin biopsy is recommended for definitive diagnosis. Mites can be difficult to find, and the extent of the skin damage is not always representative of the numbers present. Itching is often severe causing the animal to rub, bite at itself or stamp its feet. Lesions are typified by hair loss and thickened, scaly, greasy skin. Debility, weakness and poor appetite may occur in severe cases.

Species	Predilection site	Pruritus	Diagnosis	Treatment
Sarcoptes	Severe lesions starting on head neck and shoulders	Intense pruritus	Skin scrape or biopsy	Pyrethroid wash or oral ivermectin. Repeat doses/treatments at 2-week intervals for at least 3 treatments. Wash saddle and grooming equipment and treat all in-contact animals.
Psoroptes	Thickly-haired regions and ears	Pruritus	Skin scrape	Treatment as for sarcoptes
Chorioptes	Distal limbs	Pruritus, foot stamping	Skin scrape	Clip hair, treat with whole body wash with pyrethroids.
Demodex	Rare in equids, body or eyes and muzzle affected	Pruritus absent	Skin scrape	No effective treatment. Do not use amitraz as this medication can cause severe colic.

Table 17.5.1 Diagnosis and treatment of mites.

Ticks

Ticks are more common in the wet season. Predilection sites are generally protected areas such as the axilla, groin and ears (Figure 17.5.1). Tick infestations are normally mild and produce few direct clinical problems, but in many regions they are vectors for protozoal disease (see Section 17.7). Anaemia and debility only occur in very severe infestations. Remove ticks using blunt forceps (Gammons and Salam 2002).

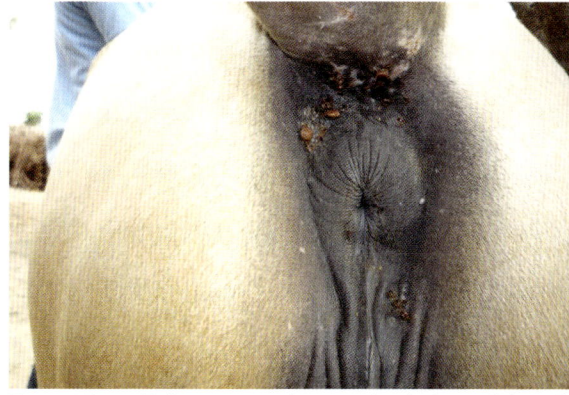

Figure 17.5.1 Ticks in a typical area under the base of the tail.

17 PARASITOLOGY

Helminth parasites

Onchocerca

Microfilariae of the nematode *Onchocerca cervicalis* are spread between equids by biting flies.

Life cycle

Adults live in long tendons, particularly the ligamentum nuchae in the neck. Inflammation is induced at these sites forming granulomatous, mineralised nodules. Onchocerca may be a factor in the development of fistulous withers (Doumbia 2011). Patent females produce microfilaria that migrate in the subcutaneous tissue to the ventral midline as well as other sites including the eye. At these locations the microfilariae initiate an inflammatory reaction which stimulates rubbing and self-trauma to these sites. Flies feed at the sites of inflammation and trauma and ingest the microfilaria. Microfilaria develop into infective stages in the fly. They are passed onto the next host when the fly feeds again.

Clinical signs

Although ocular and cutaneous lesions are seen, infection with *Onchocerca* spp. can be asymptomatic in up to 80% of cases.

Cutaneous lesions

Diffuse patchy alopecia (hair loss), erythema (redness), ulceration and scaling of the skin (Figure 17.5.2). Common sites include the ventral midline, face, base of mane, and a 'bull's-eye lesion' on the centre of the forehead.

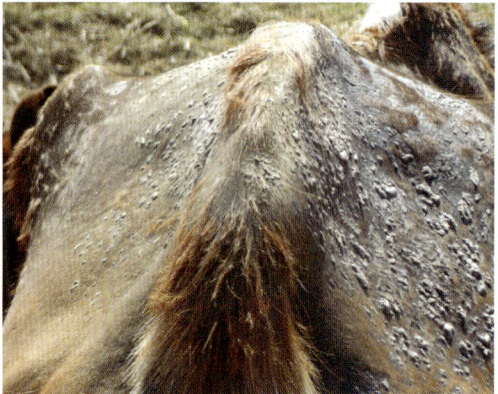
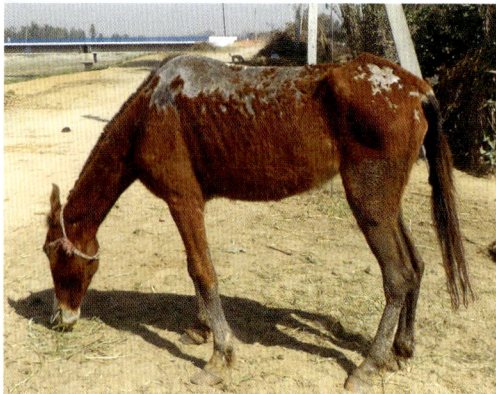

Figure 17.5.2 Clinical signs of onchocerciasis, a scaly dermatitis and patchy alopecia with an unusual presentation on the dorsal midline

Ocular lesions

Conjunctivitis and uveitis occur as an inflammatory response to dying microfilariae. Inflammation at the junction between the cornea and bulbar conjunctiva is a common clinical sign as well as de-pigmentation and inflammation at the lateral limbus of the eye. *Onchocerca cervicalis* has been implicated in the development of recurrent equine uveitis; however, this association is unclear (Moran and James 1987). *Onchocerca volvulus* causes ocular lesions known as 'river blindness' in humans. Use fluorescein dye to check that there is no corneal ulceration.

Diagnosis

The most effective method of diagnosis is by skin biopsy, preferably a full-thickness biopsy ≥ 6 mm. Mince the tissue and incubate in isotonic saline for several hours. Centrifuge the supernatant to concentrate the microfilariae. Stain with methylene blue and examine microscopically (Figure 17.5.3).

Treatment

Administer topical corticosteroids and systemic NSAIDs. Initiate this treatment 2 days prior to the ivermectin treatment and continue for a few days following. Dead microfilariae stimulate a greater immune reaction and damage than live ones. Administer systemic ivermectin (0.2 mg/kg PO). Ivermectin is not effective against the adult parasites; therefore, repeat treatment may be required after 2–4 months. Educate owners as to the importance of fly control to reduce infection rates and transmission.

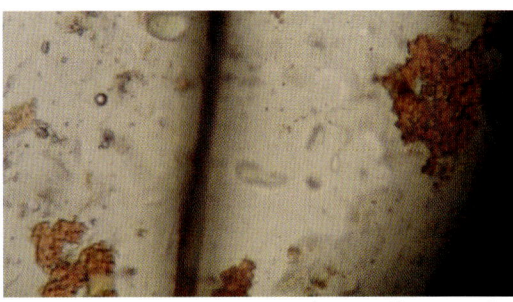

Figure 17.5.3 Microscopic view of a microfilariae. (Taken as a still from a video in which the microfilariae were very active.)

Habronemiasis

Habronema spp. are small nematodes which parasitise the stomach and the skin and also cause ocular lesions (See Section 9.6 *Common eye diseases of working equids*). Flies, intermediate hosts of *Habronema* species, deposit infective larvae around the mouth. These are then swallowed by the equid. Larvae develop into adults in the stomach. Eggs are shed in the faeces and ingested by fly larvae. *Habronema* larvae then develop into the infective stages in the flies ready for onward transmission. The ocular and cutaneous forms develop when larvae are deposited into open wounds on the skin (summer sores) or around the eye. In these cases the larvae penetrate the dermis resulting in a hypersensitivity reaction. The *Habronema* larvae cannot complete development in the skin.

Clinical signs

Habronemiasis is most commonly seen in warmer climates and seasons. Lesions are nodular and ulcerated. In the ocular form, lesions are commonly seen at the medial canthus. Other ocular sites include the conjunctival sac, the lacrimal duct and the third eyelid. Yellow caseous ocular discharge contains necrotic material which encases the infective larvae. Severe ocular problems can result as sequalae, including epiphora, chemosis, and photophobia. *Habronema* spp. can cause a catarrhal gastritis but it is generally not considered clinically significant in this organ.

Diagnosis

Clinical signs and history can provide an accurate diagnosis. Cytology on a deep skin scraping can reveal larvae.

Treatment

Systemic treatment (PO) with ivermectin (see Section 9.6). NSAIDs and, occasionally, steroids are required to treat hypersensitivity reactions associated with the lesions. Raise awareness of the life cycle of *Habronema* amongst equine owners. Highlight the importance of fly control and hygiene as a preventative measure. Clean eyes regularly and cover wounds.

Myiasis (fly strike)

Flies deposit eggs around wounds or infected areas, the larvae (maggots) hatch and burrow into the tissue. Maggot infestation causes extensive inflammation, tissue damage and secondary infection.

Treatment

Remove as many maggots as possible using forceps. The animal may need to be sedated to allow deep exploration of the wound. Open any deep tracts using a scalpel blade, following administration of local anaesthesia. Apply 1–2 ml ivermectin or permethrin ectoparasiticide topically to kill any remaining maggots. Debride and clean the wound and allow to heal by secondary intention. Cover the wound to prevent further infestation and check it daily until healing is complete.

Prevention

Check all wounds daily and keep them bandaged or covered wherever possible. Keep feet clean, dry and free from infection. Use insect repellents.

17.6 Ectoparasite medication

In the treatment of ectoparasites, only when a diagnosis has been made can the optimal therapeutic protocol be chosen and a positive treatment outcome achieved. When attempting to control lice and mites, apply treatment to all members of a group rather than just to those showing reactions. Hypersensitivity to killed parasites can result in the persistence of pruritus; this may be perceived as treatment failure. Judicious use of anti-histamines, or corticosteroids, can be employed to limit pruritus.

Pyrethroids

Pyrethroids are neurotoxin insecticides. The pyrethroids – permethrin, cypermethrin, fenvalerate and deltamethrin – are available in spot-on, spray and wash formulations. These medications are effective against lice and mites, including *Sarcoptes* and *Chorioptes*. When using as a topical wash ensure that the entire coat is covered. This treatment should be repeated 3 times, 7 days apart. Powder formulations are less likely to provide effective coverage and tend to lose potency rapidly when stored.

Macrocyclic lactones

Parenteral and per os administration of ivermectin and moxidectin is generally only effective for ectoparasites that ingest blood or live within the skin, the sucking lice and skin helminths. These medications can also be used to treat *Sarcoptes scabei* in horses. Pour-on formulations used to treat cattle are not licensed for use in equids.

Benzyl benzoate

Benzyl benzoate is often more affordable and available than permethrin products and is used as a topical treatment for lice and *Sarcoptes scabei*. There are reports of variable efficacy but this medication is used frequently in the treatment of scabies in humans, particularly in less developed countries (Mounsey and McCarthy 2013). Apply to the entire coat. Rinse the coat after 24 hours as prolonged skin contact can cause irritation.

Fipronil is used to treat fleas in small animals. Fipronil is not licensed in horses but is effective against mange mites in the spray form; however, the large volume required to treat equids is prohibitively expensive.

> Organophosphates are no longer used as for ectoparasite treatment in many countries as there is a high risk of poisoning for both the animals and owners.

Synthetic pyrethroids are significantly less toxic and have been used in preference. Organophosphates may still be available in some regions; use is not recommended.

Insect growth regulators are in development for veterinary use (Pasay *et al.* 2012).

Protozoal infections 17.7

Equine piroplasmosis

Equine piroplasmosis (EP) is a tick-borne infection caused by the haemoprotozoa *Babesia caballi* and *Theileria equi*. This disease affects all members of the *Equus* genus, including donkeys and mules (Gizachew *et al.* 2013). *B. caballi* and *T. equi* are endemic in many tropical and subtropical countries in Mediterranean Europe, Africa, the Middle East, Asia, and Central and South America. Equine piroplasmosis is a notifiable disease in many countries and is reportable to the OIE by government veterinary services.

Twelve species of ixodid ticks of the genera *Dermacentor* spp. (central Asia), *Hyalomma* spp. (Middle East and Africa), and *Rhipicephalus* spp. (Africa and South America) were listed as vectors for EP by the OIE. *T. equi* is also transmitted by contaminated needles and syringes. Although identification of EP tick vectors is possible, it is impractical as a diagnostic tool. As the incubation period can be up to 30 days for *B. caballi* and 20 days for *T. equi*, the infected tick is likely to have dropped off the host prior to the development of clinical signs of disease. Equids presenting with a tick infestation and concurrent clinical signs of anaemia and weakness should be tested for EP to confirm the suspected diagnosis.

The causative agents of EP are intracellular parasites which invade red blood cells inducing haemolysis, thereby causing a haemolytic anaemia. The severity of clinical signs relates to the parasite burden, and disease can manifest as acute or chronic, mild to severe. Fatalities may occur in the first 48 hours of infection but chronic disease often develops. Generally *B. caballi* is clinically milder than *T. equi*; severe anaemia is very rare with a *B. caballi* infection. Donkeys tend to develop the chronic form of the disease and the signs are often unspecific. **Carrier equids remain sources of infection for tick vectors for up to 4 years after infection.**

Clinical signs of *acute* EP

- Intermittent fever (> 40°C), sudden sweating
- Anaemia, icterus
- Petechial haemorrhage of third eyelid (Figure 17.8.1)
- High heart rate and respiratory rate
- Oedema of muzzle, limbs, ventral abdomen and thorax
- Hindlimb weakness, reluctance to move, tremors
- Haemoglobinuria and dry faeces
- May lead to death within a few days (mortality 5–10% in endemic areas and up to 50% in naïve horses)

Clinical signs of *chronic* EP

- Inappetance, weight loss
- Poor performance
- Difficult to detect parasites in blood

Diagnosis

The number of parasites in the blood varies throughout the course of infection. In acute cases with clinical signs the haemoparasites are readily visible on a blood film, appearing as dark dots, rings or pear-shaped marks within red blood cells. It may be difficult to detect parasites in animals in the latent or chronic stages of disease, particularly with *B. caballi*. Laboratory techniques include PCR and antibody ELISA (Rosales *et al.* 2013).

Treatment

The medications used to treat EP are toxic, so administer treatment only to animals with severe clinical signs or if parasites are present in > 50% of RBCs. Provide supportive treatment such as fluid therapy, NSAIDs, and a blood transfusion (if the facilities are available and the PCV is < 12%).

Imidocarb diproprionate Efficacy of this medication is variable (Grause *et al.* 2012), and toxic side effects are common. Administration can cause severe colic and diarrhoea; these effects may be reduced by pre-medicating with glycopyrrolate (Kutscha *et al.* 2012). Administer 2.4 mg/kg as a single deep IM injection; donkeys are more susceptible to toxic side effects so use a low dose (1–2 mg/kg). A treatment protocol of 4 injections at 4 mg/kg at 72-hour intervals has been recommended for complete elimination of *T. equi* (Grause *et al.* 2012); in endemic areas complete parasite elimination will reduce endemic stability.

Diminazine aceturate It is recommended to avoid this drug in equids unless other drugs are unavailable, as it has a low therapeutic index and toxic side effects are common. Administration of 3.5 mg/kg IM reduces the clinical signs within 24 hours. (In areas of resistance, horses require even higher doses; 2 doses 24 hours apart at 5 mg/kg for *B. caballi*, 6–12 mg/kg for *T. equi*.) However, this drug is associated with marked side effects **even at the lower dose rate**. At higher doses, the risk and severity of such side effects would be increased and is not recommended. Toxicity can be treated with calcium salts.

> **Endemic stability**
>
> 'Infected but not affected'
>
> Endemic stability is an epidemiological state in which severe clinical disease is scarce despite high levels of infection in the population. In endemic areas where equids are faced with a low level of continuous challenge, immunity develops and reduces the severity of disease. Disruption of this low-level challenge, through control (of ticks or the causative agents of EP), might result in an increase in clinical disease incidence. Under conditions of epidemiological stability, when hosts are under frequent exposure to EP, foals are protected passively by maternal antibodies acquired via colostrum. This protection can last for up to 9 months. Infections of foals in this period will induce immunity without any overt signs of the disease.

Trypanosomiasis

The causative organisms of trypanosomiasis in equids are the tsetse transmitted *Trypanosoma* spp. (which cause the disease known as nagana in cattle), *T. evansi* (surra) and *T. equiperdum* (dourine). These flagellate haemoprotozoan live extracellularly in the blood. The different species have differing life cycles and transmission mechanisms.

Tsetse transmitted trypanosomiasis

Tsetse flies are distributed in a 'belt' across 37 countries in Africa; trypanosomiasis is endemic in these areas. For *T. congolense* and *T. brucei*, development within the tsetse is an essential stage in the life cycle. All domestic animals are at risk of infection in tsetse areas.
T. brucei gambiense and *rhodesiense* cause disease in humans resulting in a fatal condition known as sleeping sickness. Horses cannot be kept in tsetse areas without trypanocidal prophylaxis; however, donkeys have been kept in these areas. Although resilient, donkeys are not resistant to tsetse transmitted trypanosomiasis (Faye *et al.* 2001, Mukiria *et al.* 2010).

T. brucei Horses are particularly susceptible to this species of trypanosome and mortality usually occurs within 14–90 days if left untreated. Clinical signs include anaemia, icterus (jaundice), enlarged lymph nodes and petechial haemorrhages of the mucous membranes. Classic parasitaemic 'waves' of intermittent high fever (41°C) occur as host immunity responds to changes in the proteins on the parasite surface. *T. brucei* can cause a serious and acute disease in donkeys as well as horses.

T. congolense **and *T. vivax*** These are rarer with relatively milder and more chronic clinical signs compared to *T. brucei*, often indicated by anorexia, wasting and generalised oedema around 14 days after infection. *T. vivax* can also be transmitted mechanically, and therefore can spread beyond the tsetse belt as well as occurring in South America.

Surra

The causative agent of surra, *Trypanosoma evansi*, is transmitted mechanically by haematophagus flies. The insects which spread the disease are various types of *Tabanids* (**horse flies**) and *Stomoxys* (**stable flies**). The trypanosome parasites are mechanically transferred during feeding; there is no biological development of the trypanosome parasite within the fly. Surra is a particular problem in India, but also affects equids across Asia, North Africa, Central and South America.

The **clinical signs** of surra are **severe weight loss** (Figure 17.7.1), progressive weakness, anaemia, haemoglobinuria, intermittent fever, petechial haemorrhage of mucous membranes, oedema of limbs, lower abdomen and thorax and severe neurological signs. **The mortality rate in untreated horses is almost 100%.** The severity of the disease depends on the parasite strain and factors including stress and the health of the equid. Animals subjected to stress, such as malnutrition and physical labour, are more susceptible to the disease.

Chronic forms persist for several months up to 2 years, providing a **reservoir** of infection for other animals. There is considerable variation in host species susceptibility; severe rapidly fatal disease is common in horses, whereas donkeys and mules tend to develop chronic mild or subclinical infections.

There are rare reports of *T. evansi* infection in humans, these are thought to be anomalies as the individuals were immuno-compromised (Joshi *et al.* 2005; Powar *et al.* 2006).

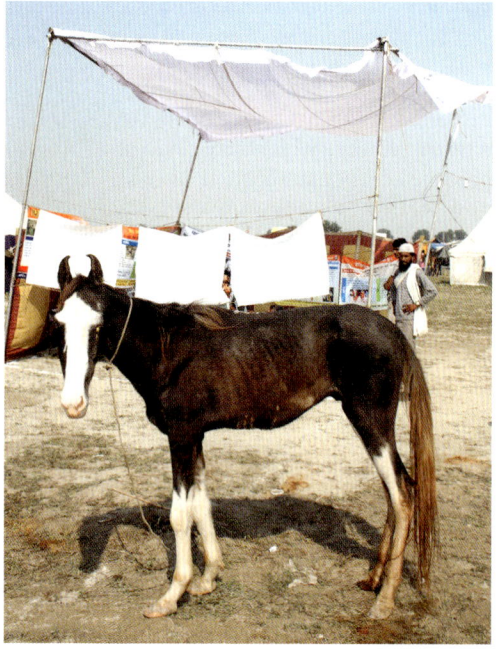

Figure 17.7.1 A horse with severe weight loss at an equine fair in India, subsequently diagnosed with a surra infection.

Prevention of surra

Control measures include early detection and treatment of infected animals and protection of all animals from biting flies. The aim is to alter attitudes (Figure 17.7.2) so that individual animals, preferably with a laboratory diagnosis, are treated with the medication at an appropriate dose. Treatment of groups of animals for a long period at sub-optimal doses is discouraged.

- Isolate infected animals by moving them away from the rest of the herd (biting flies are then less likely to transfer the disease).
- Keep other livestock, which act as a reservoir, separate from equids.
- Ensure vector control, fly repellents, dung removal, and do not house equids close to stagnant water.

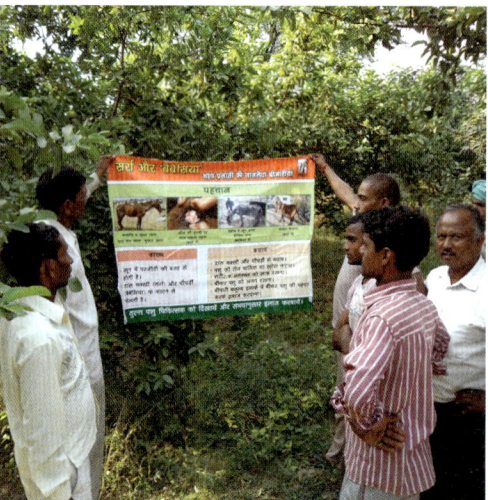

Figure 17.7.2 Developing a health plan to reduce surra within a community in India.

Prophylactic treatment is not recommended. Although in the short term this may reduce the number of clinical cases, it will ultimately lead to resistance. There are very few alternative drugs to treat surra and, if resistance develops, then there will be no effective treatment.

Dourine

Dourine is a venereal disease of equids caused by *T. equiperdum* and transmitted mechanically when mating. *T. equiperdum* is the only trypanosome that is not transmitted by an invertebrate vector. The pathogenesis of dourine differs from other trypanosomes in that it is primarily a tissue parasite which rarely invades the blood. There is no known natural reservoir of the parasite other than infected equids (Claes *et al.* 2005). Dourine was previously widespread; it is now limited to confined parts of Africa, Asia, Central and South America.

> *T. equiperdum* may persist for years in donkeys and mules without showing clinical signs; mortality can be high in untreated horses.

A mucopurulent discharge from the penis or vulva, and oedema around the area, is the most common initial presenting sign. Generalised clinical signs can include fever, oedema, anaemia and wasting. Approximately a month following inoculation, urticarial reactions erupt all over the body. Progressive paralysis is a possible sequel and these cases are frequently fatal. Abortion is also common.

Diagnosis of trypanosomiasis

A clinical diagnosis of trypanosomiasis must be confirmed by a laboratory test; however, the standard techniques for the detection of trypanosomes are not sufficiently sensitive. The infection is not always detected by microscopic examination of the blood; the trypanosomes must be at a high level to be detected by this method, and in chronic or latent infections the number of parasites will be low. The detection rate can be improved by centrifuging the blood sample to concentrate the parasites. Serologic tests (CFT and ELISA) and trypanosome antigen detecting tests (PCR) have been developed. Diagnosis is challenging as clinical signs are similar to other diseases, such as babesiosis, equine infectious anaemia and African Horse Sickness.

Collect blood samples from capillaries using an ear prick. Examine as a wet smear or as a thick or thin stained smear (Figure 17.8.2). Alternatively centrifuge the sample in a capillary tube and look at the tube under the microscope. The organisms are flagellate-protozoa free in plasma, moving with a whip-like motion just above the buffy coat. This is a relatively simple and efficient technique (75% sensitive). However, the fresh blood sample (EDTA or lithium heparin tube) must be examined within 7–12 hours of collection. Parasitaemia is intermittent, so it is good practice to take a number of samples at 4-day intervals. In chronic infections parasites in the blood are very rarely found, making diagnosis difficult. In these cases clinical signs, the presence of anaemia and acanthocytes, can be useful in diagnosis.

T. equiperdum rarely produces haemoparasitism so blood smear detection is not usually effective. Microscopy of direct smears from the fluid of infected genitalia may detect parasites; however, serology is the most reliable test for dourine. When using the CFT, cross reactions with *T. brucei* are common so this test is not applicable in tsetse zones.

Treatment of trypanosomiasis

As the result of overuse of medication in cases of misdiagnosis and prophylaxis, there is widespread resistance to trypanocides. In addition to concerns regarding resistance, these drugs have **narrow safety margins**. The availability of trypanocidal medication and resistance patterns will vary according to geographical area. Attempts to develop a vaccine have been thwarted as the parasite is able to override immune defences by rapidly changing the surface proteins. Each time an antibody response is mounted, the coat changes and the defences are useless.

Treatment is **not recommended for dourine** as it is never 100% effective; recovered animals can still infect others. Castration may be an option in males; however, euthanasia should be discussed with the owner. It is important to reiterate that infected animals should not be used for breeding.

Quinapyramine salts For infections of *T. evansi* use 3–5 mg/kg of a 5% solution split between three injection sites. Quinapyramine dimethylsulphate is recommended as a treatment whereas quinapyramine chloride is thought to have a longer duration of action (prophylaxis is not recommended). There are formulations where these drugs are delivered together (Triquin) with the aim to provide a depot at the injection site.

These medications are often poorly tolerated (particularly in horses) and now have widespread resistance. Only administer via deep IM injection using a long narrow-gauge needle, as SC injection results in sloughing and may take many months to resolve.

Phenanthridinium compounds

Homidium bromide Purple tablets (250 mg) dissolved in sterile water, prepared as 1–2.5% solution for SC or IM injection at 1 mg/kg. With both prophylactic and curative properties, this is most effective against *T. vivax*; however, there is widespread resistance in tsetse areas. Isometamidium is structurally similar to homidium, therefore there is the potential for cross-resistance with these drugs.

Pyrithidium bromide Red tablets (500 mg) dissolved in boiling water to make a 2.5% solution. Give via deep IM injection, 2–2.5 mg/kg will provide 4 months' protection in non-resistant areas. Severe local reactions can occur and resistance is common.

Isometamidium chloride The current recommended dose rates are *T. vivax* (0.5 mg/kg IM), and *T. brucei, T. congolensis* (0.5–1mg/kg). Administer a 1–2% solution as a deep IM injection. Resistance is common in areas where this drug is widely used for prophylaxis.

Diminazene aceturate This compound was discussed previously with reference to EP; however, in equids at therapeutic doses against trypanosomiasis, there are severe side effects which can be fatal so **do not use!**

Suramin This is considered the drug of choice for the early stages of Human African Trypanosomiasis. In domestic animals it has predominantly been used as a curative drug against *T. evansi* in camels and horses.

The standard prophylactic dose in horses is 7–10 mg/kg IV. Complexes of suramin with quinapyramine have found to be effective prophylactically but they are expensive and have severe tissue reactions. The safety margins of suramin are low and horses/donkeys are considered more susceptible than camels.

Melarsenoxide Although not widely available, this is used for treatment of *T. evansi* infections in camels and horses. Efficacy is also reported against *T. brucei* in horses. Melarsomine has no prophylactic activity. The dose rate is 0.25 mg/kg IM/SC. The introduction of this compound has been seen as a clinical breakthrough in the treatment of *T. evansi* in camels. Unlike other trypanocidal drugs, the therapeutic index of this drug is high. Melarsenoxide crosses the blood-brain barrier.

Resistance

The development of resistance to trypanocidal drugs is a growing concern. It has been speculated that drug resistance in trypanosomes is likely to occur under the same circumstances as for many other parasites as a result of the following factors:

- Large scale drug use as (preventive treatments)
- Treatment with inadequate dose
- Use of medication that is slowly eliminated from the body
- The phenomenon of cross-resistance has been well established. For instance, quinapyramine usage has been shown to induce resistance to isometamidium, homidium and diminazene

Equine protozoal myoencephalitis
See Chapter 16 *Disorders of the neurological system*.

Case study – Surra 17.8

Area India

Attending veterinarians Dr Nidhish Bhardwaj and Dr Kamlesh

History
A working horse was presented with a 4-day history of anorexia, dullness and depression.

Clinical findings
The temperature was high (38.8°C). Other vital parameters were also elevated. Petechial haemorrhages were seen on third eyelid and mucous membrane were pale (Figure 17.8.1). Oedema of the lower limbs was observed and the animal was walking with a stiff gait.

Diagnosis
A blood smear was prepared and examined in the laboratory for confirmation (Figure 17.8.2). This case was diagnosed as surra, based on the symptoms and laboratory findings.

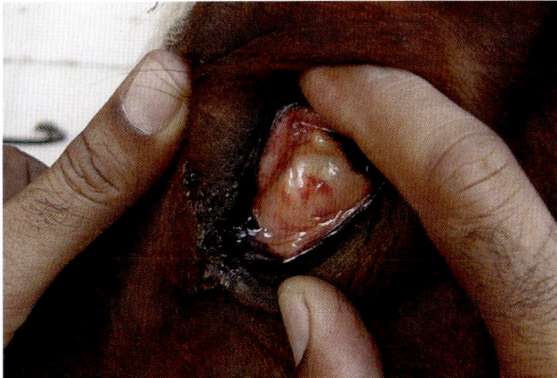

Figure 17.8.1 Petechial haemorrhage of the third eyelid.

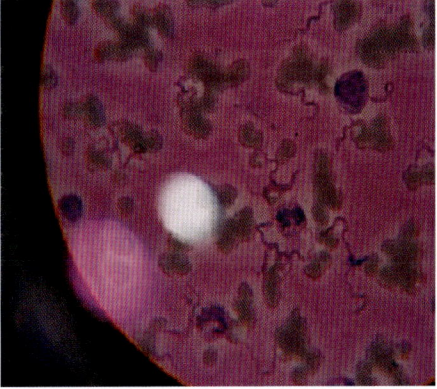

Figure 17.8.2 Trypanosomes in a blood smear.

Treatment

- Ketoprofen 2.2 mg/kg (NSAID)
- Pheniramine maleate 0.25 mg/kg (anti-histamine)
- Fluid therapy
- Quinapyramine sulphate 3 mg/kg

Outcome
The animal was showing signs of recovery after 2 days.

Discussion
Prevention is the best policy to control surra in an endemic area. Continuous owner education, generating awareness of the necessity of fly control, and identification of early signs of surra can be a key in managing this disease.

17.9 References

Andersen, U.V., Howe, D.K., Dangoudoubiyam, S., Toft, N., Reinemeyer, C.R., Lyons, E.T., Olsen, S.N., Monrad, J., Nejsum, P., Nielsen, M.K. (2013) SvSXP: a Strongylus vulgaris antigen with potential for prepatent diagnosis. *Parasites Vector*. 4 (6) 84.

Binev, R., Kirkova, Z., Nikolov, J., Russenov, A., Stojanchev, K., Lazarov, L., Hristov, T. (2005) Efficacy of parenteral administration of ivermectin in the control of strongylidosis in donkeys. *J. S. Afr. Vet. Assoc.* 76 (4) 214–216.

Claes, F., Büscher, P., Touratier, L., Goddeeris, B.M. (2005) *Trypanosoma equiperdum*: master of disguise or historical mistake? *Trends Parasitol*. 21 (7) 316–321.

Clayton, H.M., Neave, R.M.(1979) Efficacy of mebendazole against *Dictyocaulus arnfieldi* in the donkey. *Vet. Rec*. 104 (25) 571–572.

Doumbia, A. (2011) Onchocerciasis in working donkeys in Mali, Africa. 12th Congress of the World Equine Veterinary Association, Hyderabad, India.

Duncan, J.L., Bairden, K., Abbott, E.M. (1998) Elimination of mucosal cyathostome larvae by five daily treatments with fenbendazole.*Vet. Rec*. 142 (11) 268–271.

EMEA European Agency for the Evaluation of Medicinal Products (1999) Piperazine Summary Report. Available online at: *http://www.ema.europa.eu/docs/en_GB/document_library/Maximum_Residue_Limits_-_Report/2009/11/WC500015672.pdf*

Eysker, M., Boersema, J.H., Kooyman, F.N. (1992) The effect of ivermectin treatment against inhibited early third stage, late third stage and fourth stage larvae and adult stages of the cyathostomes in Shetland ponies and spontaneous expulsion of these helminths. *Vet. Parasitol*. 42 (3–4) 295–302.

Eysker, M., Pandey, V.S. (1989) Small Strongyle Infections in Donkeys from the Highveld in Zimbabwe. *Vet. Parasitol.* 30 (4) 345–349.

Faye, D., Pereira de Almeida, P.J., Goossens, B., Osaer, S., Ndao, M., Berkvens, D., Speybroeck, N., Nieberding, F., Geerts, S. (2001) Prevalence and incidence of trypanosomosis in horses and donkeys in the Gambia. *Vet. Parasitol.* 101 (2) 101–114.

French, D.D., Torbert, B.J., Chapman, M.R., Klei, T.R., Pierce, M.S. (1983) Comparison of anti-strongyle activity of a micellar formulation of ivermectin given parenterally or per os. *Vet. Med. Sm. Anim. Clin.* 78, 1778–1780.

Gammons, M., Salam, G. (2002) Tick Removal. *Am. Fam. Physician.* 4 (66) 643–645.

Getachew, A.M., Innocent, G., Proudman, C.J., Trawford, A., Feseha, G., Reid, S.W., Faith, B., Love, S. (2013) Field efficacy of praziquantel oral paste against naturally acquired equine cestodes in Ethiopia. *Parasitol Res.* 112 (1) 141–146.

Getachew, A.M., Innocent, G., Trawford, A.F., Reid, S.W.J., Love, S. (2012) Gasterophilosis: a major cause of rectal prolapse in working donkeys in Ethiopia. *Trop. Anim. Health Pro.* 44 (4) 757–762.

Getachew, M., Innocent, G.T., Trawford, A.F., Reid, S.W., Love, S. (2010a) Epidemiological features of fasciolosis in working donkeys in Ethiopia. *Vet. Parasitol.* 169 (3–4) 335–339.

Getachew, M., Trawford, A., Feseha, G., Reid, S.W. (2010b) Gastrointestinal parasites of working donkeys of Ethiopia. *Trop. Anim. Health Pro.* 42 (1) 27–33.

Gizachew, A., Schuster, R.K., Joseph, S., Nissy, R.W., Georgy, A., Elizabeth, S.K., Asfaw, Y., Regassam, F., Wernery, U. (2013) Piroplasmosis in Donkeys—A Hematological and Serological Study in Central Ethiopia. *J. Equine Vet. Sci.* 33 (1) 18–21.

Gokbulut, C., Cirak, V.Y., Senlik, B., Aksit, D., Durmaz, M., McKellar, Q.A. (2010) Comparative plasma disposition, bioavailability and efficacy of ivermectin following oral and pour-on administrations in horses. *Vet. Parasitol.* 170 (1–2) 120–126.

Grause, J.F., Ueti, M.W., Nelson, J.T., Knowles, D.P., Kappmeyer, L.S., Bunn, T.O. (2012) Efficacy of imidocarb dipropionate in eliminating Theileria equi from experimentally infected horses. *Vet. J.* 196 (3) 541–546.

Haridy, F.M., Morsy, T.A., Gawish, N.I., Antonios, T.N., Abdel Gawad, A.G. (2002) The potential reservoir role of donkeys and horses in zoonotic fascioliasis in Gharbia Governorate, Egypt. *Journal of the Egyptian Society of Parasitology.* 32 (2) 561–570.

Hearn, F.P., Peregrine, A.S. (2003) Identification of foals infected with *Parascaris equorum* apparently resistant to ivermectin. *J. Am. Vet. Med. Assoc.* 223 (4) 482–485.

Johnson, P.J., Mrad, D.R., Schwartz, A.J., Kellam, L. (1999) Presumed moxidectin toxicosis in three foals. *J. Am. Vet. Med. Assoc.* 214 (5) 678–680.

Joshi, P.P., Shegokar, V.R., Powar, R.M., Herder, S., Katti, R., Salkar, H.R., Dani. V.S., Bhargava, A., Jannin, J., Truc, P. (2006) A rare case of human trypanosomiasis caused by *Trypanosoma evansi*. *Indian Journal of Medical Microbiology.* 24 (1) 72–74.

Kaplan, R.M., Nielsen, M.K. (2010) Equine veterinary education An evidence-based approach to equine parasite control: It ain't the 60s anymore. *Equine Vet. Educ.* 22, 306–316.

Klei, T.R., Chapman, M., French, D.D. (1993) Evaluation of ivermectin at an elevated dose against encysted equine cyathostome larvae. *Vet. Parasitol.* 47, 99–106.

Kutscha, J., Sutton, D.G., Preston, T., Guthrie, A.J. (2012) Equine piroplasmosis treatment protocols: specific effect on orocaecal transit time as measured by the lactose 13C-ureide breath test. *Equine Vet. J. Supplement.* 44 (43) 62–67.

Kuzmina, T.A., Kharchenko, V.O. (2008) Anthelmintic resistance in cyathostomins of brood horses in Ukraine and influence of anthelmintic treatments on strongylid community structure. *Vet. Parasitol.* 154 (3–4) 277–288.

Kyvsgaard, N.C., Lindbom, J., Andreasen, L.L., Luna-Olivares, L.A., Nielsen, M.K., Monrad, J. (2011) Prevalence of strongyles and efficacy of fenbendazole and ivermectin in working horses in El Sauce, Nicaragua. *Vet. Parasitol.* 181 (2–4) 248–254.

Leaning, W.H.D. (1983) The efficacy and safety evaluation of ivermectin as a parenteral and oral antiparasitic agent in horses. *P. Am. Assoc. Equine Prac.* 29, 319–328.

Lyons, E.T., Tolliver, S.C., Collins, S.S. (2011) Reduced activity of moxidectin and ivermectin on small strongyles in young horses on a farm (BC) in Central Kentucky in two field tests with notes on variable counts of eggs per gram of feces (EPGs). *Parasitol Res.* 108 (5) 1315–1319.

Marchiondo, A.A., White, G.W., Smith, L.L., Reinemeyer, C.R., Dascanio, J.J., Johnson, E.G., Shugart, J.I. (2006) Clinical field efficacy and safety of pyrantel pamoate paste (19.13% w/w pyrantel base) against *Anoplocephala* spp. in naturally infected horses. *Vet. Parasitol.* 137 (1–2) 94–102.

Meana, A., Luzon, M., Corchero, J., Gómez-Bautista, M. (1998) Reliability of coprological diagnosis of Anoplocephalaperfoliata infection. *Vet. Parasitol.* 74 (1) 79–83.

Molento, M.B., Nielsen, M.K., Kaplan, R.M. (2012) Resistance to avermectin/milbemycin anthelmintics in equine cyathostomins – Current situation. *Vet. Parasitol.* 185 (1) 16–24.

Monahan, C.M., Chapman, M.R., Taylor, H.W., French, D.D., Klei, T.R. (1996) Comparison of moxidectin oral gel and ivermectin oral paste against a spectrum of internal parasites of ponies with special attention to encysted cyathostome larvae. *Vet. Parasitol.* 63 (3–4) 225–235.

Moran, C.T., James, E.R. (1987) Equine ocular pathology ascribed to Onchocerca cervicalis infection: a re-examination. *Ann. Trop. Med. Parasit.* 38 (4) 287–288.

Mounsey, K.E., McCarthy, J.S. (2013) Treatment and control of scabies. *Curr. Opin. Infect. Dis.* 26 (2) 133–139.

Mukiria, P., Mdachi, R., Thuita, J., Mutuku, J., Wanjala, K., Omolo, J., Getachew, M., Trawford, A.F., Ouma, J., Murilla, G. (2010) Semi-longitudinal study of trypanosomiasis and its vectors in donkeys (Equus africanus asinus, fitzinger) in the Lamu archipelago. Presented at 12th *KARI Biennial Scientific Conference.* 8–12 November. Nairobi, Kenya.

Owen, J., Slocombe, D. (2004) A modified critical test for the efficacy of pyrantel pamoate for Anoplocephalaperfoliata in equids. *Can. J. Vet. Res.* 68 (2) 112–117.

Pasay, C., Rothwell, J., Mounsey, K., Kelly, A., Hutchinson, B., Miezler, A., McCarthy, J. (2012) An exploratory study to assess the activity of the acarine growth inhibitor, fluazuron, against *Sarcoptes scabei* infestation in pigs. *Parasite Vector* 5:40.

Powar, R.M., Shegokar, V.R., Joshi, P.P., Dani, V.S., Tankhiwale, N.S., Truc, P., Jannin, J., Bhargava, A. (2005) Human trypanosomiasis caused by *Trypanosoma evansi* in India: the first case report. *Am J Trop Med Hyg.* 73 (3) 491–495.

Presland, S.L., Morgan, E.R., Coles, G.C. (2005) Counting Nematode eggs in equine faecal samples. *Vet. Rec.* 156, 208–210.

Reed, S.M. (1983) Ivermectin and CNS signs. *Mod. Vet. Pract.* 64, 783–784.

Reinemeyer, C.R., Prado, J.C., Nichols, E.C., Marchiondo, A.A . (2010) Efficacy of pyrantel pamoate and ivermectin paste formulations against naturally acquired *Oxyuris equi* infections in horses. *Vet. Parasitol.* 171 (1–2) 106–110.

REFERENCES 17.9

Reinemeyer, C.R. (2009) Diagnosis and control of anthelmintic-resistant Parascaris equorum. *Parasite Vector*. 25 (2) Suppl 2:S8.

Rosales, R., Rangel-Rivas, A., Escalona, A., Jordan, L.S., Gonzatti, M.I., Aso, P.M., Perrone, T., Silva-Iturriza, A., Mijares, A. (2013) Detection of *Theileria equi* and *Babesia caballi* infections in Venezuelan horses using Competitive-Inhibition ELISA and PCR. *Vet. Parasitol*. (In press).

Rossano, M.G., Smith, A.R., Lyons, E.T. (2010) Shortened strongyle-type egg reappearance periods in naturally infected horses treated with moxidectin and failure of a larvicidal dose of fenbendazole to reduce fecal egg counts. *Vet. Parasitol*. 173 (3–4) 349–352.

Rubilar, L., Cabreira, A., Giacaman, L. (1988) Treatment of *Fasciola hepatica* infection in horses with triclabendazole. *Vet. Rec*. 123 (12) 320–321.

Singh, G., Soodan, J.S., Singla, L.D., Khajuria, J.K. (2012) Epidemiological studies on gastrointestinal helminths in horses and mules. *Vet. Pract*. 13 (1) 23–27.

Skotarek, S.L., Colwell, D.D., Goater, C.P. (2010) Evaluation of diagnostic techniques for *Anoplocephala perfoliata* in horses from Alberta, Canada. *Vet. Parasitol*. 172 (3–4) 249–255.

Slocombe, J.O., Coté, J.F., de Gannes, R.V. (2008) The persistence of benzimidazole-resistant cyathostomes on horse farms in Ontario over 10 years and the effectiveness of ivermectin and moxidectin against these resistant strains. *Can. Vet. J*. 49 (1) 56–60.

Slocombe, J.O., Cote, J.F. (1977) Small strongyles of horses with cross resistance to benzimidazole anthelmintics and susceptibility to unrelated compounds. *Can. Vet. J*. 18 (8) 212–217.

Slocombe, J.O., Heine, J., Barutzki, D., Slacek, B. (2007) Clinical trials of efficacy of praziquantel horse paste 9% against tapeworms and its safety in horses. *Vet. Parasitol*. 144 (3–4) 366–370.

Soulsby, E.J.L. (1982). Helminth, Arthropod and Protozoa of Domestic Animals. 7th Ed. Baillere Tindall, London, UK. 809.

Steinbach, T., Bauer, C., Sasse, H., Baumgartner, W., Rey-Moreno, C., Hermosilla, C., Damriyasa, I., Zahner, H. (2006) Small strongyle infection: Consequences of larvicidal treatment of horses with fenbendazole and moxidectin. *Vet. Parasitol*. 139 (1–3) 115–131.

Tavassoli, M., Dalir-Naghadeh, B., Esmaeili-Sani, S. (2010) Prevalence of gastrointestinal parasites in working horses. *Pol. J. Vet. Sci*. 13 (2) 319–324.

Traversa, D., von Samson-Himmelstjerna, G., Demeler, J., Milillo, P., Schürmann, S., Barnes, H., Otranto, D., Perrucci, S., di Regalbono, A.F., Beraldo, P., Boeckh, A., Cobb, R. (2009) Anthelmintic resistance in cyathostomin populations from horse yards in Italy, United Kingdom and Germany. *Parasite Vector*. 2 Suppl 2:S2.

Trawford, A.F., Tremlett, J.G. (1996) Efficacy of triclabendazole against *Fasciola hepatica* in the donkey *(Equus asinus)*. *Vet. Rec*. 139 (6) 142–143.

Valdez-Cruz, M.P., Hernandez-Gil, M., Galindo-Rodriguez, L., Alonso-Diaz, M.A. (2006) Gastrointestinal parasite burden, body condition and haematological values in equines in the humid tropical areas of Mexico. *The Fifth International Colloquium on Working Equines*. Addis Adaba, Ethiopia. 30 October–2 November. 62–72.

Valdéz-Cruz, M.P., Hernández-Gil, M., Galindo-Rodríguez, L., Alonso-Díaz, M.A. (2013) Gastrointestinal nematode burden in working equids from humid tropical areas of central Veracruz, Mexico, and its relationship with body condition and haematological values. *Trop. Anim. Health Pro*. 45 (2) 603–607.

Further Reading

Bergvall, K. (2005) Advances in Acquisition, Identification, and Treatment of Equine Ectoparasites. *Clin. Tech. Equine P.* 4 (4) 296–301.

Brady, H.A., Nichols, W.T. (2009) Drug Resistance in Equine Parasites: An Emerging Global Problem. *J. Equine Vet. Sci.* 29 (5) 285–295.

Corning, S. (2009) Equine cyathostomins: a review of biology, clinical significance and therapy. *Parasite Vector.* 2(Suppl 2):S1

Crane, M.A., Khallaayoune, K., Scantlebury, C., Christley, R.M. (2011) A randomized triple blind trial to assess the effect of an anthelmintic programme for working equids in Morocco. *BMC Vet. Res.* 7:1.

Lyons, E.T., Drudge, J.H., Tolliver, S.C. (1986) Pyrantel pamoate: evaluating its activity against equine tapeworms. *Vet. Med.* 81, 280–285.

Mathews, J.B. (2011) Facing the threat of equine parasitic disease. *Equine Vet. J.* 43 (2) 126–132.

Nielsen, M.K., Fritzen, B., Duncan, J.L., Guillot, J., Eysker, M., Dorschies, P., Laugier, C., Beugnet, F., Meana, A., Lussot-Kervern, I., Samson-Himmelstjerna, G.V. (2010) Practical aspects of equine parasite control: a review based upon a workshop discussion consensus. *Equine Vet. J.* 42 (5) 460–468.

OIE terrestrial manual on equine piroplasmosis. Available online at: *http://www.oie.int/fileadmin/Home/eng/Health_standards/tahm/2.05.08_EQUINE_PIROPLASMOSIS.pdf*

Proudman, C., Mattews, J. (2000) Control of intestinal parasites in horses. *In Practice.* 22: 90–97.

Royal Veterinary College/Food and Agriculture Organisation. Guide to Veterinary Pathology. McMaster egg counting technique. Available online at: *http://www.rvc.ac.uk/review/parasitology/EggCount/Step2.htm*

Trawford, A., Mulugeta, G. (2008) Parasites. In: The Professional Handbook of the Donkey. 4th Edn. Eds: Duncan, J. and Hadrill, D. Whittet, Yatesbury, UK. 82–110.

Uhlinger, C., Johnstone, C. (1984) Failure to re-establish benzimidazole susceptible populations of small strongyles after prolonged treatment with non-benzimidazole drugs. *Equine Vet. Sci.* 4, 7–9.

von Samson-Himmelstjerna, G. (2012) Anthelmintic resistance in equine parasites – detection, potential clinical relevance and implications for control. *Vet. Parasitol.* 185 (1) 2–8.

Foal diseases

18

Foal diseases **18.1**
References **18.2**

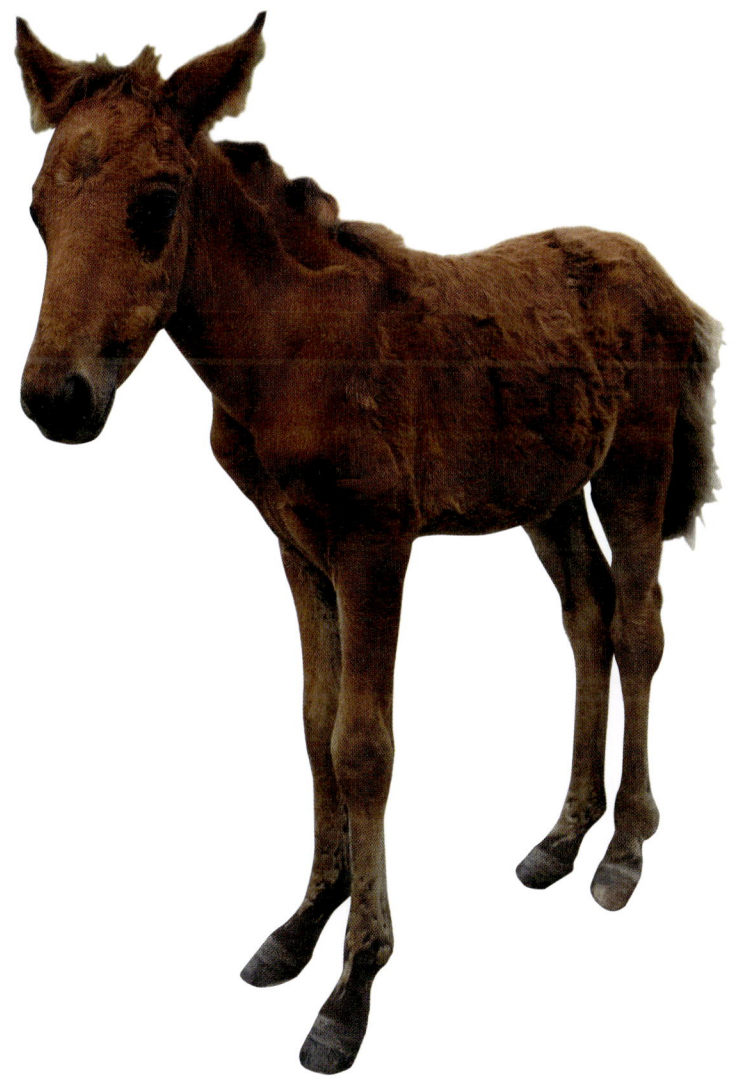

18.1 Foal diseases

Most conditions in foals require intensive, long-term treatment undertaken in specialist facilities, with varying success. Secondary complications and septicaemia are a common sequel to many foal conditions, resulting in death particularly in the first weeks of life. Often quite simple measures can be very effective in avoiding disease in the first few weeks of life, such as ensuring foals receive **adequate colostrum**.

Failure of passive transfer

All neonatal equids are born without circulating immunoglobulin and initial immune protection is passed from the mare via the colostrum through intestinal absorption. Antibodies are absorbed from the intestine for the first 12–18 hours after birth. **Failure of passive transfer** (FPT) is the result of insufficient absorption of immunoglobulin from colostrum. Without circulating immunoglobulin, foals are vulnerable to a wide range of secondary opportunistic infections which can be severe or even fatal.

Causes

- Delayed colostrum intake
- Leakage of colostrum from the udder before the foal can drink
- The mare not allowing the foal to drink, e.g. in cases of mastitis or if a maiden mare rejects the foal
- Poor colostrum quality

Following FPT a foal is likely to develop a bacteraemia (bacteria in the bloodstream) leading to: depression, weakness, respiratory distress, inappetance, diarrhoea, congested/septic mucous membranes and joint ill.

> **Ensure all foals receive their first meal of colostrum within the first 2–4 hours of birth.**

If a foal cannot drink, either support the foal every hour to allow suckling, or milk the mare and feed the foal. If there is insufficient colostrum production, supplement with milk from another mare.

Foal diarrhoea

Diarrhoea (scour) is common in foals. In most cases it is self-limiting and resolves with **fluid therapy** rather than medication. Foals become dehydrated rapidly; correct the fluid deficit if present. If a foal stops feeding, more aggressive treatment may be necessary as the foal will soon become dehydrated and hypoglycaemic.

Nutritional diarrhoea

Changes in milk composition, excessive milk intake, or ingestion of foreign material can cause mild and transient nutritional diarrhoea.

Treatment

Allow the foal to suckle little and often to prevent excessive intake, keep standing areas clean and pick up faeces. **Avoid antibiotics** as this will disrupt the balance of intestinal bacteria. Offer oral glucose/electrolyte solutions in drinking water.

Infectious diarrhoea

Knowledge of the most common pathogens at certain age groups will aid diagnosis and effective treatment.

Pathogens which can affect all age groups of foals
Clostridium difficile
Clostridium perfringens types A and C
Salmonella spp.
These bacterial infections can be severe in foals less than 1 week old.

Pathogens that can affect foals from 1 week to 2 months
Rotavirus (Diarrhoea is often benign but has the potential to progress to life-threatening disease.)
Cryptosporidium (Frequently causes mild, self-limiting diarrhoea. Crypto is most common within the first 3–4 weeks. Foals over 6 months can develop chronic diarrhoea.)

Pathogens that can affect foals older than 2 months
Large parasite burdens have the potential to cause diarrhoea in all foals older than 1 or 2 months.
Cyathostomiasis should be considered as a cause of diarrhoea in foals from 2 months of age onwards.
Lawsonia intracellularis causes proliferative enteropathy with diarrhoea and hypoproteinaemia in weanlings from 3 months of age.

Diagnosis

Without access to laboratory facilities, diagnosis of the aetiology of foal diarrhoea can be difficult. Cryptosporidia and cyathostomes can be diagnosed by microscopic faecal examination, although encysted cyathostomes may not be producing eggs. An acid fast stain must be used to detect cryptosporidium in a faecal smear. Local laboratories may have access to further testing facilities, e.g. faecal culture testing for bacterial diarrhoea. Diagnosis based only on clinical signs is likely to be inaccurate; however, profuse watery faeces with blood, mucus and a foul smell is typical of bacterial diarrhoea.

Treatment

The most important aspect of the treatment of foal diarrhoea is to **maintain hydration** (see *Fluid therapy* on page 504). If systemic illness is severe use a penicillin (20,000 IU/kg) and gentamicin (3.5 mg/kg; Crisman et al. 1997) combination, trimethoprim-sulphonamide is also acceptable. Antibiotic use in non-bacterial diarrhoea can make the symptoms worse. Good nursing care is essential. To reduce the helminth burden keep the environment clean and pick up faeces daily. Determine the frequency of anthelmintic use with a FEC of mare and foal. Salmonella and cryptosporidium are zoonotic; strict hygiene and isolation are essential. Unfortunately, the prognosis for severe systemic illness is poor as death can result from enterotoxaemia, dehydration and circulatory collapse.

Fluid therapy in foals

Successful fluid therapy in foals relies upon early diagnosis of hypovolaemia and rapid fluid replacement. Clinical signs of hypovolaemia are less obvious in foals than in adult equids. Moreover, foals are less able to adapt physiologically to hypovolaemia so can deteriorate quickly. The clinical signs of hypovolaemia include increased heart rate, increased respiratory rate, reduced pulse strength, reduced jugular filling, and cold extremities (distal limbs, ears, and nose). Attempts should be made to maintain hydration, using oral electrolytes, in foals with diarrhoea. A small stomach tube can be used for administration in foals that are not drinking. Check that the tube is in the oesophagus by feeling the tube in the neck.

Intravenous fluid therapy

When working in a field clinic, maintaining foals on intravenous fluids can be problematic; if left unattended risks include a fluid overdose or thromboembolitis. **Fluid boluses** can be given quickly with minimal complications.

Foals are usually recumbent with hypovolaemia, and almost always lethargic/dull.

Administer 0.5 litres (15-kg foal) or 1 litre (50-kg foal) of isotonic electrolyte solution via a 16–18 gauge jugular catheter. In cases of diarrhoea use Lactated ringer's/Hartmann's solution, as saline is mildly acidifying.

Wait 15 minutes and monitor the response.

- If the bolus of fluids is sufficient, then the foal will become brighter and attempt to get up.
- Urination is a useful indication of improvement; however, foals will continue to urinate in the face of hypovolaemia/dehydration as the kidneys are immature.
- Monitor clinical signs.
- If the foal remains recumbent and depressed, a second bolus can be given as above (no more than three boluses should be given).

Pulmonary oedema is a rare complication which results from over-hydration. Listen to the thorax with a stethoscope before, during and after fluid therapy. Fine crackles will be heard across the lung fields if pulmonary oedema develops, and a frothy watery discharge can be seen at the nostrils. If this occurs, fluid therapy should be stopped and frusemide (0.25–1 mg/kg IV) administered.

Gastric ulceration

The aetiology of gastric ulceration in foals differs from that in adults. In foals less than thirty days old the predominant cause is reduced perfusion of the mucosa, particularly during illnesses such as sepsis. Neonatal foals are at significant risk of developing **perforating** peptic ulcers, until they are several weeks old because their gastric mucosa is not developed to full thickness at birth. Weaning, intermittent starvation, NSAID therapy, prolonged transportation and other stressful factors have also been implicated in foal gastric ulcer aetiology.

Clinical signs

- May be asymptomatic (clinical signs become apparent when the ulceration is widespread or severe)
- Reduced appetite
- Diarrhoea (a common sign in younger foals)
- Teeth grinding and hypersalivation
- Dorsal recumbency with abdominal pain
- Differential diagnoses include septicaemia, peritonitis or oesophageal obstruction.

Treatment

Treat concurrent illness, avoid the use of NSAIDs. Gastric ulceration can be treated or prevented with oral antacids and gastric protectants.

Proton pump inhibitor – **omeprazole** 1 mg/kg PO every 24 hours

Histamine receptor antagonist – **cimetidine/ranitidine** 6–8 mg/kg PO every 8 hours

Gastric protectant – **sucralfate** 30 mg/kg PO every 6–8 hours

Colic in foals

Colic can be quite common in neonates, and clinical signs of abdominal pain can be slightly different from those shown by adult equids.

Clinical signs

Rolling, pawing the ground, abnormal position when recumbent (lying on back), abdominal distension, teeth grinding, abdominal straining (arched back, raised tail, attempting to defecate), depression, not suckling, increased heart and respiratory rate.

Diagnosis

Meconium impaction is a common cause of colic in the newborn foal; the meconium is usually passed in the first 24 hours. If this does not occur an impaction develops; this can be diagnosed by careful rectal digital palpation.

Other less common causes of colic include the following:

- **Gastroduodenal ulceration**
- **Ileus** Secondary to gastrointestinal (GI) hypoxia associated with dystocia (foaling problems) and septicaemia
- **Intussusception** Euthanasia is indicated on welfare grounds. Ultrasound is used for diagnosis, and surgical correction is the only treatment option. Neither of these is feasible in the working equid context.
- **Intestinal volvulus** As in adult equids, this is only correctable with immediate surgery as there is severe ischaemic gut injury. This surgery is not possible in field conditions; therefore, euthanasia is indicated on welfare grounds.

Treatment

To treat a meconium impaction, use an enema to soften the faeces. Insert a small catheter or feeding tube into the rectum to deliver 50 ml of warm soapy water or warm water mixed with rectal lubricant. Analgesics are essential; administer Flunixin meglumine 0.5–1.0 mg/kg IV every 24–36 hours, but use sparingly due to ulcerogenic effect. Alternatively, administer ketoprofen 1–2 mg/kg IV every 24 hours. If treating with NSAIDs, consider concurrent omeprazole treatment to reduce ulcerogenic side effects. To treat ileus, administer pain control and ensure that the foal continues to feed.

Cleft palate

This is a congenital condition where the palate has not fused, leaving an opening between the oral cavity and the nasal cavity. Aspiration pneumonia is a sequalae as the foal is unable to swallow effectively. Assess the size of the defect and the foal's body condition to determine whether euthanasia is necessary.

Clinical signs

Milk can been seen flowing from the foal's nostrils when it is feeding.

Treatment

If the fissure is small the animal may learn to cope and reach maturity. However, if the growth rate is poor, or secondary aspiration pneumonia develops, recommend euthanasia.

Septicaemia

Septicaemia, a systemic inflammatory condition in response to infection, is a major cause of equine neonatal morbidity and mortality. The presence of bacteria in the blood stream is termed 'bacteraemia'. Gram-negative bacteria are the predominant causal organisms. There is a positive correlation between FPT and septicaemia in foals (Robinson *et al.* 1993).

Clinical signs

- The foal is depressed, not sucking (the mare's udder remains distended).
- Body temperature is not an accurate indicator.
- Lung sounds may still be normal despite major pathology.
- Diarrhoea is common.
- Sudden onset lameness (joint ill) occurs.

Diagnosis

Blood culture is the optimal diagnosis. Take blood aseptically from a surgically-prepared site before beginning any antibiotic therapy. In field situations this may not be possible, so treat according to clinical signs.

Treatment

- Penicillin 20,000 IU/kg plus gentamicin 3.5 mg/kg every 12 hours. (The dose for foals is lower as gentamicin (aminoglycoside) toxicity is a risk in immature kidneys.)

- The treatment duration depends on the clinical response but may be as long as 2 weeks.
- Administer low-dose flunixin meglumine (concurrent omeprazole will reduce risk of gastric ulcers).
- Provide instructions for owners to manage the nursing care for sick foals. Foals should be kept in a clean, warm environment and have access to milk meals every hour (hand-feed weak foals).

Rhodococcus equi

Rhodococcus equi causes a severe bacterial pneumonia in foals. Clinical signs are slowly progressive, and respiratory difficulties may not become obvious until much of the lung is affected by a suppurative pneumonia. The combination of erythromycin (25 mg/kg, PO QID) and rifampin (510 mg/kg PO BID) is effective treatment. The survival rate is high with appropriate therapy.

Joint ill

Joint ill, or synovitis, usually presents as a polyarticular septic arthritis, secondary to systemic infection/septicaemia.

Clinical signs

- Joint enlargement, with heat and pain on palpation/manipulation
- Joint effusion, distension, or thickening of capsule
- Reluctance to move with varying lameness
- Depression, inappetance and fever

Treatment

Use a combination of drugs such as penicillin 20,000 IU/kg IM and gentamicin 3.5 mg/kg. Irrigation of joints may be necessary (see *Flushing an infected joint* in Section 14.7). If the joint has become damaged the prognosis for work is poor.

Angular limb deformities

Deviations of the limbs medially (varus) or laterally (valgus) (Figure 18.1.1) from the long axis is relatively common in foals. Foals may be born with a mild degree of angular deformity (3–5°) which corrects itself by the time the foal is a 1-year-old. The young growing foal is responsive to interventions. Once the physes have closed (6–24 months depending on the joint) the angulation of the limb cannot be altered by manipulating the growth direction of the limb.

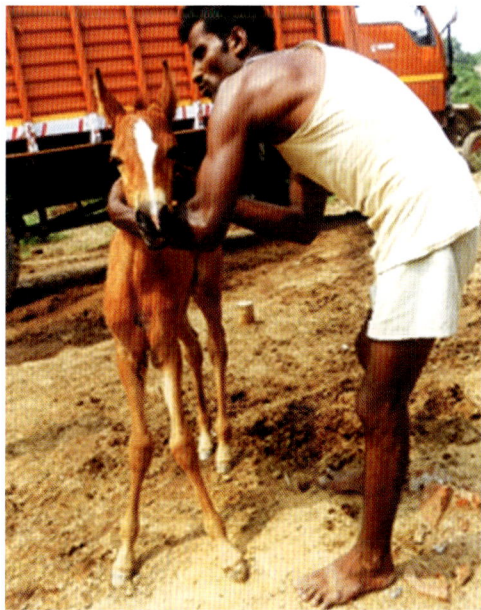

Figure 18.1.1 A foal with valgus angular limb deformity. With restricted exercise this foal showed improvement within 8 days.

Treatment

In the majority of cases, minimal interventions are required to correct angulations.

- Restrict exercise. (Provide a small patch of land for free exercise only.)
- Shoe-extensions can be employed successfully. (Plastic can be glued to the side of the hoof extending for approximately 3 cm, e.g. apply dorsomedial hoof extensions to correct carpal valgus.)
- Recommend euthanasia in severe cases that show no sign of improvement over the course of several weeks.

Flexural limb deformities

Flexural limb deformities limit the foal's ability to extend a limb to its full extent, and can affect the pastern, fetlock and/or carpus (Figure 18.1.2). The condition may be congenital or acquired, arising secondary to reduced weight bearing in the limb as a result of lameness.

Treatment

- Mild conditions resolve spontaneously.
- Rest in a small enclosure (the size of a stall or stable) provided that the foal is able to stand and suck.
- Straighten and massage the limb several times a day.
- Severe cases may improve with high-dose oxytetracycline administered slow IV (44 mg/kg diluted in 1 litre of sterile saline) (Lokai *et al*. 1985).
- If secondary to lameness, provide analgesia and treat the inciting cause.
- Lower the heels. (Elevating the heel provides temporary comfort, but will not correct the problem in young foals.)

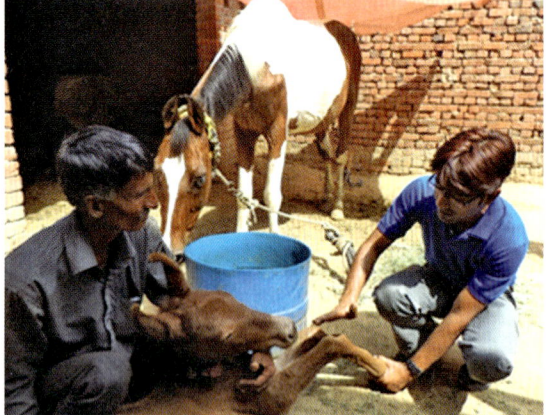

Figure 18.1.2 Bilateral carpal flexural deformity preventing full extension of both limbs.

- Protect the toe or dorsal portion of the lower limb from excessive wear.
- Splinting and casting should be used with caution.
- Consider euthanasia for severe cases that don't show improvement.

Flexor tendon laxity

Foals, particularly when premature, can be born with very weak tendons.

Clinical signs

Flexor tendons are weak so the foal stands on the plantar/palmar aspect of the pastern/fetlock. This condition is more common in the hindlimbs.

Treatment

Rest in a small enclosure. Ensure the foal is stable enough to be able to suckle, or get the owner to support the foal for suckling every hour. Splinting or casting the legs is not recommended as, in the long term, it will make the tendons weaker and could result in permanent damage. Very light bandages, which do not provide support, can be applied to protect the legs from injury if the foal is weight bearing on the plantar/palmar skin of the fetlock/pastern.

References

Crisman, M.V., Wilcke, J.R., Wallace, M.A., Friedlander, M.A. (1997) Clinical Application of Aminoglycoside Therapy in Neonatal Foals. *Am. Assoc. Equine Prac. Proceedings*. 43.

Lokai, M.M., Meyer, R.J. (1985) Preliminary-observations on oxytetracycline treatment of congenital flexural deformities in foals. *Mod. Vet. Prac.* 66 (4) 237–239.

Robinson, J.A., Allen, G.K., Green, E.M., Fales, W.H., Loch, W.E., Wilkerson, C.G. (1993) A prospective study of septicaemia in colostrum-deprived foals. *Equine Vet. J.* 25 (3) 214–219.

Further Reading

Dunkel, B., Wilkins, P.A. (2004) Infectious foal diarrhoea: pathophysiology, prevalence and diagnosis. *Equine Vet. Educ.* 16 (2) 94–101.

Hepburn, R. (2007) Management of diarrhoea in foals up to weaning. *In Practice*. 29 (6) 334–341.

Hepburn, R. (2011) Gastric ulceration in horses. *In Practice*. 33, 116–124.

Hollis, A., Corley, K. (2007) Practical guide to fluid therapy in neonatal foals. *In Practice*. 29 (3) 130–137

Lokai, M.D. (1992) Case selection for medical-management of congenital flexural deformities in foals. *Equine Practice*. 14 (4) 23–25.

Smith L. (2010) Treatment of angular limb deformities in foals. *In Practice*. 32 (4) 156–162.

Index

Page numbers in **bold** refer to tables

abdomen
   examination 12–13, 258–9
   pain 59, 61
   rupture 441-2
     see also colic
abdominocentesis 269–70
abortion
   infectious causes 343
   investigation 340–2
   treatment 344
abscess
   hoof 376–8
   skin 440–1
   tooth root 217
acepromazine (ACP) 134, **135**
   combination therapy **140**
   pre-anaesthetic use 148
acetylsalicylic acid (aspirin) 113, **114**
acute renal failure 336–7
adrenaline injection 126
African horse sickness (AHS) 307–9
   donkeys 307
ageing 10, **11**, 227–9
   donkeys 229
air embolism 82
allergic respiratory disease 318–19
allodynia 54
alpha2-adrenoreceptor agonists 135, **136**, 154
   combination therapy 139, **140**
   donkeys and mules 136
   pre-anaesthetic use 148, 150
aminoglycosides 107
anaesthesia *see* general anaesthesia; local anaesthetics; topical anaesthesia
analgesia 63–5, **66**
   alpha2-adrenoreceptor agonists 135
   donkeys 65–6
   neuroleptanalgesia 139–40, **140**
   opioid analgesics 137–9, **138**
   pre-emptive 54
   response to 64
   surgical procedures and 154, 157
   see also specific drugs
animal welfare 24–33
   advocate role 3
   ethics 33

five freedoms 26–32, **33**
   mental welfare 33
   naturalness 33
   physical welfare 33
anterior chamber of the eye 181
anthelmintics 476–9
   de-worming programme 479–81, **481**
   resistance to 480–1
     measurement 483–4
   see also specific drugs
anthrax 19, 275
antibiotics 104–10, **109**
   eye conditions 196
   rational use 104–5
   resistance 104
   side effects 105
     antibiotic-associated diarrhoea (AAD) 276, 278
   see also specific drugs
anuria 122–3
aorta severance 167
arthritis, septic 398–9
arthropod parasites 475, 484–5, 488
aseptic scrub 93–4
aspiration pneumonia 323–5
   nasogastric tube complication 75
aspirin 113, **114**
ataxia, alpha2-adrenoreceptor agonist effects 136
atropine 153, 196, 206
auriculopalpebral nerve block 192
auscultation
   abdomen 12–13, 258–9
   heart 11
   larynx/trachea 297
   lungs 11–12, 297–8
azotaemia 332, 336

babesiosis 335
   see also equine piroplasmosis
bacterial infections 104
   notifiable infections 315–17
   respiratory disease 309–17
   urinary tract infections (UTIs) 334–5, 347–8
   see also antibiotics; *specific infections*
bandaging 449–52, **450**, **451**
   maintenance 452
   materials 449

INDEX

barbiturates 168
bastard strangles 11, 314
behaviour 34
   equid traits 34–7
   flight or fight response 35
benzimidazoles 477–8
   resistance to 478
benzodiazepines 137
benzyl benzoate 489
beta-lactam antibiotics 105–6
bilirubin 92
biohazard waste management 4–5
biopsy 431
bladder
   catheterisation 331
   prolapse 336
blepharoedema 198–9
blindness 177, 191
blood sampling 85
blood smears 86–7, 89
   staining techniques 87–8
body condition scoring (BCS) 254–5
   donkeys 255
   horses 255
body weight calculation 98
bone conditions 387–94
   fractures 388–92
botulism 461–2
bradycardia, alpha2-adrenoreceptor agonist effects 136
brucellosis 343
bucked shins 392
bupivacaine hydrochloride 141, **142**
buprenorphine 137, **138**
Burkholderia mallei infection see glanders
burns, case study 67–9
bursitis 413–15, **414–15**
butorphanol 137, **138**, 154
   combination therapy 139, **140**
   drug interaction 99

calculi 338–9
canine teeth 225
canker 380
capillary refill time (CRT) 10
capped elbow **414**, 415
capped hock **414**, 415
captive bolt 166–7
carcass disposal 4
carpal hygroma **414**
carprofen **66**, 113
castration 344–5

cataracts 208–9
catheterisation
   bladder 331
   venous 80–2
caudal epidural anaesthesia 143–4
cellulitis 444
cephalosporins 106, **109**
chemical restraint 44–5, 191–3
   see also sedation
chest percussion 298
chloral hydrate 153, 169
chloramphenicol 196
chlorpromazine 134
choke 262–3
cinchocaine 169
cleft palate 506
clinical examination 8–15
   abdomen 12–13
   head and neck 9–11
   history taking 6-7
   musculoskeletal system 14, 353–9
   observation 8–9
   rectal 267–9, 340
   respiratory system 296–9
   thorax 11–12
   urogenital system 13, 330–1, 339
   see also ophthalmic examination; oral examination
clinical governance 4–5
clinical pathology 83–4
clostridial myonecrosis 410–11
   case study 416–17
Clostridium perfringens 277
club foot 375–6
colic 59, 264–72
   case study 287–8
   clinical examination 267–70
   clinical signs 265–6
      donkeys 265
      horses 265
   diagnosis 272
   foals 505–6
   history 265
   prevention 274–5
   risk factors 275
   treatment 272–4
      colonic displacement 273–4
      decision guidelines 271, **271**
      impaction 272–3, 287–8
   see also abdomen
colitis, acute 275–6
colonic displacement 273–4

INDEX

communication 4, 18
   case study 20–1
   equid communication 37
conjunctiva 179
conjunctivitis 201–2, 486
consultation 2
continuous rate infusion (CRI) sedation 157–8
   protocol 158
cornea 179–80
   colour changes **180**
   injury 189
   ulceration 202–5
      melting ulcer 204
corneal response 187
corns 379
corticosteroids 115–16, **117**
   eye conditions 196
   side effects 115–16
   see also specific drugs
cortisol levels 58
Corynebacterium pseudotuberculosis 436
cramping 410
creatinine 92
cryptorchidism 345
Cyathostomes 472–3, 477
cyclo-oxygenase 111
cystitis 334–5

dazzle response 186
de-worming programme 479–81, **481**
debility 256–8
debridement 426
degenerative joint disease (DJD) 395–8
dehydration 126–7
   NSAID effects 111
   treatment 127–8
dental charts 224
   see also teeth
dental equipment 233–6, **237**
   motorised equipment 236, **237**
   rasping blades 235–6
   speculum 232–3
dental pain 59
   see also teeth
dental records 233
dental terminology 224
dental treatment 245–50
   nerve blocks 249–50
   rasping 246–8
   tooth removal 248–9
   see also dental equipment; teeth
dentine star 228–9

dermatitis, heels 382, 433–4
dermatophilosis 433
dermatophytosis 434–5
desmitis 408
detomidine 135, **136**
   combination therapy 140
   drug interactions 99
dexamethasone 115, **117**, 196
diagnostic tests 16–17, 83–4
diarrhoea 275–9
   acute colitis 275–6
   antibiotic-associated (AAD) 276, 278
   chronic 277–9
   Clostridium perfringens 277
   drug side effects 107, 111
   fluid therapy 276, 503–4
   foals 502–4
   NSAID toxicity 278
   parasitic enteritis 277, 472
   salmonellosis 276–7
diastemata 242–3
diazepam 137, **137**
diclofenamic acid (diclofenac) 113, 196–7
Dictyocaulus arnfieldi (lungworm) 320
Diff-quick staining technique 87
differential cell count 89
digital nerve blocks 360
diminazine aceturate 490
dipyrone 112–13, **114**
diuretics 123–4
dourine 493–4
drenching 73
drug storage 103
drug use 98–103
   administration routes 72–83, 99, **100–1**
      injections 76–83, **100–1**
      liquids 73–5
      ocular therapies 193–6
      topical **101**
   dispensing 4
   dosage 103
   drug interactions 99
   drugs not licensed for equids 103
   food chain considerations 103
   instructions to owner 102, **102**
   owner compliance 101–2
   pharmacokinetics 98–100
   see also specific drugs
dystocia 342–3

ears
   cutting 447, 448
   examination 10

INDEX

pain 59
Eastern equine encephalitis (EEE) 463–4
EDTA blood collection tubes 197
embolisation 82
empyema 322
entropion 197–8
epistaxis 321–3
   nasogastric tube insertion and 75
epizootic lymphangitis 436
equine herpesviruses 306
equine influenza 306
equine piroplasmosis (EP) 91, 489–90
equine protozoal myeloencephalitis (EPM) 464–5
equine recurrent uveitis (ERU) 205–7
erythromycin 108, **109**
euthanasia 164–5
   agents that should not be used 170
   aorta severance 167
   case study 171–2
   confirmation of death 169–70
   free bullet 165–6
   penetrating captive bolt 166–7
   pharmacological 167–9
examination approach 39–40
   see also clinical examination
exercise-induced pulmonary haemorrhage (EIPH) 323
exertional rhabdomyolysis (ER) 409
exhaustion 410
eye drops 194
eyelids 178–9
   conditions 197–9
   lacerations 199–200
eyes
   anatomy 178–83
   common diseases 197–217
      parasitic conditions 211–15, 217–19
   discharge 184
   drug administration routes 193–6
   examination 10
   local anaesthesia 143
   pain 60, 184, 185
   therapeutic preparations 196–7
   see also ophthalmic examination; vision

facial nerve paralysis 459
faecal egg count (FEC) 482–4
faecal examination 259
failure of passive transfer (FPT) 502
farcy 315–16
farriery

shoeing 370–2
trimming the foot 367–70
feeding
   foals 257–8
   lactating mares 258
   sick animals 62, 256–7
fenbendazole 477
'fight or flight' response 35
filariasis, intraocular 214–15
fine needle aspirate (FNA) 430
fipronil 489
firing 46, 406, 447, 448
   case study 47–8
five freedoms 26–32, 33
flexor tendon laxity, foals 508–9
fluid therapy 126–31, **128**
   administration route 129–31
   diarrhoea 276
   fluid composition 129–30
   foals 504
   monitoring 131
flunixin meglumine **66**, 112, **114**
   drug interaction 99
fluorescein test 187–8
fly strike 488
foals
   cleft palate 506
   colic 505–6
   diarrhoea 502–4
   failure of passive transfer (FPT) 502
   feeding 257–8
   flexor tendon laxity 508–9
   fluid therapy 504
   fractures 389
   gastric ulceration 504–5
   limb deformities 507–9
   Rhodococcus equi infection 507
   septicaemia 506–7
foot
   conditions affecting 373–87
      brushing and over-reaching 383
      see also heel conditions
   conformation 362–6
      hoof pastern axis (HPA) 362–5
      medial lateral balance 364–5
   donkeys 366
   examination 355–7
   hoof anatomy 361–2
   internal structure 362
   pain 61
   see also hoof
four principle ethics 33

INDEX

fractures 388–92
   bone healing 388–9
   foals 389
   long bones 389
   non-displaced 390–1, **390**
   orbital 200–1
   periosteal regrowth 392
   sequestra 391
frontal sinuses 297, 302
Frusemide 123
fundus 182–3

gait abnormalities *see* lameness
Galvayne's groove 229
gastric reflux, nasogastric tubes and 74–5, 260
gastric ulceration, foals 504–5
gastrointestinal tract (GIT) 254
   diagnostic aids 258–60
   drug side effects
      alpha2-adrenoreceptor agonists 135
      corticosteroids 116
      NSAIDs 111
   faecal examination 259
   parasitic infections 277, 470–5, **470**
general anaesthesia (GA) 137, 145–58
   adverse reaction 154–6
   choice of anaesthetic agent 145
   drugs used 150–3, **151**, **152**
   environment for 148
   equipment 147
   induction 149, 153–4
   maintenance 149, 156
   monitoring 154–6, **155**
   phases of 148
   planes of 149
   positioning the animal 154
   pre-operative examination 147
   preparation for 146–8
   recovery 149, 156–7
   total intravenous anaesthesia (TIVA) 145–6
   unsuitable conditions 148
gentamicin 107, **109**, 196
   drug interaction 99
glanders 315–17, 436
   clinical signs 315–16
   diagnosis 316–17
   treatment 317
glaucoma 207–8
glucose absorption test 260–1
gluteal injections 77
Gram staining technique 88
granulation tissue 380, 428

greasy heel 382
guaifenesin 153
gum disease 243
guttural pouch
   bleeding from 321–2
   infections 303–4
      mycosis 321–2

habronemiasis 335, 345, 435, 487
   case study 217–19
   ophthalmic 211–12, 217–19
haematology 88–91, 332
haematoma 442–3
haematuria 333, 335
haemoglobinuria 333, 335
halter 40–1
handling 38
   dangers 38
head
   examination 9–11, 296
   pain 59
   trauma 458–9
headcollar 40–1
heart auscultation 11
heart rate, reported values **15**
heat stress 124–6
   treatment 125–6
heaves line 12
heel conditions 381–2
   contracted heels 381
   dermatitis 382, 433–4
   sheared heels 382
   traumatic wounds 381
hepatitis 286
hernias 441–2
herpesviruses 306
histoplasmosis, lacrimal 216–17, 436–7
history taking 6–7
   direct and indirect questions 6
homidium bromide 494
hoof
   anatomy 361
   conditions affecting 373–87
      avulsion 375
      cracks 374
      overgrowth/over wear 373–4
      puncture wounds and abscesses 376–8
   shoeing 370–2
   trimming 367–70
      laminitic foot 387
   see also foot
hoof pastern axis (HPA) 362–5

515

broken back 363–4
broken forward 364
Horner's syndrome 322
hydrocoele 345–6
hygroma 413–15, **414–15**
hyperalgesia 54
hyperthermia 124
hypoalbuminaemia 92
hypocalcaemia 411–12

imidocarb diproprionate 490
impaction colic 272–3
   case study 287–8
incisors 225
   abnormalities 242
   ageing 10, **11**, 227–9
      donkey 229
   examination 10–11
   fracture case study 251
inflammation 110–11, 422
   management 110–11
   see also corticosteroids; non-steroidal anti-inflammatory drugs (NSAIDs); *specific conditions*
influenza 306
infraorbital nerve block 250
infratrochlear nerve block 193
infundibular cup 228
injections 76–83
   intra-articular 82–3, 116
   intramuscular 77–8, **100**, 140
   intravenous 79–80, **101**
      catheter placement 80–2
   subcutaneous 76, **100**
insect hypersensitivity 435
integrated consultation 2
intra-arterial injection 80
intra-articular injection 82–3, 116
intramuscular drug administration 77–8, 99, 100, 140
intraocular pressure (IOP) 187
intravenous drug administration 79–82, 99, 101
   catheter placement 80–2
   complications 80, 82
   general anaesthesia 148
   see also total intravenous anaesthesia (TIVA)
intravenous fluid therapy 130–1
iris 181
isotonic fluid 130
ivermectin 476

joints 394
   conditions affecting 394–404
   dislocation 402–3
   examination 358
   flexion tests 358–9
   flushing 400–1
   injection *see* intra-articular injection
   joint ill 507
   sprains 402–3

kanamycin **110**
ketamine 150, **151**, 156
ketoprofen 66, 113, **114**
kidneys, biochemical tests 92

lacrimal nerve block 193
lacrimal system 179
   duct obstruction 184
   histoplasmosis 216–17, 436–7
lactation
   drug excretion in milk 99
   feeding during 258
lameness 352
   diagnosis 143
   examination 353–9
   flexion tests 358–9
   grading 359
   history 353
   nerve blocks 359–60
laminitis 384–7
   diagnosis 384–5
   pathogenesis 384
   prevention 387
   prognosis 386
   treatment 385–6, 387
lampas 261
larynx 297
lavage
   eye preparations 194–6
   joints 400–1
leg lift 41–2
lens 182
   conditions 208–9
leptospirosis 335, 343
leukocytes *see* white blood cells (WBCs)
lice 484
lignocaine hydrochloride 141, **142**
limb pain 60, 61
   see also foot; lameness
lip lesions 262, 446
liver

INDEX

biochemical tests 91–2
disease 284–6
  acute 284–6
  chronic 286
  clinical signs 284
  prevention 286
liver fluke 475
local anaesthetics 63, 141–4, **142**
  caudal epidural anaesthesia 143–4
  eye examination or treatment 192–3
  local infiltration 142–3
  nerve blocks 143
  side effects 141
  topical 142
locking stifle 403–4
lumpectomy 431
lungs 297–8
  abnormal sounds 298
  auscultation 11–12, 297–8
  bleeding from 323
  see also respiratory disease
lungworm 320
luxations 402–3

macrocyclic lactones 476–7, 488
  resistance to 477
macrolides 108
magnesium sulphate 169
malignant oedema 410–11
  case study 416–17
mallein test 316–17
mandibular nerve block 250
manual cell count 89
massage therapy 62–3
maxillary nerve block 250
maxillary sinuses 297, 302
mebendazole 477
meclofenamic acid 113
melanoma 439
melarsenoxide 494
menace response 186–7
mental nerve block 250
mepivacaine hydrochloride 141, **142**
methylprednisolone 115, **117**
metronidazole 108, **109**
miotics 196
mites 485, **485**
molars 225
Monday morning disease 409
moon blindness 205, 341
morphine 137, **138**
mouth conditions 261–2

trauma 262
ulceration 261–2
see also oral examination
moxidectin 476–7
mucous membrane colour 9, **9**, 296
mud fever 433–4
muscle
  atrophy 412
  biochemical tests 93
  conditions affecting 408–12
  cramping 410
muscle relaxants 169
musculoskeletal system 352
  examination 14
  see also bone conditions; joints; lameness; muscle
mycosis, guttural pouch 321–2
mydriatics 196
myiasis 488
myogloby, following general anaesthesia 157

nasal cavity conditions 300–1
  epistaxis 321
nasal discharge 10, 297
nasogastric tube insertion 73–5, **75**
  colic investigation 260, 267
  complications 75, **75**
  fluid therapy 129
  gastric reflux detection 74–5, 260
  removal 75
nasolacrimal lavage 195
navicular syndrome 393
neck
  examination 9–11, 296
  intramuscular injection 77
nephritis, verminous 335
nerve blocks 143, 157
  dental treatment 249–50
  eye examination or treatment 192–3
  lameness 359–60
neuroleptanalgesia 139–40, **140**
neuropathy, following general anaesthesia 157
nictitating membrane 179
nociceptors 53, 54
nomogram 98
non-steroidal anti-inflammatory drugs (NSAIDs) **66**, 110–13, **114**
  eye conditions 196–7
  pre-anaesthetic use 148, 154
  side effects 111–12
    diarrhoea 278
  see also specific drugs

517

INDEX

nosebleed *see* epistaxis
nostrils
   discharge 10, 297
   examination 297
   slitting 46–7, 447, 448
notifiable diseases
   bacterial respiratory infections 315–17
   viral respiratory infections 307–9

obturator nerve paralysis 460
oedema 443–4
   malignant 410–11
      case study 416–17
oesophageal obstruction 262–3
oliguria 122
Onchocerca 212–13, 486–7
ophthalmic examination 183–93, **185**
   chemical restraint 191–3
   diagnostic tests 187–8
   history 183
   intraocular pressure (IOP) 187
   ocular discharge 184
   ophthalmoscopy 189–90
   reflex testing 186–7
   signs of disease 184
   see also eyes; vision
opioid analgesics 63, 137–9, **138**
   controlled drug status 139
   pre-anaesthetic use 148
optic disc 183
optic nerve disease 210–11
oral drug administration 72–3, 99, **100**
   drenching 73
oral examination 230–3
   dental speculum 232–3
   extra-oral examination 231
   see also mouth conditions; teeth
orbit 178
   fracture 200–1
organophosphates 489
osteitis 393–4
osteoarthritis (OA) 395–8, **396**
   case study 20–1
   treatment 397–8
osteochondrosis 401–2
osteomyelitis 393–4
oxfenbendazole 478
oxibendazole 478
oxybuprocaine 141
oxytetracycline 107–8, **109–10**

packed cell volume (PCV) 89

pain 52
   acute 54
   aggression and 57
   assessment 56–60
      donkeys 60–1
      objective 57–8
      practical 58–60
      subjective 57
   breakthrough 55
   central mechanisms 54
   chronic 55
      case study 67–9
   coping mechanisms 55
   diagnosis 52
   management 62–3
      assisted feeding/drinking 62
      donkeys 65–6
      physiotherapy and massage 62–3
      rest 62
      warmth and comfort 62
      see also analgesia
   peripheral mechanisms 53–4
   pre-emptive analgesia 54
   responses 56
   welfare promotion 65
palmar digital nerve block 360
palpebral blink reflex 186
papillomatosis 438
paracentesis 269–70
Parascaris equorum 320, 473
parasitic conditions 470–96
   external parasites 484–9
      medication 488–9
   eye 211–15
      case study 217–19
   gastrointestinal parasites 277, 470–5, **470**
      anthelmintics 476–9
      de-worming programme 479–81, **481**
      faecal egg count (FEC) 482–4
   protozoal infections 489–95
   respiratory disease 320
   see also specific parasites
pastern dermatitis 433–4
patella, upward fixation 403–4
pectoral muscle injection 77
pedal osteitis 383, 393–4
Pen-Strep 107
penetrating captive bolt 166–7
penicillins 105–6, **109–10**
   adverse reactions 106
penis
   examination 135, 339

paralysis 346
pentobarbitone sodium 168
peri-vascular injection 80
periapical infection 244
perineural anaesthesia 143
   see also nerve blocks
periodontal disease 243
periostitis 392
peripheral nerve trauma 459–60
peritoneal fluid 270, **270**
peritoneal tap 269–70
peritonitis 283
pethidine 137, **138**
pharmacokinetics 98–100
   absorption 99
   distribution 99
   drug interactions 99
   excretion 99
   metabolism 99
   see also specific drugs
phenanthridium compounds 494
phenothiazines 134–5
phenylbutazone (PBZ) 65, **66**, 112, **114**
phlebitis 80
photosensitisation 444–5
physiotherapy 62–3
pilocarpine 196
pinworms 474
piperazine 478
piroplasmosis 91, 489–90
pithing 166, 167
plantar digital nerve block 360
platelet estimation 90
pleuropneumonia 311
pneumonia
   aspiration 323–5
   bacterial 309–11
poll evil 414
postpartum haemorrhage 343–4
potassium chloride 168–9
praziquantel 479
pre-anaesthetic medication 148, 150
pre-breeding tests 339
prednisolone 115, **117**, 196
pregnancy
   abortion investigation 340–2
   alpha2-adrenoreceptor agonist side effects 136
   complications 342–4
   corticosteroid side effects 116
   diagnosis 340
premolars 225

procaine penicillin 105–6, **109–10**
   intramuscular injection 78
prognosis determination 10
   case study 20–1
propofol 153
prostaglandin (PG) 111
protozoal infections 489–95
proxymetacaine 141
pruritus 432–5
pulse 10
   reported values **15**
pupil 182
pupillary light reflex (PLR) 186
purpura haemorrhagica 314
pyelonephritis 334–5
pyoderma 432–3
pyrantel emboate 478
pyrethroids 488
pyrimidines 478–9
pyrithidium bromide 494

quinalbarbitine 169
quinapyramine salts 494

rabies 462–3
rain scald 433
re-breathing bag 298–9
record keeping 4
rectal examination 267–9, 340
rectal prolapse 279–81
rectal tears/perforation 281–2
rectal temperature 14–15
   reported values **15**
red blood cell (RBC) count 89
registration 4
reproductive system diseases 339–46
   abortion investigation 340–2
   examination 339
   pregnancy complications 342–4
respiratory disease 294
   allergic disease 318–19
   bacterial infections 309–17
   clinical signs 299–300
   donkeys 299
   dust and pollution effects 295
   examination 296–9
   guttural pouch infections 303–4
   nasal passage conditions 300–1
   parasitic disease 320
   sinusitis 302
   transmission 295–6
   viral infections 304–9

INDEX

respiratory rate, reported values 15
responsibilities of an animal health provider 3–5
restraint
    chemical 44–5, 191–3
    physical 40–4
retained foetal membranes (RFM) 344
retina 182
    disease 209–10
return to work prognosis 19
rhabdomyolysis 336, 409
Rhodococcus equi infection 507
ringworm 434–5
romifidine 135, **136**
    combination therapy 140
rope halter 40–1
Rose Bengal stain 188
roundworms 473, 477
ruptures 441–2

saline autoagglutination 91
salmonellosis 276–7
sarcoids 439–40
Schirmer tear test 188
scrotal swelling 345
sedation 134–9
    continuous rate infusion (CRI) 157–8
    dental treatment 245, **246**
    neuroleptanalgesia 139–40, **140**
    pre-anaesthetic 148, 150, **151, 152**
sentience 24
septic arthritis 398–9, 424
septicaemia, foals 506–7
seroma 443
serum
    biochemistry 332
    eye disease treatment 197
    proteins 93
sesamoid nerve block 360
sesamoiditis 392
setaria 214–15
setonism 30, 447, 448
shear mouth 240–1
shoeing 370–2
shooting 165–6
sight limitation using cupped-hand 44
sinusitis 302
skin
    diseases 429–45
        diagnosis 429–31
        parasitic infections 484–9
    pain 59

sterile preparation 93–4
skin twitch 43–4
sleeping sickness 491
smear preparation 86–7, 430–1
smooth mouth 241
spinal cord trauma 458
splints 392, **451**
sporotrichosis 436
sprains 402–3
squamous cell carcinoma 438–9
standing surgery 157–8
step mouth 240, 248
steroidal anti-inflammatory drugs *see* corticosteroids
stomach bot 475
strangles 11, 312–14
    clinical signs 312
    complications 314
    diagnosis 313
    management 313–14
    transmission 312
streptomycin 107
stress leukogram 90
strongyles 470–3, **470**
    large 470–1
    small 472–3, 477
Strongylus edentatus 471
Strongylus vulgaris 470–1
sub-luxations 402–3
subcutaneous drug administration 76, **100**
submandibular lymph nodes 11
subpalpebral lavage 196
sulphonamides 107
    drug interactions 99, 136
sunburn 444–5
supraorbital nerve block 192
supraspinous fistulous withers 415, **415**
suramin 494
surgical drains 427–8
surra 491–2
    case study 495–6
suturing 426–7
suxamethonium 169
sweeny 459
sweet itch 435
synovial bursal conditions 413–15, **414–15**
synovial fluid sampling 399–400, **400**
synovitis 398, 507

tail-base lesions 446
tapeworms 474
teeth

ageing 10, **11**, 227–9
  anatomy 225
  dental charts 224
  dental pain 59
  dental records 233
  diastemata 242–3
  donkeys 226, 229
  examination 10–11
  problems due to mastication and wear 238–41
    excessive transverse ridges (ETRs) 239
    hooks 238–9
    sharp enamel points 238, 246–7
    shear mouth 240–1
    smooth mouth 241
    step mouth 240, 248
    wave mouth 240
  rasping 246–8
  removal 248–9
  retained deciduous crowns (caps) 241–2
  structure 226
  trauma 243–4
    case study 251
  see also oral examination
tendonitis 405–6
tendons 404
  examination 357
  flexor tendon laxity, foals 508
  rupture 406–7, **407**
  strains 405–6
tenosynovitis 405–6
testicular torsion 346
tetanus 460–1
  case study 465–7
tetracyclines 107–8
thalaziasis 213–14
thermocautery 46
thiopentone 150, **152**, 168
thorax examination 11–12
thrombocytopaenia 91
thrombophlebitis 80, 82
thrush 379–80
ticks 485
togaviral encephalitis 463–4
tongue trauma 262
tooth root abscess 217
topical anaesthesia 142, 191–2
topical drug administration **101**
  eye examination and treatment 191–2, 194
total intravenous anaesthesia (TIVA) 145–6
  advantages and disadvantages 146
  adverse reaction 154–6
  maintenance 156
  monitoring 154–6, **155**
  recovery 156–7
  see also general anaesthesia (GA)
triamcinolone acetonide 115, **117**
triclabendazole 478
trimethoprim-sulphur 107, **109**
trypanosomiasis 91, 491
  dourine 493–4
  surra 491–2
    case study 495–6
  treatment 493–5
    resistance 494–5
tsetse flies 491
tumours
  gastrointestinal 278–9
  ocular 216
  oral 244
  see also specific tumours
twitch
  skin 43–4
  upper lip 42–3
tying up 336, 409
tylosin 108

ulceration
  corneal 202–5
  gastric, foals 504–5
  oral 261–2
upper lip twitch 42–3
urea 92
urethral concretion 337–8
urinalysis 332–3
urinary tract diseases 334–9
  case study 347–8
  examination 330–1
  history 330
urolithiasis 338
uterine prolapse 343
uterine rupture 343
uterine torsion 343
uveitis 205–7, 486

Venezuelan equine encephalitis (VEE) 463–4
venous catheterisation see intravenous drug administration
verminous enteritis 277, 472–3
verminous nephritis 335
vesicular stomatitis 261
viral infections
  respiratory disease 304–9
    notifiable disease 307–9

INDEX

prevention 305–6
treatment 305
see also specific infections
vision 176
testing 191
see also eyes; ophthalmic examination

warts 438
waste management 4–5
wave mouth 240
weightloss 256-8
West Nile virus (WNV) 464
Western equine encephalitis (WEE) 463–4
wheezing 298
white blood cells (WBCs) 89, 90–1
toxic changes 90
white line disease 378
withers lesions 415, **415**, 447
case study 453
wolf teeth 225
wounds
eyelid 198–200
factors affecting healing 423–4
healing phases 422–3
management 424–8
antibiotic use 104
case study 453
closed wounds 426–8
open wounds 425–6
proud flesh 428
see also bandaging
prevention 445–8

xylazine 135, **136**
combination therapy **140**
continuous rate infusion (CRI) 157–8

zoonotic disease 19
zygomatic nerve block 193